Food Additive
Toxicology

Food Additive Toxicology

edited by

Joseph A. Maga
Anthony T. Tu
Colorado State University
Fort Collins, Colorado

MARCEL DEKKER   NEW YORK

Library of Congress Cataloging-in-Publication Data

Food additive toxicology / edited by Joseph A. Maga and Anthony T. Tu.
　　p.　cm.
　　Includes bibliographical references and index.
　　ISBN 0-8247-9245-9 (alk. paper)
　　1. Food additives—Toxicology.　I. Maga, Joseph A.　II. Tu,
Anthony T.
　TX553.A3F563　1994
　664'.06—dc20

94-27241
CIP

The publisher offers discounts on this book when ordered in bulk quantities. For more information, write to Special Sales/Professional Marketing at the address below.

This book is printed on acid-free paper.

Marcel Dekker
270 Madison Avenue, New York, New York 10016

Current printing (last digit):
10　9　8　7　6　5　4　3

PRINTED IN THE UNITED STATES OF AMERICA

Preface

It is generally accepted that a food additive can be defined as a single compound or mixture of substances, other than a basic foodstuff, which finds its way into a food during any aspect of its production, processing, storage, packaging, or preparation for consumption. By applying this definition to our food supply, it is quite obvious that food additives have been used for centuries to enhance and preserve the quality of numerous foods.

Some individuals have a preconceived notion that food additives are restricted to various forms of synthetic and perhaps toxic compounds that are indiscriminately added to every commercial food. However, it should be remembered that compounds such as smoke, alcohol, vinegar, and spices, have traditionally been used to extend the shelf life of foods and, as such, are also considered to be food additives.

Continued consumer demand for modified or entirely new types of foods having improved flavor, color, convenience, stability, or nutritional qualities has resulted in the introduction and utilization of both natural and synthetic compounds, in the form of food additives, during the last 50 years. As a result, today there are approximately 2800 compounds approved for food use in the United States that can be legally incorporated into over 20,000 different food items.

Individual and consumer group concern over the safety associated with the excessive use of various food additives has a long history that has led to the enactment of various national and international laws and regulations governing their use. In the United States, these include the 1906 Pure Food and Drug Act, the 1938 Federal Food, Drug and Cosmetic Act, the 1958 Food Additives Amendment, and the 1960 Color Additives Amendment. However, a better understanding of toxicology and the lack of any recently passed legislation in the area of food additives has been interpreted by some that both the food industry and government are not treating consumer safety as a major concern. Others counter that our food supply is quite safe and that the proper authorities continue to monitor the safe use of food additives, using the concept of benefits-to-risk assessment. As a result, a process has been established to introduce safe additives and to remove from use additives that are deemed unsafe.

Europe and other parts of the world rely on the E system, which was developed by the European Economic Community, to list food additives that, based on current knowledge, are permitted to be utilized as food additives. The counterpart in the United States is the Food and Drug Administration (FDA) and its Generally Recognized as Safe (GRAS) list.

Most would agree that numerous potential benefits can be derived from the use of certain food additives. High on the list of benefits is increased food safety via the utilization of antimicrobial agents that minimize the risk of certain types of food poisoning.

The use of antioxidants and nutritional additives also have a positive effect relative to nutrition. For example, without added antioxidants, essential unsaturated fatty acids and certain vitamins can be degraded with processing and storage, thereby lowering the overall nutritional value of certain foods.

The inclusion of certain additives is also useful in extending the shelf life of various seasonably available foods and provides the basis for the development of a wider variety of foods. For example, the vast array of breakfast cereals, low-calorie foods, and numerous convenience foods would not be possible without the intentional inclusion of various food additives.

It can also be argued that the use of food additives has resulted in overall lower food prices since factors such as spoilage during processing, distribution, and storage and the use of lower-cost packaging can be utilized when additives are used.

On the other hand, obvious risk factors associated with the intentional use of a wide array of food additives include the fact that the potential long-term risk associated with the extensive use of food additives has not been completely studied in humans per se from a scientific standpoint. Since most additives are incorporated at relatively low levels in most foods, one can assume that direct toxicological effects are not going to be apparent. However, there can still be significant physiological and perhaps life-threatening effects from some additives for certain sensitive individuals. The setting of maximum usage levels for certain additives is problematical from both a moral and legal standpoint when "safe" levels nevertheless have the potential to cause adverse reactions in these individuals.

The ultimate concern is that certain food additives have potential toxicological implications based on data obtained from nonhuman models, and thus the legal aspects of food additive use will be debated long into the future. Therefore, the toxicological properties of food additives have become the objective of this book. Specific areas covered include: types of food additives, food acidulants, antioxidants, food colors, curing agents, flavoring agents, flavor potentiators, salts, modified food starches, incidental food additives, and antimicrobial agents.

Joseph A. Maga
Anthony T. Tu

Contents

Contributors

S. S. Deshpande, Ph.D.[1] Department of Nutrition and Food Science, Utah State University, Logan, Utah

Usha S. Deshpande, M.S.[2] Department of Plant Science, University of Manitoba, Winnipeg, Canada

V. M. Ghorpade, Ph.D.[3] Department of Nutrition and Food Science, Utah State University, Logan, Utah

D. L. Madhavi, Ph.D.[4] Department of Nutrition and Food Science, Utah State University, Logan, Utah

Joseph A. Maga, Ph.D. Professor of Food Science, Department of Food Science and Human Nutrition, Colorado State University, Fort Collins, Colorado

S. Raharjo, M.S., Ph.D.[5] Department of Food Science and Human Nutrition, Colorado State University, Fort Collins, Colorado

D. K. Salunkhe, Ph.D. Professor Emeritus, Department of Nutrition and Food Science, Utah State University, Logan, Utah

---

[1]*Current affiliation*: Senior Scientist, Research and Development, Idetek, Inc., Sunnyvale, California
[2]*Current affiliation*: Research Associate, COR Therapeutics, Inc., South San Francisco, California
[3]*Current affiliation*: Research Associate, Industrial Agricultural Products Center, University of Nebraska, Lincoln, Nebraska
[4]*Current affiliation*: Research Associate, Department of Horticulture, University of Illinois, Urbana, Illinois
[5]*Current affiliation*: Research Staff, Food and Nutrition Development and Research Center, Gadjah Mada University, Yogya Karta, Indonesia

John N. Sofos, Ph.D. Professor, Departments of Animal Sciences, and Food Science and Human Nutrition, Colorado State University, Fort Collins, Colorado

Robert Leslie Swaine, Jr., M.S., R.Ph. Research Fellow, Department of Flavor Technology, The Procter & Gamble Company, Cincinnati, Ohio

Otto B. Wurzburg, M.S.[1] Consultant, National Starch and Chemical Company, Bridgewater, New Jersey

[1]Retired: Formerly Vice President of Research—Starch Division

1
Types of Food Additives

Joseph A. Maga
Colorado State University
Fort Collins, Colorado

I. INTRODUCTION

There are approximately 2800 compounds approved for food-additive use in the United States. Since the approved list is continually changing due to additions and deletions, it is not a priority to provide a current listing of all approved food additives.

Interestingly, the E list of additives permitted in Europe approaches only 400 compounds, and the fact that many fewer food additives are permitted in European than in American foods has been a rallying point for consumers opposing the use of additives. However, it is interesting to note that approximately 1300 of the 2800 compounds on the American list are food-flavoring compounds that are used at quite low levels due to their low flavor thresholds. Also, most food flavors are composed of a multitude of compounds, and very seldom is only one compound utilized as a food flavorant.

According to the federal Food, Drug and Cosmetic Act, there are five broad categories of compounds associated with human food. These include generally recognized as safe (GRAS), which represents approximately 1600 substances, pesticide residues, unavoidable contaminants, color additives, prohibited substances, and intentional food additives.

Since one of the prerequisites for food-additive approval is effectiveness of function in a food system, one practical way in attempting to classify nearly 2800 compounds would be by their technical effect or functionality in foods. Thus, the following represents a generalized attempt to classify food additives using this approach. In addition, where appropriate, certain compounds are listed as typical of most of the categories listed.

II. CLASSES OF FOOD ADDITIVES

Anticaking and Free Flow Agents

These are compounds that are added to dry ingredients such as salt, powdered sugar, and finely ground spice blends to keep the product free flowing during storage and use. The compound added, such as calcium stearate, has the ability to preferentially tie up moisture, therefore maintaining the free flow properties of the dry product and minimizing the problems of caking, lumping and agglomeration.

Antioxidants

Traditionally, these food additives have been added to fats, oils, and fat-containing foods to prevent oxidation from occurring, which in turn can result in product rancidity. Both naturally occurring compounds such as vitamins A and C as well as synthetic antioxidants typified by butylated hydroxyanisole (BHA) and butylated hdyroxytoluene (BHT) have been utilized due to their ability to tie up free oxygen before it can react with the unsaturated portion of fatty acids. Due to the potency of some synthetic antioxidants, maximum usage levels are enforced. It should be noted that antioxidants are intended to retard but not prevent product deterioration and discoloration.

Antibrowning Agents

Certain foods can darken in color during processing or storage. These reactions can be enzymatically or nonenzymatically controlled. The reactions are potential problems with dried fruits and vegetables. The rate of reaction can be slowed by the addition of compounds such as vitamin C, citric acid, and sodium sulfite since these compounds interfere with dark color pigment formation.

Sulfiting agents have received special attention because their use in the manufacture of wine and salad bar presentations have resulted in reported adverse reactions, especially among asthmatics. Current law requires the use and presence of sulfites in food-processing operations to be noted on packaging or displayed in a prominent location relative to salad bars.

Antimicrobial Agents

These compounds are commonly called chemical preservatives and function by controlling the growth of bacteria, yeast, and molds in various food systems, thereby extending product shelf life. Common additives in this category include sodium benzoate, calcium propionate, and sorbic acid. These compounds basically retard microbial activity, which if left unchecked would result in accelerated food spoilage.

The use of chemical preservatives in various food systems has resulted in the successful widespread distribution of numerous normally highly perishable foods that are very susceptible to microbial attack. Some opponents of chemical preservatives argue that their use minimizes the need for good manufacturing procedures with special attention to the proper storage conditions for food. In certain countries the use of chemical preservatives is viewed as an alternative to the inactivation of microorganisms via traditional heat-processing techniques such as pasteurization and sterilization.

Coloring Agents and Adjuncts

Color changes associated with food processing and storage present major acceptance problems to the consumer. Therefore, various natural and synthetic coloring agents can be added to food systems to enhance product appearance. Synthetic colorants (dyes) are generally more effective and stable that most natural colorants such as grape skin extract. In addition, substances used to preserve or enhance the color of foods such as fixatives, color retention agents, and color stabilizers fall into this category.

Curing and Picking Agents

These are associated with the curing of certain meats, resulting in a characteristic pink color. A typical compound is sodium nitrite, which has the ability to interact with meat pigments to fix processed meat color.

The levels of added nitrites in various foods is dictated by law due to the fact that free nitrites have the potential to form nitrosamines during the heat processing of foods. Interestingly, nitrites can also occur naturally in foods that have received high levels of nitrate fertilizer during agricultural production. A classical example would be the application of nitrogen fertilizer just prior to the harvesting of green leafy vegetables such as spinach. The fertilizer produces a product that is dark green in color, which is desired by the consumer. However, naturally occurring microflora have the ability to convert nitrate to nitrite, which is then capable of reacting with naturally occurring free amino acids to produce a series of carcinogenic nitrosamines.

It is interesting to note that certain human water sources derived from agricultural water runoff high in nitrates due to fertilization can result in the same situation as described above. In addition, poor oral hygiene can result in the presence of microflora that have the ability to convert residual nitrate to nitrites in the mouth. When swallowed in saliva, the nitrites have the ability to produce nitrosamines in the human digestive tract.

Dough Conditioners or Strengtheners

These include various inorganic and organic compounds that have the ability to modify protein and starch in cereal-based foods, which can result in improved properties such as reduced mixing time and increased loaf volume. Compounds in this category range from various phosphates and sulfates to enzymes. Compounds in this category have the ability to produce more uniform bakery products due to naturally occurring compositional variations in wheat flour.

Drying Agents

These are similar to anticaking agents in that they have the ability to absorb moisture from other food ingredients. Dried cornstarch can be considered a drying agent.

In certain food systems, the use of drying agents is a very effective way of controlling water activity, which in turn directly influences the ability of various microbes to grow. This can influence both microbial food safety and subsequent product shelf life.

Emulsifiers

These can be both natural, such as lecithin and mono- and diglycerides, or synthetic, and they provide a means to obtain stable mixtures of systems that normally do not mix. For example, they are used to uniformly disperse certain flavors and oils throughout a food.

Emulsifiers function by effectively lowering the surface tension among ingredients, thereby establishing an emulsion. This in turn retards or prevents the separation into various phases of ingredients that normally are not miscible, such as oil and vinegar.

Enzymes

These are naturally occurring complex proteins that have the ability to degrade food lipids, proteins, and carbohydrates. For example, a pectinase can be used to naturally degrade pectin, which can cause cloud formation in fruit juices. A wide range of enzymes exist that have the ability to improve the efficiency of food processing and the overall quality of various foods. Certain enzymes can be used to improve the nutritional quality of foods by effecting complete or nearly complete degradation of proteins, thereby aiding in the digestion and assimilation of amino acids. This technique is utilized in certain infant and geriatric formulations.

Firming Agents

These compounds have the ability to add or maintain desirable crispness or texture in various food systems. Examples include the use of alum in pickles and the addition of various calcium salts to maintain firmness in canned whole tomatoes. The use of these agents results in products that can be heat processed to ensure microbial safety and that have textural properties very similar to the original raw product, which results in greater consumer acceptability.

Flavor Enhancers

These are also known as flavor intensifiers or potentiators and have the ability to intensify certain existing food flavors, especially in meats and vegetables. Classical examples include monosodium glutamate (MSG) and certain 5-nucleotides such as inosine monophosphate (IMP) and guanosine monophosphate (GMP). In addition, these compounds can be used to supplement, augment, or modify the original flavor of certain foods, thereby expanding the original flavor profile of the product in question.

The use of MSG has been under recent scrutiny due to the belief that a certain portion of the population experiences various adverse reactions, historically called the Chinese Restaurant Syndrome (CRS). However, there can be relatively high levels of naturally produced MSG in certain foods such as well-aged cheeses and concentrated tomato-based products such as tomato paste. In these food systems naturally occurring glutamic acid is produced due to protein hydrolysis. The free glutamic acid then has the ability to chemically react with the sodium portion of sodium chloride to produce the monosodium salt of glutamic acid, namely, MSG. Therefore, the basic scientific question remains as to why individuals who claim to experience adverse reactions to intentionally added MSG apparently do not experience similar reactions to naturally occurring MSG.

Flavor Adjutants

These compounds possess no characteristic flavor of their own but are used to improve the dispersability of various liquid and semi-liquid flavorants. These include compounds such as ethanol and propylene glycol.

Flavoring Agents

This class represents the most diverse group of food additives and is composed of both natural and synthetic compounds. Typical compounds include esters, lactones, and numerous heterocyclics. Numerous combinations are used to intensify or mimic flavors found in nature. They are the basis for the formulation of a wide variety of foods that have characteristically different flavors.

For the most part, the compounds primarily responsible for the characteristic flavor of most foods have been isolated, quantitated, and identified. These specific compounds in turn can be synthesized to the exact structure of their naturally occurring counterpart. In some cases, the organic flavor chemist has been able to improve on nature by modifying the chemical structure of a flavor compound to produce a more potent flavorant than is naturally occurring. Some of these compounds are extremely potent and thus can contribute specific and characteristic odors in the ppb range.

For certain food flavors, the world supply of natural flavorants is not sufficient to meet the needs of the food processing industry and thus the synthesis of the same compounds augments the natural supply. Some countries do not permit the use of synthetic flavorants whereas others do if they are so noted on the food ingredient label.

Flour-Treating Agents

These are similar to dough conditioners in that they improve the mixing properties and loaf volume of bread products. Certain of these compounds both bleach flour, giving a white flour, and modify flour protein, thereby improving flour functionality.

Formulation Aids

These compounds permit the compounding and blending of various food ingredients in an effective manner. An example would be the incorporation of an antidusting compound during the mixing of dry seasoning blends. This category of additives includes numerous compounds, all of which promote or produce a desired or modified physical or textural state in processed foods. Other examples include carriers, binders, fillers, plasticizers, film-formers, and tableting aids.

Fumigants

Most consumers ignore the fact that various insects are attracted to agricultural crops during their production, processing, and subsequent storage. For example, various insects, such as aphids, can be present in wheat at the time of harvest. In addition, the aphids may have layed eggs to ensure their next generation in the wheat. These eggs in turn have the ability to hatch at a later date into larva, which later change into mature insects and thus can be present in a bag of flour that a consumer opens. In this situation, most consumers blame the food processors for the manufacture of a contaminated product. Therefore, the use of fumigants ensures that any naturally occurring insect contamination, at any stage of its growth cycle, is inactivated.

Humectants

Consumers expect certain foods to have a uniform level of moistness associated with them. Via storage and possible moisture migration and loss, some foods can essentially "dry out," thereby seriously decreasing their overall acceptability. These compounds are used to maintain uniform moisture in semi-moist foods, thereby not permitting the food to dry out. An example would be the inclusion of propylene glycol to shredded coconut to keep it moist.

Leavening Agents

The acceptability of a wide range of baked goods relies on the formation of the gas carbon dioxide. This gas causes product expansion resulting in light, fluffy baked goods instead of heavy, dense products. This in turn adds to product appearance and eating enjoyment. These include both inorganic compounds (baking powder) used for the chemical leavening of foods and yeast for yeast-leavened products.

Lubricants and Release Agents

These represent lipid or food-grade oil-based compounds added to make the production of certain foods more efficient. An example would be spraying bread pans with a release agent so that loaves of bread can be easily removed after baking. This would be analogous to the greasing of a bread pan at home so the baked loaf will fall out of the pan after baking.

Nonnutritive Sweeteners

These include both naturally occurring and synthetic compounds that have elevated sweetening power as compared to sucrose. As a result, they are usually incorporated at low levels into various foods as a replacement for sugar. These compounds make possible the manufacture of a wide range of low- or reduced-calorie foods to serve the needs of people who have a need or desire to reduce their caloric intake. In the United States, the use of a specific nonnutritive sweetener requires preapproval for each food system for which it is intended. The economic and functional properties of this class of additives is quite interesting. Compounds hae been naturally identified and synthesized that have thousands of times the sweetening power of sucrose, for example. However, the levels found in certain natural sources are extremely low, which has a significant economic impact. Some of these compounds are rather easily denatured during product processing or with subsequent storage, therefore minimizing their effective use as a replacement for products such as sucrose.

Some of these products serve a specific need in the diabetic market, thereby providing the person with diabetes with a wider range of foods that have sweet taste properties without the deleterious heath effects of sucrose. Some of the sugar alternatives have anticariogenic properties and some are used as a means of effectively lowering total caloric intake in numerous formal and informal weight-reduction programs.

Nutrient Supplements

Typical compounds in this category include vitamins, minerals, and amino acids. They permit the food processor to restore certain nutrients that can be lost during normal processing operations. They also provide a means by which products can be fortified with nutrients to levels higher than are normally available in foods.

Certain consumer advocate groups claim that this food-additive group would not be necessary if the American food supply were not so overprocessed. However, our entire food supply cannot be consumed entirely in the raw state due to the presence of numerous antinutritional components such as urease and trypsin inhibitors. Heat processing of various foods results in the inactivation of certain antinutritional components, thereby improving these foods' overall nutritional profile.

Nutritive Sweeteners

These have been defined as products that have greater than 2% of the caloric value of sucrose per equivalent unit of sweetening capacity. Typical of this food-additive class is high-fructose corn syrup (HFCS), which is used as a replacement for sucrose in carbonated beverages. After an effective means was found to enzymatically convert the glucose in cornstarch to fructose, it became practical to use HFCS in numerous food applications. Not only is HFCS sweeter than sucrose, it also adds body or thickness to liquid preparations. In addition, HFCS serves as a humectant in semi-moist food systems, thereby maintaining product freshness.

Oxidizing and Reducing Agents

This class of additives has functional properties similar to dough conditioners in that they have the ability to chemically oxidize or reduce other food ingredients, thereby resulting in a more stable product.

pH Control Agents

These include compounds that can serve as buffers, acids, alkalis, and neutralizing agents. A typical compound would be citric acid, which can be used to acidify foods, thereby minimizing heat-processing requirements and limiting the growth of toxin-producing bacteria. Some of these compounds are used in conjunction with other food-additive classes. For example, buffering agents are used in conjunction with various chemical leavening systems to prolong or extend the effectiveness of the overall leavening system.

Processing Aids

These compounds assist in making various food-processing steps faster, easier, or simpler. An example would be the use of activated charcoal to remove unwanted color in a liquid food. Other functional agents in this category include clarifying agents, clouding agents, catalysts, floculents, filter aids, and crystallization inhibitors, all of which enhance the acceptability or utility of various foods.

Propellants, Aerating Agents, and Gases

These represent gases that are added to foods in pressurized cans such as whipped topping.

Sequestrants

A typical seqestrant is ethylenediaminetetraactic acid (EDTA), used in salad dressings. These compounds have the ability to tie up trace minerals, such as iron and copper, that can cause color changes in certain foods if present in their free state. The presence of trace amounts of polyvalent metal ions can also serve as catalysts to rancidity. These can be inactivated via the addition of EDTA.

Solvents

These compounds are used to effectively extract and concentrate functional food ingredients such as spice oleoresins. A practical example is the use of hexane to effectively and selectively extract the lipid portion from soybeans in the manufacture of soybean oil. After initial extraction, the solvent/oil mixture is heated under vacuum to volatize the hexane, which is then condensed and reused. Another example is the use of selective solvents to decaffeinate coffee.

Stabilizers and Thickeners

These include numerous starches and hydrocolloids that, when added to foods, produce a thickening action that limits subsequent product separation. They are used to control the consistency of liquid and semi-liquid foods and prevent the separation of food components during processing and storage.

Other specific functional properties provided by this class of compounds include suspending, setting, gelling, and bulking properties. For the most part, they are used in conjunction with other additive classes. For example, if a nonnutritive sweetener is used by the consumer to sweeten a cup of coffee, the actual amount of sweetener needed is extremely small. Therefore, a bulking agent is added to the sweetener to provide a larger mass of product, which is more easily used by the consumer.

Surface-Active Agents

These compounds permit the rapid wetting and rehydration of dry foods when reconstituted with liquids. Other compounds in this class can be used to either encourage or discourage foam formation in various foods. In addition, these compounds can be used to solubilize and disperse other ingredients in a formulation such as added protein to an infant formulation.

Surface Finishing Agents

These compounds basically serve to increase palatability by preserving the original gloss or shine associated with certain foods and inhibiting the discoloration of other foods. Specific compounds utilized include food-grade glazes, polishes, waxes, and protective coatings normally applied to the intact surfaces of foods such as apples and cucumbers. For example, the waxing of a cucumber retards moisture loss during the transportation and storage of an intact cucumber, thereby extending its practical shelf life to the consumer.

CONCLUSION

From the brief presentation above, it can be appreciated that food additives are an intricate part of our food supply, and if most were banned from use, dramatic changes in our food supply and subsequent eating habits would occur.

Another logical way to classify food additives is as intentional and unintentional additives. The first category represents direct additives that have a specific function, such as those outlined at the beginning of this chapter. Their functional properties can be consolidated into four rather broad categories: nutritive, freshness maintenance, sensory, and as processing aids.

The presence of unintentional food additives is a significant emotional issue, since their purpose is not evident at the time of consumption. This category includes compounds utilized during the production, processing, or storage of food. Most of these compounds—insecticides, pesticides, herbicides, and fungicides—are associated with efficient agricultural production. The vast majority of these compounds have legal maximum permissible levels, but some consumers would prefer to have zero levels in their food supply. Other types of compounds in this category include sprout inhibitors for potatoes and onions, plant hormones that increase fruit cluster yields, animal pest control agents such as rodenticides, the use of antibiotics to control disease in domesticated animals, and animal growth stimulants.

It should be noted that not all unintentional additives are synthetic compounds. For example, naturally occurring radionucleotides associated with deep well-water sources and certain soils that have naturally high levels of selenium can result in the production of various agricultural crops with measurable levels of these potentially dangerous compounds. Also to be considered in this category is the presence of insects and insect fragments that naturally become entrapped in a crop during harvest.

Packaging materials can also be a potential source of unintentional food additives finding their way into various foods. For example, with certain foods that are high in fat or alcohol, some plasticizers, pigments, and labeling inks may be partially solubilized into the food. Packaging abuse by the consumer can also result in the formation of unintentional food additives. This can be typified by the microwave heating of foods in containers that were not originally designed to be microwave processed.

According to certain consumer groups, the use of radiation in food processing may result in the formation of certain unintentional food additives. In spite of the fact that it has been scientifically documented that such foods do not actually become radioactive, some believe this to be the case. The level of radiation utilized is a significant factor to consider; for example, if low levels are used to retard microbial growth, little or no chemical changes have been documented. However, if foods are sterilized via radiation, certain chemical and flavor changes do occur, with the resulting compounds being considered unintentional additives.

2
Food Acidulants

S. S. Deshpande* and D. K. Salunkhe
*Utah State University
Logan, Utah*

Usha S. Deshpande[†]
*University of Manitoba
Winnipeg, Canada*

I. INTRODUCTION

Besides flavor and antimicrobial activities, acids contribute a variety of functional properties that lead to the enhancement of quality, palatability, nutritive value, and sensory appeal of processed foods. They are most commonly used for flavor and tartness, while their salts can act as buffering agents to modify and smooth out these sensory qualities. Several acids, because of their metal chelating ability, are also excellent synergists for use with antioxidants to retard the rancidity of fat-based foods and to prevent oxidation and browning reactions in several food products.

Acidulants are excellent antimicrobial agents. They play an important role in the preservation of various food systems, either by controlling the growth of food pathogens by maintaining an appropriate pH or by directly interfering with microbial metabolism. In several foods, the incorporation of acids into the product at sufficiently high levels can ensure a commercially sterile product (Doores, 1983). The judicious use of an acidulant for its antimicrobial properties is counterbalanced by sensory characteristics that predicate the amount of acid that can be used.

Acids also stabilize food colors, reduce turbidity, modify melt characteristics, prevent splattering, or enhance gelling (Gardner, 1966, 1972). They are also used as leavening or inversion agents, emulsifiers, nutrients, and dietary supplements. Food acidulants thus make up an extremely versatile chemical group, which may account for their extensive use as food additives.

In this chapter, the production, functionality, applications, and toxicological aspects of the inorganic and organic acids commonly used in the food industry are described.

**Current affiliation*: Idetek, Inc., Sunnyvale, California
†*Current affiliation*: COR Therapeutics, Inc., South San Francisco, California

II. GENERAL FUNCTIONS IN FOODS

Acidulants serve several important functions in food processing and preservation. The judicious selection of the proper acid for a particular food product requires knowledge of the physical and chemical properties of each acid and the functions it is capable of performing. Some of the important functions of food acidulants are described below.

A. pH Control Agents

Acidulants are important food additives for controlling pH during the processing of different food systems. Optimum pH is essential for processing or stabilizing a food system. It is particularly essential in gel-type products such as gelatin desserts, jams, jellies, and jellied candies (Gardner, 1972; Liebrand, 1978). Proper adjustment of pH is essential for optimum development of gel character and strength. This is particularly true in case of pectin gels where, depending on the pectin type, a pH range between 2.9 and 3.4 is critical, and even slight variation can have a profound effect on product quality. In formulating food products of this type, the amount of acid required to give the desired physical properties is the determining factor. Where sucrose is used as the sweetening agent, consideration must be given to the rates of inversion catalyzed by the various acidulants at different temperatures.

Acidifying agents are also important additives in leavening agents, where their reaction with the baking soda is essential for the leavening action of the carbon dioxide produced in the process. The reaction is the basis of chemical leavening in the baking industry as well as effervescence in some confectionery tablets and beverage powders. The rate of reaction is dependent upon the absolute solubility of the acid, its rate of solution, and the temperature of the environment. Acidulants are also important ingredients in maintaining the acidic pH and the tartness of carbonated beverages.

Alkaline salts of acidulants such as phosphoric acid are important food ingredients in the preparation of pasteurized, process cheese to produce the slightly alkaline pH necessary for optimum protein dispersion. These salts also react with proteins to improve their emulsification and water-binding capacities.

B. Preservatives

A proper pH control is extremely important in foods where benzoates, sorbates, and propionates are used as preservatives. These additives are often added as their salts. Their microbicidal action requires the maintenance of pH between 3.0 to 5.0. Unless the product contains sufficient natural acids, acidulants need to be added to produce the acids of these preservatives. Acidulants themselves can exert a preservative effect by lowering the pH of a product. Acidulants serve both as sterilizing acids and as antibrowning agents to maintain the normal flavor, color, and texture of several canned fruits and vegetables. An acidic pH often permits a shortening of sterilization time, which in turn results in a better quality, more nutritious product. Although fruits normally contain large amounts of organic acids, addition of acidulants may be required for proper sterilization during canning since drought, growing conditions, and the plant variety often lead to a lowered acid content. The use of acidulants in such cases, however, is not a means for overcoming poor sanitary or processing conditions.

Acidulants play a key role as antibrowning aids in preserving the quality of fruits and vegetables during canning and dehydration processes. Prior to further processing, the cut and peeled fruits and vegetables are often soaked in an acid solution containing salts. In such cases, acidulants tend to inhibit the oxidation reactions, which lead to enzymatic and nonenzymatic browning reactions by displacing any redox equilibrium in the direction of reduction.

Acidulants themselves perform a bacteriostatic function in processed foods such as salad dressings and syrups. The reproduction and growth of bacteria and other microorganisms are inhibited in an acidified medium. This helps to improve the shelf life of foods, which otherwise would be spoiled in a short period of time.

C. Chelating Agents/Antioxidant Synergists

The presence of trace metals in any food process or product can often produce undesirable reactions such as discoloration, rancidity, and instability of nutrients. These effects are often the result of oxidation, which is promoted by the catalytic action of certain metallic ions such as iron, nickel, manganese, cobalt, chromium, copper, and tin. Certain acidulants, especially the citrates and phosphates, are capable of chelating these metals. This chelating function of acidulants is also useful in retarding the enzymatic browning of fruits and vegetables. The chelating ability of acids in itself is a form of antioxidant activity. When combined with antioxidants such as BHA, BHT, and ascorbates, the acidulants are often referred to as synergists. In such cases, the combined activity of the two antioxidants is greater than their additive function. Acidulants are, therefore, widely employed as synergists for antioxidants used in the preservation of fats and oils and in food products containing fatty compounds. The synergistic effect, although in part due to their lowering the redox potential, is primarily related to their sequestering metal ions.

The sequestering ability of the acidulants, especially the phosphates, is often used in the treatment of water used in food processing. The mineral constituents of natural waters can have devastating effects on the foods processed with those natural waters. It is, therefore, a common practice to treat the waters in such a way as to "soften" them. The treatment generally involves the addition of a phosphate, alkali, shorter-chain polyphosphates, and, in some cases, orthophosphates or mixtures of these in order to complex the heavy metal ions such as iron and copper and the alkaline-earth metal ions calcium and magnesium.

D. Flavor Adjuncts

Food acidulants play an important role in the enhancement of food flavors. Without them, foods such as hard candies, gelatin desserts, carbonated and noncarbonated beverages, jellies, preserves, toppings, and many other products would taste flat. Acidulants add the tartness required to balance the excessive sweetness of these products. Until the proper balance of tartness and sweetness is achieved, the flavor cannot develop to its fullest potential. Even near the balance point, the ratio of sweetness to tartness can be fine-tuned to pronounce the primary flavor and enhance the secondary flavor notes, which otherwise would be masked by excessive sweetness or tartness (Sausville, 1974). The ratio of sweetness to tartness is commonly known as the "brix acid ratio."

The influence of an acid on overall flavor is governed by its own characteristic flavor and the degree of tartness it imparts. The characteristic flavor of some acids make them particularly useful with certain flavors. For example, tartaric acid in combination with grape flavor and phosphoric acid with cola flavors are often used. Others such as citric, fumaric, and malic acids have a broader spectrum of utility, as they are compatible with most fruit and berry flavors.

The degree of tartness of each acid also has a marked effect on the flavor of a product and governs the level at which it is used in a given product. Each individual acidulant has a slightly different tartness. Among the organic acids, the tartness of citric acid is described as clean, that of malic as smooth, fumaric as metallic, adipic as chalky, vinegar as astringent, tartaric as sharp or bitter, and lactic as sour. The inorganic phosphoric acid tends to have a flat sourness (Gardner, 1972; Sausville, 1974; Liebrand, 1978).

E. Fortification

The nutritive value of certain foods is also enhanced by the addition of acidulants when they contain ascorbic acid as one of their components. Unless present in appreciable amounts, ascorbic acid is preferentially oxidized to dehydroascorbic acid with rapid loss of vitamin activity. High acidity tends to reverse this reaction by maintaining a low redox potential, especially during the initial stages of oxidation (Gardner, 1972). The addition of food acids, therefore, tends to preserve in part some of the nutritive value of these products.

Certain dietary essential nutrients such as iron and calcium and vitamins such as vitamin D and choline are often used as supplements as salts or esters of various acidulants.

F. Viscosity and Melting Modifiers

Acidulants can markedly influence the rheological properties of dough when specifically added for this purpose or contained in the leavening agents. Succinates and acetates can react with gluten proteins to modify their plastic behavior, thereby influencing the shape and texture of baked goods. Acidulants can also influence the softening point, melt properties, and texture when added to foods such as cheese, margarines, and the mixtures used in manufacturing hard candy.

In addition, acidulants are also used for dispersing food constituents; stabilizing different emulsion systems; as meat curing agents together with other curing components in enhancing color, flavor, and preservative action; for preventing caking of dry mixes; to improve the peelability of frankfurters prior to or after smoking; as ingredients of preservatives incorporated in food wrappings of various types; and in acidic dairy cleaners for their bactericidal properties and their ability to attack milkstone through chelation. It is quite apparent that, because of their diverse valuable functions, acidulants are an important group of food additives. As a group, they are exceeded in volume of consumption only by the emulsifying agents (Sanders, 1966; Gardner, 1972).

III. CLASSIFICATION

The different acids used in the food industry can be broadly classified into two groups: inorganic and organic (Fig. 1). Among the inorganic acids, phosphoric acid and its derivatives are the most widely used food acidulants. Phosphoric acid is also the highest-value inorganic acid marketed in the United States and the second largest in terms of volume after sulfuric acid. Hydrochloric and sulfuric acids are seldom used as direct food acidulants. Nevertheless, they are used indirectly in the chemical synthesis of several food-grade chemicals. They are also used in the cornstarch-processing industry to manufacture corn syrups.

As a group, the organic acids constitute the most widely used acidulants in the food industry. The carboxylic acids, depending on the number of carboxyl groups they carry, could be further classified as mono-, di-, or tricarboxylic acids (Fig. 1). Of these, citric acid alone commands over 60% of the market share of all the acidulants used in food processing. The phenolic benzoic acid and the fatty sorbic acid are primarily used as preservatives, while other fatty acids such as butyric and caprylic acids find limited use as acidulants and flavoring ingredients.

The lactones ascorbic acid and glucono δ-lactone are both used as acidulants. Ascorbic acid is also an excellent antioxidant synergist. Both are capable of chelating metal ions that are responsible for enhancing the rancidity of fat-rich foods. Lysine, glutamic acid, and cysteine are amino acids that find limited uses as acidulants. Of these, cysteine and its derivatives are primarily used as dough conditioners in the baking industry, while the sodium salt of glutamic acid is used as flavor enhancer in numerous products. Lysine is primarily used to fortify wheat-

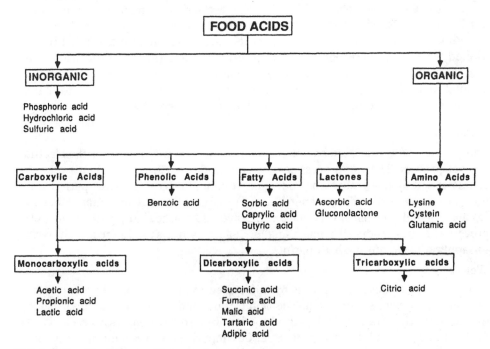

Fig. 1 Classification of acidulants.

based products to enhance their protein nutritional value. Other essential amino acids are primarily used as nutrients, especially in parenteral nutrition formulations.

IV. COMMONLY USED FOOD ACIDULANTS

A. Phosphoric Acid and Phosphates

The discovery of phosphorus by Brandt in 1669 was soon followed by characterization of its combustion product, phosphorus pentoxide. In 1694, Boyle prepared phosphoric acid by dissolution of the oxide in water (Hudson and Dolan, 1978). During the first half of the nineteenth century, the value of phosphates as fertilizers was recognized, and, by the end of the century, fertilizers had become, along with matches, the most important commercial use for phosphorus compounds. On a tonnage basis, fertilizers still remain the single largest application for phosphorus derivatives. In addition, phosphoric acid and the phosphates are widely used in detergents, human foods, animal feed supplements, metal treating, water softening, and fire retardants.

Phosphates may be defined very broadly as compounds containing four phosphorus-oxygen (P—O) linkages in which the phosphorus atom is surrounded by a tetrahedron of four oxygen atoms (Fig. 2). By sharing oxygen atoms between tetrahedra, chains, rings, and branched polymers of interconnected PO_4, tetrahedra can be formed. Since each tetrahedron can share up to three of its corners in polyphosphate formation, one-, two-, or three-dimensional networks can result (Ellinger, 1972; Hudson and Dolan, 1978). Compounds containing discrete, i.e., monomeric $(PO_4)^{3-}$, ions are known as orthophosphates or simply phosphates (Fig. 2A), its dimers produced by dehydration as pyrophosphates (Fig. 2B), linear P—O—P chains as polyphosphates (Fig. 2C), cyclic rings as metaphosphates (Fig. 2D,E), and branched polymeric materials and cage anions as ultraphosphates.

Phosphoric acid (H_3PO_4) is the highest-value inorganic acid marketed in the United States and the second largest in terms of volume (after sulfuric acid). It is also the only inorganic acid extensively used as a food acidulant, and accounts for about 25% of the weight of all the acids used in foods, compared to 60% for citric acid and 15% for the rest of the food acidulants (Gardner, 1972).

Manufacture

Phosphoric acid is produced commercially by either the wet process or the electric furnace process. The wet-process acid, produced directly from phosphatic ores, is characterized by relatively high production volume, low cost, and low purity. It is used worldwide for fertilizer manufacture. Furnace or thermal acid, manufactured from elemental phosphorus, is more expensive and considerably purer than wet-process acid. It is produced in much smaller quantities and is used almost exclusively for applications requiring high purity.

Wet Process

In this method, phosphoric acid is manufactured by digestion of phosphate rock (apatite forms) with sulfuric acid. The acid is separated from the resultant calcium sulfate slurry by filtration. Unless used for fertilizer applications, it is necessary to further purify the acid slurry to remove various impurities such as fluorides, calcium, iron, vanadium, aluminum, arsenic, and sulfates. Chemical precipitation and sol-

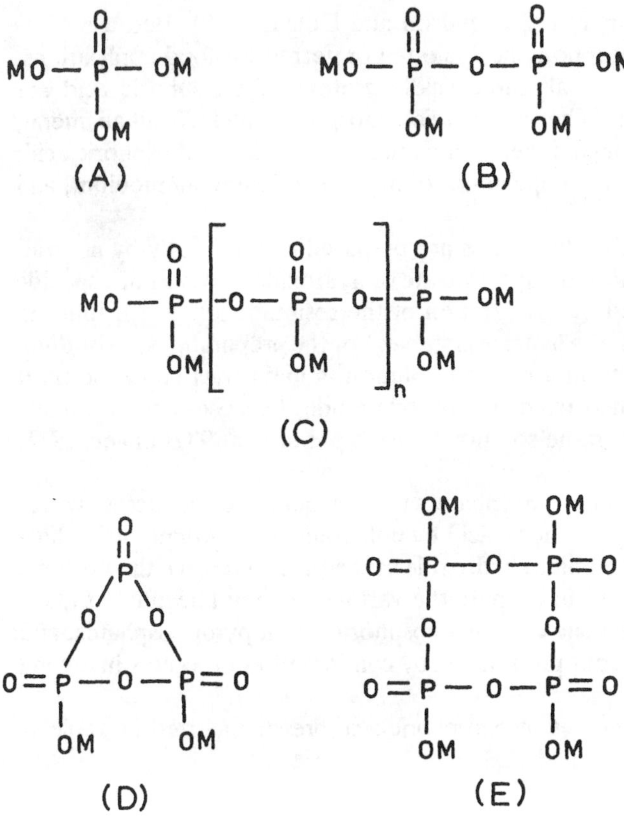

$$\begin{array}{c}
\text{O} \\
\parallel \\
\text{MO}-\text{P}-\text{OM} \\
\mid \\
\text{OM}
\end{array}
\qquad
\begin{array}{c}
\text{O} \qquad\quad \text{O} \\
\parallel \qquad\quad \parallel \\
\text{MO}-\text{P}-\text{O}-\text{P}-\text{OM} \\
\mid \qquad\qquad \mid \\
\text{OM} \qquad\quad \text{OM}
\end{array}$$

(A)   (B)

$$\text{MO}-\overset{\overset{\textstyle O}{\parallel}}{\underset{\underset{\textstyle OM}{\mid}}{P}}-\left[\!-\text{O}-\overset{\overset{\textstyle O}{\parallel}}{\underset{\underset{\textstyle OM}{\mid}}{P}}-\text{O}-\!\right]_{n}\!-\overset{\overset{\textstyle O}{\parallel}}{\underset{\underset{\textstyle OM}{\mid}}{P}}-\text{OM}$$

(C)

(D)   (E)

Fig. 2 Structures of phosphate acids and salts commonly used in foods. (A) Phosphoric or orthophosphoric acid. All orthophosphate salts will share this common structure. (B) Pyrophosphoric acid, a dimer produced by the dehydration of two orthophosphoric acid molecules. All pyrophosphate salts will have this common structure. (C) Linear chain polyphosphates. (D) Cyclic trimetaphosphates. (E) Cyclic tetrametaphosphates. The letter M in these structures can be hydrogen or a cationic ion such as sodium, calcium, potassium, or iron.

vent extraction are the main methods for purifying wet-process acid, although crystallization and ion exchange also have been used (Hudson and Dolan, 1978). During concentration with superheated steam, much of the fluorine, most of the calcium, and some of the iron, aluminum, and sulfate impurities are removed as precipitates. The remaining iron and vanadium are removed by potassium ferrocyanide treatment and the arsenic with hydrogen sulfide (Gardner, 1972).

Furnace Process

In the manufacture of phosphoric acid from elemental phosphorus, the phosphate rock is reduced to elementary phosphorus in an electric or blast furnace, the white (yellow) phosphorus is then burned in excess air, the resulting phosphorus pentoxide is hydrated, the heats of combustion and hydration are removed, and the phosphoric acid mist is collected. The product is purified further with hydrogen sulfite to remove arsenic. Oxidation and hydration are carried out as either a one-

or a two-step process (Gardner, 1972; Hudson and Dolan, 1978). Because of its purity, the furnace-grade phosphoric acid is often preferred for food applications.

In phosphate salts, any or all three acidic protons of phosphoric acid are replaced by cationic species. The commercial phosphates include alkali metal, alkaline earth, heavy metal, mixed metal, and ammonium salts of phosphoric acid; sodium phosphates are the most important, followed by calcium, ammonium, and potassium salts.

Both mono- and disodium phosphates are prepared commercially by neutralization of phosphoric acid with sodium carbonate or hydroxide. Crystals of a specific hydrate can then be obtained by evaporation of the resultant solution within the temperature range over which the hydrate is stable. For the preparation of trisodium phosphate by crystallization from a wet-mix solution, a main fraction of the third sodium atom must be obtained from sodium hydroxide, because carbon dioxide cannot be stripped readily from the solution above a pH of near 9 (Ellinger, 1972; Hudson and Dolan, 1978).

Mono-, di-, and tripotassium phosphate salts are obtained by successive replacement of the protons of phosphoric acid by potassium ions. Ammonium phosphates are prepared using ammonium hydroxide as the base to replace the protons, while calcium hydroxide is used to prepare the various calcium phosphate salts.

The condensed phosphates such as polyphosphoric acids, pyrophosphates, and polyphosphates are derived from phosphates by condensation processes involving the loss of water.

Data on the physical properties of phosphoric acid are summarized in Table 1.

Food Uses

The U.S. FDA in its Code of Federal Regulations (CFR, 1988) lists orthophosphoric and polyphosphoric acids and their calcium, potassium, sodium, and ammonium salts as GRAS food additives. The various groups are listed in Table 2. Each food additive is listed under functional categories for its applications. The straight-chain polymeric phosphates are also allowed since they are hydrolyzed to orthophosphate.

Table 1   Physical Properties of Phosphoric Acid

Chemical name	Orthophosphoric acid
Molecular formula	H_3PO_4
Molecular weight	98.00
Appearance	Unstable, orthorhombic crystals, or clear, syrupy liquid, pleasing acid taste when suitably diluted
Melting point	42.35°C
Boiling point	Loses 1/2 H_2O at 213°C
Specific gravity	1.864 to 25°C
pK_1:	2.12
pK_2:	7.21
pK_3:	12.32
Solubility	Miscible with water, alcohol

Source: Budavari, 1989; Lewis, 1989.

Table 2 Phosphate Food Additives Recognized as GRAS by the FDA

Miscellaneous and/or General Purpose Food Additives
  Phosphoric acid
  Ammonium phosphate (mono-, dibasic)
  Sodium acid pyrophosphate
  Sodium aluminum phosphate
  Calcium phosphate (mono-, di-, tribasic)
  Sodium phosphate (mono-, di-, tribasic)
  Sodium tripolyphosphate

Sequestrants
  Calcium hexametaphosphate
  Calcium phosphate (monobasic)
  Dipotassium phosphate
  Disodium phosphate
  Sodium acid phosphate
  Sodium hexametaphosphate
  Sodium metaphosphate
  Sodium phosphate (mono-, di-, tribasic)
  Sodium pyrophosphate
  Tetrasodium pyrophosphate
  Sodium tripolyphosphate

Nutrients and/or Dietary Supplements
  Calcium glycerophosphate
  Calcium phosphate (mono-, di-, tribasic)
  Calcium pyrophosphate
  Ferric phosphate
  Ferric pyrophosphate
  Ferric sodium pyrophosphate
  Magnesium phosphate (di-, tribasic)
  Manganese glycerophosphate
  Manganese hypophosphite
  Potassium glycerophosphate
  Sodium phosphate (mono-, di-, tribasic)

Emulsifying Agents
  Monosodium phosphate derivatives of mono- and diglycerides

Source: CFR, 1988.

Although doubts were cast earlier on the use of cyclic metaphosphates as GRAS additives, subsequent studies have shown that little, if any, cyclic metaphosphates are absorbed through the intestinal wall when they are administered orally (Ellinger, 1972). The metaphosphates must first be hydrolyzed to tripolyphosphate and next to orthophosphate, which then can be absorbed. Sodium metaphosphate is allowed as a GRAS additive, provided it meets the Food Chemicals Codex specifications. The ammonium, calcium, and potassium salts are also equally acceptable.

Phosphoric acid is the least expensive of all the food-grade acidulants; it is also the strongest, giving the lowest attainable pH (Gardner, 1972). The bulk of the acid is used in cola, root beer, sarsaparilla, and similar flavored carbonated beverages. It is also used in cheeses and in brewing to adjust pH. Besides its major use in soft drinks, phosphoric acid is also used to enrich and preserve fodder, as an ingredient of bread dough, as a yeast stimulant, to neutralize the caustic in peeling of fruits, to clarify and acidify collagen in the production of gelatin, in the purification of vegetable oils, and, to a small extent, in the manufacture of jams and jellies (Gardner, 1972).

The salts of phosphoric acid, such as monocalcium phosphate, dicalcium phosphate, sodium aluminum phosphate, and sodium acid pyrophosphate, are ingredients of baking powders and other leavening mixtures.

The monosodium phosphate derivatives of mono- and diglycerides of edible fats or oils or edible fat-forming fatty acids are included under emulsifying agents.

Several phosphate derivatives are also listed in the Standards of Identity for a wide variety of food products. Disodium phosphate is allowed as an optional ingredient in ice cream and frozen custards where chocolate or cocoa is added for flavor (CFR, 1988). Phosphoric acid is also an optional ingredient in both the fruit-flavored noncarbonated beverage standard and the nonalcoholic carbonated beverage standard. Calcium, magnesium, potassium, or sodium phosphates are included as buffering agents. The Standards of Identity for artificially sweetened fruit jellies allow the use of sodium phosphate, disodium phosphate, and trisodium phosphate.

Phosphates are optional emulsifying agents in the pasteurized process cheese standard, while phosphoric acid is listed as one of the permitted acidulants. Monocalcium phosphate is a permitted acidulant in cereal flours, and calcium phosphate, sodium acid pyrophosphate, or sodium aluminum phosphate are optional ingredients for self-rising flour (CFR, 1988).

Toxicology

The toxicity of various phosphate derivatives commonly used in foods has been extensively investigated by several researchers. Similar to other inorganic salts, phosphates in excess quantities can be toxic. Excessive amounts of inorganic salts not only upset mineral balance in the body, but they also affect the osmotic pressure of body fluids (Ellinger, 1972). The Food and Agriculture Organization, in collaboration with the World Health Organization, has published two extensive reports on the toxicology of various phosphates (FAO/WHO, 1967; FAO, 1974). The following comments on the toxicity of phosphates are primarily based on these two reports, and an extensive review on this topic was compiled by Ellinger (1972).

Data summarized in Table 3 on the acute toxicity of various phosphates indicate that orthophosphates and the shorter-chain polyphosphates are more toxic than sodium chloride when given orally, while the longer-chain and the cyclic polyphosphates are less toxic. In general, all phosphates are significantly more toxic when introduced into the body in a manner that circumvents the digestive system. Intraperitoneal or intravenous injection of the phosphates, including the higher polyphosphates, produces only small differences in the LD_{50} levels, probably due to rapid enzymatic hydrolysis of the polyphosphate chains to orthophosphate in the blood (Ellinger, 1972).

The introduction of phosphate salts into the body by other than oral methods is meaningless in evaluating the toxicity of phosphates as food ingredients. These studies do not take into consideration the changes that salts undergo prior to or during absorption through the intestinal wall. The feeding studies, in contrast,

Table 3 Acute Toxicity Levels of Phosphates in Animals

Phosphate	Animal	Route	LD_{50} (mg/kg)	Approx. lethal dose (mg/kg)
H_3PO_4	Rabbit	i.v.		1010
NaH_2PO_4	Mouse	oral		>100
NaH_2PO_4	Guinea pig	oral		>2000
NaH_2PO_4	Rat	i.p.		>36
Na_2HPO_4	Rabbit	i.v.		>985, ≤1075
$NaH_2PO_4 + Na_2HPO_4$	Rat	i.v.	>500	
$Na_2H_2P_2O_7$	Mouse	oral	2650	
$Na_2H_2P_2O_7$	Mouse	s.c.	480	
$Na_2H_2P_2O_7$	Mouse	i.v.	59	
$Na_2H_2P_2O_7$	Rat	oral	>4000	
$Na_4P_2O_7$	Rat	i.p.	233	
$Na_4P_2O_7$	Rat	i.v.	100-500	
$Na_4P_2O_7$	Mouse	i.p.		ca. 40
$Na_4P_2O_7$	Mouse	oral	2980	
$Na_4P_2O_7$	Mouse	s.c.	400	
$Na_4P_2O_7$	Mouse	i.v.	69	
$Na_4P_2O_7$	Rabbit	i.v.		ca. 50
$Na_5P_3O_{10}$	Mouse	oral	3210	
$Na_5P_3O_{10}$	Mouse	s.c.	900	
$Na_5P_3O_{10}$	Mouse	i.v.	71	
$Na_5P_3O_{10}$	Rat	i.p.	134	
$Na_6P_4O_{13}$	Rat	oral	3920	
$Na_6P_4O_{13}$	Rat	s.c.	875	
$(KPO_3)n$ + pyro	Rat	oral	4000	
$(KPO_3)n$ + pyro	Rat	i.v.	ca. 18	
Hexametaphosphate[a]	Rabbit	i.v.		ca. 140
Hexametaphosphate	Mouse	oral		>100
Hexametaphosphate	Mouse	oral	7250	
Hexametaphosphate	Mouse	s.c.	1300	
Hexametaphosphate	Mouse	i.v.	62	
$(NaPO_3)\eta = 6$[b]	Rat	i.p.	192	
$(NaPO_3)\eta = 11$	Rat	i.p.	200	
$(NaPO_3)\eta = 27$	Rat	i.p.	326	
$(NaPO_3)\eta = 47$	Rat	i.p.	70	
$(NaPO_3)\eta = 65$	Rat	i.p.	40	
$(NaPO_3)_3$ cyclic	Mouse	oral	10,300	
$(NaPO_3)_3$ cyclic	Mouse	s.c.	5,940	
$(NaPO_3)_3$ cyclic	Mouse	i.v.	1,165	
NaCl (table salt)	Mouse	oral	5,890	
NaCl (table salt)	Mouse	s.c.	3,000	
NaCl (table salt)	Mouse	i.v.	645	

i.p. = Intraperitoneal; i.v. = intravenous; s.c. = subcutaneous; oral = by mouth (in diet, by stomach tube, etc.).
[a]Average chain lengths (η) were not given.
[b]Polyphosphate preparations for which η was determined.
Source: Ellinger, 1972; FAO, 1974.

reflect more accurately on the toxicity of phosphates as food ingredients. Even then, definitive conclusions are difficult to draw, because in most studies, optimum ratios of dietary essential minerals were either not used or mentioned in detail. The interrelationship between calcium and phosphorus in human nutrition is well established. A proper ratio of these two minerals in the human diet is essential to maintain proper bone system. While the short-term studies, sometimes conducted at concentrations as high as 2–4% in the diet, generally do not indicate any adverse effects of phosphates, most long-term feeding studies indicate some retardation of growth rates, calcium deposition in various tissues and organs, and, more noticeably, heart and kidney damage in test animals (Table 4). Toxic symptoms may also manifest over a period of time as a result of chelation of calcium, iron, magnesium, copper, and similar ions essential to human metabolism by the phosphate anion.

The results of animal-feeding studies reported in the scientific literature indicate that levels of 0.5% of the phosphates could be tolerated in the diet without any adverse physiological effects. Higher levels could possibly be tolerated if a proper balance of other ions, particularly calcium, magnesium, and potassium, is maintained (Ellinger, 1972; FAO, 1974). Few, if any, applications for phosphates require a concentration of >0.5% to obtain the desired effect. In fact, higher levels of phosphates often produce adverse physical and chemical effects and off-flavors in food products. According to Ellinger (1972), a 0.5% phosphate level is highly unlikely ever to appear in the total human diet.

While setting the dietary intake guidelines for phosphoric acid and its salts additives, the FAO (1974) has taken into consideration the important role phosphates play in human metabolism, especially in bone, teeth, and many enzyme systems. Phosphorus is also a key element in carbohydrate, fat, and protein metabolism and is the primary source of energy store in the plant and animal kingdom.

FAO (1974) estimated that adult humans require a minimum of 0.88 g of phosphorus in their daily diet. The blood serum of human adults normally carries 2.5–4.5 mg phosphorus per 100 ml, while that of children carries a higher level. While setting the guidelines for phosphorus intake in the diet, in addition to the available toxicological data on various phosphates, the FAO (1974) has also taken into consideration the levels of calcium and other minerals in the human diet that affect the levels of phosphates that will produce the earliest signs of adverse effects. The Committee has recommended an unconditional acceptance level for total dietary phosphorus of <30 mg/kg body weight/day in the human nutrition. This level is considered safe under all conditions of diet. The FAO (1974) has also suggested a conditional acceptance level of 30–70 mg/kg body weight/day when the dietary calcium level is high.

B. Hydrochloric Acid

Hydrochloric acid is rarely used as an acidulant by the classical definition. Nevertheless, it finds many applications in the food industry.

Manufacture

Hydrochloric acid is produced industrially by the interaction of NaCl and H_2SO_4; from NaCl, SO_2, air, and water vapor; by controlled combination of the elements; or as a byproduct of the synthesis of chlorinated hydrocarbons (Rosenberg, 1980).

Food Uses

Hydrochloric acid is permitted as a food acidulant by the FAO (1974). Indirectly, it also finds several applications in the food industry. It is used to produce the chloride salts of several important food additives. Hydrochloric acid is also used in processes that require hydrolysis of starting materials such as proteins and starches. It can be used in the production of corn syrups of varying degrees by controlled acid hydrolysis of corn starch.

Toxicology

The constituent ions of hydrochloric acid are normal participants in animal and human metabolism and, per se, of no toxicological significance. Toxicological considerations are involved either in the purely local action of the corrosive acid or in the effects of the addition of large quantities of either hydrogen or chloride ions to the electrolyte pool of the body (FAO, 1974).

The hydrolytic action of hdyrochloric acid on food substances is similar, in principle, to that of the acid occurring in normal gastric juice. In addition, it also regulates the pepsin activity of the gastric juice (Lehninger, 1972). Physiologically, hydrochloric acid is also important in controlling the tone of the pylorus, and thus the rate of gastric emptying, as well as the amount of acid secretion in the stomach.

Concentrated solutions of hydrochloric acid cause severe burns; permanent visual damage may also occur. Prolonged exposures also result in dermatitis and photosensitization. Inhalation of acid vapors results in cough, choking, and inflammation and ulceration of the respiratory tract. Ingestion of the strong solutions of the acid corrodes mucous membranes, esophagus, and stomach and causes dysphagia, nausea, vomiting, intense thirst, and diarrhea. In extreme cases, circulatory collapse and death may occur (Budavari, 1989).

Because of its physiological role, the FAO (1974) concluded that in concentrations approaching the physiological pH of the gastric juice, hydrochloric acid is probably of no toxicological significance. It also found no need to limit its use on toxicological grounds when used in accordance with good manufacturing practice.

C. Sulfuric Acid

In terms of volume, sulfuric acid is the most important inorganic acid marketed in the United States and is second in terms of commercial value after phosphoric acid. Similar to hydrochloric acid, it is not directly used as an acidulant in foods but finds several applications in the manufacture and synthesis of various additives used in foods.

Manufacture

Sulfuric acid is prepared by the Contact process (Lowenheim and Moran, 1975) according to the reactions

$$2\,SO_2 + O_2 \rightarrow 2\,SO_3$$

and

$$SO_3 + H_2O \rightarrow H_2SO_4$$

Table 4 Short-Term and Long-Term Feeding Studies with Phosphates

Phosphate	Test animal	Length of test[a]	Maximum level tolerated	Effect of excess phosphate
Orthophosphoric Acid				
H_3PO_4 (36.4%)	Humans	Variable	17–26 g/d	No adverse effects[b]
H_3PO_4 (36.4%)	Rats	>12 mo	>0.75%	No adverse effects
H_3PO_4 (36.4%)	Rats	44 d	<2.94%	Kidney damage
Na and K Orthophosphates				
MSP	Humans	Variable	5–7 g/d	No adverse effects
MSP	Rats	42 d	>3.4 g/kg/d	Kidney damage
MSP	Guinea pigs	200 d	>2.2%, <4.0%	Calcium deposits, reduced growth
MSP	Guinea pigs	12–32 wk	4–8%[c]	Calcium deposits, reduced growth
MSP + DSP	Rats	3 generations	>0.5%, <1.0%	Kidney damage
DSP	Rats	6 mo	>1.8%, <3.0%	Kidney damage
DSP	Rats	1 mo	<5.0%	Kidney damage
DKP	Rats	150 d	>5.1%	No adverse effects
Pyrophosphates				
TSPP	Rats	6 mo	>1.8%, <3.0%	Kidney damage
TSPP	Rats	16 wk	<1.0%	Kidney damage
SAPP + TSPP + $(KPO_3)n$	Rats	3 generations	>0.5%, <1.0%	Kidney damage
Tripolyphosphates				
STP	Rats	6 mo	>1.8%, <3.0%	Kidney damage
STP	Rats	1 mo	>0.2%, <2.0%	Kidney damage
STP	Rats	2 y	>0.5%, <5.0%	Kidney damage
STP	Dog	1 mo	>0.1 g/kg/d	No adverse effects
STP	Dog	5 mo	<4.0 g/kg/d	Kidney, heart damage

Polyphosphates

SHMP	Rats	150 d	>0.9%,	<3.5%	Slight growth reduction
SHMP	Rats	1 mo	>0.2%,	<2.0%	Kidney damage
SHMP	Rats	3 generations	>0.5%,	<5.0%	Kidney damage
SHMP	Dog	1 mo	>0.1 g/kg/d		No adverse effects
SHMP	Dog	5 mo	<2.5 g/kg/d		Kidney, heart damage
Graham's salt	Rats	6 mo	>1.8%,	<3.0%	Kidney damage
(KPO$_3$)n + SAPP + TSPP	Rats	3 generations	>0.5%,	<1.0%	Kidney damage

Cyclic Phosphates

(NaPO$_3$)$_3$	Rats	1 mo	>2.0%,	<10.0%	Kidney damage
(NaPO$_3$)$_3$	Rats	2 y	>0.1%,	<1.0%	Retarded growth of males
(NaPO$_3$)$_3$	Rats	3 generations	>0.05%		No adverse effects
(NaPO$_3$)$_3$	Dog	1 mo	>0.1 g/kg/d		No adverse effects
(NaPO$_3$)$_3$	Dog	5 mo	<4.0 g/kg/d		Kidney, heart damage
(NaPO$_3$)$_4$	Rats	1 mo	>2.0%,	<10.0%	Kidney, heart damage
(NaPO$_3$)$_4$	Dog	1 mo	>0.1 g/kg/d		No adverse effects
(NaPO$_3$)$_4$	Dog	5 mo	<4.0 g/kg/d		Kidney, heart damage

MSP = Monosodium phosphate; DSP = disodium phosphate; DKP = dipotassium phosphate; TSPP = trisodium pyrophosphate; SAPP = sodium acid pyrophosphate; TSPP = trisodium pyrophosphate; STP = sodium tripolyphosphate; SHMP = sodium hexametaphosphate.
[a]Some studies did not give definite time periods.
[b]No adverse effects = no physiological damage noticeable at any level of phosphate tested.
[c]Guinea pigs tolerated higher levels of phosphate only when increased levels of Mg^{2+} and K$^+$ were present in diets.
Source: Ellinger, 1972; FAO; 1974.

and by the Chamber process according to the reactions

$$2 \, NO + O_2 \rightarrow 2 \, NO_2$$

and

$$NO_2 + SO_2 + H_2O \rightarrow H_2SO_4 + NO$$

Sulfuric acid of commerce contains 93–98% H_2SO_4.

Food Uses

Sulfuric acid is used in the chemical synthesis of several compounds intended for food applications. Phosphoric acid manufacture by the wet-acid process also requires the digestion of phosphate rock with sulfuric acid. It is also used in the hydrolysis of cornstarch for the production of corn syrups. The various sulfate derivatives used in food applications are also prepared using sulfuric acid.

Toxicology

Sulfuric acid is corrosive to all body tissues. Inhalation of concentrated vapors of the acid causes serious lung damage, while its contact with eyes results in total loss of vision. Skin contact with strong sulfuric acid solutions produces severe necrosis, while frequent skin contact with dilute solutions causes dermatitis (Gosselin, 1984).

D. Acetic Acid and Its Salts

Acetic Acid (Vinegar)

Acetic acid (CH_3COOH) is a colorless, waterlike liquid that has a piercingly sharp, vinegary odor and a burning taste. Vinegar, its dilute aqueous solution, has been used since the earliest recorded human history. Theophrastus (327–287 B.C.) studied the use of vinegar in white lead and verdigris manufacture (Wagner, 1978). This work was later closely followed by the Roman encyclopedist, Plins (A.D. 27–79), and the architect Vitruvius (ca. 25 B.C.) The term "acetic acid" appears to have been introduced by Libavius (A.D. 1540–1600). Kolbe was credited with the preparation of acetic acid from its elements in 1847 (Wagner, 1978). In contrast, the literal meaning of vinegar is "sour wine."

Very little pure acetic acid is used in foods, although it is classified by the FDA in its Code of Federal Regulations (CFR, 1988) as a GRAS material. Consequently, it may be used in products not covered by the Definitions and Standards of Identity.

Manufacture

Virtually all acetic acid produced commercially is made by one of three routes: acetaldehyde oxidation, liquid phase hydrocarbon oxidation, and methanol carbonylation (Faith et al, 1957; Miller, 1969; Wagner, 1978). Its use in food, however, is not permitted by the law. The ancient method of ethanol fermentation is still applied to the production of vinegar.

Vinegars are produced from cider, grapes (or wine), sucrose, glucose, or malt by successive alcoholic and acetous fermentations (Gardner, 1972). In the first step, sugar in the plant material is converted into alcohol and carbon dioxide through the action of enzymes produced by yeasts. The next step involves the conversion of alcohol into vinegar by *Acetobacter*. This bacteria provides the enzymes to convert the alcohol first to acetaldehyde and then to acetic acid.

Three distinct approaches are used in vinegar fermentation. In all three, the air supplies the oxygen needed for the conversion of alcohol into vinegar. They differ primarily in the manner in which the raw materials (mash, bacteria, and air) are brought together. These methods are described briefly below.

Open Vat Method. The open vat method was used for vinegar production until the beginning of the nineteenth century (Mayer, 1963). It consists of exposing fermented grape, apple, or other fruit juices to the action of airborne vinegar bacteria. Vinegar made by such primitive methods naturally contains other acids, such as lactic and propionic, by the action of wild bacteria. Such vinegars, therefore, show an aroma of high degree of esterification and a characteristic taste pattern.

Trickle Method. In the trickle method, the stock solution is trickled over twigs or wood shavings to increase the contact surface with the air, rather than let the product stand in shallow pans. It increases the speed of vinegar production and reduces excessive losses from overoxidation and evaporation. The process also produces vinegars of a higher grain strength, generally in excess of 6–7%. The process is still used for the production of white vinegar.

Most trickle generators are filled with beechwood shavings. Most recirculating generators hold about 2000 cubic feet of shavings. The flow rates for the mash and the supply of air are controlled by rotameters, while the temperature is controlled through a cooling system with water and a heat exchanger. Such generators produce 500–1000 gallons of 100 grain vinegar during a 24-hour period. Batch sizes generally vary from 2000 to 4000 gallons.

Bubble Method. Submerged fermentation processes in which the aeration of the bulk liquid is obtained by bubbling air through it are now routinely used for vinegar production. Most processes are continuous systems in which an exactly measured amount of fresh mash is fed continuously through a metering pump, while an equal amount of finished vinegar is discharged continuously into a receiving tank. It is essential to maintain the maximum number of vinegar bacteria to avoid periods of low vinegar production.

Data on the physical properties of acetic acid are summarized in Table 5.

Food Uses

Vinegar is used as an acidifier, flavor enhancer, flavoring agent, pH control agent, pickling agent, solvent, and for its antimicrobial properties. Vinegars are extensively used in the preparation of salad dressings, mayonnaise, sour and sweet pickles, sauces and catsups, cheese, chewing gum, dairy products, baked goods, rendered fats, gravies, and oils. They are also used in the curing of meat and in the canning of certain vegetables (Meat Inspection Division, 1966; Gardner, 1966). Because of its low cost and antimicrobial action, vinegar is often added to infant feeding formulas to replace lactic acid (Doores, 1983).

Acetic acid is more effective in limiting yeast and bacterial growth than mold growth. It probably works by lowering the pH below the optimum levels for growth. *Acetobacter* and certain lactic acid bacteria can tolerate acetic acid, since they are often associated with it in fermented products such as pickles, sauerkraut, and vinegar (Doores, 1983, 1989). It is also an effective antifungal agent at pH 3.5 against bread molds.

Toxicology

Acetic acid enters naturally into the metabolism of the body. It is absorbed from the gastrointestinal tract and is completely utilized in oxidative metabolism or in

Table 5   Physical Properties of Acetic Acid

Chemical names	Monocarboxylic acid, ethanoic acid
Molecular formula	CH_3COOH ($C_2H_4O_2$)
Molecular weight	60.06
Appearance	Clear, colorless liquid, pungent odor
pK_a	4.75
pH of aqueous solutions	
1.0 M	2.4
0.1 M	2.9
0.01 M	3.4
Ionization constant, K_1	8×10^{-5}
Melting point	16.7°C
Boiling point	118.1°C
Flash point	43°C (closed cup), 57°C (open cup)
Lower explosive level	5.4 vol % at 100°C
Upper explosive limit	16.0 vol % at 100°C
Specific gravity	1.049 at 20°/4°C
Surface tension	27.57 dyne/cm at 20.1°C
Autoignition temperature	465°C
Vapor pressure	11.4 mm at 20°C
Vapor density	2.07
Solubility	Miscible in water, alcohol, glycerol, and ether

Source: Gardner, 1972; Budavari, 1989; Doores, 1989; Lewis, 1989.

anabolic syntheses. Isotope experiments have shown acetates to be utilized in the formation of glycogen, intermediates of carbohydrates and fatty acid synthesis, as well as cholesterol synthesis (FAO, 1974). Acetic acid also participates in the acetylation of amines and may be converted to alanine by transamination and, therefore, incorporated into proteins of plasma, liver, kidney, gut mucosa, muscle, and brain (Anonymous, 1970).

Acetic acid solutions in water or organic solvents can be very strongly corrosive to the skin and can cause irreparable scarring of tissues of the eyes, nose, or mouth. Any solution containing >50% acetic acid should be considered a corrosive acid (Wagner, 1978). Its action is insidious because there is no immediate burning sensation upon applying the strong acid to the unbroken skin, and blisters appear within 30 minutes to 4 hours. When sensory nerve receptors are attacked, severe and unremitting pain is felt. After the blisters appear, washing with water or bicarbonate seldom alleviates the pain.

Acetic acid causes a variety of adverse effects in humans. These range from allergic-type symptoms such as canker sores (Tuft and Ettelson, 1956), cold sensitivities (Wiseman and Adler, 1956), and epidermal reactions (Weil and Rogers, 1951) to death (Palmer, 1932). Humans ingesting acetic acid in high concentrations at a low pH have exhibited burned lips, stomach, and intestinal mucosa, corroded lung tissue, and subsequent pneumonia resulting from the inhalation of vapors (Gerhartz, 1949). Acidosis and renal failure, reduction of clotting efficiencies, and interference in blood coagulation have also been reported (Paar et al., 1968; Fin'ko, 1969).

In short-term feeding studies, Sollman (1921) fed groups of three to six rats 0.01, 0.1, 0.25, and 0.5% acetic acid in drinking water for periods of up to 9–15 weeks. Although mortality rate was unaffected, rats given 0.5% acetic acid showed a progressive reduction in body weight gain, loss of appetite, and a 27% decrease in food consumption. In other studies, Okabe et al. (1971) observed ulceration of gastric mucosa at 10% level in rat diets, while a 20% concentration was required for the same effect in cats.

Takhirov (1969) studied the effects of vapor levels of acetic acid in air. Rats exposed to levels of 0.2 or 0.5 mg/m^3 acetic acid vapors showed muscle imbalance. The human olfactory thresholds to acetic acid vapors were 0.60 mg/m^3. Levels of 0.48 mg/m^3 altered sensitivity to light, and 0.29 mg/m^3 caused changes in electroencephalograms. Based on these studies, Takhirov (1969) suggested that the levels of acetic acid vapors in air should not exceed 0.06 mg/m^3.

In other human studies, Parmeggiani and Sassi (1954) reported that workers exposed for 7–12 years to acetic acid vapors in the production of acetyl cellulose displayed corrosion of the hands, eyes, teeth, pharynx, and lungs with an air concentration of 0.2–0.65 mg/L. Men having 7–25 years of exposure displayed blood abnormalities (Cesaro and Granata, 1955).

Since acetic acid occurs naturally in plant and animal tissues and is involved in fatty acid and carbohydrate metabolism as acetyl CoA, and because humans consume about 1 g/day acetic acid in vinegar and other foods and beverages, the FAO has set no limit on its acceptable daily intake for humans (FAO, 1974).

Acetate Salts and Derivatives

Certain salts of acetic acid, such as sodium, calcium, or potassium acetate, are often substituted for acetic acid for certain food applications. According to the Code of Federal Regulations (CFR, 1988), their use in food is subject to good manufacturing practices. Some of the regulatory uses of acetate salts and derivatives for food applications are summarized in Table 6.

Compared with acetic acid, comprehensive data on the toxicity of various acetate salts and their derivatives are lacking. The LD$_{50}$ for sodium acetate when injected intravenously in mouse was reported to be 380 mg/kg body weight (Spector, 1956). A short-term study with chickens fed diets supplemented with 5.44% sodium acetate (equivalent to 4% acetic acid) showed reduced growth rates, depressed appetite, and increased mortality rates compared to those fed control diets (Waterhouse and Scott, 1962). These effects, however, were attributed to the sodium rather than the acetate moiety.

The FAO (1974) concluded that, similar to acetic acid, acetate is a normal metabolite with rapid turnover in humans, and, hence, no guidelines were set for its acceptable daily intake in human diets.

Sodium and Calcium Diacetate

Sodium and calcium diacetates are effective antifungal agents. They are used primarily to retard mold growth in cheese spreads at 0.1–2.0% levels and in malt syrups at 0.5% levels (Doores, 1989). Butter wrappers can also be treated with sodium diacetate to prevent mold growth (Chichester and Tanner, 1972). At acidic pH of 3.5 to 4.5, they were also proven effective in controlling mold growth in animal feeds and silage (Glabe and Maryanski, 1981). Sodium diacetate has been

Table 6 Food Applications of Acetate Salts and Derivatives

Salt/Derivative	Applications
Sodium acetate	pH control agent, flavoring agent, adjuvant, boiler water additive for food grade steam, GRAS compound
Calcium acetate	Firming agent, pH control agent, processing aid, sequestrant, texturizer, stabilizer, thickener, stabilizer when salts migrate from food-packaging material, GRAS compound
Ethyl acetate	Solvent for decaffeination of tea and coffee
α-Tocopherol acetate	Dietary supplement
Vitamin A acetate	Dietary supplement
Polyvinyl acetate	Chewing gum base
Trisodium nitriloacetate	Boiler feedwater additive at less than 5 ppm levels with the exception of processing of dairy products
Miscellaneous	As indirect food additive in adhesives, resinous and polymeric coatings, plasticizers, paper and paperboard packaging material, as closures with sealing gaskets for food containers

Source: CFR, 1988.

used in the baking industry to inhibit bread molds and the "rope-forming" bacteria, primarily because it is ineffective against the yeasts used in the bread-making process (Doores, 1989).

The Code of Federal Regulations (CFR, 1988) allows the use of sodium and calcium diacetate as antimicrobial or pH control agents, flavoring agents, and adjuvants. They are approved for use in cheese spreads, malt syrups, salad dressings, pickled products, butter, and wrapping materials. In combination with malic acid, the diacetates can also be used in the manufacture of synthetic dry vinegars. Both sodium and calcium diacetate are GRAS substances.

Comprehensive toxicological data for the diacetates are not available. Although they do not occur naturally in plants and animals, they are presumed to be metabolized in a manner similar to that of acetic acid (FAO/WHO, 1962, 1963). The FAO (1974) has limited the use of sodium diacetate in the human diet to a level of 15 mg/kg body weight/day.

Dehydroacetic Acid

Dehydroacetic acid, because of its high pKa value of 5.27, is an effective antifungal agent at higher pH ranges than most other acidulants. It is also shown to be twice as effective as sodium benzoate at pH 5.0 against *Saccharomyces cerevisiae* and 25 times more effective against *Penicillium glaucum* and *Aspergillus niger* (Banwart, 1979).

The Code of Federal Regulations (CFR, 1988) has approved the use of dehydroacetic acid and its sodium salt as a preservative for cut and peeled squash up to levels not exceeding 65 ppm. It is also allowed for use as a fungistatic agent in cheese wrappers.

Spencer et al. (1950) have reported extensive toxicological studies on dehydroacetic acid. It did not show any adverse effects in rats fed diets containing 10,

30, or 100 mg acid/kg body weight/day for a period of 34 days. However, at higher levels (>300 mg/kg/day), the animals showed severe weight loss and damage to internal organs. A similar 2-year feeding study with male and female rats fed 0.02, 0.05, and 0.1% acid in the diet showed no adverse changes in growth rates, mortality, appearance, hematology, or histopathology. Spencer et al. (1950) did not observe any toxic effects in monkeys when dehydroacetic acid was given at 50 and 100 mg/kg body weight five times a week for up to one year, although 200 mg/kg dose led to growth and organ changes. These authors also reported that the sodium salt of the acid was nonirritating to rabbit skin, even after prolonged exposure.

E. Propionic Acid and Its Salts

Propionic acid, a monocarboxylic acid, is an oily liquid with a slightly pungent, disagreeable rancid odor. Its salts are white, free-flowing powders with a slight cheeselike flavor. Propionic acid is normally found in cheese and as a metabolite in the ruminant gastrointestinal tract (Doores, 1983). Swiss cheeses may contain up to 1% acid due to the growth and metabolism of the genus *Propionibacterium*, associated with the manufacture of this cheese and the development of its characteristic cheesy flavor. This naturally produced acid also acts as a preservative in Swiss cheese.

Manufacture

Propionic acid and its salts can be manufactured using the Reppe process from ethylene, carbon monoxide, and steam and using the Larson process from ethanol and carbon monoxide using boron trifluoride as a catalyst (Goos, 1953; Gardner, 1972). It can also be produced by the oxidation of propionaldehyde, as a byproduct in the Fischer-Tropsch process for the synthesis of fuel, and in wood distillation. Fermentation processes can also be used for the production of propionic acid.

Data on the physical properties of propionic acid are summarized in Table 7. The acid is readily miscible in water, alcohol, ether, and chloroform, while its sodium salt is more soluble than the calcium salt.

Table 7 Physical Properties of Propionic Acid

Chemical names	Methylacetic acid, ethylformic acid
Molecular formula	CH_3CH_2COOH ($C_3H_6O_2$)
Molecular weight	74.09
Appearance	Oily liquid, pungent, rancid odor
Specific gravity	0.998 at 15°/4°C
Melting point	−21.5°C
Boiling point	141.1°C
Refractive index	1.3848 at 25°C
pK_a	4.87
Vapor pressure	10 mm at 39.7°C
Vapor density	2.56
Autoignition temperature	513°C
Solubility	Miscible in water, alcohol, ether, and chloroform

Source: Goos, 1953; Gardner, 1972; Budavari, 1989; Lewis, 1989.

Food Uses

The FDA, in its Code of Federal Regulations (CFR, 1988), lists propionic acid and its sodium, potassium, and calcium salts as preservatives in their summary of permitted GRAS additives when used at a level not in excess of the amount reasonably required to accomplish the intended effect. Calcium and sodium propionates are also listed as antimycotics when migrating from food-packaging materials.

Propionic acid and its salts are used primarily in baked products to suppress bacteria causing "rope" in the center of bread and the growth of mold on both bread and cakes (Goos, 1953; Matz, 1960; Gardner, 1972). It also acts as a mold inhibitor in cheese foods and spreads.

Propionates may be added to bread dough without interfering with leavening, since they do not inhibit yeast. Sodium propionate is recommended for use in chemically leavened products, because the calcium ion interferes with the leavening action (Doores, 1983). Calcium propionate, however, is preferred for use in bread and rolls, since it contributes to the enrichment of the product. The use of propionates in bakery products is regulated by the Standards of Identity, which set a limit of 0.32% in flour and in white breads and rolls, 0.38% in whole wheat products, and 0.3% in cheese products.

Toxicology

Propionic acid is not a normal constituent of edible fats and oils. It is, however, produced in the intermediary metabolism as the terminal three-carbon fragment in the form of propionyl CoA during the oxidation of odd-number carbon fatty acids. The oxidation of the side chain of cholesterol by rat liver mitochondria also produces propionate as the immediate product of cleavage (Lehninger, 1972). Propionates are metabolized and utilized in the same way as normal dietary fatty acids. Even after large doses, no significant amounts of propionic acid are excreted in the urine (FAO, 1974). In vitro propionic acid is completely oxidized by liver preparations to carbon dioxide and water.

Propionic acid is a poison if taken by the intraperitoneal route (Lewis, 1989). It is moderately toxic by ingestion, skin contact, and intravenous routes, while being a corrosive irritant to eyes, skin, and mucous membranes.

In short-term feeding studies using mice and rats, the calcium and sodium salts of propionic acid produced no adverse effects on growth, mortality, hematology patterns, or histopathology (Harshbarger, 1942; Graham et al, 1954; Graham and Grice, 1955; Hara, 1965). In adult humans, daily oral doses of up to 6 g of sodium propionate produced no toxic effects; however, it did produce local antihistaminic activity (Heseltine, 1952; FAO, 1974). Similarly, solutions of propionate applied to the eye in concentrations of up to 15% in humans and up to 20% in rabbits had no irritating effects (FAO, 1974).

Since propionic acid is a normal constituent of food and an intermediary metabolite in humans and ruminants, the FAO (1974) has not established any guidelines on the acceptable daily intake for humans.

F. Lactic Acid and Its Derivatives

Lactic acid (Fig. 3) is one of the most widely distributed organic acids in nature. It was also one of the earliest used as a food additive (Gardner, 1972). Lactic acid

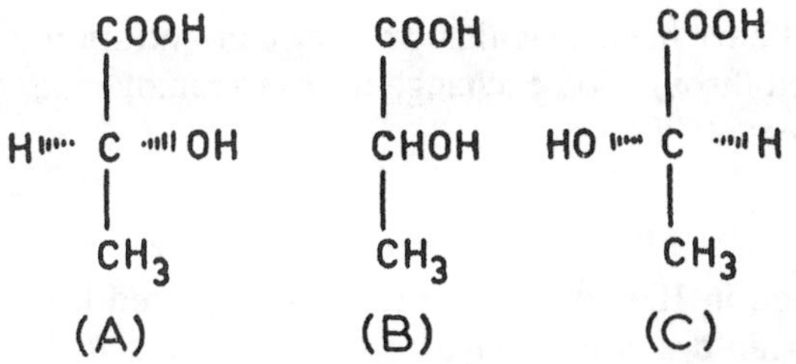

COOH   COOH   COOH

$$H\cdots C \cdots OH \qquad CHOH \qquad HO\cdots C \cdots H$$

$$CH_3 \qquad\qquad CH_3 \qquad\qquad CH_3$$

(A)   (B)   (C)

Fig. 3 (A) D-(−)Lactic acid, (B) DL-lactic acid, and (C) L-(+)lactic acid.

is present in many foods. It is a primary acid component in sour milk and also occurs naturally in sauerkraut, pickles, beer, buttermilk, and cheese. It is also a normal constituent of animal blood and muscle tissue. Lactic acid has been identified in yeast fermentations, and is a major component of corn steep liquor, a byproduct of the corn wet-milling industry.

Manufacture

Lactic acid is manufactured commercially either by fermentation or by synthesis. In the United States, more than 85% of lactic acid is made by a synthetic route, while in Japan all of it is made by organic synthesis. Lactic acid from the European Economic Community, whose combined capacity is approximately half of the estimated world capacity, is produced by fermentation processes. The world capacity is estimated at over 30,000 metric tons per year (Van Ness, 1978).

Fermentation Processes

Two types of microorganisms produce lactic acid. The heterolactic fermentation organisms, which produce some lactic acid as well as other fermentation products including carbon dioxide, ethyl alcohol, and acetic acid, are of little use for commercial production of lactic acid. In contrast, the homolactic fermentation bacteria, namely, *Lactobacillus delbrueckii*, *L. bulgaricus*, and *L. leichmanii*, form lactic acid exclusively or predominantly from carbohydrates and are used commercially for the production of lactic acid. Products containing starch such as cornstarch, potato starch or rice starch, whey, cane sugar, beet sugar, molasses, and sulfite lyes are the preferred substrates for lactic acid production, while the ammonium salts serve as nitrogen sources.

The process involves fermentation of a carbohydrate with suitable mineral and proteinaceous nutrients in the presence of an excess of calcium carbonate. A thermophilic strain of *L. delbrueckii* type, which exhibits its optimum activity at about 50°C and at a pH of 5.0–5.5, is often preferred, since it eliminates most contamination problems and permits the use of a growing medium that only needs to be pasteurized. This process converts all of the lactic acid to calcium lactate. After filtration of the fermentation broth, calcium lactate is acidified with sulfuric acid to regenerate the lactic acid and to precipitate the calcium as calcium sulfate. The resulting filtrate consists of about a 10% solution of crude lactic acid, which is concentrated to over 50% and then further refined.

Refining of lactic acid includes treatment with activated vegetable carbon to remove organic impurities, use of sodium ferrocyanide to remove heavy metals, and filtration to remove impurities that have been coagulated during concentration. The solution is then filtered and passed through ion exchange resins to remove the final traces of contamination (Van Ness, 1978).

Synthetic Processes

Lactic acid synthesis was first described in 1863 by Wislicenus who prepared lactonitrile from acetaldehyde and hydrogen cyanide and hydrolyzed it to lactic acid:

$$CH_3CHO + HCN \rightarrow CH_3CHOHCN$$

$$CH_3CHOHCN + 2 H_2O + HCl \rightarrow CH_3CHOHCOOH + NH_4Cl$$

The same reactions are used commercially. Lactic acid is isolated and purified by esterification with methyl alcohol. The resulting methyl lactate is purified by distillation and hydrolyzed with a strong acid catalyst to produce a semirefined lactic acid. Further purification is achieved by a combination of steaming, carbon treatment, and ion exchange (Anonymous, 1964; Gardner, 1972; Van Ness, 1978).

Synthetic lactic acid is produced in three grades—technical, food, and USP—and in two concentrations—50 and 88%. Synthetic lactic acid is water-white and has excellent heat stability.

Other possible chemical syntheses of lactic acid include the degradation of sugars (preferably sucrose with sodium hydroxide); interaction of acetaldehyde, carbon monoxide, and water at elevated temperatures and pressures; hydroformylation of vinyl acetate, oxidation, and hydrolysis; hydrolysis of a chloropropionic acid; nitric acid oxidation of propylene; and continuous hydrolysis of lactonitrile in an aqueous sulfuric acid solution (Van Ness, 1978).

Lactic acid is a viscous, nonvolatile, hygroscopic liquid (Table 8). Its aqueous solutions are colorless and practically odorless. Lactic acid is very soluble in water and has a moderately strong acid taste.

Table 8   Physical Properties of Lactic Acid

Chemical names	2-Hydroxypropanoic acid, 1-hydroxyethane 1-carboxylic acid
Molecular formula	$CH_3CH(OH)COOH$ ($C_3H_6O_3$)
Molecular weight	90.08
Appearance	Yellow to colorless crystals or syrupy, nonvolatile liquid with acrid taste
pK$_a$	3.862 at 25°C
Ionization constant	1.37×10^{-4} at 25°C
Melting point	16.8°C
Boiling point	122°C at 15 mm
Specific gravity	1.249 at 15°C
Solubility	Very soluble in water, alcohol, furfural, less soluble in ether, practically insoluble in chloroform, volatile with superheated steam

Source: Gardner, 1972; Van Ness, 1978; Budavari, 1989; Lewis, 1989.

Food Uses

Lactic acid is used as an acidifier, antimicrobial agent, curing agent, flavor enhancer, flavoring agent, pH control agent, pickling agent, solvent, and carrier. The FDA classifies it as a GRAS food additive when used at a level not exceeding the amount reasonably required to accomplish the intended effect.

Lactic acid is used in the manufacture of jams, jellies, sherbets, confectionery products, and beverages. It is the preferred acidulant for adjusting acidity and ensuring the clarity of brines for pickles and olives (Gardner, 1972; Doores, 1983, 1989). Lactic acid is also used in certain frozen desserts to provide a mild, tart flavor without masking that of the natural fruit.

The calcium salt of lactic acid is primarily used to preserve the firmness of apple slices during processing, to inhibit the discoloration of fruits and vegetables, as a gelling agent for dehydrated pectins, and to improve the properties of dry milk powders, condensed milk, and baked food products (Hansen, 1951a,b,c; Johnston and Thomas, 1961).

Several derivatives of lactic acid have also found a wide variety of applications in the food industry. Its ethyl esters are used as flavoring agents. The monosodium salt of lactic acid is used as a cooked-out juice retention agent, emulsifier, flavor enhancer, flavoring agent, hog scald agent, humectant, lye peeling agent, pH control agent, and washing agent (Lewis, 1989). Ferrous lactate is allowed for food use as a dietary and nutrient supplement. Lactylic esters of fatty acids and the lactylated fatty acid esters of glycerol and propylene gycol are used as emulsifiers, plasticizers, stabilizers, and surface-active and whipping agents.

Toxicology

Lactic acid is a normal intermediate in mammalian metabolism. It arises from glycogen breakdown, amino acids, and dicarboxylic acids. Abnormally high lactic acid content has been observed in human blood in cases of pneumonia, tuberculosis, and heart failure (Van Ness, 1978).

Lactic acid is moderately toxic by ingestion and rectal routes and is a severe skin and eye irritant (Lewis, 1979). It was found to be lethal in infants who consumed milk that has been acidified with an unknown quantity of lactic acid. Hemorrhaging, gangrenous gastritis, and esophageal burning were discovered upon autopsy (Pitkin, 1935; Young and Smith, 1944; Trainer et al., 1945).

Granados et al. (1949) have carried out long-term studies on hamsters fed a carcinogenic diet in which lactic acid was added either to the drinking water (40 mg/100 mL) or to the feed (45.6 mg/100 g). The growth rates of the test animals did not differ from those of the control group. However, some enamel decalcification was apparent in the experimental animals, although no significant differences were noted in the content of carious lesions among the different groups.

The isomeric forms of lactic acid differ in their toxicological properties. Feeding trials with premature infants have shown that the groups fed acidified milk containing D($-$) or DL forms acquired acidosis, lost weight, became dehydrated, and vomited (Ballabriga et al., 1970). These researchers concluded that only the L($+$)-lactic acid should be used in feeding premature infants. Substitution of acetic acid for lactic acid as an acidulant in infant formulas appeared to be an effective preservative with none of the deleterious side effects (Seymour et al., 1954).

In evaluating the acceptable daily intake of lactic acid in the human diet, the FAO/WHO (1967) has taken into consideration its well-established metabolic pathway after normal consumption in humans. It does not allow the use of D(−) or the DL-lactic acid in infant foods. Although no limits were set for the consumption of L(+)-lactic acid, the FAO/WHO (1967) has set a conditional daily intake for D(−) isomer at 100 mg/kg body weight/day in adult humans.

G. Succinic Acid and Succinic Anhydride

Succinic acid (Fig. 4A) is a normal constituent of almost all plant and animal tissues. Succinic anhydride (Fig. 4B) is the dehydration product of the acid. Succinic acid was first obtained as the distillate from amber (Latin, *Succinum*) for which it is named. It occurs in beet, broccoli, rhubarb, sauerkraut, cheese, meat, molasses, eggs, peat, coal, fruits, honey, and urine (Gardner, 1972; Winstrom, 1978; Doores, 1989). It is formed by the chemical and biochemical oxidation of fats, by alcoholic fermentation of sugar, and in numerous catalyzed oxidation processes. Succinic acid is also a major byproduct in the manufacture of adipic acid.

Succinic acid, a dicarboxylic acid, is a relatively new nonhygroscopic product approved for food uses. Its apparent taste characteristics in foods appear to be very similar to the other acidulants of this type, although pure aqueous solutions tend to have a slightly bitter taste (Monsanto Chemical Co., 1970; Gardner, 1972). Succinic anhydride, in contrast, is the only commercially available anhydride for food uses (Gardner, 1972).

Manufacture

Succinic acid and its anhydride can be manufactured in a number of different ways. The choice often depends upon the raw materials available, labor costs, energy considerations, and technology. It is obtained primarily as a byproduct of adipic acid synthesis. Various techniques are available for its recovery, including separation as the urea adduct, formation of succinimide, extraction, selective crystallization or distillation to recover succinic anhydride, and esterification followed by distillation (Winstrom, 1978). The ester mixture may be used as such or separated by fractionation. The methyl ester can be converted to the anhydride by a catalytic process, in addition to saponification techniques for reclaiming the acid.

Succinic acid can also be manufactured by catalytic hydrogenation of malic or fumaric acids. It has also been produced commercially by aqueous acid or alkali

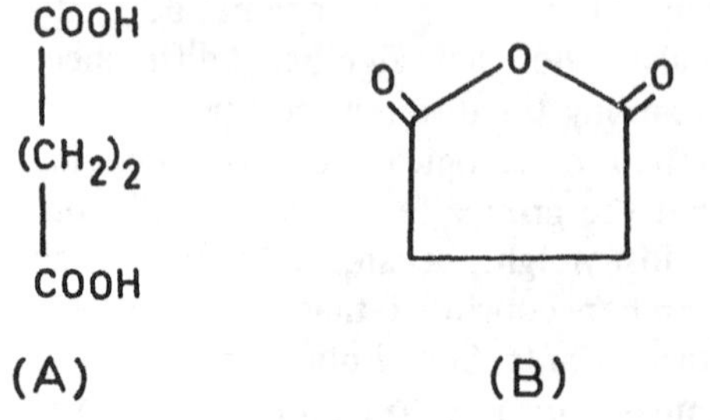

```
COOH
 |
(CH2)2
 |
COOH

 (A)                    (B)
```

Fig. 4 (A) Succinic acid and (B) succinic anhydride.

hydrolysis of succinonitrile derived from ethylene bromide and potassium cyanide (Gergel and Revelise, 1952; Gardner, 1972).

The preparation of succinic acid by fermentation has been studied extensively in Japan. Normal paraffins, sucrose, acetone, and isopropyl alcohol are among the feedstocks utilized. The acid can be separated from the fermentation broths using lead salt precipitation and ion exchange (Winstrom, 1978). The use of a cheap, renewable raw material such as sucrose or an inexpensive petroleum feedstock could make this route attractive to producers employing fermentation technology.

Succinic anhydride is made from the acid by removing the water using azeotropic distillation or by using a hydrophilic solvent that condenses at a temperature above that of the water vapor. In either case, the anhydride is purified by fractionation.

Data on the physical properties of succinic acid and the anhydride are summarized in Table 9. The acid is odorless and has a sour, acid taste. This nonhygroscopic acidulant has a slow taste build-up. Since it is more soluble in water at room temperature than other nonhygroscopic food acids, it offers somewhat greater latitude in formulating powdered foods and beverages (Gardner, 1972). In contrast, the thermal stability and low melting point of succinic anhydride permits its easy incorporation in products at comparatively low temperatures.

Food Uses

The FDA has approved succinic acid as a flavor enhancer, miscellaneous and general purpose food chemical, neutralizing agent, and pH control agent (CFR, 1988). It is a GRAS chemical when used at levels not exceeding good manufacturing practice. Although it is listed as a GRAS additive for miscellaneous and/or general purpose use, succinic acid is not mentioned specifically in any of the Definitions

Table 9 Physical Properties of Succinic Acid and Succinic Anhydride

Property	Succinic acid	Succinic anhydride
Chemical names	1,4-Butanedioic acid, ethylenesuccinic acid	Dihydro-2,5-furandione, succinic acid anhydride, succinyl oxide, 2,5-diketotetrahydrofuran, butanedioic anhydride
Molecular formula	$C_4H_6O_4$	$C_4H_4O_3$
Molecular weight	118.09	100.07
Appearance	Colorless or white monoclinic prism crystals, burning acid taste	White orthorhombic prism crystals, odorless with acid taste
Melting point	185–188°C	119.6°C
Boiling point	235°C, with partial conversion to anhydride	261°C
Specific gravity	1.564 at 20°/4°C	1.503 at 20°/4°C
pK_1	4.16	
pK_2	5.61	
Solubility	1 g/13 mL cold water or 1 mL boiling water	Very slightly soluble in water

Source: Gardner, 1972; Winstrom, 1978; Budavari, 1989; Lewis, 1989.

and Standards of Identity. It is, however, covered under "other edible organic acids" as optional ingredients.

The reactions of succinic acid with proteins are often used for modifying the plasticity of bread doughs (Gardner and Flett, 1954; Gardner, 1972; Doores, 1989). Succinoyl monoglycerides are optional ingredients of the amended Bakery Products Standards of Identity (FDA, 1966).

The derivatives of succinic acid can be used as flavoring agents or in combination with paraffin as a protective coating for selected fruits and vegetables. Succinylated gelatin can be used in the manufacture of capsules for flavoring substances at levels not to exceed 4.5–5.5% of the gelatin content and 15% of the total weight of the capsule and the flavoring compounds (Doores, 1989). Dioctylsodium sulfosuccinate is permitted as a flavoring compound at levels not exceeding 75 ppm in dry cocoa beverage mixes (CFR, 1988). It is also used as a wetting agent in fumaric acid-acidulated foods, a processing aid in sugar manufacture, a solubilizing agent on gums and hydrophilic colloids, or an emulsifying agent for cocoa fat in noncarbonated beverages.

Succinostearin, yet another lipid derivative of succinic acid, is also used as an emulsifier in or with shortenings and edible oils intended for use in cakes, cake mixes, fillings, icings, pastries, and toppings consistent with good manufacturing practices. Succinylated monoglycerides are also used as emulsifiers in liquid and plastic shortenings and as dough conditioners in bread at up to 0.5% levels by weight of the flour.

The Code of Federal Regulations (CFR, 1988) also allows several derivatives of succinic acid as components of adhesives, resinous and polymeric coatings, adjuncts for epoxy resins, surface-active agents, or adjuvants in coatings for polyolefin films. They are used as components of paper and paperboard in contact with aqueous, fatty, and dry foods or as defoaming agents. They can also be used as components of single and repeated-use food contact surfaces and in closures with sealing gaskets for food containers.

Succinic anhydride is an ideal leavening agent for baking powders (Allied Chemical Co., 1961; Gardner, 1966, 1972). Its slow rate of hydrolysis to the acid is especially advantageous during mixing of the dough, since one of the requirements of a leavening acidulant is not to react with the soda in the mixture until the product reaches the baking stage. The increased rates of hydrolysis at the elevated temperatures during baking ensures a steady evolution of carbon dioxide, leaving behind a salt residue with nutrient properties. Succinic anhydride is also an effective dehydrating agent to remove small amounts of water in various dry food mixtures; the acid formed often serves as a useful flavoring agent in these foods.

Toxicology

Succinic acid is moderately toxic by subcutaneous route (Lewis, 1989). It is also a severe eye irritant. When heated to decomposition, succinic acid emits acrid smoke and irritating fumes.

Dye et al. (1944) conducted short-term studies on rats who received daily subcutaneous injections of 0.5 mg succinic acid. These doses were increased gradually up to 2.0 mg/day at 4 weeks, and the studies continued at this level for 100 days. When compared with the control animals, the test animals did not show any abnormalities in reproduction, hair appearance, tooth eruption, or eye opening.

Dye et al. (1944) also found no abnormalities in the development of chick embryos when comparable dosages were administered into the air sacs.

Since it occurs naturally in small amounts in several fruits and vegetables and as an intermediate in the Krebs cycle, no limit has been set on the acceptable daily intake of succinic acid in the human diet.

H. Fumaric Acid and Its Salts

Fumaric acid (Fig. 5) is a polyfunctional chemical of significant commercial interest worldwide. It is found naturally in many plants and is named after the genus *Fumaria*. Fumaric acid is a normal constituent of tissues as an intermediate in the Krebs cycle.

Manufacture

Essentially all of the fumaric acid in commerce is derived as a byproduct in the manufacture of phthalic acid and maleic anhydride or by the catalytic isomerization of maleic acid (Flett and Gardner, 1952; Gardner, 1972; Robinson and Mount, 1978). Several catalysts can be used for isomerization, including mineral acids (e.g., HCl), peroxy compounds with bromides and bromates, and sulfur-containing compounds such as thioureas. The processing is greatly simplified when maleic anhydride is used as the raw material. High-purity fumaric acid is produced by cooling the reaction mixture and then separating, washing, and drying the crystals. Several decolorizing and crystallization techniques are available to prepare high-grade fumaric acid from impure maleic liquors (Robinson and Mount, 1978). Fumaric acid can also be produced by the fermentation of glucose and molasses with certain strains of *Rhizopus nigricans* and *R. japonicus* (Gardner and Flett, 1952; Gardner, 1972).

Data on the physical properties of fumaric acid are summarized in Table 10. It is a nonhygroscopic unsaturated dicarboxylic acid with a strong tart, acidic taste. Compared with most acidulants, it has a relatively low solubility in water.

Food Uses

Fumaric acid imparts a sour taste to foods and is one of the most acidic solid acids (Doores, 1989). It blends very well with other food acidulants without giving a "burst" to the taste. The FDA has approved its use in foods as an acidifier, curing accelerator, and flavoring agent.

Fumaric acid is used extensively in fruit juice drinks, gelatin desserts, pie fillings, refrigerated biscuit doughs, maraschino cherries, and wines (Anonymous, 1964; Gardner, 1972). It is also used in preparing various edible coatings for candy, water-in-oil emulsions, reconstituted fats, and dough conditioners. Fumaric acid

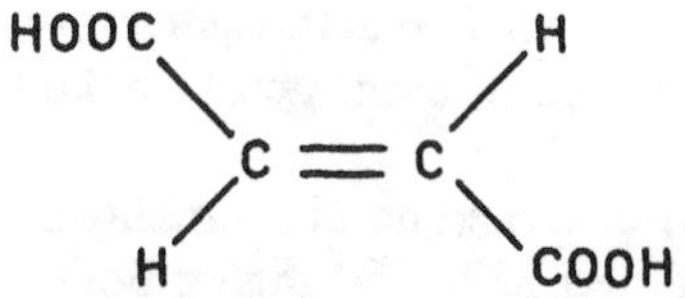

Fig. 5 Fumaric acid.

Table 10 Physical Properties of Fumaric Acid

Chemical names	*Trans*-2-butenedioic acid, *trans*-1,2-ethylenedicarboxylic acid, allmaleic acid, boletic acid
Molecular formula	$C_4H_4O_4$
Molecular weight	116.07
Appearance	White, monoclinic crystals, odorless with tart taste
Specific gravity	1.635 at 20°/4°C
Melting point	287°C
Boiling point	290°C, sublimes
pK$_1$	3.03
pK$_2$	4.77
Solubility in water, g/100 mL	
25°C	0.63
40°C	1.07
60°C	2.4
100°C	9.4

Source: Gardner, 1972; Robinson and Mount, 1978; Budavari, 1989; Lewis, 1989.

eliminates extensive hardening and rubbery texture in alginate-based desserts. Its limited solubility coupled with an extremely low rate of moisture absorption makes fumaric acid a valuable ingredient for extending the shelf life of powdered dry mixes.

Fumaric acid has good antioxidant properties. It is often used to prevent the onset and development of rancidity in lard, butter, powdered milk, sausage, bacon, nuts, and potato chips (Gardner, 1972; Doores, 1989; Lewis, 1989). It also complements sodium benzoate as a preservative in green foods and fish products.

The Code of Federal Regulations (CFR, 1988) also allows the use of fumaric acid and its salts as special dietary and nutritional additives. Ferrous fumarate is often used as a source of available iron in human nutrition.

Several derivatives of fumaric acid have also been approved for food uses. Sodium stearyl fumarate is used as a dough conditioner in yeast-leavened bakery products at levels not exceeding 0.5% by weight of the flour, as a conditioning agent in dehydrated potatoes and processed cereals for cooking at up to 1% level, in starch- or flour-thickened foods at not exceeding 0.2% by weight of the food, and as a stabilizing agent in non–yeast-leavened bakery products at up to 1% by weight of the flour. Other derivatives are also used as components of adhesives, resinous and polymeric coatings, paper and paperboard in contact with dry foods, and in single-use and repeated-use food contact surfaces.

Toxicology

Fumaric acid is poisonous by intraperitoneal route (Lewis, 1989). It is mildly toxic by ingestion and skin contact and is a skin and eye irritant. It reacts vigorously with oxidizing materials, and when heated to decomposition, it emits acrid smoke and irritating fumes.

In short-term feeding trials, Packman et al. (1963) observed no abnormalities in the normal blood and urine components of rabbits fed 320–2080 mg/kg body weight disodium fumarate (equivalent to 6.9% salt or 5% of the free acid).

Levey et al. (1946) have conducted extensive long-term feeding studies in rats. Eight groups of 14 weanling rats were fed diets containing 0, 0.1, and 1.0% fumaric acid and 1.38% sodium fumarate for one year (half of the groups) or 2 years. No adverse effects were noted on the rate of weight gain, hemoglobin, normal blood constituents, calcium balance as studied by bone histology, or on the histology of liver, kidney, spleen, and stomach.

In another study, five groups of 12 male and 12 female rats were fed diets containing 0, 0.1, 0.5, 0.8, and 1.2% fumaric acid for 2 years without noticing any toxic effects on growth or food consumption (Fitzhugh and Nelson, 1947). In the same study, when a further four groups of 12 male rats were kept for 2 years on diets containing 0. 0.5, 1.0, and 1.5% fumaric acid, only the group on the 1.5% fumaric acid diet showed a "very slight increase" in mortality and testicular atrophy. Further gross and microscopic examination of other major organs revealed no abnormalities, while the tumor incidence was not significantly different among the groups.

In the only human study conducted thus far, Levey et al. (1946) gave 75 chronically disabled subjects, ranging in age from 29 to 91 years, 500 mg fumaric acid daily for one year without any toxic manifestations in hemoglobin level, red and white blood cell counts, nonprotein nitrogen and creatinine levels, and bromosulfonphthalein and phenosulfonphthalein excretion. Based on their observations, Levey et al. (1946) recommended an LD_{50} of 8000 mg/kg for fumaric acid and its disodium salt.

Based primarily on the 2-year study of Fitzhugh and Nelson (1947), the FAO/WHO (1967) established the level causing no toxicological effects in rats at 1.2% or 12,000 ppm of fumaric acid in the diet (equivalent to 600 mg/kg body weight/day) and for sodium fumarate at 1.38% or 13,800 ppm (equivalent to 690 mg/kg/day).

Similar levels for humans were established at 500 mg/day, equivalent to 10 mg/kg/day. The FAO/WHO (1967) has also approved the use of fumaric acid and its salts at 0–6 mg/kg body weight/day as an unconditional acceptable daily intake for humans, and conditionally at 6–10 mg/kg/day.

I. Malic Acid and Malic Anhydride

L-Malic acid (hydroxysuccinic acid, Fig. 6C), which was isolated from apples by Scheele in 1785 (Robinson and Mount, 1978), is widely distributed in small amounts, especially in several fruits and vegetables. It is the predominant acid in apples, apricots, bananas, cherries, grapes, orange peels, peaches, pears, plums, quinces, broccoli, carrots, peas, potatoes, and rhubarb (Gardner, 1966, 1972). It is the second-largest acid in citrus fruits, many berries, figs, beans, and tomatoes.

Manufacture

DL-Malic acid (Fig. 6B) is manufactured by hydrating maleic and fumaric acids in the presence of suitable catalysts and then separating the malic acid from the equilibrium product mixture (Irwin et al., 1967). In the United States, the acid is now produced by a continuous process, which is much more economical than the older batch process (Gardner, 1972).

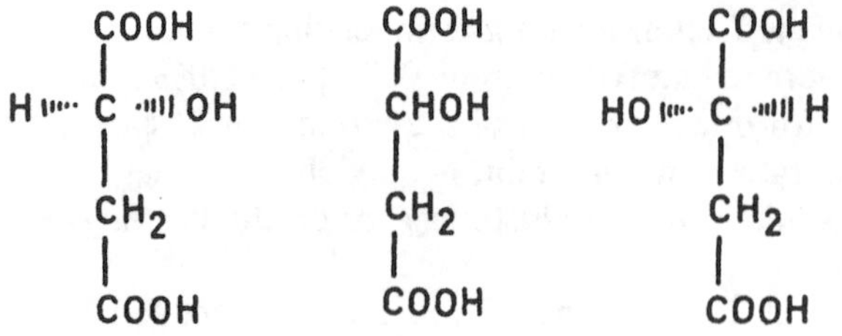

$$
\begin{array}{ccc}
\text{COOH} & \text{COOH} & \text{COOH} \\
| & | & | \\
\text{H---C---OH} & \text{CHOH} & \text{HO---C---H} \\
| & | & | \\
\text{CH}_2 & \text{CH}_2 & \text{CH}_2 \\
| & | & | \\
\text{COOH} & \text{COOH} & \text{COOH} \\
\end{array}
$$

(A)   (B)   (C)

Fig. 6 (A) D-(+)-Malic acid, (B) DL-malic acid, and (C) L-(−)-malic acid.

Table 11 Physical Properties of Malic Acid

Chemical names	Hydroxybutanedioic acid, hydroxysuccinic acid, 1-hydroxy-1,2-ethane dicarboxylic acid
Molecular formula	$C_4H_6O_5$
Molecular weight	134.09
Appearance	White or colorless triclinic crystals, odorless with smooth, tart taste, exists as DL, L, and D isomers
Melting point	100°C (D or L), 128°C (DL)
Boiling point	140°C (D or L, decomposes), 150°C (DL)
Specific gravity	1.595 at 20°/4°C (D or L), 1.601 (DL)
pK_1	3.40
pK_2	5.11
Solubility, g/100 mL at 20°C	55.8 (DL), 36.3 (L) in water
	45.5 (DL), 86.6 (L) in alcohol

Source: Robinson and Mount, 1978; Budavari, 1989; Lewis, 1989.

Data on the physical properties of malic acid are summarized in Table 11. It is a white, triclinic crystalline powder with no detectable odor and a smooth tart, acidic taste. It is nonhygroscopic under normal humidity conditions, with high water solubility.

Food Uses

The Code of Federal Regulations (CFR, 1988) allows the use of malic acid in foods as an acidifier, flavor enhancer, flavoring agent, pH control agent, and synergist for antioxidants. It is one of the miscellaneous and/or general purpose food additives in the FDA list of GRAS chemicals. It is an optional ingredient in the FDA standards for sherbets and water ices, fruit butters, preserves, jams and jellies, nonalcoholic carbonated beverages, and fruit-flavored noncarbonated beverages. The following limits have been set for its use in different food products: 3.4% in nonalcoholic beverages, 3.0% in chewing gum, 0.8% in gelatins, puddings, and fillings, 6.9% in hard candy, 2.6% in jams and jellies, 3.5% in processed fruits and fruit juices, 3.0% in soft candy, and 0.7% in all other foods when used in accordance with good manufacturing practice.

Generally, less malic acid than citric acid is required to impart the same degree of acidity. Malic acid provides excellent antibrowning properties in fruits (Gardner, 1972). It is also used as a synergist at levels not to exceed 0.01% with antioxidants in a wide variety of foods to prevent fats and oils from becoming rancid and as an agent for releasing oil from gum contaminants in the refining of edible fatty oils.

The ethyl and isopropyl esters of malic acid are recommended for improving the whipping properties of egg white and of gelatin in foamed types of desserts, while the fatty alcohol monoesters are useful antispattering agents in cooking fats (Conrad and Stiles, 1954; Harris, 1959).

Toxicology

Malic acid is moderately toxic by ingestion and is a skin and severe eye irritant (Lewis, 1989). Upon decomposition, it emits acrid smoke and irritating fumes.

Long-term studies using rats fed 500 and 5000 ppm malic acid in their basal diets showed no reduction in growth rates and abnormal changes in hematology, urine analysis, and histology. Diets containing 50,000 ppm malic acid, however, significantly decreased food consumption and growth (Hazleton Laboratories, 1971a). Dogs fed the same three levels of malic acid showed no effects using the same parameters (Hazleton Laboratories, 1971b). Reproductive experiments using rats fed 1000 and 10,000 ppm malic acid prior to mating showed no significant differences from the controls (Hazleton Laboratories, 1970).

According to a FAO/WHO (1967) report, the need to impose a severe limitation on the content of maleic acid in malic acid arises from the established nephrotoxicity of maleic acid. Male rats fed diets containing 1% or more maleic acid showed growth retardation, increased mortality, and changes in the renal proximal convoluted tubules (Fitzhugh and Nelson, 1947). Intraperitoneal administration of 0.1 M sodium maleate in daily doses of 1–2 mL/kg for 2–3 weeks produced glucosuria, phosphaturin, and aminoaciduria. The lethal doses by the oral route were established at 5000 mg L(+)-malic acid/kg for rabbits and at 1000 mg sodium malate/kg body weight for dogs.

In evaluating the acceptance of malic acid, the FAO/WHO (1967) has placed emphasis on its well-established metabolic pathway. It has not set any limits for the acceptable daily intake of the L(+)-isomer of malic acid, while the D(−)-isomer is conditionally recommended at 0–100 mg/kg body weight/day in the human diet. Excepting therapeutic purposes, the FAO/WHO (1967) does not allow the use of D(−) and DL-malic acids in baby food formulas.

J. Tartaric Acid and Its Salts

Tartaric acid is dihydroxy dicarboxylic acid with two chiral centers. It exists as the dextro- and levorotatory acid, the *meso*-form (which is inactive owing to internal compensation), and the racemic mixture (Fig. 7). This enantiomer occurs naturally in grapes as its acid potassium salt (cream of tartar). In the fermentation of wine, this salt deposits in the vats; free crystallized tartaric acid was first obtained from such fermentation residues by Scheele in 1769 (Berger, 1978).

Manufacture

Tartaric acid and cream of tartar are manufactured as the byproducts of the wine industry. Crude tartars are recoverable from the following sources.

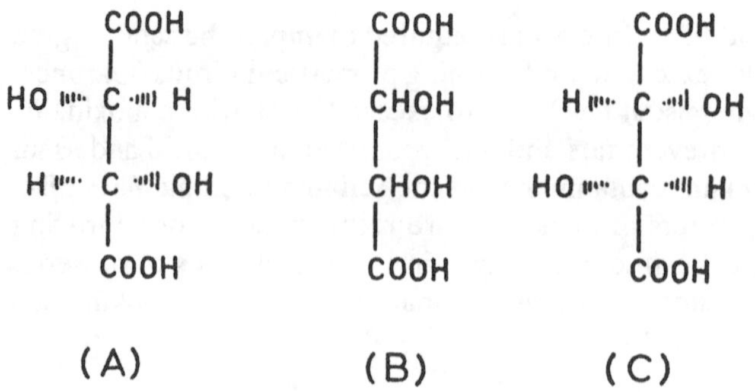

Fig. 7   (A) D-(−)Tartaric acid, (B) DL-tartaric acid, and (C) L-(+)tartaric acid.

1. The press cakes from grape juice (unfermented "marcs" or the partly fermented "pomace") are boiled with water, and alcohol, if present, is distilled. The hot mash is settled, decanted, and the clear liquor is cooled to crystallize. The recovered high-test crude cream of tartar (vinaccia) has an 85–90% cream of tartar content.
2. Lees, which are the dried slimy sediments in the wine fermentation vats, consist of yeast cells, pectinous substances, and tartars. Their content of total tartaric acid equivalent ranges from 16 to 40%.
3. Argols, the crystalline crusts that form in the vats in the secondary fermentation period, contain more than 40% tartaric acid; they are high in potassium hydrogen tartrate and low in the calcium salt.

It usually is advantageous to combine the manufacture of tartaric acid, cream of tartar, and the Rochelle salt in one plant. This permits the most favorable disposition of the mother liquors from the three processes. The following chemical reactions are involved.

1. Formation of calcium tartrate from crude potassium tartrate

$$2KHC_4H_4O_6 + Ca(OH)_2 + CaSO_4 \rightarrow 2\ CaC_4H_4O_6 + K_2SO_4 + 2H_2O$$

2. Formation of tartaric acid from calcium tartrate

$$CaC_4H_4O_6 + H_2SO_4 \rightarrow H_2C_4H_4O_6 + CaSO_4$$

3. Formation of Rochelle salt from argols

$$2\ KHC_4H_4O_6 + Na_2CO_3 \rightarrow 2\ KNaC_4H_4O_6 + CO_2 + H_2O$$

4. Formation of cream of tartar from tartaric acid and Rochelle salt liquors

$$2\ H_6C_4O_6 + 2\ KNaC_4H_4O_6 + K_2SO_4 \rightarrow 4\ KHC_4H_4O_6 + Na_2SO_4$$

The oldest calcium tartrate preparation procedure is the decantation process, in which fresh, wet lees or finely ground dry lees are treated with sufficient hydrochloric acid to dissolve all tartrates. The acidified magma is diluted with sufficient water to obtain at least 50% supernatant solution after settling. The acidic liquor is drawn off, and the insolubles are washed by repeated suspension in water and decantation. The combined extracts are neutralized with ground limestone or hydrated lime, which leaves the end reaction slightly acidic. Tartar recovery from winery still residues may be accomplished by exchange adsorption on an ion exchanger in the chloride form (Berger, 1978). The calcium tartrates are then decomposed with 70% sulfuric acid to obtain tartaric acid.

Data on the physical properties of tartaric acid are summarized in Table 12. It exists as colorless to translucent crystals or white powder. Tartaric acid is odorless with a strong, tart acid taste. It is the most soluble of the solid acidulants.

Food Uses

The Code of Federal Regulations (CFR, 1988) allows tartaric acid for use in foods as an acidifier, firming agent, flavor enhancer, flavoring agent, humectant, pH control agent, and sequestrant. Tartaric acid, sodium and sodium-potassium tartrates, and choline bitartrate are GRAS food additives when used in accordance with good manufacturing practice. Tartaric acid is listed as an optional ingredient in standards for fruit butters, fruit jellies, preserves and jams, in artificially sweetened jellies and preserves, and in fruit sherbets.

Tartaric acid is widely used in grape- and lime-flavored beverages of all types because of its effect on the flavor. It also enhances the optical properties of the deep purple colored grape-flavored products (Gardner, 1972). For similar reasons, it is often the choice acidulant for grape-flavored and for tart-tasting jams, jellies, and candies. Blends of tartaric acid with citric acid are used in hard candies to obtain the popular sour apple, wild cherry, and other especially tart-tasting varieties.

Both tartaric acid and its acidic monopotassium salt (cream of tartar) are common ingredients of baking powders and leavening systems. The limited solubility of cream of tartar in cold water prevents premature leavening, as is required during the dough mixing stage. Various amounts of the acid are incorporated to accelerate the leavening reactions during baking (Gardner, 1972; Doores, 1989). Tartaric acid also acts as a synergist with antioxidants in preventing rancidity in fat-based products.

Choline bitartrate is often used as a dietary supplement and nutrient, while the diacetyl tartaric acid esters of mono- and diglycerides of edible fats or oils or edible fat-forming fatty acids are used as emulsifying agents.

Table 12 Physical Properties of Tartaric Acid

Chemical names	2,3-Dihydroxybutanedioic acid, 2,3-dihydroxysuccinic acid
Molecular formula	$C_4H_6O_6$
Molecular weight	150.09
Appearance	Colorless to translucent crystals or white powder, odorless with an extremely tart, acid taste, commercial acid is L isomer but dextrorotatory
Melting point	168–170°C
Specific gravity	1.7598 at 20°/4°C
pK_1	2.98
pK_2	4.34
Solubility, g/100 mL in water	139 at 20°C, 217 at 60°C, 343 at 100°C

Source: Budavari, 1989; Lewis, 1989.

Toxicology

Tartaric acid is moderately toxic by intravenous route and mildly toxic by ingestion (Lewis, 1989). Similar to other acids, when heated to decomposition, it emits acrid smoke and irritating fumes.

In short-term studies, rats fed 7.7% sodium tartrate (5.0% free acid) did not show any adverse effects on food consumption, growth, mortality, and gross history (Packman et al., 1963). In a long-term feeding study, 21 day-old weanling rats were fed diets containing 0, 0.1, 0.5, 0.8, and 1.2% tartaric acid (Fitzhugh and Nelson, 1947). No significant differences were observed in weight gain, mortality, histopathological effects, and tumor incidence. However, subcutaneous administration of 0.25–1 g tartaric acid to rabbits produced abnormalities in blood chemistry, including increased nonprotein nitrogen, sugar, and cholesterol levels (Rose, 1924). In teratogenic testing, no abnormalities were observed in mice, rats, hamsters, or rabbits at levels of 274, 181, 225, and 215 mg/kg body weight, respectively (Food and Drug Research Laboratories, 1973a). Humans working in a manufacturing plant that produced the acid and exposed to tartaric acid dust of up to 32 mg/m^3 displayed skin eruptions, which disappeared after removal from the worksite (Barsotti et al., 1954).

The FAO (1974) has set an unconditional acceptable daily intake limit of 30 mg/kg body weight for tartaric acid as the L(+) form or its salt in human nutrition.

K. Adipic Acid

From a commercial viewpoint, adipic acid is the most important of all the aliphatic dicarboxylic acids, with a worldwide annual production of over 2 million metric tons. Its primary use is in the manufacture of nylon-6,6, the polyamide formed by its reaction with 1,6-hexamethylenediamine. Its uses were subsequently extended to the manufacture of other synthetic fibers such as polyester, acrylic, polyolefin, and other polyamide fibers. Since 1960, it has found a wide variety of uses in the food industry.

Manufacture

The predominant commercial route to adipic acid synthesis is via oxidation of cyclohexane in two processing steps (Danly and Campbell, 1978). The first step involves oxidation of cyclohexane with air to form a mixture of cyclohexanone and cyclohexanol [termed ketone-alcohol (KA) or ol-one], followed by oxidation of the KA mixture with nitric acid to produce adipic acid. The balance of adipic acid is made from phenol by hydrogenation to cyclohexanol, followed by similar nitric acid oxidation.

When a high-purity KA or cyclohexanol feedstock is employed, yields of adipic acid range from 1.35 to 1.40 kg/kg KA (92–96% of the theoretical maximum). The major byproducts are glutaric acid and succinic acid, produced to the extent of about 6 and 2%, respectively, of the adipic acid synthesized. Use of an impure KA feed, by air oxidation of cyclohexane without KA refining, lowers adipic and increases glutaric and succinic acid yields (Danly and Campbell, 1978).

Data on the physical properties of adipic acid are summarized in Table 13. It is a white, crystalline, nonhygroscopic powder with limited water solubility. It is four to five times more soluble than fumaric acid at room temperature and has the

Table 13 Physical Properties of Adipic Acid

Chemical names	1,4-Butanedicarboxylic acid, hexanedioic acid
Molecular formula	COOH(CH$_2$)COOH (C$_6$H$_{10}$O$_4$)
Molecular weight	146.14
Appearance	White, monoclinic crystals, odorless with tart taste
Melting point	152°C
Boiling point	337.5°C
Specific gravity	1.360 to 25°/4°C
pK$_1$	4.43
pK$_2$	5.41
Solubility, g/100 mL	1.4 at 20°C, 160 at 100°C in water, very soluble in alcohol

Source: Danly and Campbell, 1978; Budavari, 1989; Lewis, 1989.

lowest acidity of any of the food acids (Gardner, 1972; Doores, 1983). Adipic acid has no odor and has a tart taste.

Food Uses

The Code of Federal Regulations (CFR, 1988) allows the use of adipic acid as a flavoring agent, leavening agent, neutralizing agent, and a pH control agent. The FDA has classified adipic acid as a miscellaneous and/or general purpose food additive and has set the following limitations on its use in different food categories: 0.05% in baked goods, 0.005% in nonalcoholic beverages, 5.0% in condiments and relishes, 0.45% in dairy product analogs, 0.3% in fats and oils, 0.0004% in frozen dairy desserts, 0.55% in gelatin and puddings, 0.1% in gravies, 0.3% in meat products, 1.3% in snack foods, and 0.02% in other food categories when used in accordance with good manufacturing practice.

Adipic acid imparts a smooth, tart taste to foods. In grape-flavored products, it adds a lingering supplementary flavor and gives an excellent set to food powders containing gelatin (Pintauro and Hall, 1962; Gardner, 1972). Adipic acid is extensively used in gelatin desserts, powdered and bottled fruit beverages, as a leavening acidulant in baking powders, candies, refrigerated rolls, to improve the melting characteristics and texture of processed cheese and cheese spreads, as an agent for increasing the whipping quality of products containing egg white, as a gel-inducing agent in imitation jams and jellies, in the canning of vegetables, as a sequestrant in edible oils, and in biscuits where a smooth, mildly acidic flavoring is required (Gardner, 1972; Doores, 1983, 1989).

Toxicology

Adipic acid is a poison by intraperitoneal route, while it is moderately toxic by other routes (Lewis, 1989). It is also a severe eye irritant.

The capacity of humans and animals to metabolize adipic acid appears to be limited to a relatively small amount (FAO/WHO, 1967). While summarizing the acute toxicity data by various routes of administration of adipic acid in rats and mice, Doores (1983) noted that the acid caused hemorrhaging in the small intestine in conjunction with distention of the stomach by administration of the acid via the oral route. Both intravenous and intraperitoneal injections produced hemorrhaging in the lungs, in addition to acidosis by the former route and adhesions of the intestines by the latter. Extensive studies conducted by Enders (1941) in rabbits showed similar symptoms as seen in mice and rats, with marked obstruction in the liver and kidneys by the peroral route and polyurea by intravenous administration, resulting in the loss of up to 20% of the body weight.

In short-term studies, groups of 18 young male rats were fed diets containing 0, 200, 400, and 800 mg adipic acid per day for up to 5 weeks. The highest level produced decreased growth, diarrhea and altered behavior (Lang and Bartsch, 1953). These researchers also did not observe any adverse effects with offspring from treated female rats fed 40 mg adipic acid per day for up to 28 days. When rats were fed protein-deficient diets and dosed at 400 mg/day, significant inhibition of growth occurred. However, as compared with the control group, only slight anemia was noted in the test animals.

In the long-term feeding studies conducted by Horn et al. (1957), groups of 20–39 male and female rats were fed diets containing 0, 0.1, 1, 3, and 5% adipic acid for up to 2 years. In the beginning, the body weight was depressed significantly in male rats receiving 3 and 5% adipic acid, the latter showing the lowest weights and a slightly reduced food consumption. There was, however, no significant difference in survival among the various test groups from controls. Autopsy findings and tumor incidence were also not significantly different from controls, while the histopathological examination revealed normal organs. Sodium adipate fed at the 5% level also decreased the rate of weight gain in rats (Anonymous, 1943).

Teratological studies involving mice, rats, and hamsters fed doses of adipic acid at 263, 288, and 205 mg/kg body weight, respectively, showed no differences from the controls (Food and Drug Research Laboratories, 1973b). Inhalation of adipic acid for 6 hours at a rate of 126 μg/L produced no abnormal findings (Gage, 1970).

The FAO/WHO (1967) has established the level causing no toxicological effect of adipic acid in rats at 10,000 ppm in the diet, equivalent to 500 mg/kg body weight/day. They have also set a conditional daily intake of 0–5 mg adipic acid/kg body weight/day for humans.

L. Citric Acid and Its Salts

Citric acid (Fig. 8), a natural constituent and common metabolite of plants and animals, is the most versatile and widely used organic acid in foods and pharmaceuticals. It is also widely used in several industrial applications to sequester ions, neutralize bases, and act as a buffer. Esters of citric acid are used commercially as plasticizers in the preparation of polymer compositions, protective coatings, and adhesives.

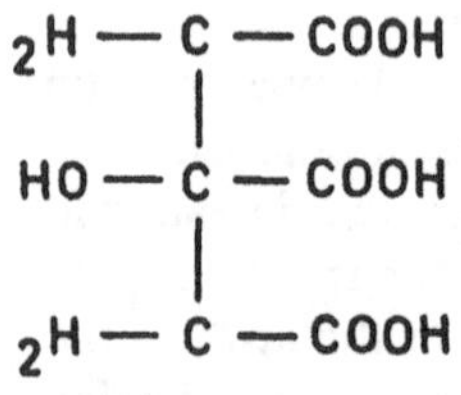

$$_2H - C - COOH$$
$$|$$
$$HO - C - COOH$$
$$|$$
$$_2H - C - COOH$$

Fig. 8   Citric acid.

Citric acid was first isolated in the crystalline form by Scheele in 1784 from lemon juice (Lockwood and Irwin, 1964). Liebig in 1838 recognized citric acid as a hydroxy tribasic acid. Subsequently, Grimoux and Adam synthesized citric acid in 1880 from glycerol, while Wehmer was the first to recognize that certain fungi produce citric acid when grown on sugar solutions. Citric acid plays a vital role in the Krebs or the tricarboxylic acid cycle in human metabolism. It occurs in the terminal oxidative metabolic system of all but a very few organisms.

Citric acid occurs widely in both the plant and animal kingdoms (Table 14). It is the major acid constituent in the fruits of the citrus family. As the free acid or a salt, it is also found in the seeds and juices of a wide variety of flowers and seeds. The total circulating citric acid in the human serum is approximately 1 mg/kg body weight, while the normal daily excretion in the urine is about 0.2–1.0 g.

Manufacture

The traditional method of preparing citric acid was by extraction from the juice of certain citrus fruits, such as limes and lemons, and later from pineapple wastes. It is recovered from the pineapple waste by first washing and peeling the fruit. It is then shredded and pressed to obtain the juice. The juice is then subjected to a spontaneous fermentation from natural yeast to destroy pectin, sugar, and proteinaceous materials, clarified, and the citric acid precipitated with lime to "citrate of lime" (Lockwood and Irwin, 1964; Gardner, 1972). With pineapple canning wastes, some sucrose and bromelin are obtained as byproducts.

Table 14 Distribution of Citric Acid in Fruits and Vegetables and Various Animal Tissues and Fluids

Fruits and Vegetables	% Citrate	Animal Tissues/Fluids	ppm
Lemon	4.0–8.0	Human whole blood	15
Grapefruit	1.2–2.1	Blood plasma	25
Tangerine	0.9–1.2	Red blood cells	10
Orange	0.6–1.0	Milk	500–1250
Black currant	1.5–3.0	Urine	100–750
Red currant	0.7–1.3	Semen	2000–4000
Raspberry	1.0–1.3	Cerebrospinal fluid	25–50
Gooseberry	0.9–1.0	Mammary gland	3000
Strawberry	0.6–0.8	Thyroid gland	750–900
Apple	0.008	Kidney	20
Potato	0.3–0.5	Bone	7500
Tomato	0.20–0.25	Amniotic fluid	17–100
Asparagus	0.08–0.2	Saliva	4–24
Turnip	0.05–1.1	Sweat	1–2
Pea	0.05	Tears	5–7
Butternut squash	0.007–0.025	Skeletal muscle, liver, brain	2–100
Corn	0.02	Total circulating in human	1 mg/kg body
Lettuce	0.016	serum	weight
Eggplant	0.01	Urinary excretion	0.2–1.0 g/day

Source: FDA, 1973, 1974; FAO, 1974.

Commercial production of citric acid, however, is derived almost exclusively from fermentation processes. Several different processes are employed for this purpose.

Surface Process

The microbial production of citric acid on a commercial scale was first begun by Pfizer Inc. in 1923. The process uses certain strains of *Aspergillus niger*, which when grown on the surface of a sucrose and salt solution produces significant amounts of citric acid. Variations of this surface culture technique still account for a substantial portion of the world's production of this acid.

The surface process involves inoculating sugar solutions along with sources of assimilable nitrogen, phosphate, magnesium, and various trace minerals with spores of *A. niger* in shallow aluminum or stainless steel pans. The mold grows on the solution surface producing a rubbery, convoluted mycelial mass. Air is circulated over the surface to provide oxygen and control temperature by evaporating cooling.

Because of their relatively low cost, molasses are often the preferred source of sugar for this fermentation process. However, since it is a byproduct of sugar refining, molasses vary considerably in composition, and not all types are suitable for citric acid production. Beet molasses is generally preferred to cane (Lockwood and Irwin, 1964).

Submerged Process

In this process *A. niger* is grown dispersed through a liquid medium. The fermentation vessel usually consists of a sterilizable tank of thousands of gallon capacity and equipped with a mechanical agitator and a means of introducing sterile air. The inoculum is transferred aseptically to the production fermenter containing the proper media.

Citric acid can also be produced by submerged process fermentation using certain species of yeast (*Candida guilliermondii*). The process, patented by Miles Laboratories, requires shorter fermentation times than with *A. niger* fermentation.

Citric acid is generally recovered from a fermented aqueous solution by first separating the microorganisms, generally by rotary filtration or centrifugation, and then precipitating the citrate ion as the insoluble calcium salt. If fermented solutions are of sufficiently high purity, it may be possible to recover crude citric acid by direct crystallization; however, commercial success with this method has not been reported (Gardner, 1972).

The recovery of citric acid via calcium salt precipitation is a highly complex process. The clarified fermentation broth is treated with a calcium hydroxide slurry in two stages. The first removes oxalic acid when present as a byproduct, and the second precipitates the citrate. The citrate is formed by adding a lime slurry to obtain a neutral pH. After filtration, the resulting calcium citrate is acidified with sulfuric acid, which converts the salt to calcium sulfate and citric acid. The calcium sulfate is filtered and washed free of citric acid solution. The clear citric acid solution then undergoes a series of crystallization steps to achieve the physical separation of citric acid from the remaining trace impurities. The finished citric acid is dried and sifted in conventional rotary drying equipment. Because anhydrous citric acid is hygroscopic, care must be taken to reach the final moisture specification during drying and to avoid storage under high-temperature and high-humidity conditions.

The citric acid yield from fermentation processes range from 50 to 70% based on the sugar conversion (Gardner, 1972).

Data on the physical properties of citric acid are presented in Table 15. It exists as colorless, odorless monoclinic holohedra crystals and has a pleasant sour taste. Citric acid is highly soluble in water.

Food Uses

Citric acid has approved for food uses as an acidifier, curing accelerator, dispersing agent, flavoring agent, sequestrant, and as a synergist for antioxidants. Citric acid and its sodium and potassium salts are classified by the FDA as GRAS food additives when used in accordance with the good manufacturing practice. Sodium citrate is listed as an optional ingredient in ice cream, while the acid is listed as an ingredient for fruit sherbets and water ices.

Citric acid and its salts are widely used in ice cream, sherbets and ices, beverages, salad dressings, fruit preserves, and in jams and jellies. It is also used as an acidulant in canned vegetables, while calcium citrate is permitted for firming peppers, potatoes, tomatoes and lima beans during processing. Citric acid is also used in enzyme preparations for clarifying fruit juices, in dry dough, baked farinaceous and crusty bakery products, and in antioxidants for chocolate and cocoa.

Citric acid is an important acidulant for use in dairy products (Gardner, 1972). It is used extensively in creamed cottage cheese, pasteurized process cheese and cheese spreads, and as a flavoring agent and acidifier in dry cured cottage cheese. Sodium citrate is used in processed cheese as an emulsifying and aging agent. Citric acid is a precursor of diacetyl and, therefore, indirectly improves the flavor and aroma of a variety of cultured dairy products.

Citric acid is one of the major acidulants in carbonated beverages, imparting to them a tangy citrus flavor (Gardner, 1966, 1972). It also acts as a preservative, both in the syrup and in finished beverage products. Sodium citrate is preferred

Table 15 Physical Properties of Citric Acid

Chemical names	2-Hydroxy-1,2,3-propanetricarboxylic acid, β-hydroxytricarballylic acid
Molecular formula	$C_6H_8O_7$
Molecular weight	192.14
Appearance	Colorless, translucent orthorhombic crystals from cold water; anhydrous, colorless translucent monoclinic holohedra crystals, odorless with tart test
Melting point	153°C (anhydrous)
Boiling point	Decomposes
Specific gravity	1.665 at 20°/4°C (anhydrous), 1.542 at 20°/4°C (monohydrate)
pK_1	3.14
pK_2	4.77
pK_3	6.39
Solubility, g/100 mL in water	59.2 at 20°C, 73.5 at 60°C, 84.0 at 100°C

Source: Gardner, 1972; Budavari, 1989; Lewis, 1989.

in club soda to impart a cool, saline taste and to enhance retention of carbonation. Citric acid is also one of the most popular acidulants for artificially flavored non-carbonated or "still" drinks and for beverage powders. In wines, it is added to adjust acidity, prevent cloudy precipitates, and to inhibit oxidation.

Commercially, citric acid is widely used as a synergist for antioxidants and as a retardant of browning reactions. Sodium citrate is also used as a chelating agent in conjunction with phosphate buffers to prepare noncaking meat-salt mixtures (Gardner, 1966). Other approved citrate-based sequestrants include isopropyl citrate at levels not to exceed 0.02%, monoisopropyl citrate, and stearyl citrate. Stearyl monoglyceridyl citrate can be used as an emulsion stabilizer in or with shortening-containing emulsifiers. Monoglyceride citrate is also used in antioxidant formulations for addition to fats and oils not to exceed 200 ppm of the combined weight of the additive and fat or oil (CFR, 1988).

An iron–choline–citrate complex may be used as a source of iron in foods for special dietary use (CFR, 1988). Iron ammonium citrate can be used as an anti-caking agent in salt for human consumption when the level of the additive does not exceed 25 ppm in the finished product.

Toxicology

Citric acid is a poison by intravenous route. It is moderately toxic by subcutaneous and intraperitoneal routes and by ingestion (Lewis, 1989). It is a severe eye and moderate skin irritant, and has some allergenic properties.

In short-term feeding studies, three dogs given a daily oral dose of 1380 mg citric acid/kg body weight for 112–120 days produced no symptoms or evidence of renal damage (FAO, 1974). Similar studies with rats fed 0, 0.2, 2.4, and 4.8% citric acid in a commercial diet showed a depressed food intake with a concurrent lowering of body weight and slight blood chemistry abnormalities at the 4.8% level as compared with the control group (Yokotani et al., 1971). Test animals in this group also showed a slight atrophy of thymus and spleen. In contrast, Packman et al. (1963) did not observe any abnormal blood or urine analyses and histopathological changes in rabbit fed 7.7% sodium citrate (equivalent to 5% citric acid) for up to 60 days.

Bonting and Jansen (1956) conducted long-term studies involving three generations of rats fed diets containing 1.2% citric acid. The test animals did not show any acidosis, abnormal serum composition, or any abnormalities in the reproductive system. In a 2-year chronic feeding study using male rats fed a basal diet containing 3 or 5% citric acid, Horn et al. (1957) found no adverse effects in survival rates and histopathology as compared with the control animals. Weight gains in the treated groups, however, were significantly lower than control, while food consumption was greatly lowered in the 5% group.

Cramer et al. (1956) investigated the relationship of the intake of sodium citrate and citric acid in rats fed vitamin D–free diets containing low levels of phosphorus but adequate levels of calcium. In the absence of the vitamin in diets, the citrates completely prevented the absorption of calcium, although there was no adverse effect on weight gain. The calcium was excreted as calcium citrate in the urine. Based on their studies, Cramer et al. (1956) concluded that citrates had a rachitogenic effect on the test animals.

Dalderup (1960) evaluated the effects of 1.5, 4.5, and 12 g citric acid per kilogram of food in a noncarcinogenic diet on the formation of dental caries in rats. No differences were noted in the number of cavities formed, although animals in the highest dosage group did show more enamel erosion when compared with the control group.

In other studies evaluating the effects of citrates on calcium metabolism, dogs given subcutaneous injections of 320–1200 mg of sodium citrate per kg body weight showed decreased blood calcium levels, while showing an increased excretion of urinary calcium (Gomori and Gulyas, 1944). Gruber and Halbeisen (1948) suggested that several of the symptoms produced through the use of high levels of citrates in the diets resembled calcium deficiency. They concluded further that such effects may have been due to the chelation of calcium by the acid moiety rather than the salt itself.

Martindale's Extra Pharmacopoeia (1972) summarizes the effects of citric acid in human beings. The ingestion of citric acid frequently or in large doses may cause erosion of teeth and local irritation, probably because of the low pH. Such effects are also seen with lemon juice that contains 7% citric acid and has a pH of less than three.

Citric acid is an important intermediate in the oxidative metabolic pathway of the Krebs cycle. Moreover, potassium and sodium citrates in doses of up to 4 g have been routinely used in medical practice for years without giving rise to ill effects. Both compounds are used as mild diuretics, and to render the urine less acid in daily doses of up to 10 g (*Martindale's Extra Pharmacopoeia*, 1972). Based on these facts, the FAO (1974) concluded that citric acid and its sodium and potassium salts do not constitute a significant toxicological hazard to humans and, hence, no limits were set on their acceptable daily intake in the human diet.

M. Benzoic Acid and Its Salts

Benzoic acid (Fig. 9A) is not a food acidulant. It is, however, included here by virtue of its acidic nature. It is one of the oldest chemical preservatives used in cosmetic, drug, and food industries. Its antimicrobial properties were first described in 1875 (Lueck, 1980). Difficulties in large-scale manufacturing prevented its use in foods prior to 1900. Since then, synthetic benzoic acid, because of its low cost,

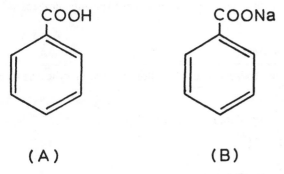

Fig. 9 (A) Benzoic acid and (B) sodium benzoate.

ease of incorporation into products, lack of color, and relatively low toxicity, has become one of the most widely used preservatives in the world.

Benzoic acid occurs naturally in free and combined forms in cranberries, prunes, greengage plums, apples, cinnamon, and ripe cloves (Dunn, 1968, Bykova et al., 1977; Chipley, 1983). Gum benzoin contains as much as 20% benzoic acid.

Manufacture

Benzoic acid is synthesized in a variety of ways. The manufacturing processes include the air oxidation of toluene, the hydrolysis of benzotrichloride, and the decarboxylation of phthalic anhydride (Williams, 1978).

Benzoic acid occurs in pure form as colorless or white needles or leaflets (Table 16). It has only a limited solubility in water. Its sodium salt is a white granular or crystalline powder and is more soluble in water. It is, therefore, preferred for use in several applications.

Food Uses

The Code of Federal Regulations (CFR, 1988) allows the use of benzoic acid and sodium benzoate up to a maximum permitted level of 0.1%. They may also be used in certain standardized foods. Benzoic acid and its sodium salt are most suitable for preserving foods and beverages that naturally are in a pH range below 4.5 or that can be brought into that range by acidification. The narrow pH range of its activity limits wider applications of this preservative in foods. It has a wide spectrum of action in foods effectively inhibiting bacteria belonging to Bacillaceae, Enterobacteriaceae, Micrococcaceae, and a wide variety of fungi and yeast.

Benzoic acid and sodium benzoate are used to preserve carbonated and noncarbonated beverages, fruit pulps and juices, jams and jellies, whole or liquid egg yolk, margarine, mayonnaise, mustards, pickles, bakery products, salad dressings, relishes, and sauces and ketchups (Chichester and Tanner, 1972; Lueck, 1980). The levels of applications in different food products are summarized in Table 17.

The undissociated moiety of benzoic acid is responsible for its antimicrobial activity. There is no general consensus regarding its mechanisms of action. However, inhibition of microorganisms by interfering with the permeability of the microbial cell membranes, uncoupling of both substrate transport and oxidative phosphorylation from the electron transport system, inhibition of membrane transport of amino acids resulting in starvation, inhibition of enzyme systems, inhibition of passive anion transport, and its scavenging of free radicals are the mechanisms

Table 16 Physical Properties of Benzoic Acid

Chemical names	Benzenecarboxylic acid, phenylformic acid, dracylic acid
Molecular formula	$C_7H_6O_2$
Molecular weight	122.12
Appearance	Colorless or white needles or leaflets
Melting point	122.4°C (begins to sublime at ~100°C)
Boiling point	249.2°C
Specific gravity	1.266–1.321 at 20°/4°C
Solubility, g/L water	2.9 at 20°C, 12.0 at 60°C, 68.0 at 95°C

Source: Budavari, 1989; Lewis, 1989.

Table 17 Food Uses and Levels of Incorporation of Benzoic Acid

Products	% Levels
Beverages	
Carbonated[a]	0.03–0.05
Noncarbonated	0.1
Beverage syrups[b]	0.1
Fruit drinks	0.05–0.1
Fruit juices	0.1
Purees and concentrates	0.1
Cider	0.05–0.1
Margarine, salted	0.1
Bakery products, pie and pastry fillings, icings	0.1
Miscellaneous	
Soy sauce[c], mincemeat	0.1
Salads, salad dressings	0.1
Fruit salads, relishes, pickles	0.1
Fruit cocktails, olives, and sauerkraut	0.1
Preserves, dried fruits, jams and jellies	0.1

[a]A maximum level of 0.1% sodium benzoate may be used for all product listed. A maximum level of 0.2% sodium benzoate may be used in orange juice manufacturing. Orange juice not for manufacturing may not contain a preservative (Federal Standards of Identity).
[b]Additional preservative must be added to the final diluted product.
[c]In Japan, benzoic acid can be legally added to refined soy sauce.

proposed by different researchers (Web, 1966; Freese et al., 1973; Hunter and Segel, 1973; Freese, 1978; Harvath, 1979, Chipley and Uraih, 1980; Corlett and Brown, 1980; Eklund, 1980; Chipley, 1983).

A broader spectrum of microbicidal activity in foods is often achieved by using a combination of benzoic acid and sorbic acid as food preservatives. For example, combinations of these two acids inhibit several bacterial strains better than either sorbic acid and benzoic acid alone (Rushing and Senn, 1963). Synergistic effects have also been reported using combinations of benzoate and sulfur dioxide, carbon dioxide, sodium chloride, boric acid, or sucrose (Rehme, 1960; Chichester and Tanner, 1972; Lueck, 1980).

Toxicology

The toxicological properties of benzoic acid and its salts have been extensively studied. Short-term feeding studies with mice fed 3 g sodium benzoate for 10 days showed a 10% reduction in their creatine output, probably due to depletion of the glycine pool (FAO, 1974). Shtenberg and Ignatev (1970) fed groups of 50 male and 50 female mice 80 mg benzoic acid/kg body weight/day, sodium bisulfite at 160 mg/kg/day, and a mixture of these two at the same levels by gavage. The highest mortality rates (60%) were observed in mice given the combination dose compared with the acid alone (32%). A 5-day period of food restriction after 75 days produced 85% mortality in both groups. Similarly, rats fed sodium benzoate at 16–1090 mg/kg/day over a 30-day period showed no adverse effects on body weight, appetite, or morphology, nor any histopathological abnormalities in the internal organs (FAO, 1974).

The results of several long-term feeding studies were summarized in a report prepared by the FAO (1974). In one study, three groups of 20 male and 20 female rats were pair fed for 8 weeks on diets containing 0, 0.5, and 1.0% benzoic acid and thereafter fed *ad libitum* over four generations. Two generations were fed for their entire life span; the third and fourth generations were autopsied after 16 weeks. No adverse effects were observed during the course of this study on growth rates, fertility, lactation, and life span. The postmortem examination also did not reveal any abnormalities. In yet another experiment, 20 male and 30 female rats were fed a diet containing 1.5% benzoic acid with 13 male and 12 female rats as controls for 18 months. The mortality rates were five times higher in the test group. The test animals also showed reduced body weights and food intake. Repeat experiments on groups of 20 test animals and 10 controls taken from another strain of rat also showed similar findings.

Minor and Becker (1971) have also shown that sodium benzoate has no teratogenic effect following peroral administration. Similarly, no carcinogenic activity was observed when rabbits were given benzoic acid by subcutaneous or intravenous routes, or when rats were given sodium benzoate as 5% of their diet (Hartwell, 1951). These results were later confirmed by Sodemoto and Enomoto (1980), who fed sodium benzoate to rats for 18–24 months at concentrations of 1 and 2% of their diet. No adverse clinical signs directly attributable to this compound were observed in test animals. Differences in average body weights and mortality rates between treated and control groups were also negligibile. Sodium benzoate does not appear to be mutagenic (Njagi and Gopalan, 1980), although Ishidata and Odashima (1977) reported positive results in chromosomal aberration tests conducted in Chinese hamster cells grown in culture. There is also no apparent additive toxicity from simultaneous ingestion of more than one preservative such as benzoic acid and sorbic acid (Ohno et al., 1978).

The results of extensive human feeding studies conducted during the early part of this century suggest that sodium benzoate is not deleterious to human health (Chittenden et al., 1909; Dakin, 1909). Benzoates do not appear to be accumulated in the body. They are absorbed from the intestine and detoxified and excreted as hippuric acid via the formation of benzoyl CoA intermediate (White et al., 1964). With the exception of fowls, almost all vertebrates excrete benzoic acid via hippuric acid pathway. Kao et al. (1978) found that different animal species differ markedly in their ability to metabolize benzoic acid. Hippuric acid formation was detected in hepatocytes and renal tubules from omnivores but was not detectable in hepatocytes from carnivores. These researchers postulated that species differences in patterns of benzoic acid conjugation were apparently related to differences in the ability of liver and kidney cells to carry out glycine and glucuronic acid conjugation.

Based on the overwhelming data and considering the metabolic and the large toxicological margin of safety in animals and humans, the FAO established the levels of benzoate causing no toxicological effect at 1% level in the diet, or equivalent to 500 mg/kg body weight. The acceptable daily intake for total benzoates in the human diet is established at 0–5 mg/kg body weight.

N. Sorbic Acid and Its Salts

Similar to benzoic acid, sorbic acid is not a food acidulant. It is, however, one of the most widely used food preservatives worldwide. Sorbic acid was first isolated in 1859 by a German chemist, A. W. von Hoffmann, by hydrolysis of the oil distilled from unripe rowanberries of the mountain ash tree (Keller et al., 1978; Sofos and Busta, 1981, 1983). The name was derived from the scientific name of the tree, *Sorbus aucuparia* Linne. In 1900, Doebner performed the first synthesis. Interest in this compound was minimal until its antimicrobial effects were discovered in 1940s. High manufacturing costs prohibited expanded use until its applicability as a food preservative was approved in 1953. It is now widely used in moist foods below pH 6.5 where control of bacteria, molds, and yeasts is essential to obtain safe and economical extended storage life.

Manufacture

The first synthesis of sorbic acid was from crotonaldehyde and malonic acid in pyridine (Keller et al., 1978). One of the first commercial methods involved the reactions of ketene and crotonaldehyde in the presence of boron trifluoride in ether at 0°C, giving a 70% yield. At present most commercial sorbic acid is produced by a modification of this route.

Ketenes can produce a condensation adduct in excess of such solvents as crotonaldehyde, or aliphatic, alicyclic and aromatic hydrocarbons and their derivatives to form compounds of molecular weights of 1000–5000. This polyester adduct, after the removal of unreacted components and solvents, is decomposed in acidic media or by controlled pyrolysis to pure *trans,trans*-2,4-hexadienoic acid. Sorbic acid thus produced is separated by distillation and purified further using carbon treatments and recrystallization from aqueous or other solvent systems to meet food-grade specifications.

Data on the physical properties of sorbic acid are summarized in Table 18. It is an almost odorless, white, crystalline powder with a slightly acidic taste. The carboxyl group of sorbic acid is highly reactive and can form various salts and

Table 18   Physical Properties of Sorbic Acid

Chemical names	(2-Butenylidene) acetic acid, crotylidene acetic acid, hexadienic acid, 2,4-hexadienoic acid, 1,3-pentadiene-1-carboxylic acid, 2-propenylacrylic acid
Molecular formula	$CH_3CH=CH-CH=CH-COOH$ ($C_6H_8O_2$)
Molecular weight	112.14
Appearance	Colorless needles, or white crystalline powder, odorless with slightly acidic taste
Melting point	134.5°C
Boiling point	228°C (decomposes)
Solubility, g/100 mL	
water, 20°C	0.16
ethanol, 25°C	14.8

Source: Gardner, 1972; Budavari, 1989; Lewis, 1989.

esters. Commercially available salts include calcium, sodium, and potassium sorbates. Sorbic acid has only very limited solubility in water at room temperature; however, its potassium salt is very soluble.

Food Uses

Sorbic acid and its salts, collectively known as sorbates, are used primarily in a wide range of foods and feed products and, to a lesser extent, in certain cosmetics, pharmaceuticals, and tobacco products. Although the calcium and sodium salts have been used in limited applications, the acid and its potassium salt are used almost exclusively (Keller et al., 1978).

Sorbates are classified as GRAS food additives, with no upper limit set for foods that are not covered by the Standards of Identity. They are used in more than 70 food products that have federal standards of identity. They can be applied to foods by any of several methods including direct addition into the product in the form of a powder or a solution, dipping in or spraying with an aqueous sorbate solution, dusting with sorbate powder, or impregnating the food-packaging material (Chichester and Tanner, 1972; Lueck, 1976, 1980; Keller et al., 1978; Sofos and Busta, 1983). The potassium salt is used in applications where high solubility is desired. The particular method of application depends on the form of sorbate used, the objectives to be accomplished, and the physical, chemical, and morphological properties of the product to be preserved.

Sorbates exhibit inhibitory activity against a wide spectrum of yeasts, molds, and bacteria, including most foodborne pathogens (Gardner, 1972; Lueck, 1976, 1980; Keller et al., 1978; Sofos and Busta, 1983). As bacterial inhibitors, they are, however, least effective against lactic acid bacteria. Because of this fact, they can be used effectively to suppress yeasts during lactic fermentations.

The inhibitory activity of sorbates is attributed to the undissociated acid molecule and, hence, is pH dependent. The upper limit for its activity is at about pH 6.5 in moist applications, and the activity increases with decreasing pH. The upper pH limit can be extended higher in low-water-activity solutions (Keller et al., 1978). Thus sorbates have one distinct advantage over the two other most commonly used preservatives—benzoic and propionic acids—since the upper pH limits for activity of these compounds are approximately pH 4.5 and 5.5, respectively. Sorbates are generally recognized as microbial growth retardants rather than microbicidals.

The exact mechanism of inhibition by sorbates has not been thoroughly understood. It has been postulated that they exert their activity by inhibiting various microbial enzyme systems (Sofos and Busta, 1981). Dehydrogenases and sulfhydral-containing enzymes including fumarase and aspartase are suggested to be inhibited by sorbates (Melnick et al., 1954; Whitaker, 1959; York and Vaughn, 1964). Other postulated mechanisms include a possible uncoupling of oxidative phosphorylation through inhibition of enzymes within the cell, inhibition of amination of α-ketoglutarate, formation of stable complexes with sulfhydral-containing enzymes through a thiohexenoic acid derivative, formation of covalent bonds between sulfur or the zinc oxide of the enzyme and the α and/or β carbons of sorbate, inhibition of enolase, proteinase, and catalase, and the inhibition of respiration through a competitive action with acetate on the site of acetyl CoA formation (Whitaker, 1959; York and Vaughn, 1960, 1964; Azukas et al., 1961; Troller, 1965; Dahle and Nordal, 1972; Sofos and Busta, 1981, 1983).

The lack of consensus suggests that no single mechanism can explain the action of sorbates under all conditions and in all situations. It is quite possible that the microbial inhibition by sorbates may result from one or more mechanisms under different conditions and circumstances of use.

Sorbic acid and its salts are widely used as fungistats and preservatives for pickles and pickled products, mayonnaise, margarine, delicatessen salads, condiments, spices, sherbet bases, fruit pulps and juices, jams and jellies, dried fruits, refrigerated salads, soft drinks, fruit syrups, beer, wine, confections, cottage cheese, yogurt, sour cream, seafoods, meat and poultry products, and a variety of bakery products (Gardner, 1972; Keller et al., 1978; Sofos and Busta, 1983). Their uses and levels of incorporation in different food products are summarized in Table 19.

Toxicology

Sorbic acid is one of the least harmful preservatives allowed for food use. Short-term feeding studies conducted with groups of 25 male and 25 female mice given 40 mg/kg body weight/day sorbic acid by oral intubation for 2 months showed no harmful effects (Shtenberg and Ignatev, 1970). Similar feeding studies in rats fed diets containing 1 or 2% sorbic acid for 80 days indicated no adverse effects on growth rates or any histopathological abnormalities in internal organs. Only the liver was enlarged slightly as compared with the controls (FAO, 1974).

Sorbic acid was shown to produce local sarcomas in rats when given by repeated subcutaneous injections at the same site in either peanut oil or in aqueous solutions. The potassium salt when administered under similar conditions, however, failed to produce any tumors (Dickens et al., 1968). Sorbic acid in the drinking water (10 mg/100 ml) for 64 weeks and the potassium salt given either in the drinking water (0.3%) or in the diet (0.1%) for 100 weeks failed to produce any tumors. Other rat feeding studies have indicated that a dosage of 10% sorbic acid in the diet can be tolerated for 40 days (Lueck, 1980). Upon extending the feeding period to 120 days, however, the growth rate and liver weight of test animals increased (Demaree et al., 1955). Additional studies with rats and dogs have shown no damage with feeding 5% sorbic acid for 90 days, while 8% sorbic acid resulted in

Table 19 Food Uses and Levels of Incorporation of Sorbic Acid

Dairy (cheese, cheese spreads and dips, cheese products, cottage cheese, yogurt, sour cream)	0.05–0.30
Bakery (cakes, cake mixes, pies and fillings, baking mixes, doughs, icings, fudges, toppings)	0.03–0.30
Vegetables (fresh salads, fermented vegetables, pickles, olives, relishes)	0.02–0.20
Fruits (dried fruits, fruit juices, fruit salads, jams and jellies, syrups)	0.02–0.25
Beverages (wines, carbonated and noncarbonated beverages, fruit drinks)	0.02–0.10
Miscellaneous (salad dressings, smoked and salted fish, margarine, confections, mayonnaise)	0.05–0.20

Source: Sofos and Busta, 1983.

a slight increase in liver weight (Deuel et al., 1954; Demaree et al., 1955; Lueck, 1976).

Chronic toxicity feeding studies with rats and mice over a period of two generations with sorbic acid concentrations as high as 90 mg/kg body weight showed no abnormalities. In some instances, the growth rate of test animals increased significantly, apparently due to an increased caloric intake resulting from the metabolizable sorbic acid. No carcinogenic or mutagenic effects have been observed with sorbates alone (Dickens et al., 1968; Litton Biometrics, 1974, 1977; Food and Drug Research Laboratory, 1975; Gaunt et al., 1975; Hendy et al., 1976; Lueck, 1980; Sofos and Busta, 1981).

As a preservative for cosmetics and pharmaceutical products, sorbates have been extensively examined for skin tolerance (Lueck, 1976). Average sorbic acid concentrations for skin irritation are in the range of 1.0%. Considering the average use levels of 0.10–0.30% in food processing, the potential for such interactions to occur in real life is minor. Thus, sorbates appear to be one of the safest food preservatives available.

Under normal metabolic conditions, sorbates are completely oxidized to carbon dioxide and water in the same way as other fatty acids, releasing 6.6 kcal/g energy. As a result of the extensive favorable toxicological and physiological aspects of sorbic acid, the FAO (1974) has allowed for its highest acceptable daily intake of all food preservatives at 25 mg/kg body weight.

O. Caprylic Acid

Caprylic acid is an eight-carbon saturated fatty acid. It occurs as a normal constituent of fats and oils in various foods. Along with butyric and lauric acids, it constitutes a major proportion of naturally occurring saturated fats and oils.

Manufacture

Caprylic acid is commercially manufactured by the oxidation of octanol. It can also be synthesized from 1-heptene.

Caprylic acid (MW 144.2, pK_a 4.89) is an oily liquid with a slightly unpleasant, rancid taste. It has only a very limited solubility in water. Caprylic acid, however, is freely soluble in alcohol, chloroform, ether, carbon disulfide, and glacial acetic acid.

Food Uses

Caprylic acid is approved as a GRAS food additive for miscellaneous and general purpose when used in accordance with the good manufacturing practices. It is used as a flavoring adjuvant in levels not to exceed 0.013% in baked goods; 0.04% for cheese; 0.005% for fats and oils, frozen dairy desserts, gelatins and puddings, meat products, and soft candy; 0.16% for snack foods; and 0.001% or less for other food categories (CFR, 1988).

Caprylic acid imparts a "sweatlike" odor and a cheesy and buttery taste to foods (Doores, 1989). It occurs naturally in conjunction with dairy-based flavors. It is also used as an antimicrobial agent for indirect use in cheese wraps. Other derivatives of caprylic acid, such as cobalt, iron and manganese caprylates, are classified as driers when migrating from food-packaging material (CFR, 1988).

As an antimicrobial compound, caprylic acid is ineffective against many gram-positive and gram-negative bacteria or yeasts in concentrations as high as 7.8 μmol/ml (Kabera et al., 1972). However, its minimum inhibitory concentration (MIC), when compared with that of acetic and propionic acids at pH 6.0, is 4–23 times lower. It is, therefore, more inhibitory to a broad group of microorganisms at a lower concentration at around neutral pH. The MIC of caprylic acid, unlike most other acid preservatives, is not significantly affected with changes in pH.

Toxicology

Caprylic acid is a normal constituent of several foods and is metabolized as a fatty acid. Hence, no limit has been set for its acceptable daily intake in the human diet.

P. Butyric Acid

Butyric acid was discovered by Lieben and Rossi in 1869 (Budavari, 1989). It is present in butter as an ester at a level of 4–5%. It also occurs as a normal constituent of dietary fats and oils, especially those with a high degree of saturation.

Manufacture

Butyric acid can be obtained by suitable fermentation of carbohydrates. Since it is a volatile fatty acid, it can also be obtained by fractional steam distillation of cream fat after acid hydrolysis. Chemically it is synthesized from n-propanol and carbon monoxide at 200 atm pressure in the presence of $Ni(CO)_4$ and NiI_2.

Butyric acid ($C_4H_8O_2$, MW 88.10) is an oily liquid with an unpleasant, rancid odor. It is miscible with water, alcohol, and ether. Its calcium salt is less soluble in hot than in cold water.

Food Uses

Butyric acid esters are used as bases of artificial flavoring ingredients in certain liqueurs, soda water, syrups, and candies. It also occurs naturally in conjunction with dairy-based flavors. Butyric acid is an important chemical reactant in the manufacture of shortening, emulsifying, and other edible additives employed in a wide variety of foods (Gardner, 1972).

Toxicology

Butyric acid is a major constituent of milk fat and other fats and oils. It is metabolized as a fatty acid. No limits have been set for its acceptable daily intake in the human diet.

Q. Ascorbic Acid (Vitamin C)

Ascorbic acid (Fig. 10) is widely distributed in the plant and animal kingdom. Citrus fruits, hip berries, acerola, and fresh tea leaves are particularly excellent sources of vitamin C.

Manufacture

Commercially, ascorbic acid is synthesized from simple sugars. D-Glucose is the most important sugar used as a starting material for the synthesis of L-ascorbic

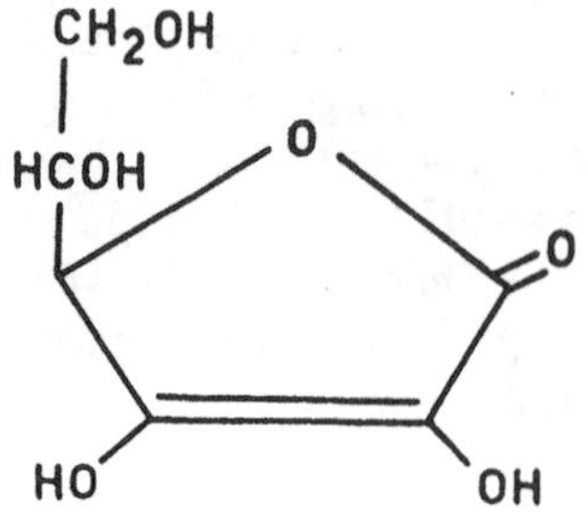

CH_2OH
|
HCOH

Fig. 10 Ascorbic acid (vitamin C).

acid. It contains the requisite six carbon atoms, some or all of the appropriate chiral centers (depending on the approach used), and an attractively low cost.

D-Glucose can be converted into L-ascorbic acid by two different procedures (Seib and Tolbert, 1982). In the first approach, C1 of glucose becomes C1 of ascorbic acid. This method requires that C1 and C2 be oxidized and the stereochemistry at C5 be inverted. In the second procedure, the carbon chain of D-glucose is inverted. In this method, the C1 of glucose must be reduced, and C5 and C6 oxidized, with the chirality at C4 and C5 of L-ascorbic acid coming from that at C3 and C2, respectively, in D-glucose.

Of the two, the second approach is commercially the most often preferred synthesis. The D-glucose is first reduced to D-glucitol, which is then fermentatively oxidized to L-sorbose. On treatment with acetone and acid, a mixture of mono- and diprotected derivatives of L-sorbose are formed and separated. The 2,3:4,6-di-*o*-isopropylidene-L-*xylo*-2-hexulofuranose thus obtained is oxidized to its corresponding acid. When the acid is heated in water, L-*xylo*-2-hexulosonic acid (2-keto-L-gulonic acid) is obtained, which upon heating at 100°C is converted with 13–20% yield into L-ascorbic acid. Alternatively, 2-keto-L-gulonic acid could be esterfied to obtain methyl-L-*xylo*-2-hexulosonate (methyl-2-keto-L-gulonate), which, after treatment with sodium methoxide in methanol followed by acidification, produces L-ascorbic acid in 73% yield.

In succeeding year, each step in this synthesis was optimized so that each individual step can now be carried out in greater than 90% yield providing L-ascorbic acid in greater than 50% overall yield from glucose. As a result of these process improvements, this synthesis became, and remains, the industrial method for the production of L-ascorbic acid (Seib and Tolbert, 1982). All other efforts to develop a less expensive synthesis of L-ascorbic acid have been unsuccessful to date.

Ascorbic acid occurs as a crystalline (usually plates, sometimes needles, monoclinic) powder (Table 20). It has a pleasant, sharp acidic taste. In impure preparations and in many natural products, it is readily oxidized to dehydroascorbic acid on exposure to air and light, although it is stable to air when dry.

Ascorbic acid is readily soluble in water, but insoluble in organic solvents, fats, and oils. It possesses relatively strong reducing power. Its aqueous solutions are rapidly oxidized by air. The reaction is accelerated by alkalies, iron, and copper. Its sodium salt is relatively stable.

Table 20 Physical Properties of Ascorbic Acid

Chemical names	L-Xyloascorbic acid, L-3-Ketothreo-hexuronic acid lactone
Molecular formula	$C_6H_8O_6$
Molecular weight	176.12
Appearance	Monoclinic needle or plate crystals, pleasant, sharp acidic taste
Melting point	190–192°C (some decomposition)
Specific gravity	1.65 at 20°/4°C
pK_1	4.17
pK_2	11.57
Solubility, g/100 mL water	33 at 20°C, 40 at 45°C, 80 at 100°C

Source: Budavari, 1989; Lewis, 1989.

Food Uses

Ascorbic acid is used as an antimicrobial and antioxidant in foods. It is preferentially oxidized in place of other substrates and complements very well as a synergist to other antioxidants, such as BHA and BHT, in polyphase food systems.

Ascorbic acid is used as an adjunct to meat-curing systems. Ascorbate or isoascorbate reduces nitrite, forming dehydroascorbic acid and nitric oxide. The latter reacts with myoglobin under reducing conditions to yield nitrosomyoglobin, the customary red pigment associated with cured meat products (Doores, 1989). Ascorbic acid also accelerates the color development and promotes color uniformity and stability.

Ascorbic acid and its sodium and calcium salts are used as nutritive additives (CFR, 1988). Whenever there is a need to preserve the vitamin content in fortified foods, the D isomer of ascorbic acid, isoascorbate or erythrobate, is incorporated with ascorbic acid. The D isomer has no vitamin activity. However, since it is more rapidly oxidized than ascorbic acid, the D isomer protects the vitamin C from oxidation, thus retaining its vitamin activity (Gardner, 1966). The use of other acidulants such as citric or malic acid also inhibits the oxidation of vitamin C and tends to reduce vitamin loss. In multivitamin preparations, nicotinamide–ascorbic acid complex serves as a source of both niacin and vitamin C (CFR, 1988).

Ascorbic acid is also used as an acidulant to adjust pH to prevent the enzymatic browning of fruits and vegetables by polyphenol oxidase enzyme system (Doores, 1989).

Toxicology

Ascorbic acid occurs in nature in its reduced form or as L-dehydroascorbic acid, its readily oxidized form. Its biological activity is confined only to its L isomer (Gardner, 1972). Plants and mammals except humans, monkeys, and guinea pigs can synthesize ascorbic acid. Those three mammalian species, therefore, require external sources, such as citrus fruits and vegetables, in their daily diet.

High doses of ascorbic acid are often advised as a treatment for cancer or common colds. Unlike the fat-soluble vitamins A and D, ascorbic acid exerts no adverse effects when given at very high concentrations. Since it is an essential nutrient in the human diet and appears to be nontoxic even at large doses, no acceptable daily intake limits are given for ascorbic acid.

R. Glucono-δ-Lactone

Glucono-δ-lactone (D-gluconic acid-δ-lactone, δ-gluconolactone, Fig. 11) is a derivative of glucose. It is prepared by the oxidation of glucose with bromine water or in *Acetobacter suboxydans* (Budavari, 1989).

Glucono-δ-lactone has been found useful in the processed-meat industry. In fermented sausages, it is used as a replacement for bacterial starter cultures and as a curing accelerator where slowly lowered pH will speed up curing without shorting the emulsion (Liebrand, 1978). It is also used in leavening agents.

Glucono-δ-lactone is used as a component of many cleaning compounds because of the sequestering ability of the gluconate radical, which remains active in alkaline solutions, in the dairy industry to prevent milk stones, in breweries to prevent beerstone, and as a latent acid catalyst for acid colloid resins, particularly in the textile industry.

Data on the toxicity of glucono δ-lactone are not available. It ionizes to form gluconic acid, an oxidation product of glucose, which is the normal dietary carbohydrate and the principal energy source in human nutrition. It is, therefore, not expected to pose serious health hazards to humans.

S. Amino Acids

Although amino acids are included here by virtue of their acidic nature, they are not used as acidulants, nor do they share similar functional and antimicrobial properties of other organic acids. Several essential amino acids, however, are used for fortification to enhance the nutritive value of food products. Lysine, in particular, is used for supplementation of wheat-based foods to improve the protein quality.

Cysteine and its derivatives have found applications as dough conditioners in the baking industry. Glutamic acid is the only amino acid that is used as a flavor enhancer in the food industry. Only its L isomer has food-flavor-enhancement qualities. It is primarily used as sodium salt to impart a meat flavor to foods, while its hydrochloride is used to improve the taste of beer. Data on essential amino acids and their manufacture and uses are summarized in Table 21.

Toxicological aspects of amino acids in human nutrition were recently reviewed by Deshpande and Sathe (1991). Amino acid toxicity, amino acid imbalance, and

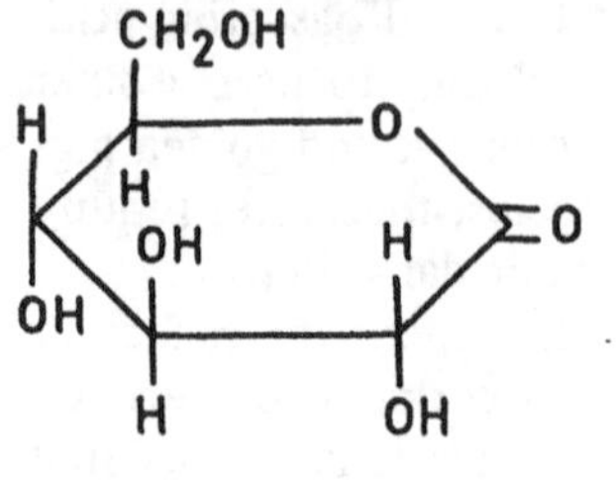

Fig. 11 Glucono-δ-lactone.

Table 21 Production and Uses of Essential Amino Acids

Amino acid	Production	Uses
Valine	Hydrolysis of fish proteins, Strecker synthesis by the action of ammonia and hydrogen cyanide on isobutyraldehyde followed by hydrolysis, action of ammonia on α-bromoisovaleric acid	Nutrient
Leucine	From gluten, casein, and keratin; action of ammonia on α-bromoisocaproic acid; and from hydantoin	Nutrient
Isoleucine	From beet sugar mother liquors, casein, ovalbumin, blood fibrin, and yeast proteins; from tiglaldehyde and hydantoin	Nutrient
Threonine	From oat protein and casein	Nutrient
Glutamic acid[a]	Fermentation of carbohydrates using *Micrococcus glutamicus* or by acid hydrolysis of gluten, casein, soybean cake, or beet molasses; condensation of sodium derivative of ethyl bezamidomalonate with ethyl α-bromopropionate; from methyl acrylate and phthalimidomalonate; from 2-cyclopentenylamine	Only the L(−) form has food flavor enhancement qualities; mainly used as Nasalt to impart a meat flavor to foods, hydrochloride used to improve the taste of beer
Lysine	Acid hydrolysis of casein, fibrin, or blood corpuscle paste	Food enrichment, to improve protein quality of wheat-based foods
Histidine	From blood corpuscles by an electrical transport method, by precipitation with mercuric chloride	Dietary supplement
Arginine	From gelatin; L-ornithine and cyanamide in aqueous solution in the presence of barium hydroxide	Dietary supplement
Phenylalanine	From ovalbumin, lactalbumin, zein and fibrin, from L-tyrosine	Nutrient
Tryptophan	From casein; from β-indolylaldehyde and hippuric acid; from hydantoin, 3-indoleacetonitrile, and α-ketoglutaric acid phenylhydrazone	Nutrient, antidepressant
Cysteine[a]	Acid hydrolysis of proteins, from electrolytic reduction of cystine	Dough conditioner
Methionine	Casein digestion with pancreatin, industrial synthesis with β-methylmercapto propionaldehyde	Nutrient, lipotropic agent, used to regulate urinary pH

[a]Nonessential amino acid in human nutrition.
Source: Budavari, 1989.

amino acid antagonism are examples of some problems encountered. Although humans can tolerate large intakes of protein and amino acids in a well-balanced pattern, excessive consumption sometimes leads to liver and kidney damage. This suggests that an increase in the metabolic load of these nutrients increases the demand for metabolic capacity and regulatory mechanisms.

Of the three most widely used amino acids in the food industry described above, the sodium salt of glutamic acid is often associated with the so-called Chinese Restaurant syndrome (Kwok, 1968). Higher-than-normal blood levels of glutamate can result in a feeling of weakness, palpitation, and numbness of the neck and back, and symptoms may last up to 2 h.

Available acute toxicity data, expressed as LD_{50} values, for various acidulants and their derivatives are summarized in Table 22.

V. GENERAL APPLICATIONS IN FOODS

The use of various acidulants in food products is primarily determined by the desired end product. Because of a variety of functional properties, their use in different food systems often leads to the enhancement of food quality. The proper selection of a food-grade acid is determined by the property or a combination of properties of the acid as well as its cost.

Acidulants are most commonly used for flavor and tartness and as antimicrobial agents to extend the shelf life of food products by maintaining the appropriate pH control. In turn, the salts of some acids can also be used as buffering agents to modify these properties. Several acidulants are also excellent antioxidants. In fat-based food products, they prevent or retard lipid oxidation by complexing the metal ions. Depending upon the food system, acidulants are used to stabilize color, reduce turbidity, modify melt characteristics, prevent splattering, and enhance gelling. They are also used as leavening or inversion agents, emulsifiers, nutrients, and supplements (Gardner, 1966). In the following sections, the applications of acidulants in the processing of foods and food ingredients are described briefly according to the general food categories.

A. Beverages

The beverage industry utilizes a major portion of food acids manufactured globally. A proper selection of acid(s) is essential for flavor balance and tartness, to extend shelf life through microbiological inhibition, and to chelate metal ions harmful to color and flavor in several alcoholic, carbonated, powdered, and nutritional beverages. Some of these applications are described below.

Alcoholic Beverages

In brewing, salts of several acids are used to maintain a buffering system to obtain maximum conversion of humulon to *iso*-humulon in the preparation of dried hops extract. Heyer (1957) first reported that the boiling hops suspension must be buffered between pH 8.0 and 8.3 for maximum conversion and yields. Acidulants are also essential to control bacterial contamination of brewer's yeast. The yeasts are often washed with a solution of phosphoric acid and sodium persulfate at 5°C to increase their viability and resistance towards contaminating bacteria.

Acidulants such as polyphosphates are especially useful in alcoholic beverage production because of their ability to form stable, soluble complexes with heavy metal and alkaline earth metals. The formation of such complexes with iron, copper, and calcium inactivates them effectively and precludes the need for their removal from beverages. The formation of metal complexes in the presence of acidulants also prevents clouding and haze formation in beer and wine.

Acidulants play an important role in wine making. The control of acidity of grape must is essential for optimum fermentative action of yeast and for enhancing the resistance of the wine to microbial spoilage (Liebrand, 1978). In some crop years, the natural acid content of wine grapes is high enough not to require adjustment of the acid content of the wine must. In other years, when the natural acidity is too low, the necessary adjustment in grape wine must can be made with citric, fumaric, lactic, malic, and tartaric acids. The choice and use of acidulants in this case is governed by federal regulations and state laws of the wine-producing states.

Acidulants are also used in flavoring some wines. For example, citric acid may be used for adjusting the acidity of citrus fruit wine and malic acid for apple wine. Because of its low solubility, the use of fumaric acid in this regard is rather limited. Acidulants also enhance the storage quality of wines by sequestering iron and other metal ions that are capable of complexing with tannins. Metal–tannin complexes are insoluble and can give rise to turbidity in wines.

Carbonated Beverages

Carbonated beverages are made by preparing a concentrated syrup, which is subsequently diluted with carbonated water. Because of their solubility, citric, malic, phosphoric, and tartaric acids are widely used in carbonated beverages. The acid contents of variously flavored carbonated beverages are summarized in Table 23.

Phosphoric acid is used in many bottled soft drink beverages. These include the leaf-, root-, or nut extract–flavored carbonated cola beverages. Since it is a natural constituent of many fruits, phosphoric acid blends well with flavors in these drinks. It is generally sold as 75–85% solutions and can be used as such to make each batch of beverage syrup. The quantity used, however, is often determined by the type of fruit flavor. It generally varies according to the degree of tartness and acidity desired.

Citric acid is used in most other flavors. In contrast, the high cost and periodic shortages limit the use of tartaric acid generally to only grape-flavored products. These acids are sold as dry powders and are added to each batch of beverage syrup as a previously prepared 50% stock solution.

Buffering agents such as sodium citrate often are added to carbonated beverages to reduce the sharpness of the acid taste, if the quantity of the acid is relatively large (Liebrand, 1978). Buffer salts tend to mellow the flavor in lemon-lime type drinks. In club soda, sodium citrate imparts a cool, saline taste and aids in the retention of carbonation.

Noncarbonated (Still) Beverages

This category includes fruit drinks, nectars, and cocktail mixes. Since these beverages are not usually prepared in carbonated form, solubility is less of a factor in

Table 22 LD_{50} Values for Various Acidulants Used in the Food Industry

Acidulant	Test animal	Route of administration	LD_{50} (mg/kg body weight)
Phosphoric acid	Rat	Oral	1530
	Rabbit	Subcutaneous	2740
Sodium hydrogen phosphate	Rat	Oral	17000
Sodium dihydrogen phosphate	Rat	Oral	8290
Trisodium phosphate	Rabbit	Intravenous	1580
Hydrochloric acid	Rabbit	Intragastric	300
Acetic acid	Mouse	Oral	4960
	Mouse	Intravenous	525
	Rat	Oral	3310–3530
	Rabbit	Rectal	1200
	Rabbit	Subcutaneous	1200
	Rabbit	Oral	1200
Sodium acetate	Rat	Oral	3530–4960
	Mouse	Oral	3310
	Mouse	Intravenous	380
Calcium acetate	Rat	Intravenous	147
	Mouse	Intravenous	52
Dehydroacetic acid	Rat	Oral	1000
Propionic acid	Rat	Oral	2600–3500
	Mouse	Intravenous	625
Sodium propionate	Mouse	Subcutaneous	2100
	Rabbit	Skin	1640
	Rat	Oral	5100
	Rat	Intravenous	1380–3200
Calcium propionate	Rat	Oral	3340
	Rat	Intravenous	580–1020
Lactic acid	Rat	Oral	3730
	Guinea pig	Oral	1810
	Mouse	Oral	4875
Sodium lactate	Rat	Intraperitoneal	2000
Ferrous lactate	Mouse	Oral	147
Succinic acid	Rat	Oral	2260
Fumaric acid	Rat	Oral	10700
Sodium fumarate	Rat	Oral	8000
Disodium fumarate	Rabbit	Oral	3600–4800
L-(+)-Malic acid	Rabbit	Oral	5000
	Rat	Oral	1600
Sodium malate	Dog	Oral	1000
Tartaric acid	Dog	Oral	5000
	Mouse	Intravenous	485

Table 22 Continued

Acidulant	Test animal	Route of administration	LD$_{50}$ (mg/kg body weight)
Adipic acid	Mouse	Oral	1900
	Mouse	Intravenous	680
	Mouse	Intraperitoneal	275
	Rat	Oral	3600
	Rabbit	Oral	2430–4860
	Rabbit	Intravenous	2430
Citric acid	Mouse	Oral	5040–5790
	Mouse	Intravenous	203–960
	Mouse	Intraperitoneal	961
	Mouse	Subcutaneous	2700
	Rat	Oral	11700
	Rat	Intraperitoneal	725–884
	Rat	Subcutaneous	5500
	Rabbit	Intravenous	330
Sodium citrate	Mouse	Intravenous	44
	Mouse	Intraperitoneal	1460
	Rat	Intraperitoneal	1210
	Rabbit	Intravenous	338
Potassium citrate	Dog	Intravenous	167
Benzoic acid	Rat	Oral	17000–40000
Sodium benzoate	Rat	Oral	2700
	Rat	Intravenous	1714
	Rabbit	Oral	2000
	Rabbit	Subcutaneous	2000
	Dog	Oral	2000
Butyl p-hydroxybenzoate (free acid)	Mouse	Oral	5000
	Mouse	Intraperitoneal	230
Butyl p-hydroxybenzoate (sodium salt)	Mouse	Oral	950
	Mouse	Intraperitoneal	230
Ethyl p-hydroxybenzoate	Mouse	Oral	8000
	Guinea pig	Oral	2000–2400
	Rabbit	Oral	5000
	Dog	Oral	5000
Methyl p-hydroxybenzoate	Mouse	Oral	8000
	Guinea pig	Oral	3000–3600
	Rabbit	Oral	6000
	Dog	Oral	6000
Propyl p-hydroxybenzoate	Mouse	Oral	8000
	Mouse	Intraperitoneal	400
Sorbic acid	Rat	Oral	7360–10,500
Sodium sorbate	Rat	Oral	4000–7160
	Mouse	Intraperitoneal	2500
Potassium sorbate	Mouse	Intraperitoneal	1300
	Rat	Oral	4920–6170
Caprylic acid	Mouse	Intravenous	600
δ-Gluconolactone	Rabbit	Intravenous	7630

Source: FAO/WHO, 1962, 1963, 1967; Ellinger, 1972; FAO, 1974; Chipley, 1983; Doores, 1983, 1989; Sofos and Busta, 1983; Lewis 1989.

Table 23   Acid Content of Carbonated Beverages

Type	Flavors	Percentage acid		
		Low	High	Average
Low acid	Cream soda	0.005	0.03	0.02
	Root beer			
	Birch beer			
	Sarsaparilla			
Medium acid	Cola types	—	—	0.08
	Ginger ale	0.10	0.20	0.13
	Fruit-flavored	0.10	0.23	0.15
High acid	Mixers	0.30	0.60	0.40

Source: Liebrand, 1978.

the choice of an acidulant. Citric, malic, and tartaric acids can be added to a batch either as 50% stock solutions or, if convenient, directly as a powder.

Fumaric acid also finds many uses in single-strength fruit drinks. It must be added directly to the batch, since its low solubility will not allow the preparation of a stock solution. In large batches, complete solution of fumaric acid can be achieved in a reasonable time by efficient agitation and the use of a powder with fine particle size.

Powdered Beverages

The acidic, crystalline phosphate salts are often included as a portion or all of the acidulant in powdered beverages. The commonly used salts include monocalcium phosphate, monosodium phosphate, and hemisodium phosphate (Van Wazer, 1958). Diller and Brout (1958) and Brout (1961) have obtained patents for a soft, carbonated drink dry mix that, upon addition to tap water, produces a prolonged effervescence. The basis for this prolonged effervescence was a combination of hemisodium phosphate, monosodium phosphate, and monoammonium carbonate.

Tricalcium phosphates are used to improve flow properties of powdered, instant beverage mixes. They act by influencing the particle size distribution of the dry mixes.

Acidic phosphates and pyrophosphates as well as other acidic inorganic and organic salts are used to neutralize histidine compounds in chickory for use in coffee-chickory blends (Stayton, 1944). Neutralizing these compounds removes the characteristic aromas and flavors of chickory, and, therefore, the blend tastes more like a high-grade coffee.

Nutritional Beverages

Beverages designed to provide improved nutrition or for special dietary purposes have become quite popular in recent years. These beverages must be fortified with various minerals and vitamins to meet the dietary requirements. Sodium iron pyrophosphate, ferric pyrophosphate, and ferric orthophosphate are often used as sources of iron in some of these beverages. Calcium phosphates also are often added to provide the proper levels of calcium and phosphorus. Polyphosphoric acids are used to complex metal ions and to stabilize ascorbic acid as well as added food coloring in vitamin C–fortified beverages (Hashimoto and Miyazaki, 1961).

B. Cereal and Baked Products

Acidulants are used as food additives in cereal products primarily as leavening acids. They are also used for pH adjustment, buffering, dough conditioning, and mineral enrichment.

Leavening Acids

The evolution of carbon dioxide through the reaction of an acid and a carbonate salt is the basis for chemical leavening. Leavening, in general, refers to the introduction and expansion of some type of gas in the batter or dough system. Mixing or kneading the batter or dough also incorporates air in proportion to the energy expended in the mixing action. These gas bubbles then expand during baking and provide part of the leavening in the baked product. The desired properties of an acidulant for use as a leavening acid include:

1. Acidification to release carbon dioxide from the baking soda to create new gas bubbles and to expand the existing bubbles
2. Buffering to provide the optimum pH in the baked product
3. Interaction with the protein constituents of flour to modify the elastic and viscosity properties of doughs and batters
4. Imparting desired volume, texture, and taste to the baked product

The commonly used acids and acid salts and their neutralizing capacity are summarized in Table 24. The neutralizing value, sometimes also called the neutralizing strength, of a leavening acid represents the number of grams of sodium bicarbonate that will be neutralized by 100 g of the leavening acid. The various acids also differ in their rate of reaction in response to changes in temperature and in the taste they impart to the finished product. All of these factors must be taken into consideration in selecting an acidulant for a particular condition. Under some conditions, a mixture of acidulants may be most suitable to achieve the desired reaction times. The various applications of leavening acids in cereal-based products are briefly described below.

Table 24 Neutralizing Value of Various Acidulants Used in Chemical Leavening

Acidulant	Neutralizing value[a]
Fumaric acid	145
δ-Gluconolactone	47
Cream of tartar	45
Sodium acid pyrophosphate	72
Anhydrous monocalcium phosphate	83
Monocalcium phosphate monohydrate	80
Sodium aluminum sulfate	100
Sodium aluminum phosphate	100
Dicalcium phosphate dihydrate	33

[a]Defined as g of sodium bicarbonate neutralized by 100 g of the leavening acid.
Source: Ellinger, 1972; Liebrand, 1978.

Baking Powders

Baking powder is a complete leavening system consisting of a mixture of the proper quantities of soda, leavening acid, and a diluent such as starch that separates these ingredients so that they will not interact with each other during storage. The baking powders in commercial use contain sufficient soda to yield not less than 12% of their weight as carbon dioxide when used.

There are two types of baking powders. The more commonly used "double-acting" baking powder contains monocalcium phosphate (MCP) and sodium aluminum sulfate (SAS). The MCP provides rapid reaction during the mixing stage, while the SAS acts only during the baking stage (Bradley and Tucker, 1964). "Single-acting" baking powder is also known as phosphate or tartrate baking powder. It contains one of the MCPs or cream of tartar and tartaric acid as the single leavening acid. Baking powders are generally intended for household baking needs, as well as commercial bakers, restaurants, and other large-volume customers.

Prepared Baking Mixes

Prepared baking mixes offer the consumer the advantages of convenience, economy, and uniform quality. These mixes contain all of the dry ingredients needed to prepare the final product and require only the addition of liquid or other speciality ingredients such as eggs and shortening.

Most modern cake mixes contain combinations of leavenings in order to obtain maximum volume, maximum uniformity of grain and texture, and optimum shape of the baked cake. The pancake and waffle mixes are usually somewhat simpler ingredient systems than prepared cake mixes. Other examples include prepared biscuit mixes, self-rising flour, and cake doughnut mixes.

Refrigerated Doughs

Refrigerated biscuits, dinner rolls, sweet rolls, pizza breads, and similar products are becoming increasingly popular in the United States. Several phosphates are used as leavening acids in these products.

Nonleavening Uses

In addition to their leavening effects, acidulants find many other applications in cereal technology. Some of the more important ones are described below.

Dough Conditioning

Acidulants such as phosphates are often used to improve gluten characteristics in doughs. The type of interaction and its effect on the final dough or batter system depend on the chemical characteristics of the phosphate and the gluten protein. Acidulants are also helpful in retarding the microbial deterioration of refrigerated doughs.

Inhibition of Enzyme Activity

Acidulants inhibit lipoxidase enzyme activity in sponge-cake batter. Inorganic phosphates can also inhibit α-amylase activity when malt flour is used in baking mixes.

Antioxidant Activity

Acidulants also inhibit oxidative rancidity in cereal products, thereby preventing the development of stale, rancid flavors.

Inhibition of Microbial Growth

Acidulants help stabilize cereal products such as doughs, batter, and baked products against microbial spoilage.

Mineral Enrichment

Calcium and iron salts of inorganic acids and often their phosphates are commonly added to baked products to provide these essential minerals.

Decreasing Cereal-Cooking Time

The addition of phosphates decreases the cooking time of several grains such as rice, barley, wheat, rye, and oats used as breakfast cereals. Several phosphates are also used to decrease the cooking time of legumes and pulses.

C. Candy Making

Most of the food acid in the confectionery industry is used in hard candy, and that only for flavoring purposes. Citric or malic acids are used because of their solubility characteristics and since they impart a tartness compatible with most hard candy flavors. Tartaric acid is used only in grape-flavored candy or in sours where its high relative tartness is an advantage (Liebrand, 1978). The acids are added "as is" to the molten candy mass after the moisture is reduced to less than 1% to minimize the addition of water and sucrose inversion. In gums and jellies made with starch or agar, acids are added after the cook, mainly as a flavoring agent. Pectin jellies require acidification for pH control. The more soluble acids are also suitable for this application.

D. Gelatin Desserts

The setting properties of gelatin are intimately related to pH. Acidulants, therefore, play a critical role in careful control of pH in gelatin-based desserts. They also contribute a desired tartness to these products. Fumaric and adipic acids, although of limited solubility, are used in gelatin desserts because the powders are dissolved in hot water. Citric acid is also used; however, its hygroscopic properties need to be overcome with appropriate packaging.

E. Jams, Jellies, and Preserves

Federal Standards of Identity permit the use of citric, malic, fumaric, and tartaric acids in jams and jellies. Food acids are used to obtain proper gelation and to bring out the fruit flavor (Liebrand, 1978).

Good pectin gels are obtained only with a narrow pH range. The acids are added after the cook to minimize sucrose inversion or hydrolysis of the pectin. Citric, malic, or tartaric acids are added as 50% solutions, but fumaric is added as a slurry because of its poor solubility. In the event that the substitution of one acid for another is desirable for purposes of evaluation, the acid levels must be adjusted relative to acid strength in order to obtain a correct pH.

F. Dairy Products

Acidulants play several important roles in the processing of dairy products. Phosphates and citrates are the major food acids used in dairy processing, although the Federal Standards of Identity have been amended to include lactic acid, hydrochloric acid, and glucono-δ-lactone in the process of direct acidification of milk and mild products. Because of their importance in dairy processing, the following discussion is primarily related to the use of various phosphates and citrates in milk processing.

Interactions with Milk Calcium

Sommer and Hart (1926) first proposed that the addition of phosphates and/or citrates changed the "salt balance" of the milk through the formation of complexes with calcium and magnesium ions. The complexing of these ions is an extremely important function of phosphates in dairy technology. Casein in milk also acts as a multivalent ion that can undergo ion exchange reactions. This also results in a reduction in the levels of free calcium ions and an increase in bound calcium or "colloidal" calcium as phosphates are added.

Interactions with Milk Proteins

Ortho-, pyro-, and longer-chain polyphosphates differ in their reactions with casein. At lower concentrations of 1–15 mM, orthophosphates cause little change in the viscosity of the milk, while at higher concentrations (>140 mM), they produce gelation. The rate of gelation is increased in proportion to the calcium ion concentration and the level of milk solids not fat.

Through ionic interactions with the positively charged casein at the normal pH value of milk, the negatively charged pyrophosphates precipitate casein to form thick gels. In contrast, the longer-chain polyphosphates can precipitate both casein and β-lactoglobulin. Because they are polyvalent anions, the polyphosphates are capable of reacting with more than one basic group to form cross-links between protein molecules to yield large micelles.

Heat Stability of Milk

The addition of orthophosphates increases the heat, rennet, and alcohol coagulation times of milk. This effect is especially useful in the manufacture of cheese and the stabilization of evaporated milk. The amount of calcium and phosphate ions absorbed on the surface of casein micelles has a direct bearing on the heat stability of milk. The degree of heat stability of milk is inversely proportional to the ratio of soluble calcium/soluble orthophosphate.

Milk Beverages

Phosphates have been used in various milk-based beverages to control viscosity and to stabilize and enhance the flavor of the finished product.

High-Butterfat Dairy Products

Food acids, including phosphoric acid, are used in the clarification of butter oil by coagulating the suspending materials that cause cloudiness, as well as to enhance the stability against oxidative spoilage during storage. The use of ammonium, sodium, and potassium salts of the various longer-chain and cyclic polyphosphates when used prior to acidification of bacterially fermented buttermilk produce enhanced flavor, viscosity, body, stability to whey-off, and the general appearance of the buttermilk. Sodium phosphates and citrates are also used in some commercial half-and-half milk products.

Condensed, Evaporated, and Sterile Concentrated Milks

Condensed and evaporated milks are prepared by concentrating the milk, then canning and sterilizing it by heating the cans to approximately 240°F (121°C). Unless the casein in the milk is stabilized against heat coagulation by the addition of disodium phosphate or sodium citrate, it tends to gel during storage. Polyphosphates and citrate salts also improve the heat and storage stability of sterile concentrated milks.

Mild Gels and Puddings

Prior to the development of instant milk puddings, the preparation of a pudding by cooking starch was a tedious process. Attempts to prepare puddings from pregelatinized starch were unsatisfactory, because the quantity of starch necessary produced starchy flavors, heavy, pasty textures, and sticky consistencies. The modern-day instant pudding mixes contain trisodium polyphosphates and calcium acetate as a source of soluble calcium ion with which to cause the milk to gelatinize. The mix, therefore, requires only a small quantity of pregelatinized starch to prepare the firm pudding gel desired.

Canned, refrigerated, and frozen ready-to-eat puddings are prepared by use of ultra–high-temperature, short-time heat treatment and, if they are to be stored at room temperature, by aseptic canning. These puddings also utilize trisodium polyphosphates to provide proper gelling of the milk proteins so that the desired firmness is obtained.

Nonfat Milk

The phosphates improve the properties of dried and liquid skim milk products through their interactions with milk proteins and their ability to complex calcium. To increase and improve the solubility of dried milk solids in water, the skim milk is often treated either before or after drying with acids or their soluble salts, which produce calcium salts less soluble in water than the tricalcium phosphate normally present in the milk. Only oxalates, fluorides, and metaphosphates are capable of producing such insoluble calcium salts. However, since the oxalates and fluorides are not acceptable food additives, only metaphosphates are used for this purpose.

Frozen Dairy Desserts

Acidulants are included in sherbets, ices, and ice creams to enhance fruit flavors. Until 1967, the Federal Standards of Identity allowed phosphates and citrates only in chocolate ice cream and similar frozen desserts, because they were necessary in maintaining stable chocolate suspensions. However, they also stabilize frozen desserts against churning. Churning is the phenomenon of agglomeration of fat particles or globules during excessive whipping, resulting in detectable particles in the ice cream.

Whey, Lactose, and Lactalbumin

Acidulants, especially polyphosphates, are routinely used to separate lactose from cheese whey, to solubilize whey proteins, and to improve the flow and functional properties of dried whey used as a replacement for skim milk in baked products. Similarly, denatured, heat-coagulated lactalbumin obtained as a byproduct of lactose production is very difficult to solubilize. Hence, it is often separated as lactalbumin phosphate. It is often used to replace part or all of the nonfat dried milk used in prepared cake mixes, biscuit mixes, self-rising flour, comminuted meats, pizza dough, refrigerated canned biscuits, and pancake, bread, and cookie mixes. Lactalbumin phosphate is also used as a direct functional and nutritional replacement for sodium caseinate in the preparation of imitation dairy products such as coffee whiteners, whipped toppings, artificial ice creams and frozen desserts, puddings, custards, frozen cream pies, imitation processed cheese, imitation sour cream, snack dips, baby foods, and instant breakfast and nutritional drinks.

Imitation Dairy Products

The high cost of production, processing, and delivery of dairy products has created intense interest in imitation dairy products. These have the taste and appearance characteristics, but do not contain the high-priced butterfat of real dairy products. Imitation dairy products such as imitation milk, coffee whiteners, whipped toppings, imitation sour cream, sour cream dressings and chip dips, imitation frozen desserts, cheese, cream cheese and cheese spreads, margarine all contain a phosphate, such as disodium or dipotassium phosphates.

Cheese Products

Acidulants such as phosphates and citrates are routinely used for the acidification of milk to produce cottage cheese. Glucono-δ-lactone is particularly interesting for this application, because it must undergo hydrolysis to gluconic acid before it can lower pH. Thus, the rate at which the pH is lowered is slowed, avoiding rapid local denaturation and producing a finished product of fine quality. Acidulants are also used to stabilize several cheese products including natural cheeses and pasteurized process cheese products.

G. Meat and Seafood Products

Acidulants play diverse and important roles in the processing and preservation of meat and fish. Through their interactions with water- and salt-soluble meat proteins and mineral ions, acidulants help in increasing the tenderness of meats, improve the binding of proteins in comminuted meat products, improve the moisture retention and color and flavor profiles in cured meat products, and prevent off-flavors and microbiological spoilage.

The ability of acidulants to enhance the activity of natural and added antioxidants and to sequester oxidation-promoting trace metals is utilized to retard rancidity in fish, shellfish, sausage, and dried meats. Under federal regulations, citric acid is permitted in conjunction with antioxidants to prevent oxidative rancidity in dry sausage (0.001%), fresh pork sausage (0.01%), and dried meats (0.01%). δ-Gluconolactone has also found several uses in the processed meat industry. In fermented sausages, it has been used as a replacement for bacterial starter cultures, and as a curing accelerator where slowly lowered pH will speed up curing without shorting the emulsion.

H. Fats and Oils

Acidulants have found many useful applications in the processing of fats and oils. They are used as aids in the extraction and refining of fats and oils, in fat stabilization, and in obtaining stable emulsions. Some of these applications are described below.

Refining

Crude fats and oils, as they are extracted or expressed from vegetable or animal matter, contain a number of impurities, including free fatty acids, phosphatides of various types, mucilaginous materials, protein from plant or animal tissues, as well as soluble proteins and similar contaminants. These impurities must be removed by refining the crude extracts.

The two general processes used in the refining of fats and oils are alkali and acid refining. A disadvantage of the alkali-refining process is that it may produce refining losses of 2% or more due to the saponification of the desirable glycerides to form soaps and glycerine. The addition of inorganic phosphate salts to the oil during the alkali-refining process or the formation of soluble inorganic phosphates by use of phosphoric acid and subsequent neutralization with alkali reduces such losses.

In the acid-refining process, sulfuric acid is most commonly used, although food-grade hydrochloric and chromic acids can also be used. By varying the proportion of the acid to oil, the concentration of the acid by dilution, and the temperature of the reaction, it is possible to obtain oils with levels of desired fatty acids within narrow ranges. Several phosphates are also used to solubilize protein, mucilagenous materials, phosphatides, and fatty acid contaminants and to greatly improve the odor, flavor, and stability to rancidity of the treated fats and oils. The phosphates have also found applications in bleaching or decolorizing fats and oils. Orthophosphoric acid is preferred, although sulfuric and metaphosphoric acid could also be added to bleaching clays.

Rearrangement

Rearrangement or interesterification requires the use of sodium methylate as a catalyst. The catalyst must be destroyed before further processing of the fat or oil can be accomplished. Phosphoric acid is often used for this purpose.

Hydrogenation

Phosphoric and citric acids have been used to remove nickel catalysts from hydrogenated fats and oils. Treatment with an acid and a neutral bleaching earth stabilizes the odor and flavor reversion in hydrogenated fats.

Monoglyceride Preparation

Monoglycerides prepared by treating the fat or oil with additional glycerine dissolved in caustic soda must be bleached again to remove undesirable compounds. Phosphoric acid is often used for this purpose.

Antioxidant Systems

Rancidity of untreated fats and oils may occur in storage. Oxidation is promoted by the catalytic action of certain metallic ions and their salts or soaps, such as iron, nickel, manganese, cobalt, chromium, copper, and tin. Minute quantities of these are inevitably picked up from the equipment during processing. Citric acid, when added to the oil, sequesters these trace ions and helps prevent the development of off-flavors. Acidulants also enhance the stability of antioxidants naturally present such as tocopherols in fats and oils. When protected oils are used as food ingredients, the foods in turn become more resistant to rancidity and the development of off-flavors.

I. Fruit and Vegetable Products

Fruits and vegetables contain significant levels of various acids. The common ones include citric, malic, phosphoric, tartaric, and fumaric acids. Acidulants are often used as food additives in fruit and vegetable processing as inhibitors of microbiological spoilage by surface applications, as stabilizers against oxidative rancidity, for stabilization of vitamins and color, and to increase and optimize the thickness, tenderization, and firming of fruit and vegetable tissues.

J. Protein and Starch Processing

Acidulants, especially phosphoric acid and its salts, are widely used in the processing of plant proteins and to prepare modified starches as food ingredients. Interactions with polyphosphates often improve protein dispersion and whipping properties and increase protein water-holding and gelling properties.

The phosphoric acid esters of corn and potato starches have found numerous applications in food industry as stabilizers for fountain syrups and ice cream toppings, ice cream, and various types of fat and water emulsions; as suspending agents for insoluble solids, including fruits in pie fillings, Chinese-type foods, and bakery mixes; as pan greases in combination with fats; as beer foam stabilizers; in instant puddings; and in various types of cheese sauces. The various starch phosphates approved for use in foods should contain no more than 0.4% residual phosphate calculated as phosphorus (*Federal Register*, 1967).

K. Sugar Processing

Phosphoric acid and its numerous salts are used in sugar refining process to remove nonsugar compounds in the clarification step. They are also used for the bleaching of sugar syrup prior to crystallization of sucrose.

The maximum levels of organic acids recommended for various food product categories in the United States are presented in Table 25.

VI. ANALYTICAL ASSAYS

The official methods for the analysis of individual acidulants form the basis for conducting chemical assays for the various acids in foods (AOAC, 1984). It is essential to determine the acidity of various food products for the following three reasons (Doores, 1989):

1. The acids, especially the organic ones, are a natural component of fruits and vegetables. Therefore, the qualitative or quantitative analysis of different acids is often a measure of their wholesomeness or lack of adulteration. It is also a confirmation of the standard of identity for that product.

Table 25 Maximum Percent Levels of Organic Acids Recommended for Various Food Product Categories in the United States

Food product category	Acetic acid	Calcium acetate	Sodium acetate	Sodium diacetate	Adipic acid	Caprylic acid	Malic acid	Succinic acid
Baked good, baking mixes	0.25	0.2		0.4	0.05	0.013		
Beverages, nonalcoholics					0.005		3.4	
Breakfast cereals			0.007					
Cheese		0.02				0.04		
Chewing gum	0.8						3.0	
Condiments, relishes	0.5				5.0			0.084
Dairy product analogs	9.0				0.45			
Fats, oils	0.8				0.3	0.005		
Frozen dairy desserts	0.5		0.5	0.1	0.004	0.005		
Gelatin, pudding, fillings		0.2			0.55	0.005	0.8	
Grain products			0.6					
Gravies and sauces	3.0			0.25		0.1		
Hard candy, cough drops			0.15				6.9	
Jams, jellies			0.12					2.6
Meat products	0.6		0.12	0.1	0.3	0.005		0.0061
Processed fruit juices							3.5	
Snack foods		0.6	0.05		1.3	0.016		
Soft candy			0.2	0.1		0.005	3.0	
Soup mixes			0.05	0.05				
Sweet sauces		0.15	0.05					

Source: CFR, 1988.

2. The acid is not normally present in the food product or is present at levels lower than that normally detected in a standard assay, and serves as a measure of adulteration through either addition of the acid or fermentation of the substrate to form acidic byproducts.
3. The acid is added to achieve a desired effect as regulated by good manufacturing practices.

The analysis of food acidulant is dependent upon the ease of separation of a specific acid from the food, the food product itself, and the desire for quantitative or qualitative results (Doores, 1989). It is often desirable to know the levels of acetic and proprionic acids in breads and cakes, eggs, and seafood; citric, malic, and tartaric acids in wines, nonalcoholic and carbonated beverages, fruit, and fruit products; phosphoric acid in cola-type beverages; and lactic acid in wines, eggs, milk and milk products, fruits, and canned vegetables. Cheese (dehydroacetic, citric, and tartaric acids), dried milk (citric acid), maple syrup (malic acid), baking powders (tartaric acid), and eggs (succinic acid) are some products that are often assayed for specific organic acid levels as a means of determining their quality.

For most inorganic and organic acids, aqueous titration with alkali, such as 1 N NaOH, remains the most popular method for assaying the pure chemical entity. Although not specific, the procedure is satisfactory in the absence of interfering substances and when conducted in conjunction with an appropriate test for identity. Acetic, citric, isocitric, lactic, malic, and succinic acids can be assayed by enzymatic methods (Bergmeyer, 1974). Acidulants can also be quantitated using spectrophotometry, paper and thin layer chromatography, gas chromatography, and high-performance liquid chromatographic (HPLC) techniques (Martin et al., 1971; Tijan and Jansen, 1971; Marsili et al, 1981; Doores, 1989; Tsjui et al., 1986).

VII. SUMMARY

Acidulants are an extremely versatile group of food additives. This versatility has led to their extensive use and application in the food industry. Among the different adiculants, citric acid alone accounts for about 60% of the weight of all the acids used in food, compared to 25% for phosphoric acid and 15% for the rest of the food acids. As a group, they are exceeded in volume of consumption only by emulsifying agents.

Most acids are natural components of several food products, especially fruits and vegetables and many traditional fermented foods. Several acids are also normal intermediates in mammalian metabolism. This, in conjunction with the extensive toxicological studies conducted with individual acidulants that have proven nontoxic under normal dietary conditions, has led to their being recognized as GRAS food additives subject to use in accordance with good manufacturing practice.

In the future, the applications and functionality of acidulants may be enhanced even further by the development of newer processing technologies, as well as better functional derivatives. Because of their antimicrobial and food-preservation properties, they are also expected to play a significant role in increasing the availability of food supplies in developing countries by enhancing the shelf life of perishable food products.

REFERENCES

Allied Chemical Corp. (1961). National® Food Acids. National Aniline Div., *Tech. Bull.* TS-*10*:8, New York.

Anonymous. (1943). The toxicity of adipic acid. In *Monograph on Adipic Acid-NAS/NRC Questionnaire.* Informatics, Inc., Rockville, MD.

Anonymous. (1964). Citric challenged as top flavor. *Chem. Week 94*(11:82)

Anonymous. (1970). *Documenta*, 7th ed. Geigy Basel.

AOAC. (1984). *Official Methods of Analysis*, 14th ed. The Association of Official Analytical Chemists, Arlington, VA.

Azukas, J. J., Costilow, R. N., and Sadoff, H. L. (1961). Inhibition of alcoholic fermentation by sorbic acid. *J. Bacteriol. 81*:189–194.

Ballabriga, A., Conde, C., and Gallart-Catala, A. (1970). Metabolic response of prematures to milk formulas with different lactic acid isomers or citric acid. *Helv. Paediatr. Acta 25*:25–34.

Banwart, G. J. (1979). *Basic Food Microbiology.* AVI, Westport, CT.

Barsotti, M. Sassi, C., and Ghetti, G. (1954). Health hazards to workers in a tartaric acid factory. *Med. Lav. 45*:239–243.

Berger, E. S. (1978). Hydroxy dicarboxylic acids. In *Encyclopedia of Chemical Technology*, R. E. Kirk and D. F. Othmer (eds). Wiley Interscience, New York, pp. 103–121.

Bergmeyer, H. U. (1974). *Methods of Enzymatic Analysis*, Vols. 1 and 2. Academic Press, New York.

Bonting, S. L., and Jansen, B. C. P. (1956). The effect of a prolonged intake of phosphoric acid and citric acid in rats. *Voeding 17*:137–140.

Bradley, W. B., and Tucker, J. W. (1964). Bakery processes and leavening agents. In *Encyclopedia of Chemical Technology*, R. E. Kirk and D. F. Othmer (eds.). Wiley Interscience, New York, pp. 41–59.

Brout, H. (1961). British Patent 883,169.

Budavari, S. (1989). *The Merck Index*, 11th ed. Merck & Co., Rahway, NJ.

Bykova, T. D., Davydova, M. A., Ozeretskovskaya, O. L., and Moiseeva, N. A. (1977). Antifungal substances in apples. *Mikol. Fitopatol. 11*:116–119.

Cesaro, A. N., and Granata A. (1955). Hematologic cytochemistry in subjects exposed to occupational risk in intoxication due to acetone and to acetic acid. *Folia Med. 38*:957–963.

CFR. (1988). *Code of Federal Regulations Title 21*. Office of the Federal Register, U.S. Government Printing Office, Washington, DC.

Chichester, D. F., and Tanner, F. W. (1972). Antimicrobial food additives. In *Handbook of Food Additivies*, 2nd ed. Vol. 1, T. E. Furia (ed.). CRC Press, Cleveland, OH.

Chipley, J. R. (1983). Sodium benzoate and benzoic acid. In *Antimicrobials in Foods*, A. L. Branen and P. M. Davidson (eds.). Marcel Dekker, New York, pp. 11–35.

Chipley, J. R., and Uraih, N. (1980). Inhibition of *Aspergillus* growth and aflatoxin release by derivatives of benzoic acid. *Appl. Environ. Microbiol. 40*:352–356.

Chittenden, R. H., Long, J. H., and Herter, C. A. (1909). *U.S. Dept. Agric. Bull. 88*, Washington, DC.

Conrad, L. J., and Stiles, M. N. (1954). *Improving the Whipping Properties of Gelatin and Gelatin Products.* U.S. Patent, 2,692,201.

Corlett, D. A., and Brown, M. H. (1980). pH and acidity. In *Microbial Ecology of Foods.* Vol. 1. Intl. Commission on Microbiological Specifications for Foods, Academic Press, New York, pp. 92–108.

Cramer, J. W., Porrata-Doria, E. I., and Steenbock, H. (1956). A rachitogenic and growth-promoting effect of citrate. *Arch. Biochem Biophys. 60*:58–63.

Dahle, H. K., and Nordal, J. (1972). Effects of benzoic acid and sorbic acid on the production and activities of some bacterial proteinases. *Acta Agric. Scand. 22*:29–34.

Dakin, H. D. (1909). The fate of sodium benzoate in the human organism. *J. Biol. Chem. 7*:103–109.

Dalderup, L. M. (1960). The effects of citric and phosphoric acids on the teeth. *J. Dent. Res. 39*:420–421.

Danly, D. E., and Campbell, C. R. (1978). Adipic acid. In *Encyclopedia of Chemical Technology*, R. E. Kirk and D. F. Othmer (eds). Wiley Interscience, New York, pp. 510–531.

Demaree, G. E. Sjogren, D. W., McCashland, B. W., and Cosgrove, F. P. (1955). Preliminary studies on the effect of feeding sorbic acid upon the growth, reproduction, and cellular metabolism of albino rats. *J. Am. Pharm. Assoc. Sci. Ed. 44*:619–627.

Deshpande, S. S., and Sathe, S. K. (1991). Toxicants in plants. In *Mycotoxins and Phytoalexins*, R. P. Sharma and D. K. Salunkhe (eds.). CRC Press, Boca Raton, FL, pp. 671–730.

Deuel, H. J., Alfin-Slater, R., Weil, C. S., and Smyth, H. F. (1954). Sorbic acid as a fungistatic agent for foods. I. Harmlessness of sorbic acid as a dietary component. *Food Res. 19*:1–9.

Dickens, F., Jones, H. E. H., and Waynforth, H. B. (1968). Further tests on the carcinogenicity of sorbic acid in the rat. *Br. J. Cancer 22*:762–766.

Diller, I.M., and Brout, H. (1958). U.S. Patent 2,851,359.

Doores, S. (1983). Organic acids. In *Antimicrobials in Foods*, A. L. Branen and P. M. Davidson (eds.). Marcel Dekker, New York, pp. 75–108.

Doores, S. (1989). pH control agents and acidulants. In *Food Additivies*, A. L. Branen, P. M. Davidson, and S. Salminen (eds.). Marcel Dekker, New York, pp. 477–510.

Dunn, C.G. (1968). Food preservatives. In *Disinfection, Sterilization, and Preservation*, C. A. Lawrence and S. S. Block (eds.). Lea and Febiger, Philadelphia, pp. 632–659.

Dye, W. S., Overholser, M. D., and Vinson, C. G. (1944). Injections of certain plant growth substances in rat and chick embryos. *Growth 8*:1–11.

Eklund, T. (1980). Inhibition of growth and uptake processes in bacteria by some chemical food preservatives. *J. Appl. Bacteriol. 48*:423–427.

Ellinger, R. H. (1972). *Phosphates as Food Ingredients*. CRC Press, Cleveland, OH.

Enders, A. (1941). Physiological compatibility and excretion of dicarboxylic acids. *Arch. Exp. Pathol. Pharmakol. 197*:597–601.

Faith, W. L., Keyes, D. B., and Clark, R. L. (1957). *Industrial Chemicals*, 2nd ed. John Wiley, New York, pp. 11–26.

FAO. (1974). *Toxicological Evaluation of Some Food Additives*. Food and Agriculture Organization, Rome, Italy.

FAO/WHO. (1962). *Evaluation of the Toxicity of a Number of Antimicrobials and Antioxidants*. 6th Report of the Joint Food and Agriculture Organization of the United Nations/World Health Organization Expert Committee on Food Additives. FAO Nutrition Meeting Report Ser. No. 31, Rome, Italy.

FAO/WHO. (1963). *Specifications for the Identity and Purity of Food Additives and Their Toxicological Evaluation: Emulsifiers, Stabilizers, Bleaching and Maturing Agents*. 7th Report of the Joint Food and Agriculture Organization of the United Nations/World Health Organization Expert Committee on Food Additives. FAO Nutrition Meeting Report Ser. No. 35, Rome, Italy.

FAO/WHO. (1967). *Specifications for the Identity and Purity of Food Additives and Their Toxicological Evaluation: Some Emulsifiers and Stabilizers and Certain Other Substances*. 10th Report of the Joint Food and Agriculture Organization of the United Nations/World Health Organization. FAO Nutrition Meeting Ser. No. 43.

FDA. (1966). Baker products. *Fed. Reg. 31*:5432 (Apr. 6).

FDA. (1973). *Scientific Literature Review on GRAS Food Ingredients*: *Citrates, PB-223-850*. National Technical Information Services, Springfield, VA.

FDA. (1974). *Scientific Literature Review on GRAS Food Ingredients*: *Citric Acid, PB-241-967*. National Technical Information Services, Springfield, VA.

Fin'ko, L. N. (1969). Blood coagulation changes in acetic acid poisoning. *Klin. Med.* (*Moscow*) *47*:84–87.

Fitzhugh, O. G., and Nelson, A. A. (1947). The comparative chronic toxicities of fumaric, tartaric, oxalic and maleic acids. *J. Am. Pharm. Assoc. 36*:217–219.

Flett, L. H., and Gardner, W. H. (1952). *Maleic Anhydride Derivatives*. John Wiley, New York.

Food and Drug Research Laboratories, Inc. (1975). *Teratologic Evaluation of Potassium Sorbate-Sorbistat in Mice and Rats. PB-245-520*. U.S. Dept. Commerce, National Technical Information Service, Washington, DC.

Food and Drug Research Laboratories. (1973a). *NAS/NRC Questionnaire on Tartaric Acid. Contract 71-75*. Food and Drug Administration, Rockville, MD.

Food and Drug Research Laboratories. (1973b). *Teratological Evaluation of FDA 71-50 (Adipic Acid) in Mice, Rats and Hamsters*. Food and Drug Administration, Rockville, MD.

Freese, E. (1978). Mechanism of growth inhibition by lipophilic acids. In *The Pharmacological Effect of Lipids*, J. J. Kabara (ed.). The American Oil Chemists Society, Champaign, IL, pp. 123–151.

Freese, E., Sheu, C. W., and Galliers, E. (1973). Function of lipophilic acids as antimicrobial food additives. *Nature 241*:321–322.

Gage, J. C. (1970). The subacute inhalation toxicity of 109 industrial chemicals. *Br. J. Ind. Med. 27*:1–11.

Gardner, W. H. (1966). *Food Acidulants*. Allied Chemical Corp., New York.

Gardner, W. H. (1972). Acidulants in food processing. In *Handbook of Food Additives*, 2nd ed., Vol. 1, T. E. Furia (ed.). CRC Press, Cleveland, OH, pp. 225–270.

Gardner, W. H., and Flett, L. H. (1952). Maleic acid, fumaric acid and maleic anhydride. In *Encyclopedia of Chemical Technology*, R. E. Kirk and D. F. Othmer (eds.). Wiley Interscience, New York, pp. 691–692.

Gardner, W. H., and Flett, L. H. (1954). Succinic acid and succinic anhydride. In *Encyclopedia of Chemical Technology*, R. E. Kirk and D. F. Othmer (eds). Wiley Interscience, New York, pp. 187–202.

Gaunt, I. F., Butterworth, K. R., Hardy, J., and Gangoli, S. D. (1975). Long-term toxicity of sorbic acid in the rat. *Food Cosmet. Toxicol. 13*:31–36.

Gergel, M. G., and Revelise, M. (1952). Nitriles and isocyanides. In *Encyclopedia of Chemical Technology*, R. E. Kirk and D. F. Othmer (eds.). Wiley Interscience, New York, pp. 356–372.

Gerhartz, H. (1949). Changes in the liver in a case of acetic acid poisoning and their significance for the timely measurement of liver regeneration and cirrhotic scar formation. *Virchows Arch. Pathol. Anat. Physiol. 316*:456–461.

Glabe, E. F., and Maryanski, J. K. (1981). Sodium diacetate: an effective mold inhibitor. *Cereal Foods World 26*:285–289.

Gomori, G. and Gulyas, E. (1944). Effect of parenterally administered citrate on the renal excretion of calcium. *Proc. Soc. Exp. Biol. Med. 56*:266–228.

Goos, A. W. (1953). Propionic acid. In *Encyclopedia of Chemical Technology*, Vol. II, R. E. Kirk and D. F. Othmer (eds.). Wiley Interscience, New York, pp. 174–193.

Gosselin, R. E. (1984). *Clinical Toxicology of Commercial Products*. Williams and Wilkins, Baltimore, MD.

Graham, W. D., and Grice, H. C. (1955). Chronic toxicity of bread additives to rats. Part II. *J. Pharm. Pharmacol. 7*:126–134.

Graham, W. D., Teed, H., and Grice, H. C. (1954). Chronic toxicity of bread additives to rats. *J. Pharm. Pharmacol. 6*:534–535.

Granados, H., Glavind, J., and Dam, H. (1949). Observations on experimental dental caries. III. The effect of dietary lactic acid. *J. Dent. Res. 28*:282–287.

Gruber, C. M., and Halbeisen, W. A. (1948). A study on the comparative toxic effects of citric acid and its sodium salts. *J. Pharmacol. Exp. Ther. 94*:65–67.

Hansen, F. F. 1951a). *Milk Powder and Its Preparation*. U.S. Patent 2,553,578.

Hansen, F. F. (1951b). *Composition for the Baking of Bread*. U.S. Patent 2,557,283.

Hansen, F. F. (1951c). *Condensed Milk Composition and Its Preparation*. U.S. Patent 2,570,321.

Hara, S. (1965). Pharmacological and toxic actions of propionates. Examination of general pharmacological actions and toxicity of sodium and calcium propionates. *Chem. Abstr. 62*:977f.

Harris, R. (1959). *Egg Products with Improved Whipping Properties*. U.S. Patent 2,902,372.

Harshbarger, K. E. (1942). Report of a study on the toxicity of several food preserving agents. *J. Dairy Sci. 25*:169–174.

Hartwell, J. L. (1951). *Survey of Compounds Which Have been Tested for Carcinogenic Activity*, 2nd ed. Federal Security Agency, Public Health Service, National Institute of Health, Bethesda, MD.

Harvath, L. (1979). Enhancement of granulocyte chemiluminescence with hydroxyl radical scavengers. *Infect. Immun. 25*:473–476.

Hashimoto, K., and Miyazaki, S. (1961). Japanese Patent 15,550.

Hazleton Laboratories. (1970). *Two Generation Reproduction Study—Rats X-5120 (Malic Acid). Project 165-128*. Final report submitted to Specialty Chemicals Div., Allied Chem. Corp., Buffalo, NY.

Hazleton Laboratores. (1971a). *24 Month Dietary Administration—Rats. Project No. 165-126 (malic acid)*. Final report submitted to Specialty Chemicals Div., Allied Chem. Corp., Buffalo, NY.

Hazleton Laboratories. (1971b). *104 Week Dietary Administration—Dogs. X-5120 (Malic Acid)*. Final report submitted to Specialty Chemicals Div., Allied Chem. Corp., Buffalo, NY.

Hendy, H. J., Hardy, J., Gaunt, I. F., Kiss, I. S., and Butterworth, K. R. (1976). Long-term toxicity studies of sorbic acid in mice. *Food Cosmet. Toxicol. 14*:381–389.

Heseltine, W. W. (1952). A note on sodium propionate. *J. Pharm. Pharmacol. 4*:120–121.

Heyer, W. (1957). U.S. Patent 2,816,032.

Horn, J. J., Holland, E. G., and Hazelton, L. W. (1957). Safety of adipic acid as compared with citric and tartaric acid. *J. Agr. Food Chem. 5*:759–761.

Hudson, R. B., and Dolan, M. J. (1978). Phosphoric acid and phosphates. In *Encyclopedia of Chemical Technology*. R. E. Kirk and D. F. Othmer (eds.). Wiley Interscience, New York, pp. 426–472.

Hunter, D. R., and Segel, I. H. (1973). Effect of weak acids on amino acid transport by Penicillium chrysogenum: evidence of a proton or charge gradient as the driving force. *J. Bacteriol. 113*:1184–1187.

Irwin, W. E., Lockwood, L. B., and Zienty, M. F. (1967). Malic acid. In *Encyclopedia of Chemical Technology*, 2nd ed., R. E. Kirk and D. F. Othmer (eds.). Wiley Interscience, New York, pp. 837–849.

Ishidata, M., and Odashima, S. (1977). Chromosome tests with 134 compounds on Chinese Hamster cells in vitro. A screening for chemical carcinogens. *Mutat. Res. 48*;337–345.

Johnston, C. D., and Thomas, M. J. (1961). *Composition and Method for Inhibiting Discoloration of Cut Organic Materials*. U.S. Patent 2,987,401.

Kabera, J. J., Swieczkowski, D. M., Conley, A. J., and Truant, J. P. (1972). Fatty acids and derivatives as antimicrobial agents. *Antimicrob. Agents Chemother. 2*:23–28.

Kao, J., Jones, C. A., Fry, J. R., and Bridges, J. W. (1978). Species differences in the metabolism of benzoic acid by isolated hepatocytes and kidney tubule fragments. *Life Sci.* 23:1221–1224.

Keller, C. L., Balaban, S. M., Hickey, C. S., and DiFate, V. G. (1978). Sorbic acid. In *Encyclopedia of Chemical Technology*, R. E. Kirk and D. F. Othmer (Eds.). Wiley Interscience, New York, pp. 402–416.

Kwok, R. H. (1968). Chinese restaurant syndrome. *N. Engl. J. Med. 284*:336–338.

Lang, K., and Bartsch, A. R. (1953). Concerning the metabolism and tolerability of adipic acid. *Biochem. Z. 323*:462–468.

Lehninger, A. (1972). *Biochemistry*. Butterworths, London.

Levey, S., Lasichak, A. G., Brimi, R., Orten, J. M., Smyth, C. J., and Smith, A. H. (1946). A study to determine the toxicity of fumaric acid. *J. Am. Pharm. Assoc. Sci. Ed. 35*:298–304.

Lewis, R. J. (1989). *Food Additives Handbook*. Van Nostrand and Reinhold, New York.

Liebrand, J. T. (1978). Acids (food). In *Encyclopedia of Food Science*, M. S. Peterson and A. H. Johnson (eds.). AVI Publ. Corp., Westport, CT, pp. 1–6.

Litton Biometric, Inc. (1974). *Mutagenic Evaluation of Potassium Sorbate. PB-245-434*. U.S. Dept. Commerce, National Technical Information Service, Washington, D.C.

Litton Biometric, Inc. (1977). *Mutagenic Evaluation of Calcium Sorbate. PB-266-894*. U.S. Dept. Commerce, National Technical Information Service, Washington, D.C.

Lockwood, L. B., and Irwin, W. E. (1964). Citric acid. In *Encyclopedia of Chemical Technology*, R. E. Kirk and D. F. Othmer (eds.). Wiley Interscience, New York, pp. 528–531.

Lowenheim, F. A., and Moran, M. K. (1975). *Industrial Chemicals*, 4th ed. Wiley Interscience, New York.

Lueck, E. (1976). Sorbic acid as a food preservative. *Int. Flavors Food Addit. 7*:122–124.

Lueck, E. (1980). *Antimicrobial Food Additives*. Springer-Verlag, New York.

Lueck, E. (1980). *Antimicrobial Food Additives: Characteristics, Uses, Effects*. Springer-Verlag, Berlin.

Marsili, R. T., Ostapenko, H. Simmons, R. E., and Green, D. E. (1981). High performance liquid chromatography determination of organic acids in dairy products. *J. Food Sci. 46*:52–57.

Martin, G. E., Sullo, J. G., and Schoeneman, R. L. (1971). Determination of fixed acids in commercial wines by gas-liquid chromatography. *J. Agr. Food Chem. 19*:995–998.

Martindale's Extra Pharmacopoeia (1972). 26th ed., The Pharmaceutical Press, London.

Matz, S. A. (1960). *Bakery Technology and Engineering*. AVI Publ. Co., Westport, CT.

Mayer, E. (1963). Historic and modern aspects of vinegar making (acetic fermentation). *Food Technol. 17*(5):64–76.

Meat Inspection Division. (1966). *Approval of Substances for Use in the Preparation of Meat Food Products*. Code of Federal Regulations, U.S. Government Printing Office, Washington, DC.

Melnick, D., Luckmann, F. H., and Gooding, C. M. (1954). Sorbic acid as a fungistatic agent for foods. VI. Metabolic degradation of sorbic acid in cheese by molds and the mechanism of mold inhibition. *Food Res. 19*:44–47.

Miller, S. A. (1969). *Ethylene and Its Industrial Derivatives*. Ernest Benn, Ltd., London, pp. 668–689.

Minor, J. L., and Becker, B. A. (1971). A comparison of the teratogenic properties of sodium salicylate, sodium benzoate and phenol. *Toxicol. Appl. Pharmacol. 19*:373–379.

Monsanto Chemical Co. (1970). Wisconsin Alumni Research Foundation Research Results. *Monsanto Food Processor's Tech. Data FPD-2*, St. Louis, MO.

Njagi, G. D. E., and Gopalan, H. N. B. (1980). Mutagenicity testing of some selected food preservatives, herbicides, and insecticides: 2. Ames test. *Bangladesh J. Bot. 9*:141–145.

Ohno, Y., Sekigawa, S., Yamamoto, H., Nakamori, K., and Tsubura, Y. (1978). Additive toxicity test of sorbic acid and benzoic acid in rats. *J. Nara. Med. Assoc. 29*:695–699.

Okabe, S. Roth, J. L. A., and Pfeiffer, C. J. (1971). Differential healing periods of the acetic acid ulcer model in rats and cats. *Experientia 27*:146–151.

Paar, D., Helmsoth, V., Werner, M., and Bock, K. D. (1968). Haemostatic failure due to consumption of coagulation factors in acute acetic acid poisoning. *Ger. Med. Mon. 13*:421–427.

Packman, E. W., Abbott, D. D., and Harrisson, J. W. E. (1963). Comparative subacute toxicity for rabbits of citric, fumaric and tartaric acids. *Toxicol. Appl. Pharmacol. 5*:163–167.

Packman, E. W., Abbott, D. D., and Harrisson, J. W. E. (1963). Comparative subacute toxicity for rabbits of citric, fumaric and tartaric acids. *Toxicol. Appl. Pharmacol. 5*:163–167.

Palmer, A. A. (1932). Two fatal cases of poisoning by acetic acid. *Med. J. Aust 1*:687–689.

Parmeggiani, L., and Sassi, C. (1954). Injury to health caused by acetic acid in the manufacture of acetyl-cellulose. *Med. Lav. 45*:319–326.

Pintauro, N. D., and Hall, B. J. (1962). *Gelatin Desserts Containing Adipic Acid*. U.S. Patent 3,067,036.

Pitkin, C. E. (1935). Lactic acid stricture of the esophagus. *Ann. Otol. Rhinol. Laryngol. 44*:842–843.

Rehm, H. J. (1960). A study on the antimicrobial activity of mixtures of agents used for the preservation of liquids. *Ann. Inst. Pasteur 11*:217–220.

Robinson, W. D., and Mount, R. D. (1978). Maleic anhydride, maleic acid and fumaric acid. In *Encyclopedia of Chemical Technology*, R. E. Kirk and D. F. Othmer (eds.). Wiley Interscience, New York, pp. 770–793.

Rose, W. C. (1924). The nephropathic action of the dicarboxylic acids and their derivatives. I. Tartaric, malic and succinic acids. *J. Pharmacol. Exp. Ther. 24*:123–129.

Rosenberg, D. S. (1980). Hydrochloric acid. In *Encyclopedia of Chemical Technology*, Vol. 12, 3rd ed., R. E. Kirk and D. F. Othmer (eds.). Wiley Interscience, New York, pp. 983–1015.

Rushing, N. B., and Senn, V. J. (1963). The effect of benzoic, sorbic, and dehydroacetic acids on the growth of citrus products spoilage organisms. *Proc. Fla. Hortic. Soc. 76*:271–277.

Sanders, H. J. (1966). Food additives. Part II. *Chem. Eng. News 44*(43):115, 118, 119.

Sausville, T. J. (1974). Acidulants. In *Encyclopedia of Food Technology*, Vol. 2, A. H. Johnson and M. S. Peterson (eds.). AVI Publ. Corp., Westport, CT, pp. 1–6.

Seib, P. A., and Tolbert, B. M. (1982). *Ascorbic Acid: Chemistry, Metabolism, and Uses*. American Chemical Society, Washington, DC.

Seymour, C. F., Taylor, G., and Welsh, R. C. (1954). Substitutes of vinegar for lactic acid as bactericidal agent in infant milk mixtures. *Am. J. Dis. Child. 88*:62–66.

Shtenberg, A. J., and Ignatev, A. D. (1970). Toxicological evaluation of some combinations of food preservatives. *Food Cosmet. Toxicol. 8*:369–373.

Sodemoto, Y., and Enomoto, M. (1980). Report of carcinogenesis bioassay of sodium benzoate in rats: absence of carcinogenicity of sodium benzoate in rats. *J. Environ. Pathol. Toxicol. 4*:87–91.

Sofos, J. N., and Busta, F. F. (1981). Antimicrobial activity of sorbate. *J. Food Prot. 44*:614–620.

Sofos, J. N., and Busta, F. F. (1983). Sorbates. In *Antimicrobials in Foods*, A. J. Branen and P. M. Davidson (Eds.). Marcel Dekker, New York, pp. 141–175.

Sollman, T. (1921). Studies of chronic intoxication on albino rats. III. Acetic and formic acids. *J. Pharmacol. Exp. Ther. 16*:463–473.

Sommer, H. M., and Hart, E. B. (1926). *Acids in Milk Processing*. Wis. Agr. Exp. Sta. Res. Bull. 67, Madison, WI.

Spector, W. S. (1956). *Handbook of Toxicology*, Vol. 1. W. B. Saunders, Philadelphia.

Spencer, H. C., Rowe, V. K., and Mccollister, D. D. (1950). Dehydroacetic acid. I. Acute and chronic toxicity. *J. Pharmacol. Exp. Ther. 99*:57–66.

Stayton, F. G. (1944). U.S. Patent 2,341,826.

Takhirov, M. T. (1969). Hygienic standards for acetic acid and acetic anhydride in air. *Hyg. Sanit. 34*:122–125.

Tijan, G. H., and Jansen, J. T. A. (1971). Identification of acetic, propionic, and sorbic acids in bakery products by thin layer chromatography. *J. Assoc. Off. Anal. Chem. 54*:1150–1151.

Trainer, J. B., Krippaehne, W. W., Hunter, W. C., and Lagozzino, D. A. (1945). Esophageal stenosis due to lactic acid. *Am. J. Dis. Child. 69*:173–175.

Troller, J. A. (1965). Catalase inhibition as a possible mechanism of the fungistatic action of sorbic acid. *Can. J. Microbiol. 11*:611–615.

Tsuji, S., Tonogai, Y., and Ito, Y. (1986). Rapid determination of mono-, di- and triisopropyl citrate in foods by gas chromatography. *J. Food Prot. 49*:914–916.

Tuft, L., and Ettelson, L. N. (1956). Canker sores from allergy to weak organic acid (citric and acetic). *J. Allergy 27*:536–540.

Van Ness, J. H. (1978). Hydroxy carboxylic acids. In *Encyclopedia of Chemical Technology*, R. E. Kirk and D. F. Othmer (eds.). Wiley Interscience, New York, pp. 80–103.

Van Wazer, J. R. (1958). *Phosphorus and Its Compounds*. Wiley Interscience, New York.

Wagner, F. S. (1978). Acetic acid and derivatives. In *Encyclopedia of Chemical Technology*. Vol. 1, R. E. Kirk and D. F. Othmer (eds.). Wiley Interscience, New York, pp. 124–147.

Waterhouse, H. N., and Scott, H. M. (1962). Effect of sex, feathering, rate of growth and acetates on chick's need for glycine. *Poult. Sci. 41*:1957–1962.

Webb, J. L. (1966). *Enzyme and Metabolic Inhibitors*, Vol. 2. Academic Press, New York.

Weil, A. J., and Rogers, H. E. (1951). Allergic reactivity to simple aliphatic acids in man. *J. Invest. Dermatol. 17*:227–231.

Whitaker, J. R. (1959). Inhibition of sulfhydral enzymes with sorbic acid. *Food Res. 24*:37–39.

White, A., Handler, P., and Smith, E. L. (1964). *Principles of Biochemistry*, 3rd ed. McGraw-Hill, New York.

Williams, A. E. (1978). Benzoic acid. In *Encyclopedia of Chemical Technology*, R. E. Kirk and D. F. Othmer (eds.). Wiley Interscience, New York, pp. 778–792.

Winstrom, L. O. (1978). Succinic acid and succinic anhydride. In *Encyclopedia of Chemical Technology*, R. E. Kirk and D. F. Othmer (eds.). Wiley Interscience, New York, pp. 848–864.

Wiseman, R. D., and Adler, D. K. (1956). Acetic acid sensitivity as a cause of cold urticaria. *J. Allergy 27*:50–55.

Yokotani, H., Usui, T., Nakaguchi, T., Kanabayashi, T., Tanda, M., and Aramaki, YI. (1971). Acute and subacute toxicological studies of Takeda—citric acid in mice and rats. *J. Takeda Res. Labo. 30*:25–31.

York, G. K., and Vaughn R. H. (1964). Mechanisms in the inhibition of microorganisms by sorbic acid. *J. Bacteriol. 88*:411–416.

York, G. K., and Vaughn, R. H. (1960). Studies on microbial inhibition by sorbic acid. *Bacteriol. Proc. 60*:47–49.

Young, E. G., and Smith, R. P. (1944). Lactic acid: a corrosive poison. *J. Am. Med. Assoc. 125*:1179–1181.

3
Antioxidants

**D. L. Madhavi* and
D. K. Salunkhe**
*Utah State University
Logan, Utah*

I. INTRODUCTION

Preservation of food products with additives is an ancient practice. In the late Nineteenth century and early Twentieth century, food preservation was mainly confined to heat sterilization, in combination with the addition of salts and spices. As society became more and more urbanized, the area of food technology including production, processing, and distribution of food products underwent a revolutionary change. Incorporation of longer shelf-life tolerance to facilitate processing and distribution of a wide variety of food products over significant time and distance has become a major challenge to the food manufacturer. Consequently, the use of various additives to extend the shelf life of food products has become widespread in food industry. Many products would not exist today were it not for the use of food additives such as antioxidants, antimicrobials, acidulants, and emulsifiers.

It is interesting to realize that apart from microbial spoilage and browning reactions, the oxidative degradation of polyunsaturated fatty acids contributes significantly to the shelf life of many products. Lipid oxidation is a complicated chemical and biochemical reaction process leading to the formation of a multitude of products. Some of the effects of lipid oxidation include development of off-flavors and odors in fats, oils, and lipid-containing foods, changes in texture due to the reaction of the lipid oxidation products with proteins, and loss of nutritive value due to the destruction of vitamins, amino acids, and essential fatty acids (Dziezak, 1986). Lipid oxidation products are also directly involved in the development of a number of diseases including coronary artery disease, atherosclerosis, and cancer, as well as the aging process.

**Current affiliation*: University of Illinois, Urbana, Illinois

Antioxidants play a significant role in retarding the lipid oxidation reactions in food products. The use of antioxidants dates back to 1940s. Gum guaiac was the first antioxidant approved for the stabilization of animal fats, especially lard. Today antioxidants are used not only to stabilize fats and oils but also in high-fat foods, cereals, and a host of other products containing very small amounts of lipids. Antioxidants are defined by the FDA as "substances used to preserve food by retarding deterioration, rancidity or discoloration due to oxidation." The addition of antioxidants is either intentional (direct addition to the food product) or incidental (migration of antioxidant from plastic packaging material to the food product). The proper and effective use of antioxidants depends on a basic understanding of the chemistry of fats and oils, mechanism of oxidation, and the function of an antioxidant in counteracting this type of deterioration (Stuckey, 1972) and also possible health hazards from the use of antioxidants. The safety assessment of antioxidants has become one of the controversial areas in recent years with conflicting experimental results, uncertainties in extrapolating from animal experiments to humans, problems in determining daily intakes, and extrapolation of data from different countries as intakes are likely to differ due to different dietary habits.

The present chapter highlights the toxicological aspects of antioxidants used in the food industry. An effort has been made to include compounds that are not being exploited commercially at present. Toxicological aspects include acute toxicity, short-term and long-term studies, biochemical changes, teratogenicity, mutagenicity, and carcinogenicity. A brief account of the mechanism of lipid oxidation and its biological significance is also presented to orient the reader.

II.   LIPID PEROXIDATION AND HEALTH ASPECTS OF DIETARY LIPID OXIDATION PRODUCTS

A.   Lipid Peroxidation

Most lipids in foods are in the form of triglycerides, which are esters of fatty acids and glycerol. The fatty acids are usually long-chain compounds with 16–20 carbon atoms, which are either saturated or unsaturated. It has been well established that the carbon chain length and degree of unsaturation of the fatty acids are most important in determining the oxidative stability of the lipids. In addition to triglycerides, foods also contain other types of lipids such as phospholipids, sphingolipids, sterols, and hydrocarbons.

Lipids deteriorate in various ways during processing, handling, and storage of food products. Some of the reactions encountered are

1.   Hydrolysis of the ester linkage resulting in the formation of free fatty acids and glycerol. This reaction is catalyzed by high temperatures, acids, lipolytic enzymes, and high moisture content in vegetable oils. However, because of modern refining techniques, hydrolytic cleavage is not of great influence in the development of off-flavors.

2.   Oxidation occurring at the unsaturated bonds in the fatty acid moiety of the triglyceride. Oxidation is generally regarded as the most frequently occurring form of lipid deterioration leading to the development of rancidity, off-flavor compounds, polymerization, reversion, as well as a number of other reactions reducing the shelf-life and nutritive value of the food product. Antioxidants

cannot reverse the process of lipid oxidation, nor are they effective in suppressing the hydrolytic rancidity but they can effectively retard the process of oxidation. The overall mechanism of lipid oxidation is presented in Figure 1 (Labuza, 1971).

Oxidation reactions can be broadly divided into two areas: Oxidation of highly unsaturated fats, particularly the polyunsaturated fats resulting in polymeric end products, and oxidation of moderately unsaturated fats resulting in rancidity, reversion, and other types of off-flavors and odors (Stuckey, 1972). Oxidation of unsaturated lipids in the food system is a chain reaction catalyzed by heat, light, ionization reactions, trace metals (especially copper and iron), metalloproteins such as heme, and also enzymatically by lipoxygenase. Many reviews have been published elucidating the mechanism of oxidation of different fatty acids like oleic, linoleic, linolenic, and arachidonic acid (Labuza, 1971; Frankel, 1984; Kappus, 1991). Only a brief outline is presented here, and the reader is referred to more detailed reviews.

The reaction of oxygen with unsaturated fatty acids involves free radical initiation, propagation, and termination reactions. Initiation reactions take place either by the abstraction of a H_2 radical from an allylic CH_2 group of an unsaturated fatty acid (LH) or by the addition of a radical to a double bond. The formation of free

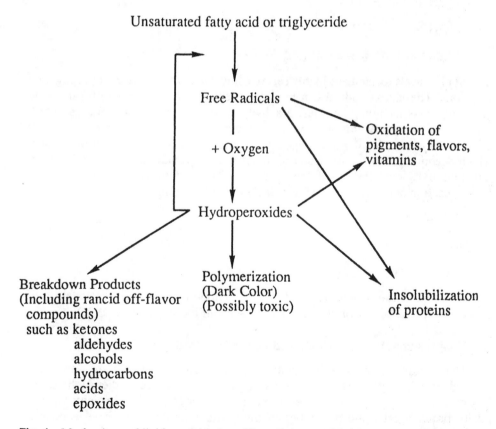

Fig. 1 Mechanisms of lipid peroxidation. (From Labuza, 1971.)

lipid radicals (L°) is usually mediated by trace metals, irradiation, light, or heat. The free radicals are very reactive with molecular oxygen and form lipid peroxy radicals (LOO°).

$$LH \xrightarrow{Initiator} L° + H°$$

$$L° + O_2 \rightarrow LOO°$$

Lipid peroxy radicals initiate a chain reaction with other lipid molecules, resulting in the formation of lipid hydroperoxides (LOOH) and free lipid radicals.

$$LOO° + LH \rightarrow LOOH + L°$$

The propagation reaction becomes a continuous process as long as unsaturated fatty acids are available. Lipid hydroperoxides may also be formed by the reaction of an unsaturated fatty acid, such as linoleic acid, with oxygen in singlet excited state or enzymatically by the action of lipoxygenase. Lipid hydroperoxides, the primary products of autoxidation, are odorless and tasteless. The hydroperoxides undergo a homolytic cleavage to form alkoxy radicals (LO°) or a bimolecular decomposition. The process is catalyzed by high temperatures, irradiation, and trace metals, especially Cu and Fe.

$$LOOH \rightarrow LO° + OH°$$

$$LOOH \rightarrow L° + HOO°$$

$$2LOOH \rightarrow LO° + H_2O + LO_2°$$

The lipid radicals formed are highly reactive and can start initiation or propagation reactions. The alkoxy radical can readily undergo C—C cleavage to form breakdown products including ketones, aldehydes, alcohols, esters, and furans, which impart undesirable flavors and odors to the food product. The peroxy radicals undergo an intramolecular rearrangement leading to a endoperoxy hydroperoxide, which decomposes in the presence of metal ions, especially iron, to form malonaldehyde and a number of breakdown products. The oxidation process is terminated by the reaction of two radicals to form stable polymeric compounds (L—L, LOOL).

$$L° + L° \rightarrow L—L$$

$$LOO° + L° \rightarrow LOOL$$

$$LOO° + LOO° \rightarrow LOOL + O_2$$

Figure 2 depicts the formation of off-flavor compounds from the autoxidation of linoleic acid, one of the predominant fatty acids in foods (Labuza, 1971).

B. Health Aspects of Dietary Lipid Oxidation Products

The health implications of lipid oxidation products formed in vivo are well documented. In recent years the possible pathological significance of dietary lipid oxidation products has attracted the attention of biochemists, food scientists, and health professionals, and a number of publications and reviews have appeared (Smith, 1981; Addis, 1986; Addis and Warner, 1991). The investigations have

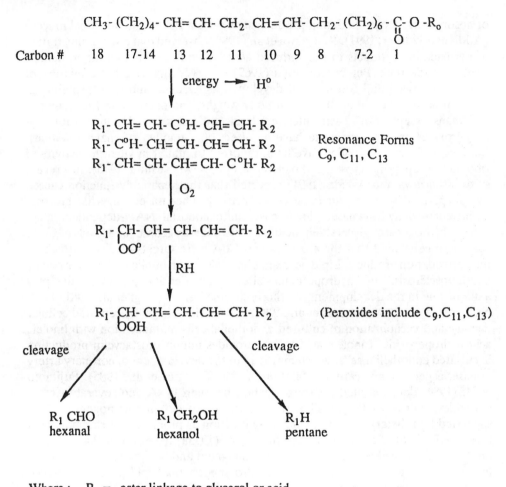

$$CH_3 - (CH_2)_4 - CH= CH- CH_2 - CH= CH- CH_2 - (CH_2)_6 - \underset{O}{\overset{\parallel}{C}} - O - R_o$$

Carbon #   18   17-14   13   12   11   10   9   8   7-2   1

$$\downarrow \text{energy} \longrightarrow H^o$$

$R_1 - CH= CH- C^oH- CH= CH- R_2$
$R_1 - C^oH- CH= CH- CH= CH- R_2$ Resonance Forms
$R_1 - CH= CH- CH= CH- C^oH- R_2$ C_9, C_{11}, C_{13}

$$\downarrow O_2$$

$R_1 - \underset{OO^o}{\overset{|}{CH}}- CH= CH- CH= CH- R_2$

$$\downarrow RH$$

$R_1 - \underset{OOH}{\overset{|}{CH}}- CH= CH- CH= CH- R_2$ (Peroxides include C_9, C_{11}, C_{13})

cleavage   cleavage

R_1 CHO R_1 CH$_2$OH R_1H
hexanal   hexanol   pentane

Where : R_o = ester linkage to glycerol or acid
          R_1 = $CH_3 - (CH_2)_4 -$
          R_2 = $CH_2 - (CH_2)_6 - \underset{O}{\overset{\parallel}{C}} - O - R_o$

Fig. 2 A typical breakdown pathway for the oxidation of linoleic acid. (From Labuza, 1971.)

focused primarily on lipid peroxides, malonaldehyde, and cholesterol oxidation products.

Lipid Peroxides

Absorption studies have established that lipid oxidation products and the secondary oxidation products are absorbed from dietary sources (Glavind et al., 1971; Naruszewicz et al., 1987). Kanazawa et al. (1985) demonstrated in rats the absorption and uptake of linoleic acid hydroperoxides and secondary oxidation products by the liver. Evidence of liver hypertrophy, increase in hepatic peroxide levels, and increased serum transaminase activities were also reported. Even in the absence of absorption, dietary oxidation products may pose a risk to the intestinal mucosa (Addis and Warner, 1991). Kanazawa et al. (1988) observed that oral administration of peroxidation products to rats induced acute toxic reaction resulting in hemorrhage and diarrhea. Peters and Boyd (1969) observed that rats fed a mixture of rancid cottonseed and cod liver oil developed listlessness, anorexia, proteinuria, oligodipsia, diarrhea, diuresis, loss in body weight, and decrease in the weight of all organs except brain, gastrointestinal tract, and the adrenal glands. Lipid hydroperoxides are also known to have an effect on a number of enzyme systems. Linoleic acid hydroperoxides have been reported to inhibit in vitro the activity of ribonuclease, pepsin, trypsin, and pancreatic lipases (Matsushita, 1975). In a recent study Kanazawa and Ashida (1991) reported that the hepatic dysfunction caused by lipid peroxides may be due to decreased activity of hepatic enzymes like glucose-6-phosphate dehydrogenase, glucokinase, mitochondrial NAD-dependent aldehyde dehydrogenase, glyceraldehyde phosphate dehydrogenase, and levels of CoA. They also concluded that the enzymes and CoA were targets of direct attack by the peroxidation products. Lipid peroxides have also been implicated in the etiology of atherosclerosis. Lipid hydroperoxides alter the low-density lipoproteins that play a major role in the development of atherosclerotic lesions (Yagi et al., 1981, 1987; Nishigaki et al., 1984; Jurgens et al., 1986). Sasaguri et al. (1984) reported cellular damage and vacuolization of cultured endothelial cells on incubation with linoleic acid hydroperoxide. Linoleic acid hydroperoxides inhibit prostacyclin production in cultured endothelial cells, which may lead to the development of coronary artery disease, especially myocardial infarction in vivo (Sasaguri et al., 1985). Fujimoto et al. (1984) demonstrated a strong reaction between DNA and several primary peroxides, indicating the possible role of the peroxides in carcinogenisis. It is suggested that dietary lipid peroxides may function as promoters of carcinogenisis (Addis, 1986). Studies of Cutler and Schneider (1973a) have shown that oxidized linoleic acid induced cervical sarcoma and malignant and benign mammary tumors in rats fed a high-fat diet. Experiments also suggest that lipid peroxides induce injection-site sarcomas in mice (Van Duuren et al., 1963, 1967). Oxidized linoleic acid increased teratogenicity in the urogenital system in rats. In mice, oxidized linoleic acid on direct application to ovaries induced fetal malformations in the first-generation and a significant increase in embryonic resorption in the second-generation litters (Cutler and Schneider, 1973b). Though studies indicate the possible role of lipid peroxides in carcinogenisis, the mechanism still remains unclear.

Cholesterol Oxidation Products

Cholesterol oxidation products have received a lot of attention because of their involvement in the development of coronary artery disease, and numerous studies have been published. Nearly 30 oxidation products have been detected in commerical cholesterol (Smith et al., 1967). Some of the typical oxidation products include cholestranetriol, enantiomeric 5,6-epoxides, 7-ketocholesterol, isomeric 7-hydroxy cholesterol, and 25-hydroxycholesterol. Cholesterol oxidation products are readily absorbed and incorporated into high-density, low-density, and very low-density lipo-proteins (Bascoul et al., 1986; Addis and Warner, 1991). Cholesterol oxides are reported to inhibit the biosynthesis of cholesterol in cultured aortic smooth muscle cells of rabbits (Peng et al., 1985a), which may result in a decrease in membrane cholesterol levels leading to impaired functionality and cellular injury. Cholesterol oxides also inhibit the activity of 5' nucleotidases and Na^+ and K^+

ATPases (Peng and Morin, 1987). Cholestranetriol and 25-hydroxycholesterol have been reported as the most atherogenic of the cholesterol oxidation products (Taylor et al., 1979). Oxysterols are also reported to affect the ion transport across membranes, particularly in calcium channels (Peng et al., 1985b; Neyes et al., 1985). Oxysterols affect membrane permeability to divalent cations and glucose (Holmes and Yoss, 1984; Theunissen et al., 1986). The toxic effects of oxysterols have been extensively reviewed by Smith and Johnson (1989). Oxysterols induce reduction in growth, loss of body weight, diminished appetite, necrosis, and acute inflammation in experimental animals. Oxysterols inhibit de novo synthesis of sterols by inhibiting 3-hydroxy-3-methylglutaryl CoA reductase activity. Several other enzymes are also affected by oxysterols including cholesterol 5,6-epoxide hydrolase, cholesterol 7α-hydroxylase, and acylcholesterol acyl CoA O-transferase. The angiotoxic effects of cholesterol oxidation products have been demonstrated both in vitro (Imai et al., 1980) and in vivo (Peng et al., 1978). Specific oxysterols and epoxides are reported to be mutagenic (Sevanian and Peterson, 1986; Smith and Johnson, 1989) and react with DNA (Blackburn et al., 1979). Cholesterol oxidation products may also have carcinogenic potential (Suzuki et al., 1986; Smith and Johnson, 1989). The studies indicate that the oxidation products of cholesterol and not pure cholesterol are responsible for the observed cytotoxic, atherogenic, angiotoxic, and enzyme effects.

Malonaldehyde

Malonaldehyde, a major secondary product of lipid oxidation, has been reported to be toxic to living cells (Addis et al., 1983; Pearson, 1983), an initiator, and a complete carcinogen and mutagen (Shamberger et al., 1974; Mukai and Goldstein, 1976; Addis et al., 1983; Basu and Marnett, 1983). Malonaldehyde can cross link with lipids and proteins (Kwon and Brown, 1965; Tappel, 1980), inactivate ribonuclease (Menzel, 1967), and bind covalently to nucleic acids (Fujimoto et al., 1984; Vaca et al., 1988; Basu et al., 1988). It has been observed that consumption of unpreserved cod liver oil increases the urinary malonaldehyde concentration in humans, indicating the absorption of malonaldehyde (Piche et al., 1988). Incubation of skin fibroblast cells with malonaldehyde resulted in cytoplasmic vacuolization, karyorrhexis, micronucleation, and a reduction in protein-synthesizing capacity of the cells (Bird and Draper, 1980). Malonaldehyde also induced chromosomal aberrations in cultured mammalian cells (Bird et al., 1982). Mukai and Goldstein (1976) have reported that malonaldehyde is mutagenic in the Ames *Salmonella* testing system. It is postulated that the fluorescent products in age pigment lipofuscin are formed by the interaction of malonaldehyde with lipids and proteins (Tappel, 1980).

III. FOOD ANTIOXIDANTS: GENERAL FUNCTIONS, CLASSIFICATION, AND SAFETY REQUIREMENTS

A. General Functions

In general, antioxidants function by reducing the rate of the initiation reactions in the free radical chain reaction both in biological systems and food products. In vivo, cells have an elaborate defense mechanism against autoxidation consisting of enzymes and low molecular weight sulfhydryls like glutathione, cysteine, and cysteinyl glycine. Natural antioxidants occur in most of the raw materials used for food manufacturing but are often depleted during processing, necessitating the addition of antioxidants. Antioxidants are generally functional at very low concentrations of 0.01% or less. At high concentrations they may become prooxidant due to their involvement in the initiation reactions (Lundberg et al., 1947; Cillard et al., 1980). Both synthetic and natural antioxidants are used in food products. Synthetic antioxidants are mostly phenolic and include butylated hydroxyanisole (BHA), butylated hydroxytoluene (BHT), tertiary butyl hydroquinone (TBHQ), and propyl, octyl, dodecyl gallates. Polymeric antioxidants like Anoxomer and Trolox C, a synthetic derivative of α-tocopherol have also been introduced, but they are not being used commerically. In general, the use of primary antioxidants is limited to 100–200 ppm of BHA, BHT, or TBHQ, or 200–500 ppm of the gallates for the stabilization of fats and oils. Commercially a number of ready-to-use antioxidant formulations containing a food-grade solvent like propylene glycol or glycerol monooleate, a synergist like citric acid, and one or more of the phenolic antioxidants are available. Some of the naturally occurring antioxidants are listed in Table 1. Of the natural antioxidants, vitamin C and tocopherols are widely used. In recent years, extensive work is being carried out to identify naturally occurring antioxidants in both plant and animal sources. Most of these compounds are not being used commercially at present. An exhaustive listing of the various sources has been compiled by Loliger (1991).

B. Classification

Based on function, antioxidants are classified as primary or chain-breaking antioxidants, synergists, and secondary antioxidants (Fig. 3). The mechanism of antioxidant activity has been reviewed by a number of investigators (Johnson, 1971; Labuza, 1971; Gordon, 1990). Primary antioxidants terminate the free radical chain reaction by acting as hydrogen or electron donors to free radicals, resulting in the formation of more stable products. Both hindered phenolic (e.g., BHA, BHT, TBHQ, and tocopherols) and polyhydroxy phenolic (e.g., Gallates) antioxidants belong to this group. Some of the naturally occurring compounds like flavonoids, eugenol, vanillin, and rosemary antioxidant also have chain-breaking properties. Primary antioxidants (AH) may either delay or inhibit the initiation step by reacting with

Table 1   Some Naturally Occurring Antioxidants

Amino acids	Phenolic acids
β-Carotene	Phytic acid
Lecithins	Rosmarinic acid
Vitamin E	Spice extracts
Vitamin C	Tannins
Soy protein hydrolysate	Flavonoids
Vanillin	Uric acid
Saponins	Nordihydroguairetic acid

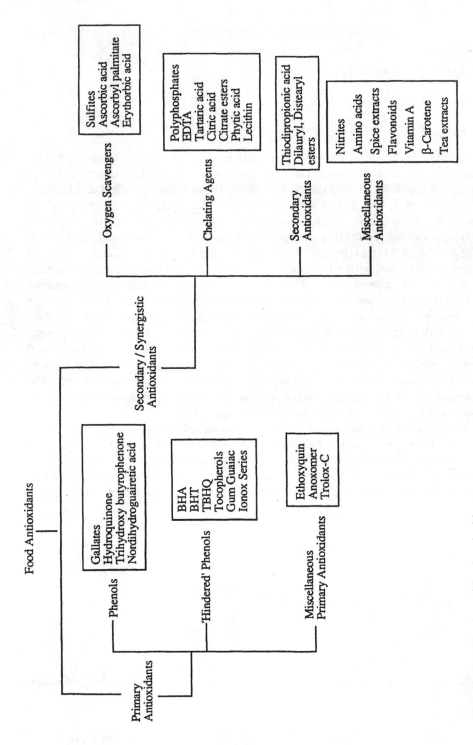

Fig. 3 Classification of food antioxidants.

a fat free radical or inhibit the propagation step by reacting with the peroxy, alkoxy radicals.

$$AH + L° \rightarrow A° + LH$$

$$AH + LOO° \rightarrow A° + LOOH$$

$$AH + LO° \rightarrow A° + LOH$$

Hindered phenolic antioxidants have substituted alkyl or electron-releasing groups in the *ortho* or *para* positions in the aromatic ring. The electron-donating groups increase the electron density on the OH group by an inductive effect and increase the reactivity with the lipid radicals. Substitution with butyl or ethyl groups at the *p*-position enhances the activity compared to methyl groups. Substitution with electron-attracting groups (e.g., nitro) or by longer-chain or branched alkyl groups at the *p*-position reduces the activity due to steric hindrance. Reaction of a hindered phenolic antioxidant with a free radical results in the formation of a free phenoxy radical (A°). The phenoxy radicals are stabilized by delocalization of the unpaired electron in the aromatic ring and undergo a dimerization reaction. Figure 4 shows the formation of the dimer 3,5,3',5'-tetra-*tert*-butyl stilbenequinone by the reaction of BHT with benzoyl peroxide. Bickel et al. (1953) also isolated some alkyl peroxy antioxidant compounds (LOOA) with the addition of the peroxide at the 4 or 6 position, which were stable in the dark but were decomposed by either light or heat. Much less is known about the chemistry of polyhydroxy phenolic antioxidants. There is a general agreement that the reaction of such an antioxidant with a peroxy radical is likely to give an orthoquinone (Johnson, 1971).

Synergistic antioxidants can be broadly classified as oxygen scavengers and chelators. Synergists function by different mechanisms. They may act as hydrogen donors to the phenoxy radical, thereby regenerating the primary antioxidant. They provide an acidic medium to improve the stability of primary antioxidants and fats and oils. Oxygen scavengers like ascorbic acid, ascorbyl palmitate, sulfites, and

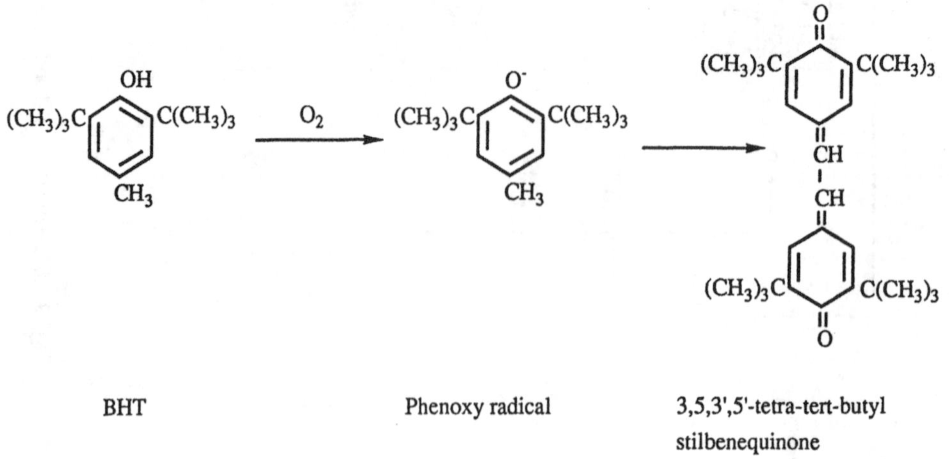

Fig. 4 Dimerization of BHT.

erythorbates react with free oxygen and can remove it in a closed system. Ascorbic acid and ascorbyl palmitate also act as synergists with primary antioxidants especially with tocopherols. Chelators like EDTA, citric acid, and phosphates are not antioxidants, but they are highly effective as synergists with both primary antioxidants and also oxygen scavengers. Chelating agents form complexes with prooxidant metals like iron and copper, which promote initiation reactions and raise the energy of activation of the initiation reactions considerably. Secondary antioxidants such as thiodipropionic acid function by decomposing the lipid peroxides into stable end products.

C. Safety Requirements

Food antioxidants should meet several requirements, as listed by Lehman et al. (1951). The antioxidant should be soluble in fats and impart no foreign color, odor, and flavor to the fat even after long storage and should be effective for at least one year at a temperature of 75–85°F (25–30°C). The antioxidant should be heat stable. The safety of the antioxidant must be established. According to Lehman et al. (1951), an antioxidant is considered safe if it fulfills two conditions. The LD_{50} must not be less than 1000 mg/kg body weight (bw), and the antioxidant should not have any significant effect on the growth of the experimental animal in long-term studies at a level 100 times the level proposed for human consumption. Approval of an antioxidant for food use also requires extensive toxicological studies including studies of mutagenic, tertatogenic, and carcinogenic effects. Even though a number of compounds have antioxidant properties, based on toxicological data only some of them have been accepted as "generally recognized as safe substances" (GRAS) for use in food products by international bodies like the Joint FAO/WHO Expert Committee on Food Additives (JECFA) and the European Commission (EC) Scientific Committee for Food (SCF) (Table 2). With the accumulation of toxicological data it has become clear that some antioxidants may have toxic effects that are very much dose dependent. Hence establishment of an acceptable daily intake (ADI) level for each compound becomes very crucial. ADIs are based on a range of toxicity tests establishing the dose-response relationship

Table 2 Antioxidants Permitted for Use in Foods

L-Ascorbic acid, Na, Ca salts	Glycine
Ascorbyl palmitate and stearate	Gum guaiac
Anoxomer	Ionox 100 (2,6-di-*tert*-butyl-4-hydroxymethylphenol
Butylated hydroxyanisole	Lecithin
Butylated hydroxytoluene	Polyphosphates
Citric acid, citrates	Tartaric acid
Erythorbic acid and Na erythorbate[a]	Tertiary butyl hydroquinone[a]
Ethoxyquin	Trihydroxy butyrophenone
Ethylenediaminetetraacetic acid,	Thiodipropionic acid, dilauryl and
Ca disodium salt	distearyl esters
Propyl, octyl, dodecyl gallates	Tocopherols

[a]Not permitted for use in European Economic Community countries.

of the toxic effect and ascertaining the maximum dose at which that effect is no longer observed (no-effect level).

IV. BIOCHEMICAL AND TOXICOLOGICAL ASPECTS OF FOOD ANTIOXIDANTS: PRIMARY ANTIOXIDANTS

A. Phenols

Gallates

The gallate group comprises the propyl, octyl, and dodecyl esters of gallic acid (3,4,5-trihydroxy benzoic acid) (Fig. 5). Of the three, propyl gallate (PG) is more effective as an antioxidant and is widely used in stabilizing animal fats and vegetable oils. It is also effective in meat products, spices, and snacks. With a melting point of 148°C, PG is unsuitable for frying applications at temperatures higher than 190°C and provides no carry-through protection in fried foods. PG is usually used in combination with antioxidants that have a carry-through effect like BHA and BHT. PG is sparingly soluble in oils and highly soluble in water. Hence in some countries octyl and dodecyl gallates (OG, DG), which are insoluble in water and freely soluble in oils, are used instead of PG. PG also chelates with iron ions, resulting in the discoloration of some food products. Hence PG is always used in combination with citric acid. In 1980 the JECFA allocated a group ADI of 0–0.2 mg/kg bw. But later studies indicated that OG and DG may have an adverse effect on reproduction. Hence in a reevaluation in 1987, an ADI of 0–2.5 mg/kg bw was allocated to PG and no ADIs were allocated to OG and DG due to insufficient toxicological information (FAO/WHO, 1987).

Biochemical Studies: Absorption, Metabolism, and Excretion

In rats nearly 70% of an oral dose of PG was absorbed in the gastrointestinal tract compared to OG and DG, which were absorbed to a lesser extent. All three esters were hydrolyzed to gallic acid and free alcohol. The free alcohols were metabolized through the Krebs cycle. Gallic acid was methylated to yield 4-*O*-methyl gallic acid, which was the main metabolite found in urine either free or conjugated with glucuronic acid. Small quantities of gallic acid were also excreted as glucuronide as well as in free form. Significant amounts of unchanged esters were excreted in the feces. Similar urinary metabolites in addition to small quantities of pyrogallol were also present in rabbits. In pigs the metabolism was similar to that observed in rats (Van Esch, 1955; Booth et al., 1959; Dacre, 1960).

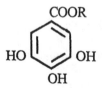

Fig. 5   Gallates. R: C_3H_7, Propyl gallate; C_8H_{17}, Octyl gallate; and $C_{12}H_{25}$, Dodecyl gallate.

Toxicological Studies

Acute Toxicity. The acute oral LD_{50} of PG in rats was 3600–3800 mg/kg bw and in mice 2000–3500 mg/kg bw (Orten et al., 1948; Lehman et al., 1951). The acute oral LD_{50} of OG in rats was 4700 mg/kg bw and for DG 6500 mg/kg bw (Sluis, 1951).

Short-Term Studies. In rats fed PG at dose levels of 0.1, 0.25, 0.3, and 0.5% for 6 weeks no adverse changes were observed in body weight, liver weight, and total liver lipid content (Johnson and Hewgill, 1961). Higher levels of 1.17 and 2.34% in the diet caused a reduction in weight gain, retarded growth, and about 40% deaths accompanied by renal damage in the first month. In the survivors no pathological changes were observed (Orten et al., 1948). In a 4-week study in rats Strik (unpublished results cited in Van Der Heijden et al., 1986) observed that at a dose level of 2.5%, PG produced growth retardation, anemia, hyperplasia in the outer kidney medulla, and an increase in the activity of cytoplasmic and microsomal hepatic drug-metabolizing enzymes. Increase in enzyme activity was also observed at 0.5% level. In mice fed 0.5 or 1% PG for 3 months, no toxic effects were observed (Dacre, 1974). PG had no adverse effects in dogs at a 0.0117% level for over a period of 12 months (Orten et al., 1948). In rats fed 0.2% DG for 70 days, no changes in body weight were observed (Tollenar, 1957). However, in weanling rats given 2.5 and 5% DG, 100% mortality was observed within 10 and 7 days, respectively (Allen and DeEds, 1951). In a 13-week study in rats fed 0.1, 0.25, and 0.5% OG, no deleterious changes were observed in body weight, food consumption, hematological studies, or urine analysis, and histopathological examination showed no compound-related effects (Hazleton Lab Inc., 1969, unpublished report, cited in FAO/WHO, 1974). In guinea pigs 0.2% of PG, OG, or DG had no demonstrable ill effects (Van Esch and Van Genderen, 1954).

Long-Term/Carcinogenicity Studies. In a 2-year study, rats fed 5% PG showed reduced food intake, growth retardation, and patchy hyperplasia of the stomach (Lehman et al., 1951). Orten et al. (1948) observed, in addition to retarded growth, lower hemoglobin levels and mottled kidneys in a 2-year study in rats at dose levels of 1.17 and 2.34%. In mice fed 0.5 and 1% PG for 21 months, no adverse effects on food intake, body weight, survival time, and hematological response were observed (Dacre, 1974). In a 103-wk chronic toxicity and carcinogenic study in F344 rats and B6C3F1 mice, PG at levels of 0.6 or 1.2% resulted in a dose-related reduction in body weight in both sexes. Male rats showed an increased incidence of hepatic vacuolization and suppurative inflammation of the prostrate gland. At lower dose levels tumors were observed at several anatomical sites, including thyroid gland, pancreas, and adrenal glands, at a higher incidence than in male controls. Also, malignant lymphoma occurred with a positive trend in males. In females, incidences of uterine polyps and mammary gland adenomas were observed (Abdo et al., 1986a). However, the control group in this experiment showed lower tumor incidence compared to the historical control groups in the same laboratory. Comparison of the experimental results with historical controls indicated that the results were not significant. Hence it was concluded that under the conditions of this study, PG was not carcinogenic to mice or rats. PG was found to have a protective effect against dimethyl benz(*a*)anthracene–induced mammary tumors in rats (King and McCay, 1980, 1983).

In a 2-year study, Van Esch (1955) observed no deleterious effects in rats fed

0.035, 0.2, or 0.5% OG or DG. In the same study, Van Esch reported that DG had no adverse effects in pigs at a 0.2% level for 13 weeks. In rats administered DG intragastrically in doses of 10, 50, and 250 mg/kg bw for 2 years, the highest dose level resulted in increased mortality, decrease in spleen weight, and morphological changes in the liver, kidneys, and spleen. The dose of 50 mg/kg bw was also toxic. Ten mg/kg was regarded as the threshold dosage for rats (Mikhailova et al., 1985).

Reproduction. In a three-generation study in rats fed 0.03, 0.2, and 0.5% PG, no adverse effects were observed (Van Esch, 1955). In a teratogenicity study, Tanaka et al. (1979) observed rats fed PG at dose levels of 0.4, 1, and 2.5% from day 0 to 20 days of pregnancy. They found maternal toxicity, and slight retardation of fetal development at higher dose levels, but no teratogenic effects were observed. In rabbits PG at dose levels of 2.5, 12, 54, or 250 mg/kg bw/day had no adverse effects on organogenesis (FDA, 1973a). In rats and rabbits PG was reported to prevent the occurrence of fetal abnormalities caused by vitamin E deficiency and hydroxyurea (King, 1964; DeSesso, 1981).

In two three-generation studies (Sluis, 1951; Van Esch, 1955), no adverse effects were observed in rats fed OG at dose levels of 0.035–0.5%. In another two-generation study in rats at dose levels of 0.1 and 0.5%, a marked reduction in weaning survival index and body weights was observed at 0.5% level. A dose-dependent reduction in the number of implantation sites as well as a reduction in the number of corpora lutea were observed (Hazelton Lab Inc., 1970, unpublished data, cited in Van der Heijden et al., 1986). In a three-generation study in rats, DG had no adverse effects at a dose level of 0.2% (Sluis, 1951). At a higher dose level of 0.5%, Van Esch (1955) observed loss of litters due to underfeeding and a slight hypochromic anemia at the 0.2% level.

Skin Toxicity. The gallates have been reported to cause allergic contact dermatitis. In three reports from Switzerland, gallates in margarine caused occupational hand dermatitis (Brun, 1964, 1970; Burkhardt and Fierz, 1964). Van Ketel (1978) reported one case of occupational hand and face dermatitis from peanut butter containing OG. In recent years a greater number of cases have been reported mainly because of topically applied products like lip balm and body lotion, in which the gallates are being used to a greater extent than other antioxidants. Sensitization did not occur when there was oral exposure. In a recent study Hausen and Beyer (1992) studied the sensitizing capacity of the three gallates using a modern sensitization procedure in guinea pigs. It was found that PG and OG were moderate sensitizers, whereas DG was the strongest sensitizer. Hausen and Beyer (1992) also observed that an increase in the side-chain length closely correlated with an increase in the sensitizing potential.

Mutagenicity. PG has been reported to be negative in a number of mutagenicity tests. In the Ames test using four tester strains of *Salmonella typhimurium* with or without metabolic activation, PG was negative (Rosin and Stich, 1980). In in vitro tests for chromosomal aberrations using human embryonic lung cells PG was negative (Litton Bionetics, 1974a). PG was a weak inducer of sister chromatid exchange in Chinese hamster ovary cells (NTP, unpublished data, cited by Abdo et al., 1986a). In vivo tests for chromosomal abnormalities in rat bone marrow cells, a dominant lethal study in rats, and a micronucleus test in mice were negative (Raj and Katz, 1984; Litton Bionetics, 1974a). PG had no clastogenic effect in rats and mice (Kawachi et al., 1980). PG inhibited the mutagenic activity of benzopyrene metabolites, pyrolysis products of albumin, and aflatoxin B in *S. typhimurium* TA98 (Lo and Stich, 1978; Rosin and Stich, 1980; Fukurhara et al., 1981). No information is available on the mutagenic potential of OG and DG.

Hydroquinone

Hydroquinone (1,4-dihydroxybenzene) (HQ) (Fig. 6) was proposed for use as a food antioxidant in 1940s, and extensive studies were conducted to determine the toxicological properties of HQ and its oxidation products quinhydrone and quinone. HQ was found to have a high level of toxicity.

HQ was rapidly absorbed from the gastrointestinal tract and eliminated in the urine as sulfate and glucuronide conjugate (Garton and Williams, 1949). Approximate oral LD_{50} in mg/kg bw in rats was 320; in mice, 400; in guinea pigs, 550; in pigeons, 300; in cats, 70; in dogs, 200; and in rats for quinhydrone, 225, and quinone, 225. Symptoms of HQ poisoning developed 30–90 minutes after oral administration. Some of the symptoms observed were hyperexcitability, tremors, convulsions, salivation in dogs and cats, and incoordination of the hind limbs in dogs. Deaths occurred within a few hours. Oral administration of HQ at 100 mg/kg bw in dogs and 70 mg/kg bw in cats produced mild to severe swelling of the area around the eye, of the nictitating membrane and of the upper lip. In dogs receiving lower doses of 25 and 50 mg/kg for 4 months, only slight involvement of the eye was observed (Woodard et al., 1949). In a chronic toxicity testing, Carlson and Brewer (1953) reported that in rats fed 0.5% HQ for 2 years and in dogs given 100 mg/kg bw for 26 weeks, no adverse effects were observed in body weight or growth rate, and no pathological changes were observed. In another 2-year chronic feeding study (FDA, 1950, unpublished data, cited by Lehman et al., 1951), HQ at 2% level increased the incidence of chronic gastrointestinal ulcerations and renal tumors in rats. In lifetime feeding studies in rats, HQ at levels 100 times that proposed for human consumption had a significant retarding effect on growth rate. Based on toxicological data HQ was considered a harmful and deleterious substance for addition to food (Lehman et al., 1951). At present HQ is used as a stabilizer in polymers and also in very small quantities in dermatological preparations as a bleach.

Trihydroxy Butyrophenone

Trihydroxy butyrophenone (2,4,5-trihydroxy butyrophenone) (THBP) (Fig. 7) is a substituted phenol listed as GRAS by the FDA for addition to foods and also food-packaging materials. THBP is effective in stabilizing vitamin A, lard, paraffin wax, mineral oil, and peanut oil (Stuckey and Gearhart, 1957). However, THBP is used only in food-packaging materials. THBP is a tan-colored powder sparingly

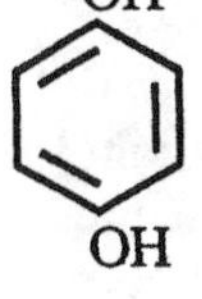

Fig. 6 Hydroquinone.

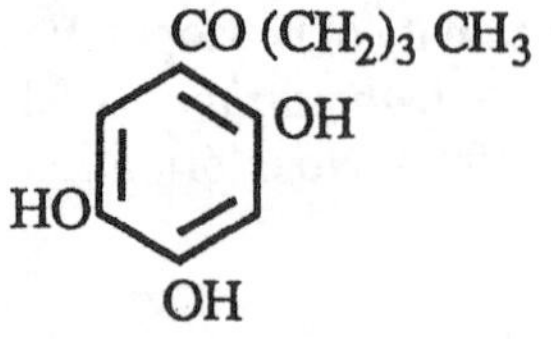

Fig. 7 Trihydroxy butyrophenone.

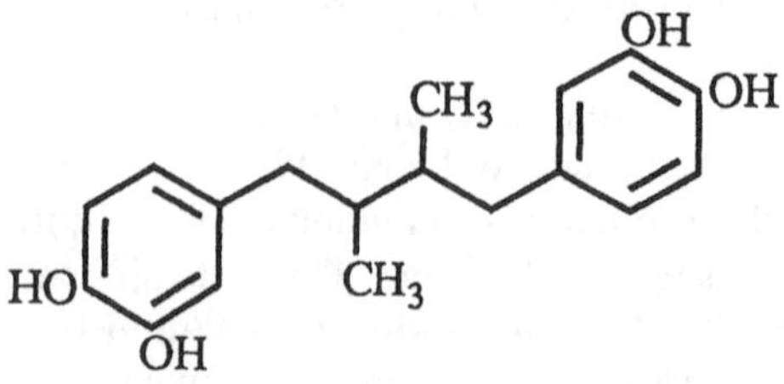

Fig. 8 Nordihydroguairetic acid.

soluble in water and soluble in fats and oils. It produces a light tan to brown color in the presence of organic metal salts.

Biochemical Studies: Absorption, Metabolism, and Excretion

The absorption, metabolism, and excretion of THBP has been studied in rats and dogs (Astill et al., 1959). Nearly 75% of a single oral dose of THBP was absorbed. In rats given single oral doses of 400 mg/kg bw, 6.3% of the dose was excreted as unchanged THBP in the urine and 1.7% in the feces, 23% as glucuronides, and 52% as etheral sulfates. In dogs given single oral doses of 300 mg/kg bw, 2.3% of the dose was excreted unchanged in the urine and 5.3% in the feces, 30% as glucuronides and 45% as etheral sulfates. The path of metabolism was largely by conjugation, and no evidence of reduction or oxidation was found. Etheral sulfate conjugation at the 5-hydroxyl group leads to 5-butyryl-2,4-dihydroxyphenyl hydrogen sulfate isolated as the potassium salt. Glucuronic acid conjugation at the 4-hydroxyl group leads to 4-butyryl-2,5-dihydroxyphenyl glucosiduronic acid, which was not isolated.

Toxicological Studies

Very little is known about the toxicity of THBP. The acute oral LD_{50} in rats was 3200–6400 mg/kg bw and in mice 800–1600 mg/kg bw (Dacre, 1960). In a long-term study in rats fed 0.1, 0.3, 1, and 3% daily for 2 years and in dogs at levels of 0.1, 0.3, and 0.5 g/kg bw/day for 1 years, no adverse effects were observed. Dogs readily tolerated 0.5 g/kg and rats 1.5 g/kg with negligible storage in body fat and various organs including liver, brain, and kidneys (Astill et al., 1959).

Nordihydroguairetic Acid

Nordihydroguairetic acid [2,3-dimethyl-1,4-bis(3,4-dihydroxy phenyl)butane] (NDGA) (Fig. 8) is a naturally occurring polyhydroxy phenolic antioxidant prepared from an evergreen desert shrub *Larrea divaricata* and has also been commercially synthesized. NDGA is effective in oils and fats and fat-containing foods.

NDGA was removed from the list of GRAS compounds (*Federal Register*, 1974) because of its toxicity at high dose levels. It is no longer used as a food antioxidant in many countries.

Biochemical Studies

Absorption, Metabolism, and Excretion. In rats NDGA was readily converted to its metabolite orthoquinone. Orthoquinone was found in all kidney extracts and urine of rats fed 0.5 and 1% NDGA. No free NDGA was observed. The orthoquinone was formed in the lower third of the ileum and cecum and was probably absorbed there. In rats after a single administration of 250 mg NDGA directly into the small intestine, 2760 μg of orthoquinone was observed in the ilium and 1620 μg in the cecum 7.5 hours after dosing (Grice et al., 1968).

Effect on Enzymes. NDGA was found to inhibit a number of enzyme systems. Tappel and Marr (1954) observed specific inhibition of peroxidase, catalase, alcohol dehydrogenase, and nonspecific inhibition of ascorbic acid oxidase, d-amino acid oxidase, the cyclophorase system, and urease. Placer et al. (1964) observed that NDGA inhibited esterase activity in liver and serum, which may have an adverse effect on fat metabolism.

Toxicological Studies

Acute Toxicity. The acute oral LD_{50} in rats was 2000–5500 mg/kg bw and in guinea pigs 830 mg/kg bw. In mice the acute oral and i.p. LD_{50} were 2000–5000 mg/kg bw and 550 mg/kg bw, respectively (Lehman et al., 1951).

Short-Term Studies. Short-term studies have been reported in mice and dogs. NDGA at dose levels of 0.25 and 0.5% for 6.5–7.5 months in mice or at levels of 0.1, 0.5, and 1% for 1 year in dogs had no deleterious effects on growth rate and food intake, and no pathological changes were observed (Cranston et al., 1947). In guinea pigs NDGA induced skin sensitivity (Griepentrog, 1961).

Long-Term Studies. Long-term studies have been conducted in rats. Cranston et al. (1947) observed in rats fed 0.1, 0.5, and 1% for 2 years a reduction in growth rate, cecal hemorrhage, and mesenteric cysts at higher dosage levels. Lehman et al. (1951) confirmed the observations and reported that 0.5% was the lowest effective dose. Grice et al. (1968) reported that at dose levels of 0.5 and 1% for 1.5 years, NDGA had a strong toxic effect in the rat and induced extensive cystic reticuloendotheliosis of the paracecal lymph nodes, increase in kidney weight, and loss of tubular function with distended tubular cells indicating an impaired kidney function. Rats fed 2% NDGA for shorter periods also showed similar pathological changes. The orthoquinone may induce loss of tubular function in the kidneys by affecting the permeability of the lysosomal membranes or by inhibiting the lysosomal enzymes (Goodman et al., 1970).

B. "Hindered" Phenols

Butylated Hydroxyanisole

Butylated hydroxyanisole (*tert*-butyl-4-hydroxyanisole) (BHA) is perhaps the most extensively used antioxidant in the food industry. BHA is used in fats and oils, fat-containing foods, confectionary, essential oils, food-coating materials, and waxes. BHA is a mixture of two isomers. 2-*tert*-butyl-4-hydroxyanisole (2-BHA) and 3-*tert*-butyl-4-hydroxyanisole (3-BHA) (Fig. 9), with the commercial compound con-

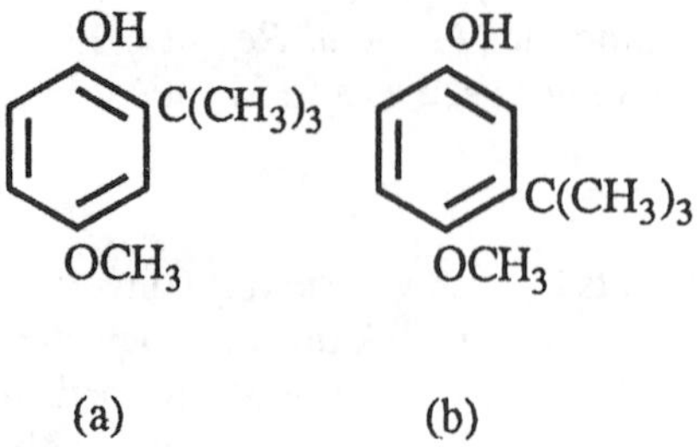

Fig. 9   Butylated hydroxyanisole: (a) 2-BHA, (b) 3-BHA.

taining 90% of the 3-isomer (Buck, 1985). BHA is readily soluble in lipids and insoluble in water. In a recent reevaluation, the JECFA allocated an ADI of 0–0.5 mg/kg bw (FAO/WHO, 1989).

Biochemical Studies: Absorption, Metabolism, and Excretion

The absorption and metabolism of BHA has been studied in rats, rabbits, dogs, monkeys, and humans. BHA was rapidly absorbed from the gastrointestinal tract in rats (Astill et al., 1960), rabbits (Dacre et al., 1956), dogs, and humans (Astill et al., 1962), rapidly metabolized, and completely excreted. No evidence of tissue accumulation of BHA was observed in rats or dogs (Astill et al., 1960; Wilder et al., 1960; Hodge et al., 1964). The major metabolites of BHA were the glucuronides, ether sulfates, and free phenols. The metabolites were excreted in the urine, and unchanged BHA was eliminated in feces. The proportion of the different metabolites varied in different species and also in different dosage levels. In rabbits dosed orally with 1 g BHA, 46% glucuronides, 9% ether sulfates, and 6% free phenols were observed in the urine (Dacre et al., 1956). In rats at lower doses, metabolism was similar to that of rabbits. Urinary excretion was 86% by 24 hours and 91% in 4 days (Golder et al., 1962). In dogs nearly 60% of a 350 mg/kg dose was excreted unchanged in the feces. The remaining was excreted as etheral sulfates, *tert*-butyl-hydroquinone (TBHQ), an unidentified phenol, and some glucuronides (Astill et al., 1962). In humans 22–72% of an oral dose of BHA at levels of 0.5–0.7 mg/kg bw was recovered as glucuronides in 24 hours, and less than 1% free BHA and very little ether sulfates were observed (Astill et al., 1962). El-Rashidy and Niazi (1983) reported substantial quantities of TBHQ glucuronide or sulfate as a metabolite of the 3-isomer. In later studies, formation of TBHQ was confirmed in rats (Armstrong and Wattenberg, 1985; Verhagen et al., 1989a). Tissue retention of BHA was greater in humans than in rats (Daniel et al., 1967). Much lower doses of BHA were required to produce a given plasma level in humans than in rats (Verhagen et al., 1989a).

Toxicological Studies

Acute Toxicity.   The acute oral LD_{50} in rats was 2200–5000 mg/kg bw and in mice 2000 mg/kg bw (Lehman et al., 1951; Dacre, 1960).

Short-Term Studies.   Short-term studies have been conducted in a number of species such as rat, rabbit, and dog. Rats administered 500–600 mg/kg bw for a period of 10 weeks showed decreased growth rate and reduced activity of the enzymes catalase, peroxidase, and cholinesterase (Karplyuk, 1962). In rabbits large doses of BHA (1 g/day) for 5–6 days administered by stomach tube caused a 10-fold increase in sodium excretion and a 20% increase in potassium excretion in the urine (Denz and Llaurado, 1957). In dogs fed 0.3, 30, and 100 mg/kg bw for 1 year, no ill effects were observed (Hodge et al., 1964).

BHA in high doses (500 mg/kg bw/day) induced an increase in the relative liver weight in rats and mice. In rats the changes follow a complex course, which depends on the mode of administration. When rats were given BHA by stomach tube, the relative liver weight increase followed a bimodal time course with maxima on days 2 and 10 and a highly significant increase on day 7. On dietary administration liver enlargement was not apparent until day 5, and a single maximum was observed by day 11 (Martin and Gilbert, 1968; Cha and Heine, 1982). A preliminary ultra-structural study by Allen and Engblom (1972) did not reveal any nucleolar abnormalities in the liver. BHA has been reported to induce a number of hepatic enzyme systems in rat and mice such as epoxide hydrolase, gluthathione-S-transferase, glucose-6-phosphate dehydrogenase, and biphenyl-4-hydroxylase (Creaven et al., 1966; Martin and Gilbert, 1968; Benson et al., 1978; Cha and Bueding, 1979; Cha and Heine, 1982). In dogs, BHA at levels of 1 and 1.3% induced liver enlargement, proliferation of smooth endoplasmic reticulum, hepatic myelinoid bodies, and increase in hepatic enzyme activity (Ikeda et al., 1986). BHA given in doses of 500 mg/kg bw to young rhesus monkeys for 28 days induced liver hypertrophy and proliferation of the smooth endoplasmic reticulum. Some differences between monkeys and rats were observed. In monkeys, the activity of microsomal glucose-6-phophatase was decreased and the nitroanisole demethylase activity increased, whereas in rats no changes were observed at similar dose levels (Creaven et al., 1966; Allen and Engblom, 1972).

Long-Term/Carcinogenicity Studies. In earlier long-term studies, BHA was found to be without any toxic effects in rats after 22 months (Wilder and Kraybill, 1948; Brown et al., 1959; Karplyuk, 1962) and in dogs after 15 months (Wilder et al., 1960). However, in later studies Ito et al. (1982, 1983a) reported that in F344 rats, administration of BHA at a 2% level resulted in a high incidence of papilloma in almost 100% of the treated animals and squamous cell carcinoma of the forestomach in about 30% of the treated animals. At lower dose levels of 0.5% no neoplastic lesions were observed, but forestomach hyperplasia was observed. Most of the changes were observed close to the limiting ridge between forestomach and glandular stomach. Verhagen et al. (1990) observed that in rats not only the forestomach but also the glandular stomach, small intestine, colorectal tissues, and possibly esophageal tissues were susceptible to the proliferative effects of BHA. Hamsters were found to be more susceptible to BHA than rats (Ito et al., 1983b). In hamsters fed 1 or 2% BHA for 24 and 104 weeks, forestomach papillomas were observed in almost all treated animals and carcinomas in 7–10% in the 104-week group. In mice fed 0.5 and 1% BHA, a lower incidence of lesions was observed (Masui et al., 1986).

In order to determine which isomer of BHA was carcinogenic or whether the isomers had a synergistic action, feeding studies were conducted with the pure isomers and crude BHA in hamsters for 1–4 weeks. Severe adverse effects were observed with crude BHA and the 3-isomer. The 2-isomer had no effect (Ito et al., 1984). In another study, Ito et al. (1986) observed that in addition to 3-BHA, two metabolites—*p-tert*-butyl phenol and 2-*tert*-butyl-4-methylphenol—also induced forestomach papillomas in the forestomach. In rats given 1 g/kg bw of the two isomers 2-BHA was also active in the induction of forestomach papillomas (Altmann et al., 1986). The forestomach hyperplasia was found to be reversible, but the time taken for recovery depended on the duration and level of treatment. In rats fed 0.1–2% BHA for 13 weeks, on cessation of treatment the forestomach reverted to normal after 9 weeks. In rats fed 2% BHA for 1, 2, or 4 weeks followed by a 4-week recovery period, the mild hyperplasia and epithelial changes observed in the 1-week group almost completely disappeared. The more severe changes observed in the 2- and 4-week groups regressed partially in the recovery period (Altmann et al., 1986).

Because of the possible relevance of these observations to humans, studies were conducted in other species like monkeys and pigs, which like humans do not have a forestomach. In female cyanomalgus monkeys BHA (0.125 or 500 mg/kg bw) given by gavage for 84 days failed to induce any histopathological changes in the stomach and esophagus. However, a 40% increase in the mitotic index was observed at the lower end of the esophagus (Iverson et al., 1986). In dogs fed BHA at levels of 0.25, 0.5, 1, and 1.3% for 6 months, no histopathological changes were noticed in the stomach, esophagus, or duodenum. Liver weights were increased without any related histopathological changes (Tobe et al., 1986; Ikeda et al., 1986). In pigs, administration of BHA at levels of 50, 200, and 400 mg/kg bw/day to pregnant pigs from mating to day 110 of the gestation period resulted in proliferation and parakeratotic changes in the esophageal epithelium in a few pigs in the two groups with the higher dose levels. But papillomas were not observed, and no changes were found in the glandular stomach (Wurtzen and Olsen, 1986a). In Japanese house musk shrews (*Sancus murinus*), which have no forestomach, BHA was fed at levels of 0.5, 1, and 2% for 80 weeks. All the animals in the 2% group died of hemorrhage in the gastrointestinal tract. Adenomatous hyperplasia in the lungs was observed in 0.5 and 1% levels at a significantly higher rate (Amo et al., 1990).

The mechanism by which 3-BHA induces carcinomas in the forestomach is not clear. Studies by De Stafney et al. (1986) suggest that two factors may be of importance. One of these entails thiol depletion. The second is an attack by the reactive metabolites of 3-BHA or secondary products produced by these metabolites on cellular constituents. Studies by Williams (1986) also indicated that BHA has an effect on membrane systems, blocking the exchange between the hepatocytes and the epithelial cells. The data strongly suggest that BHA is an epigenetic carcinogen that produces forestomach neoplasia through a promoting effect.

BHA has a promoting or inhibitory effect on the carcinogenic effects of a number of chemical carcinogens. BHA enhanced forestomach carcinogenesis initiated by either N-methyl-N'-nitro-N-nitrosoguanidine or N-methylnitrosourea (MNU) in rats. BHA had a promoting effect on the urinary bladder carcinogenesis initiated by MNU or N-butyl-N-(4-hydroxybutyl) nitrosamine and thyroid carcinogenesis initiated by MNU in rats. BHA had an inhibitory effect on the liver carcinogenesis initiated by either diethylnitrosamine or N-ethyl-N-hydroxyethylnitrosamine and mammary carcinogenesis initiated by 7,12-dimethyl-benz(a)anthracene (Ito et al., 1986).

Reproduction. BHA has not been reported to have any adverse effects on reproduction data and also in teratogenicity studies in mice, rats, hamsters, rabbits

(Clegg, 1965; FDA, 1972a, 1974a; Hansen and Meyer, 1978), pigs (Wurtzen and Olsen, 1986a), and rhesus monkeys (Allen, 1976). BHA has been reported to cause some behavioral abnormalities in mice. Weanling mice exposed to BHA via their mothers during pregnancy and lactation (0.5% level) and then directly for up to 3 weeks showed a significant increase in exploratory activity, decreased sleeping, decrease in self-grooming, slower learning, and a decrease in the orientation reflex (Stokes and Scudder, 1974). In another study Stokes et al. (1972) observed a decrease in serotonin levels and cholinesterase activity and changed noradrenaline levels in the brain of newborn mice exposed to BHA in utero, and it is postulated that these changes may have an effect on the behavioral modifications observed.

Mutagenicity. BHA was not found to be mutagenic in a number of test systems. BHA was nonmutagenic in five tester strains in the Ames *Salmonella*/microsome test at concentrations of up to 10 mg/ml (Williams, 1986). In the hepatocyte primary culture/DNA repair test, BHA was negative (Williams, 1977). In mammalian cell mutagenesis assay using adult rat liver epithelial cells (Tong and Williams, 1980) and in V79 Chinese hamster lung cells (Rogers et al., 1985), BHA was negative. BHA did not induce sister chromatid exchanges in Chinese hamster ovary cells (Williams, 1986). In tests for chromosomal aberrations, BHA was negative in Chinese hamster lung cells and in Chinese hamster DON cells (Ishidate and Odashima, 1977; Abe and Sasaki, 1977). In vivo BHA was negative in rat bone marrow cells and in the rat dominant lethal assay (Litton Bionetics, 1974b).

Butylated Hydroxytoluene

Butylated hydroxytoluene (2,6-di-*tert*-butyl-*p*-cresol) (BHT) (Fig. 10) is one of the most extensively used antioxidants in the food industry. BHT is used in low-fat food products, fish products, packaging materials, paraffin, and mineral oils. BHT is also widely used in combination with other antioxidants like BHA, propyl gallate, and citric acid for the stabilization of oils and high fat foods. BHT is a white crystalline solid readily soluble in fats and oils and insoluble in water, which is steam volatile and subject to loss during processing. ADI values for BHT have changed over the years because of its toxicological effects in different species. The latest temporary value allocated by the JECFA is 0–0.125 mg/kg bw (FAO/WHO, 1987).

Biochemical Studies: Absorption, Metabolism, and Excretion

The absorption, metabolism, and excretion of BHT has been studied in rats, rabbits, dogs, monkeys, and humans. In general, the oxidative metabolism of BHT was mediated by the microsomal monooxygenase system. In rats, rabbits, dogs, and monkeys, oxidation of *p*-methyl group predominated, whereas in humans the *tert-*

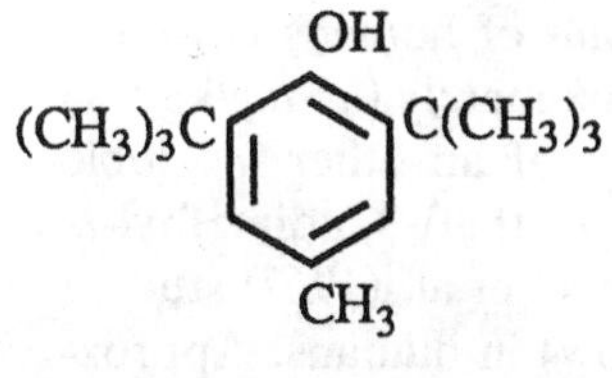

$(CH_3)_3C$ ⬡ $C(CH_3)_3$

OH

CH$_3$

Fig. 10 Butylated hydroxytoluene.

butyl groups were oxidized. In mice, oxidation of both *p*-methyl and *tert*-butyl groups was observed. The metabolism of BHT is more complicated and slower than BHA. The relatively slow excretion of BHT has been attributed to entero-hepatic circulation (Ryan and Wright, 1964; Ladomery et al., 1967; Wiebe et al., 1978).

In rats given 0.5 and 1% BHT for 5 weeks, the concentration of BHT increased rapidly in liver and body fat. Approximately 30 ppm was observed in the body fat in males and 45 ppm in females and 1–3 ppm in the liver. On cessation of treatment the concentration in the tissue decreased with a half-life of 7–10 days. In rats given single oral doses of ^{14}C BHT (1–100 mg/rat), nearly 80–90% was recovered in 4 days, with up to 40% in the urine. Approximately 3.8% was retained in the alimentary tract (Daniel and Gage, 1965; Tye et al., 1965; Ladomery et al., 1967; Daniel et al., 1968; Matsuo et al., 1984). The major urinary metabolites observed were BHT acid (both free and as ester glucuronide) and BHT mercapturic acid (di-*tert*-butyl-hydroxybenzyl acetyl cysteine) in addition to many other compounds including BHT alcohol, BHT aldehyde, and BHT dimer. Free BHT acid was the major metabolite in feces. About 10% of the dose was excreted unchanged (Yamamoto et al., 1979; Matsuo et al., 1984; Verhagen et al., 1989b). Tye et al. (1965) observed distinct sex differences in the mode of excretion. Female rats excreted about 40–60% of a single oral dose in feces and about 20–40% in the urine. Males excreted about 70–95% in the feces and 5–9% in the urine. Females showed more tissue retention, especially in the gonads. Significant biliary excretion of BHT and metabolites has also been observed. Four major metabolites have been identified, namely BHT acid, BHT alcohol, BHT aldehyde, and BHT quinone methide (2,6-di-*tert*-butyl-4-methylene-2,5-cyclohexadienone) (Daniel and Gage, 1965; Ladomery et al., 1967; Tajima et al., 1981).

In mice, the half-life of a single oral dose was found to be 9–11 hours in major tissues like stomach, intestine, liver, and kidney. The half-life was 5–10 days when daily doses were given for 10 days. The major metabolite in the urine was the glucuronide conjugate of the acid and free acid in the feces. Excretion was mainly in the feces (41–65%) and urine (26–50%). The formation of BHT quinone methide has been observed in vitro in liver microsomes and in vivo in mouse liver (Matsuo et al., 1984).

In rabbits the major metabolites observed were BHT alcohol, BHT acid, and BHT dimer. Excretion of all metabolites was essentially complete in 3–4 days (Dacre, 1961). Urinary metabolites constituted 37.5% of glucuronides, 16.7% etheral sulfates, and 6.8% free phenols. Unchanged BHT was observed only in the feces (Akagi and Aoki, 1962a; Aoki, 1962). Significant biliary excretion of BHT and metabolites has also been reported (El-Rashidy and Niazi, 1980). In dogs the metabolism was similar to that of rats and significant biliary excretion was observed (Wright et al., 1965b). In monkeys the major metabolite was the ester glucuronide of BHT acid, and the rate of excretion was similar to that of humans (Branen, 1975). Limited study in humans (single oral doses of approximately 0.5 mg/kg bw) have indicated that the major metabolite is in the form of an ether insoluble glucuronide identified as 5-carboxy-7-(1-carboxy-1-methyl ethyl)-3,3-dimethyl-2-hydroxy-2,3-dihydro benzofuran (Wiebe et al., 1978). Daniel et al. (1967) studied the excretion of single oral doses of ^{14}C BHT (40 mg/kg bw) in humans. Approximately 50% was excreted in the urine in the first 24 hours followed by a slower excretion for the next 10 days. Tissue retention was found to be greater in humans compared to rats. Studies by Wiebe et al. (1978) suggest that biliary excretion may be an important route for the elimination of BHT and also that enterohepatic circulation occurs in humans. Verhagen et al. (1989b) reported differences in the metabolism in rats and humans especially in terms of plasma kinetics and plasma concentrations and concluded that the differences were too wide to allow a hazard estimation for BHT consumption by humans on the basis of its metabolism.

Toxicological Studies

Acute Toxicity. The acute oral LD_{50} in mg/kg bw in rats was 1700–1970; in rabbits, 2100–3200; in guinea pigs, 10,700; in cats, 940–2100 (Deichmann et al., 1955); and in mice, 2000 (Karplyuk, 1959).

Short-Term Studies. In rats BHT at the level of 0.3 or 0.5% caused an increase in the level of serum cholesterol and phospholipids within 5 weeks. Brown et al. (1959) observed reduced growth rate and increase in liver weight in rats fed BHT at 0.5% in the diet. But at lower dose levels (0.1%) no adverse effects were observed (Gaunt et al., 1965). In rabbits at 2% dose level BHT caused an acute effect on electrolyte excretion similar to BHA, whereas lower levels were without any adverse effect (Denz and Llaurado, 1957). In dogs fed 0.17–0.94 mg BHT/kg bw 5 days a week for 12 months, no symptoms of intoxication and histopathological changes were observed (Deichmann et al., 1955).

BHT in high doses had a toxic effect on liver, lung, kidney, and also on blood coagulation mechanism. Early studies in rats and mice revealed that BHT at 500 mg/kg/day induced liver enlargement in 2 days and stimulated microsomal drug metabolizing enzyme activity. The effects were found to be reversible (Gilbert and Goldberg, 1965). Creaven et al. (1966) observed that in rats BHT at levels of 0.01– 0.5% for 12 days resulted in increased liver weights and induction of liver microsomal biphenyl-4-hydroxylase activity. At levels of 500 mg/kg bw for 14 days, a reduction in the activity of glucose-6-phosphatase was observed indicative of early liver damage (Gaunt et al., 1965; Feuer et al., 1965). In rats, administration of BHT by gavage at levels of 25, 250, or 500 mg/kg bw for 21 days resulted in a dose-related hepatomegaly and at the highest dose a progressive periportal hepatocyte necrosis (Powell et al., 1986). The periportal lesions were associated with proliferation of the bileducts, persistent fibrosis, and inflammatory cell reactions. At sublethal dose levels of 1000 and 1250 mg BHT/kg bw for up to 4 days, centrilobular necrosis was observed within 48 hours. At lower dose level (25 mg) no adverse effects were observed. In mice, BHT at levels of 0.75% for 12 months resulted in bileduct hyperplasia (Clapp et al., 1973). The liver hypertrophy was accompanied by a proliferation of the smooth endoplasmic reticulum, an increase in the cytochrome P-450 level, and induction of a number of enzymes including glutathione-S-transferase, glutathione reductase, thymidine kinase, nitroanisole demethylase, epoxide hydrolase, and aminopyrene demethylase. The changes were reversible after the cessation of the treatment (Botham et al., 1970; Kawano et al., 1980; Cha and Heine, 1982; Powell et al., 1986). In monkeys BHT at 500 mg/ kg bw for 14 days caused slight hepatomegaly, moderate proliferation of the smooth endoplasmic reticulum, a reduction in glucose-6-phosphatase, and an increase in nitroanisole demethylase activity. At lower dose of 50 mg/kg bw no adverse effects were observed (Allen and Engblom, 1972).

In a recent study Takahashi (1992) reported that BHT in very high doses (1.35–5% for 30 days) caused a dose-related toxic nephrosis with tubular lesions in mice. The lesions appeared as irregular patches or wedge-shaped proximal tubules, necrosis, and cyst formation. Renal toxicity has also been reported in rats (Meyer et al., 1978; Nakagawa and Tayama, 1988).

BHT was reported to cause extensive internal and external hemorrhages in rats due to a disruption of the blood coagulation mechanism, resulting in increased mortality (Takahashi and Hiraga, 1978; Takahashi et al., 1990). The minimum effective dose was found to be 7.5 mg/kg bw/day. The disruption in the blood coagulation observed was due to hypoprothrombinemia brought about by an inhibition of phylloquinone epoxide reductase activity in the liver by BHT quinone methide, one of the reactive metabolites of BHT (Takahashi, 1988). Administration of vitamin K prevented the BHT-induced hemorrhage. Takahashi and Hiraga (1979) have suggested that BHT may inhibit absorption of vitamin K in the intestines or uptake by the liver. An increased fecal excretion of vitamin K was observed in rats receiving 0.25% BHT for 2 weeks. BHT was also reported to affect platelet morphology, fatty acid composition of the platelets, and vascular permeability, which may play a role in the hemorrhage effect (Takahashi and Hiraga, 1984).

In mice, Takahashi (1992) observed that BHT at levels of 0.5, 1, or 2% for 21 days caused massive hemorrhages in the lungs and blood pooling in various organs, but only a slight reduction in the blood-coagulating activity. It was suggested that the hemorrhages may be due to a severe lung injury and not because of coagulation defect as observed in rats. BHT did not cause a significant hemorrhage in guinea pigs at dietary levels of 0–2%. The prothrombin index was slightly reduced at 1% level. BHT quinone methide was not detected in guinea pigs whereas 7–40 mg/kg liver was detected in rats. In rabbits, dogs, and Japanese quail fed BHT for 14–17 days at levels of 170 or 700 mg/kg, 173, 400, or 760 mg/kg and 1%, respectively, no hemorrhages were observed (Takahashi et al, 1980; Takahashi, 1992).

A number of studies have shown that BHT causes acute pulmonary toxicity in mice at levels of 400–500 mg/kg bw. The effects include hypertrophy, hyperplasia, and a general thickening of the alveolar walls of the lungs. A substantial proliferation of the pulmonary cells accompanied by a dose-dependent increase in total DNA, RNA, and lipids in the lungs was also observed within 3–5 days of a single i.p. injection of BHT (Marino and Mitchell, 1972; Witschi and Saheb, 1974; Saheb and Witschi, 1975). The effect was generally reversible in 6–10 days of cessation of the treatment. However, exposure to a second stress like hyperbaric O_2 after administration of BHT impeded the repair process resulting in pulmonary fibrosis (Witschi et al., 1981). Some of the morphological and cytodynamic events include perivascular edema and cellular infiltration in type I epithelial cells followed by multifocal necrosis, destruction of the air-blood barrier, and fibrin exudation by day 2 after a single i.p. injection of 400 mg/kg bw BHT (Adamson et al., 1977). Ultrastructural studies indicated that the type I cells were damaged by day 1 and cell destruction was complete within 2–3 days. Elongation of the type II cells with large nuclei and abundant cytoplasm was evident in 2–7 days (Hirai et al., 1977). It has been postulated that BHT causes cell lysis and death as a result of interaction with the cell membrane (Williamson et al., 1978). However, the mechanism of BHT toxicity still remains unclear.

Long-Term/Carcinogenicity Studies. In early studies, Deichmann et al., (1955) observed no adverse effects in rats fed 0.2, 0.5, 0.8, and 1% BHT for 2 years. In a 104-week chronic feeding study in rats, Hirose et al. (1981) reported that BHT at 0.25 and 1% levels was not carcinogenic. Treated rats of both sexes showed reduced body weight gain and increased liver weights. Only males showed increased γ-glutamyl transferase levels. Tumors were observed in different organs, but their incidence was not statistically significant compared to controls. In a two-generation carcinogenicity study with in utero exposure in rats, BHT was fed at levels of 25, 100, or 500 mg/kg bw/day from 7 weeks of age to the weaning of the F_1 generation. The F_1 generation were given 25, 100, or 250 mg/kg bw/day from weaning to 144 weeks of age. At weaning the BHT-treated F_1 rats, especially the males, had lower body weights. Dose-related increases in the numbers of hepatocellular adenomas and carcinomas were statistically significant in male F_1 rats when tested for heterogeneity or analysis for trend. In F_1 females the increases were only statistically significant for adenomas in the analysis of trend. However, all tumors were detected when the F_1 rats were more than 2 years old (Wurtzen and Olsen, 1986b). Unlike BHA, BHT had no adverse effects on the forestomach of rats and hamsters at 1% level (Altmann et al., 1986; Ito et al., 1986).

In mice, carcinogenicity studies have been conducted in different strains. In a 2-year study in B6C3F1 mice, Shirai et al. (1982) reported that BHT at levels of 0.0, 0.1, or 0.5% was not carcinogenic. A reduction in body weight gain was noticed, the effect being more pronounced in males. Nonneoplastic lesions related to BHT treatment were lymphatic infiltration of the lung in females and of the urinary bladder in both the sexes at the highest dose level. Tumors were observed in various organs, with a high incidence in the lung, liver, and lymph nodes, but the incidence was not statistically significant. In another study in the same strain at higher dose levels of 1 or 2% in the diet, a significant dose-dependent increase in hepatocellular adenomas and foci of alterations in the liver were observed in males but not in females (Inai et al., 1988). In BALB/c mice fed 0.75% BHT for 16 months, Clapp et al. (1974) reported an increase in the incidence of lung tumors and hepatic cysts. In CF1 mice, Brooks et al. (1974) reported a dose-related increase in benign and also malignant tumors in the lung in both sexes and benign ovarian tumors in females. In C3H mice, which are more prone to spontaneous liver tumors with age, BHT fed at levels of 0.05 or 0.5% for 10 months increased the incidence of liver tumors in males, which was not dose related. The incidence of lung tumors was increased in males at both dietary levels but in females only at the higher dose level (Lindenschmidt et al., 1986).

A number of studies have been conducted on the modifying effects of BHT on chemical carcinogenesis. The modifying effects of BHT depends on a number of factors including target organs, type of carcinogen, species and strain differences, type of diet used, and also the time of administration. In general, BHT inhibited the induction of neoplasms in the lung and forestomach in mice and lung, liver, and forestomach neoplasms in rats when given before or with the carcinogen. BHT had a promoting effect on urinary bladder, thyroid, and lung carcinogenesis (Ito et al., 1987).

Reproduction. In an earlier study Brown et al. (1959) reported that rats fed 0.1 or 0.5% BHT showed a 10% incidence of anophthalmia. These findings were not confirmed in any other laboratory. BHT had no adverse effects on reproduction data and was not teratogenic in single and multigeneration reproduction studies in rats, mice, hamsters, rabbits, and monkeys at lower doses, and the no-effect level was equivalent to 50 mg/kg bw (Clegg, 1965; Frawley et al., 1965; Johnson, 1965; FDA, 1972b, 1974b; Allen, 1976; Olsen et al., 1986). At higher dose levels some of the significant effects observed in rats include a dose-related response in litter size, number of males/litter, and reduced body weight gain during lactation period, and the effects were significant only at 500 mg/kg bw/day. In rabbits given 3–320 mg/kg bw/day by gavage during embryogenesis, increase in intrauterine deaths was observed at high doses. In mice at 500 mg/kg bw/day, prolonged time to birth of first litters as well as reduced pup numbers and pup weight were observed.

In a developmental neurobehavioral toxicity test, the offspring of rats fed 0.5% BHT before conception, throughout pregnancy, and during lactation showed delayed eyelid opening, surface righting development and limb coordination in swimming in males, and reduced female openfield ambulation. However, the results did not suggest any specific toxicity of BHT to the central nervous system (Vorhees et al., 1981). In another study in weanling mice fed 0.5% BHT for 3 weeks, whose parents had been maintained at the same level during entire mating, gestation, and preweaning period, showed decreased sleeping, increased social and isolation-induced aggression, and learning disabilities under the experimental conditions employed (Stokes and Scudder, 1974).

Mutagenicity. BHT was found to be negative in several strains of *S. typhimurium* with or without metabolic activation (Shelef and Chin, 1980; Hageman et al., 1988). In in vitro tests using mammalian cells, BHT was weakly positive in the test for gene mutation in Chinese hamster V79 cells (Paschin and Bahitova, 1984). In tests for chromosomal aberrations, BHT was positive in human lymphocyte cultures (Sciorra et al., 1974) and in Chinese hamster ovary cells (Patterson et al., 1987). In in vivo tests BHT was negative in tests for chromosomal damage in bone marrow cells and liver cells of rats (Harman et al., 1970; Bruce and Heddle, 1979). BHT was negative in three dominant lethal tests in mice, but in rats at high doses BHT was positive in two dominant lethal tests (Stanford Research Institute, 1972, 1977). In general, the mutagenic effects were observed only at higher levels of BHT.

Tertiary Butyl Hydroquinone

Tertiary butyl hydroquinone (TBHQ) (Fig. 11) was introduced in 1970s and was approved as a food-grade antioxidant in 1972. TBHQ is a white or light tan crystalline powder moderately soluble in fats and oils and slightly soluble in water and does not form a complex with iron and copper. TBHQ is used for the stabilization of fats and oils, confectionary, and fried foods and is regarded as the best antioxidant

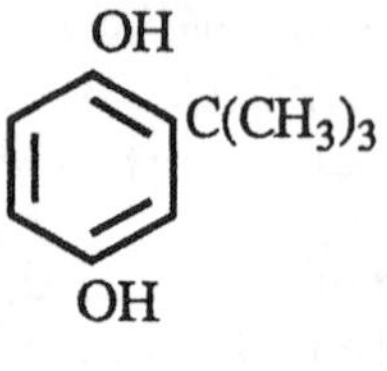

OH

$C(CH_3)_3$

OH

Fig. 11   Tertiary butyl hydroquinone.

for the protection of frying oils and the fried product (Buck, 1984). TBHQ is currently used in the United States and some other countries, but it is not permitted in EEC countries or Japan (Sherwin, 1976; EEC Commission Documents, 1982) due to lack of adequate toxicological data. In a 1987 reevaluation, the JECFA allocated a temporary ADI of 0–0.2 mg/kg bw (FAO/WHO, 1987).

Biochemical Studies: Absorption, Metabolism, and Excretion

Absorption and metabolism studies have been conducted in rats, dogs, and humans. In all three species more than 90% of an orally administered dose of TBHQ was rapidly absorbed and nearly 80% was excreted in the urine in the first 24 hours. The excretion was essentially complete within 48 hours. In the rats given single oral doses of TBHQ (100 mg/kg) about 57–80% was excreted as the 4-O-sulfate, 4% as the 4-O-glucuronide conjugate, and about 4–12% of unchanged TBHQ was observed. In long-term studies an increase in the amount of glucuronide was observed. In dogs a similar pattern was observed, but the proportion of the glucuronide was higher. No tissue accumulation of TBHQ was observed. In humans given single oral doses of 0.5–4 mg/kg in a high-fat vehicle, most of the dose was recovered in the urine within 40 hours. The proportions of the major metabolites observed were 73–88% of 4-O-sulfate, 15–22% of 4-O-glucuronide, and less than 1% unchanged TBHQ. In a low-fat vehicle, absorption was much lower, and urinary elimination accounted for less than half the intake (Astill et al., 1975).

Toxicological Studies

Acute Toxicity. The acute oral and i.p. LD$_{50}$ in mg/kg bw in rats was between 700–1000 and 300–400, respectively. In mice acute oral LD$_{50}$ was 1260 mg/kg bw, and in guinea pigs it was 790 mg/kg bw (Terhaar et al., 1968; Astill et al., 1975).

Short-Term Studies. In rats given 100 and 200 mg/kg bw TBHQ i.p. for one month or fed 1% TBHQ for 22 days, no adverse effects on growth rate, mortality, and microscopic pathology were observed (Fassett et al., 1968). TBHQ had a slight inductive effect on some of the liver microsomal mixed-function oxidases like p-nitroanisole demethylase and aniline hydroxylase in a 21-day feeding study in rats at a 0.2% level. However, the effects were slight compared to BHA and BHT. In long-term studies no effects on the enzyme system were observed (Astill et al., 1975).

Long-Term/Carcinogenicity Studies. In a 20-month study in rats at dose levels of 0.016, 0.05, 0.16, and 0.5%, TBHQ had no deleterious effects on food intake, growth rate, mortality, and organ weights. No changes were observed in hematological or biochemical analysis and extensive histological studies. In a 2-year dog study at levels of 0.05, 0.15, and 0.5%, no abnormalities were observed in histopathological studies, but at the highest dose level reductions in red blood cell counts, hemoglobin levels, and hematocrit values were observed (Astill et al., 1975).

TBHQ was also tested for its ability to induce cellular proliferation in the forestomach of rats and hamsters. In rats fed a dose level of 0.25% for 9 days, TBHQ had no significant effect but at 1% a slight but significant increase in cell proliferation was observed (Nera et al., 1984). At a 2% level TBHQ caused mild hyperplasia of the forestomach with focally increased hyperplasia of the basal cells, but no differentiation of the basal hyperplasia was observed (Altmann et al., 1986). In hamsters a 0.5% dose level for 20 weeks resulted in a slight increase in cell proliferation (Ito et al., 1986). TBHQ has also been reported to have a weak promoting effect on urinary bladder carcinogenesis induced by N-butyl-N-(4-hydroxybutyl)-nitrosamine at a dose level of 0.2% (Tamano et al., 1987).

Reproduction. In rats reproduction studies have been carried out at the highest dose level of 0.5%. The studies include a three-generation study with two litters per generation, a one-generation study, and a separate teratological study during organogenesis. At 0.5% level a reduction in food intake with a consequent decrease in the body weight of the pups was observed. TBHQ had no effect on reproduction data and was not teratogenic (Astill et al., 1975; Krasavage, 1977).

Mutagenicity. The mutagenicity of TBHQ has been studied in a number of test systems. In the Ames test for gene mutations, TBHQ was nonmutagenic in five strains of *S. typhimurium* with and without metabolic activation. In mammalian cell cultures, TBHQ was negative in CHO/HGPRT forward mutation assay and V79 Chinese hamster cells. In mouse lymphoma forward mutation assay TBHQ was slightly positive with and without a metabolic activation system. In tests for chromosomal aberrations in mammalian cells in vivo, a rat dominant lethal test and a mouse bone marrow cytogenetic assay were negative (unpublished data, cited in FAO/WHO, 1987). TBHQ was found to be slightly positive in tests for chromosomal aberrations and sister chromatid exchanges in V79 Chinese hamster lung cells and Chinese hamster fibroblast cell lines (Matsuoka et al., 1990; Rogers et al., 1992). In in vivo tests, Giri et al. (1984) reported a clastogenic effect of TBHQ in mouse bone marrow cells. Two hundred mg/kg bw of TBHQ administered i.p. resulted in a significant increase in chromosomal abnormalities like breaks, gaps, and centric fusions. A significant depression in mitotic index was also observed in treated animals. Mukherjee et al. (1989) reported sister chromatid exchanges (SCE) in mouse bone marrow metaphase cells. Six concentrations of 0.5, 2, 20, 50, 100, and 200 mg/kg of TBHQ in corn oil was injected i.p. A positive dose-response effect in SCE frequency was observed using the Cochran Armitage trend test. Two mg/kg of TBHQ was found to be the minimum effective dose. At higher concentrations of 50, 100, and 200 mg/kg, TBHQ also induced a significant delay in cell cycle. The results indicate that TBHQ may be slightly mutagenic at higher levels.

Tocopherols

Tocopherols are a group of chemically related compounds occurring naturally in plant tissues especially in nuts, seeds, fruits, and vegetables, which show both antioxidant and vitamin E activity. Vegetable oils from nuts and seeds form a rich source of vitamin E. The tocopherols include α, β, γ, and δ homologs and the corresponding tocotrienols. The basic structural unit in all the homologs is a hydroxylated benzene ring system and a isoprenoid side chain. The homologs differ in the number of methyl groups bound to the aromatic ring (Fig. 12). α-Tocopherol and its acetate have also been chemically synthesized. Synthetic products are designated as dl-α-tocopherol and dl-α-tocopheryl acetate, which are actually mixtures of four racemates. Tocopherols are insoluble in water and soluble in fats and oils and are generally considered to be the major lipid-soluble antioxidants. d-α-Tocopheryl poly (ethylene glycol) 1000 succinate (TPGS) is a synthetic water-soluble form of vitamin E prepared by the esterification of d-α-tocopheryl acid succinate with polyethylene glycol. TPGS provides 260 mg d-α-tocopherol/g and forms a clear solution in water, which is stable under normal handling and storage conditions (Krasavage and Terhaar, 1977).

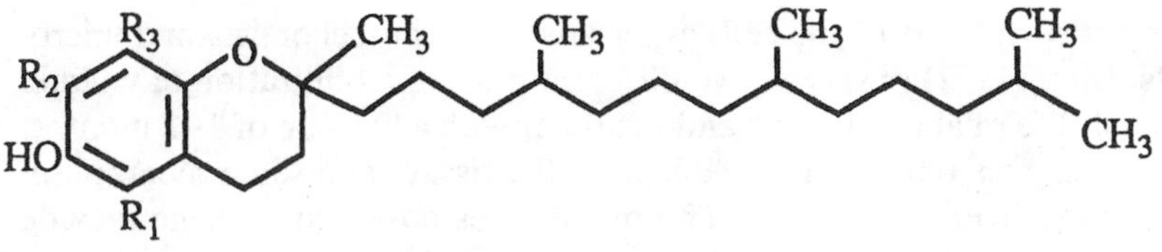

R$_1$	R$_2$	R$_3$	
CH$_3$	CH$_3$	CH$_3$	α–tocopherol
CH$_3$	H	CH$_3$	β–tocopherol
H	CH$_3$	CH$_3$	γ-tocopherol
H	H	CH$_3$	δ-tocopherol

Fig. 12 Tocopherols.

The antioxidant activity of α, β, γ, and δ homologs varies with the degree of hindering and temperature. At physiological conditions around 37°C, the antioxidant action is in the order α > β > γ > δ, similar to the biological activity. At higher temperatures of 50–100°C, a reversal in antioxidant activity is observed in the order δ > γ > β > α. α-Tocopherol is the most abundant of the homologs, and the biological activity is twice that of β and γ and 100 times that of the δ homolog (Johnson, 1971). Tocopherols are effective in a number of food products including meat products, bakery products, fats, and oils. Tocopherols show their greatest potency as antioxidants in animal fats, carotenoids, and vitamin A (Cort, 1974a). Both natural and synthetic α-tocopherol are used commercially in addition to mixed tocopherol concentrates and esters. Tocopherols as a group are permitted for use as food additives, and the JECFA has allocated an ADI of 0.15–2 mg/kg bw (as α-tocopherol) (FAO/WHO, 1987).

Biochemical Studies: Absorption, Metabolism, and Excretion

The mechanism of absorption and metabolic fate of α-tocopherol is not fully known. In mammals, the most functional absorption site was generally located in the medial small intestine. Tocopherols were partially hydrolyzed before absorption and enter the systemic circulation via the lymphatic system. In the lymph tocopherols circulate in bound form to nonspecific lipoproteins (Gallo-Torres, 1980a). In rats, Pearson and MacBarnes (1970) observed that α- and γ-tocopherol were absorbed to a greater extent (32 and 30%, respectively) than β- and δ-tocopherol (18 and 1.8%, respectively). In humans, the percent absorption of dl-α-tocopherol was inversely proportional to the dose. With a 10-mg dose, 96.9% of absorption was observed, 81.5% with a 100-mg dose, and 55.2% with a 200-mg dose (Schmandke et al., 1969). Studies with ^{14}C-labeled dl-α-tocopheryl acetate in rats revealed that absorption occurred slowly, and maximum concentration was observed after several hours of administration. High tissue levels remained for a longer period. Maximum uptake was observed in the liver, adrenals, and ovaries. Intermediate uptake was observed in heart, kidney, adipose tissue, and skeletal muscle (Wiss et al., 1962; Gallo-Torres, 1980b). In liver cell particles, nearly 85% of the α-tocopherol was located in the structural part of the cell, especially in the mitochondria and micro-somes. In rats, Bieri (1972) observed two different rates of mobilization of vitamin E, one with a half-life of about 1 week and the other with a half-life of 1–2 months. Most of the tocopherols remained unchanged in the tissue, and some metabolism was observed in the liver and kidney. The metabolites observed in urine include tocopherylquinone and dimers similar to the in vitro oxidation products of toco-pherol (Simon et al., 1956; Csallany et al., 1962). The urinary excretion of toco-pherol accounted for only 1% of the dose, whereas fecal elimination ranged from 10–75% of the dose (Simon et al., 1956; Gallo-Torres, 1980b). In humans toco-pherol is possibly metabolized via tocoquinone to tocopheronolactone (Schmandke and Schmidt, 1968).

Toxicological Studies

Acute Toxicity. The acute oral LD_{50} of α-tocopherol is not known. α-Toco-pherol was tolerated even at higher doses of 2000 mg/kg bw in rabbits, 5000 mg/kg bw in rats, and 50 000 mg/kg bw in mice (Hanck, 1986). The acute oral LD_{50} of TPGS and d-α-tocopheryl succinate were >7000 mg/kg bw in rats (Krasavage and Terhaar, 1977).

Short-Term Studies. In short-term studies in rats and mice fed α-tocopherol at dose levels of 0.4 and 5% daily for 2 months, no adverse effects were observed (Demole, 1939). Weissberger and Harris (1943) reported that in weanling rats fed 10 or 100 mg of vitamin E for 19 weeks, phosphorus metabolism was stimulated at the higher dose level. In another feeding study in weanling rats given 0.0035% and 25, 50, 100, and 1000 times of this concentration for 13 weeks, a significant reduction in feed intake and protein efficiencies were observed after 8 weeks. No changes were observed in hemoglobin levels, serum cholesterol, and urinary crea-tine levels. Serum glutamate pyruvate transaminase activity increased in the highest dose (Dysmsza and Park, 1975). Administration of TPGS at levels of 0.002, 0.2, or 2% for 90 days had no effect on body weight gain, food consumption, hema-tology, organ weights, serum constituents, or histopathology (Krasavage and Ter-haar, 1977).

In 23-day-old chicks fed 2.2 g dl-α-tocopheryl acetate/kg bw in the diet for 55 days, depression in growth, bone calcification, disturbed thyroidal function, pro-longation of prothrombin time, and increase in reticulocyte count were observed (March et al., 1973). In a 13-week study in Fischer 344 rats administered d-α-tocopheryl acetate by gavage at levels of 125, 500, or 2000 mg/kg bw/day, no adverse effects were observed in food intake or body weight. An increase in liver weight without any histopathological changes was observed in females at the highest dose level. In males high levels caused prolongation of prothrombin and activated partial thromboplastin times, reticulocytosis, and a decrease in hematocrit and hemoglobin levels. Vitamin E also caused hemorrhages in the orbital cavity of the eye and in the meninges. Also in higher doses an antagonistic effect was observed between vitamin E and vitamin K. These symptoms were reversible with supplementation of vitamin K. Vitamin E at all levels caused interstitial inflammation and adenom-atous hyperplasia of the lung. Male rats generally had more severe lesions, and also the incidence of lesions was higher compared to females (Abdo et al., 1986b).

Takahashi et al. (1990) in a recent study reported the hemorrhagic toxicity of d-α-tocopherol in rats. Dietary administration of d-α-tocopherol at levels of 0.63%

and 1% for 7 days resulted in external hemorrhages, and severe internal hemorrhages in a number of organs including the stomach, around inferior vena cava,
cranial cavity, and spinal column were observed in both test levels. The toxicity
was found to be dose dependent. Significant prolongation of prothrombin time and
kaolin-activated partial thromboplastin time were observed in both test levels.
Intraperitoneal administration of d-α-tocopherol at levels of 1.14, 1.82, and 2.91
mmol/kg for 7 days was less toxic, and in only one animal was bleeding in the
abdominal cavity found at the highest dose level. Dietary administration resulted
in a five- to eightfold increase in the concentration of tocopherol in the plasma of
rats, whereas intraperitoneal administration resulted in only a two- to fourfold
increase, indicating that the difference in the toxicity may be due to differences in
the rate of absorption of d-α-tocopherol. It has also been observed that α-toco-
pherolquinone, a metabolite of α-tocopherol, is the causative agent for hemorrhages (Olson and Jones, 1979; Bettger and Olson, 1982).

In humans, adverse effects of hypervitaminosis E include nausea, gastrointestinal disturbances, weakness, fatigue, creatinuria, and impairment of blood coagulation (Hillman, 1957; Briggs, 1974; Dahl, 1974; Tsai et al., 1978). Allergic reactions in some individuals using topical creams and sprays containing α-tocopherol
were shown by patch tests to be due to α-tocopherol (Brodkin and Bleiberg, 1965;
Minkin et al., 1973; Aeling et al., 1973). In a recent toxicological position report
on vitamin E, Kappus and Diplock (1992) observed that intakes of up to 720 mg/
day were tolerated without side effects. At levels above 720 mg and in particular
at doses of 1600–3000 mg/day, some adverse effects may be observed, which subside
rapidly on reducing the dose or discontinuation of vitamin E.

Long-Term/Carcinogenicity Studies. In rats fed 0.025, 0.25, 2.5, 10, and 25
g/kg diet of dl-α-tocopheryl acetate for 8–16 months, a reduction in body weight,
decreased bone ash content, increased heart and spleen weights, elevated hematocrit, reduced prothrombin time, increase in plasma alkaline phosphatase levels,
and increase in lipid levels in the liver were observed (Yang and Desai, 1977). In
a 2-year study in rats fed dl-α-tocopheryl acetate at levels of 500, 1000, and 2000
mg/kg bw/day, excessive hemorrhagic mortalities were observed only in males. In
female rats the increase in relative liver weight was accompanied by histopathological changes indicating liver damage. A dose-related increase in alanine ami-
notransferase activity was also observed in males. At higher doses a trend towards
mammary tumor incidence was observed (Wheldon et al., 1983). In a 10-month
study in hamsters, Moore et al. (1987) reported that α-tocopherol at a 1% level
induced forestomach lesions, although at lower levels compared to BHA.

Tocopherols show inhibitory action against some known carcinogens.
α-Tocopherol inhibited methylcholanthrene-induced buccal pouch tumors in hamsters and dimethylhydrazine-induced colonic tumors in mice (Cook and McNamara,
1980; Shklar, 1982). The anticarcinogenic properties of tocopherols have been
summarized by Tomassi and Silano (1986).

Reproduction. In a reproduction study in weanling rats fed a normal level of
dl-α-tocopheryl acetate (35 mg/kg diet) and 25, 50, 100, and 1000 times the control
amount for 8 weeks, the number of pups born alive was reduced in the highest
dose level (Dysmsza and Park, 1975). In a two-generation study in rats fed very
high levels of 2252 mg/kg bw during pregnancy and lactation, α-tocopherol induced
eye abnormalities in the progeny of both the first and second generation. Lower

levels of 90 mg/kg bw had no adverse effects. α-Tocopherol was not found to be teratogenic in rats, mice, and hamsters at dose levels of 16, 74, 250, 345, and 1600 mg/kg bw/day (FDA, 1973b). In rats fed TPGS at dose levels of 0.002, 0.2, and 2% for 90 days no adverse effects were observed on mean gestation period, litter size, sex ratio, and mortality rate. TPGS given on days 6–16 of gestation was also not teratogenic (Krasavage and Terhaar, 1977). Tocopherols also have an adverse effect on testis at high doses. In hamsters administered 75 mg of α-tocopheryl acetate for 8–30 days, significantly lower testicular weights and a transient disruption in spermatogenisis were observed (Czyba, 1966). In mice given 10 mg α-tocopheryl acetate for 20 days, an enlargement of the testicular interstitial cells and smooth endoplasmic reticulum was observed, indicating an enhanced steroid production (Ichihara, 1967). In humans, vitamin E has been reported to increase the urinary excretion of androgens and estrogens in women (Winkler, 1943; Solomon et al., 1972).

Mutagenicity.   dl-α-Tocopherol or the acetate have not been found to be mutagenic and are reported to reduce the genotoxic effect of other known mutagens. dl-α-Tocopherol reduced the mutagenic effects of dimethyl benz(a)anthracene in leukocyte cultures (Shamberger et al., 1973). In five strains of *S. typhimurium*, dl-α-tocopherol markedly reduced the mutagenic effects of malonaldehyde and β-propiolactone (Shamberger et al., 1979). Neither dl-α-tocopherol nor the acetate was mutagenic in human lymphocyte cultures in vitro and in a sex-linked lethal test in *Drosophila* (Beckman et al., 1982; Gebhart et al., 1985).

Gum Guaiac

Gum guaiac is a naturally occurring antioxidant from the wood of *Guajacum officinale* L. or *G. sanctum* L. family Zygophyllaceae. Commercial gum guaiac is in the form of brown or greenish-brown irregular lumps consisting of a mixture of about 20% α- and β-guaiconic acids, about 10% guairetic acid, and 15% guaiac yellow. It is insoluble in water and sparingly soluble in fats. Gum guaiac was used in 1940s as an antioxidant for oils and fats, especially lard, and also as a stabilizer for pastry. Though gum guaiac is an effective antioxidant, it is no longer used mainly because of availability problems and also because of its tendency to produce various undesirable colors in shortenings. In 1974 evaluation the JECFA allocated an ADI of 0–2.5 mg/kg bw.

Biochemical Studies

Very little information is available on the absorption and toxicological aspects of gum guaiac. However, gum guaiac has been used in medicine for a long time without any adverse effects and is generally considered to be a harmless substance. Absorption studies have been carried out in rats, dogs, and cats. Gum guaiac was poorly absorbed and mostly excreted unchanged in the feces, with the remainder destroyed in the colon (Johnson et al., 1938).

Toxicological Studies

The acute oral LD_{50} in rats was >5000 mg/kg bw, and in guinea pigs it was >1120 mg/kg bw. In mice both oral and i.p. LD_{50} were >2000 mg/kg bw (Lehman et al., 1951). In short-term studies in rats (0–0.5% for 4 weeks), cats (500 or 1000 mg for 34–117 weeks), and dogs (500 or 1000 mg for 62–103 weeks), no adverse effects on growth rate, general behavior, hemoglobin levels, or red and white blood cell counts were observed. The lungs, kidneys, liver, and spleen were found to be normal upon histological examination. In long-term and also lifetime studies in rats, no changes in growth rate, mortality, reproduction, or pathological examination were observed (Johnson et al., 1938; Lehman et al., 1951). In humans given 50–100 mg daily for 18–104 weeks, no adverse effects were observed (Johnson et al., 1938).

Ionox Series

The Ionox series consists of Ionox-100 [2,6-di-*tert*-butyl-4-hydroxy methyl phenol], Ionox-201 [di-(3,5-di-*tert*-butyl-4-hydroxy benzyl)ether], Ionox-220 [di-(3,5-di-*tert*-butyl-4-hydroxy phenyl)methane], Ionox-312 [2,4,6-tri-(3',5'-di-*tert*-butyl-4-hydroxy benzyl)phenol], and Ionox-330[2,4,6-tri(3',5'-di-*tert*-butyl-4-hydroxybenzyl)mesitylene] (Fig. 13). All of these compounds are derivatives of BHT. Ionox-100 is approved for use in food products, and Ionox-330 is approved for incorporation into food-packaging materials.

Biochemical Studies: Absorption, Metabolism, and Excretio⁻

The absorption, metabolism, and excretion of these compounds has been reviewed by Hathway (1966). Ionox-330 and Ionox-312 were not absorbed in the gastrointestinal tract in dogs, rats, pigs, and humans. Unchanged Ionox-330 was quantitatively eliminated in the feces. No biliary excretion was observed in rats and pigs. Rats eliminated 75% of a single oral dose of ^{14}C Ionox-330 (285.7 mg/kg bw) in 24 hours and the remainder in 48 hours. Dogs eliminated the whole dose (90 mg/kg bw) within 24 hours (Wright et al., 1965a). A similar trend was observed with Ionox-312 (Wright and Crowne, 1965, unpublished report, cited in Hathway, 1966).

Ionox-100 was completely absorbed, rapidly metabolized, and quantitatively eliminated. In rats a single oral dose (250 mg/kg bw) of ^{14}C Ionox-100 was eliminated in 11 days; 15.6–70.8% was found in the urine and 27–72.2% in the feces. Dogs showed a similar pattern of elimination. No unchanged Ionox-100 was found. The major metabolites were 3,5-di-*tert*-butyl-4-hydroxybenzoic acid and its glucuronide (Wright et al., 1965b). In addition, in rabbits, 3,5-di-*tert*-butyl-4-hydroxybenzaldehyde and unchanged Ionox-100 were also reported (Akagi and Aoki, 1962b).

Ionox-220 and -201 were found to have intermediate rates of absorption, metabolism, and elimination. In rats 89.4–97.5% of a single oral dose (10 mg/kg bw) was eliminated in the feces in 20 days. Approximately 20% of a single oral dose of Ionox-220 was absorbed, and part of it was metabolized. Some of the metabolites identified were 3,5-di-*tert*-butyl-4-hydroxybenzoic acid and its glucuronide, quinone methide, and 2,6-di-*tert*-butyl-*p*-benzoquinone. Most of the dose was in the form of unchanged Ionox-220 (Wright et al., 1966). A similar pattern was observed with Ionox-201. Approximately 32% of a single oral dose was absorbed in the rats, and about 65% was eliminated unchanged. The major metabolites were 3,5-di-*tert*-butyl-4-hydroxybenzoic acid and its glucuronide, 3,3',5,5'-di-*tert*-butyl-4-stilbenequinone, and 3,5-di-*tert*-butyl-4-hydroxybenzaldehyde (Wright et al., 1967).

Toxicological Studies

Toxicological studies have been conducted with Ionox-100 and Ionox-330.

Ionox-100. The acute oral LD$_{50}$ in rats and mice was found to be greater than 7 g/kg bw. In a 2-year study in rats at dose levels of 0.2 or 0.35%, no significant differences in survival rate, organ weights, histopathology, hematology, and serum

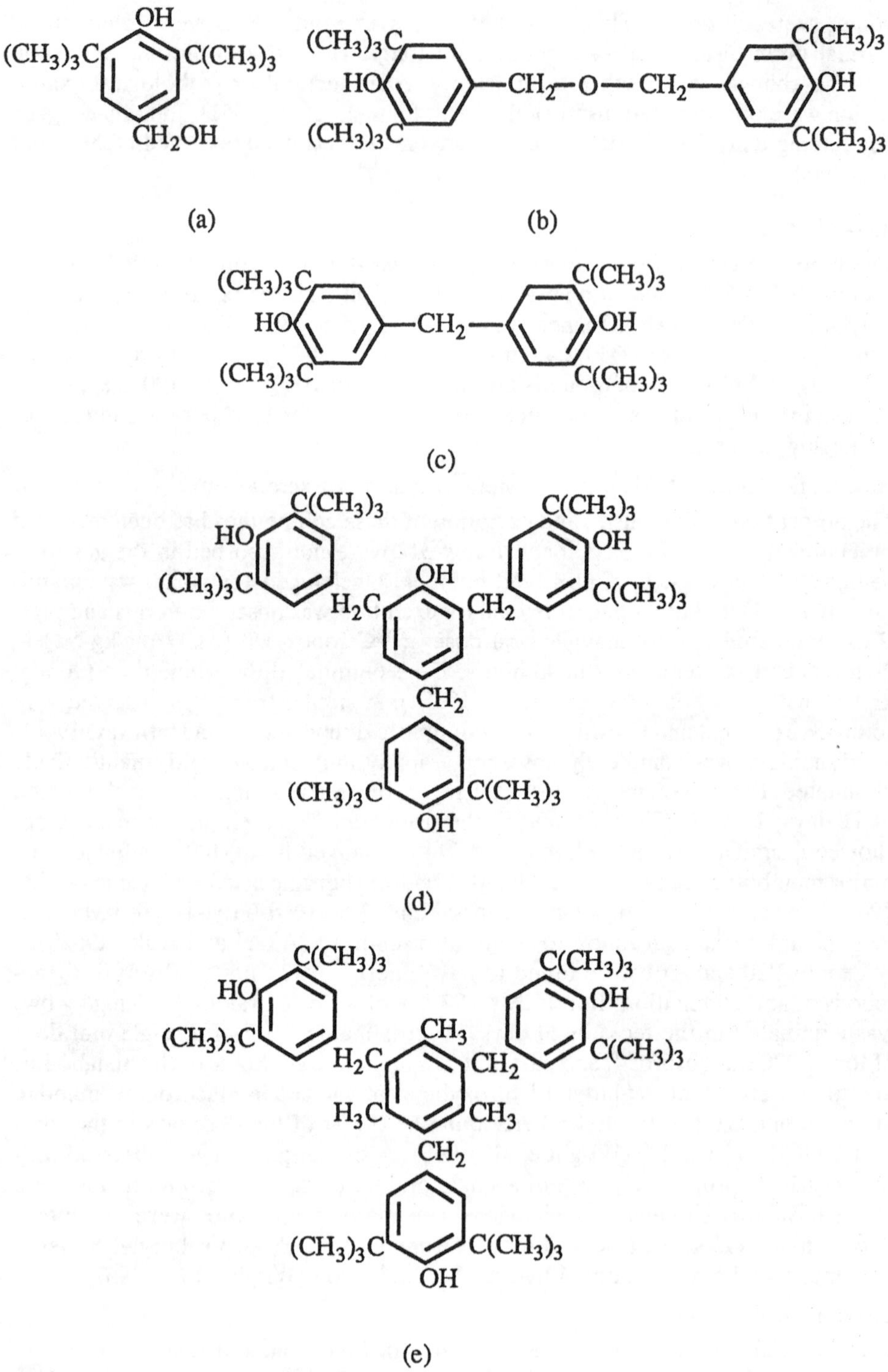

Fig. 13 Ionox series: (a) Ionox-100, (b) Ionox-201, (c) Ionox-220, (d) Ionox-312, (e) Ionox-330.

enzyme levels were found between treated and control animals. In a three-generation reproduction study in rats at a 0.35% level, Ionox-100 had no adverse effects (Dacre, 1970).

Ionox-330. The acute oral LD_{50} in rats was >5000 mg/kg bw. In a 90-day study in rats with various dosage levels, Ionox-330 had no adverse effects except for a slight suppression in growth at the highest dosage level (3.1%) (Stevenson et al., 1965).

C. Miscellaneous Primary Antioxidants

Ethoxyquin

Ethoxyquin (6-ethoxy-1,2-dihydro-2,2,4-trimethylquinoline) (EQ) (Fig. 14) was first permitted for use in the United Kingdom for the prevention of scald in apples and pears. EQ is effective as an antioxidant in feeds, particularly for the stabilization of carotenoids in dehydrated alfalfa (Bickoff et al., 1954) and in fish meals, squalene, and fish oils (Olcott, 1958; Weil et al., 1968; Atkinson et al., 1972;). EQ readily undergoes oxidation to form a stable free radical ethoxyquin nitroxide, which is more effective as an antioxidant than ethoxyquin (Weil et al., 1968; Lin and Olcott, 1975). An ADI of 0–0.06 mg/kg bw has been allocated in the Joint FAO/WHO meetings on pesticide residues (FAO/WHO, 1969).

Biochemical Studies: Absorption, Metabolism, and Excretion

EQ was readily absorbed and metabolized rapidly following the pattern of a non-physiological substance. Studies on the metabolism and metabolites of EQ have been carried out by Skaare (1979), Skaare and Solheim (1979), Wilson et al. (1959), and Wiss et al. (1962). In rats given a single oral dose of ^{14}CEQ at 100 mg/kg level, nearly 67–80% was recovered after 24 hours in urine and feces. Nearly 50% of the radioactivity was recovered from the urine and 20% from the feces. Approximately 95% of the dose was excreted in 6 days. The major metabolite in urine was 6-hydroxy-2,2,4-trimethyl-1,2-dihydroquinoline and an oxidation product, 2,2,4-trimethyl-6-quinoline. Other metabolites observed were hydroxylated EQ and dihydroxy EQ (Skaare and Solheim, 1979). In another study in rats, Skaare (1979) observed 28 and 36% of biliary excretion of a single oral dose of ^{14}C EQ (100 mg/kg bw) in 12 and 24 hours, respectively. However, EQ was not metabolized extensively before biliary excretion, and 75–85% of the ^{14}C excreted was identified as unchanged EQ. Some of the metabolites identified were 2,2,4-trimethyl-6-quinoline, hydroxylated EQ, and dihydroxylated EQ. In rats, the highest concentration of EQ was observed in the liver and the kidneys. Heart, skeletal muscles, and brain showed the least concentrations and eliminated the material rapidly. Spleen, blood,

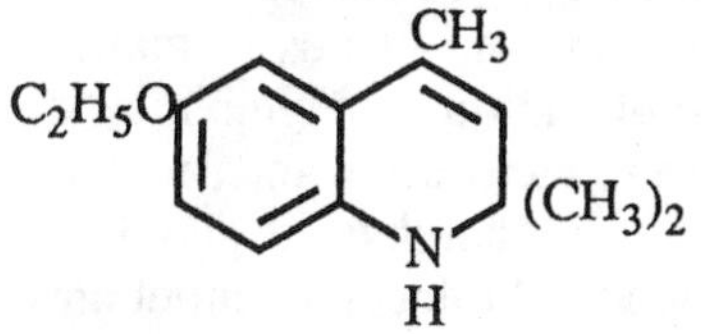

Fig. 14 Ethoxyquin.

and abdominal fat had intermediate concentrations and eliminated the material at a slower rate. A small fraction of the injected EQ was observed in the milk indicating an in utero transfer of the compound (Wilson et al., 1959). In liver cell particles, EQ was located primarily in the supernatant rather than in the structural part of the cell (Wiss et al., 1962). In the cow, of the 155 mg of ^{14}C EQ administered, 45.3 mg was recovered in the feces and 107.9 mg in the urine. In the milk the highest concentration of 0.036 ppm was found 33 hours after ingestion (Wilson et al., 1959).

Toxicological Studies

Acute Toxicity. The acute oral LD_{50} in rats and mice was found to be 178 mg/kg bw (Wilson and DeEds, 1959).

Short-Term Studies. Short-term studies have been conducted in rats and mice. In rats fed EQ at levels of up to 0.4% for 20 days, no adverse effects were observed (Wilson and DeEds, 1959). In another study in rats fed EQ at a 0.5% level, a reduction in food intake and growth rate was observed over a 60-day period. By the 14th day, a 50% increase in liver weight was observed. Concentrations of hepatic microsomal proteins, cytochrome P-450, and cytochrome b_5 were markedly reduced. Induction of hepatic drug-metabolizing enzymes like biphenyl-4-hydroxylase and ethylmorpholine-N-demethylase and a reduction in the activity of glucose-6-phosphatase was observed. A 25% increase in total hepatic DNA was observed, suggesting that the liver enlargement may have resulted both from cellular hypertrophy and hyperplasia (Cawthorne et al., 1970; Parke et al., 1972, 1974). However, the effects were found to be reversible on cessation of treatment. In rats given a single oral dose of 500 mg EQ/kg bw by stomach tube or 0.015% in drinking water (37.5 mg/kg bw/day) for 60 days, a significant increase in plasma glutamic oxalacetic transaminase activity and hepatic lesions were observed (Skaare et al., 1977). When EQ was given by gavage, ultrastructural changes observed in the liver were a proliferation of the smooth endoplasmic reticulum, dilatation of the perinuclear space, a disorganization of the mitochondrial membrane, desquamation, and fragmentation of the cells. In oral treatment, a slight proliferation of the endoplasmic reticulum was observed (Nafstad and Skaare, 1978). In a recent study Kim (1991) observed that in mice fed EQ at 0.125 and 0.5% for 14 weeks, relative liver weights and hepatic glutathione levels significantly increased. A 2-fold increase in the hepatic mitochondrial glutathione levels was observed at the 0.5% level, which may be of significance in various cellular and subcellular activities.

Long-Term/Carcinogenicity Studies. In a chronic toxicity study in rats, EQ was administered at dose levels of 0.0062, 0.0125, 0.025, 0.05, 0.1, 0.2, and 0.4% for 200, 400, and 700 days. In the 200-day group, the kidneys were significantly heavier at the 0.2 and 0.4% levels. In the males significantly heavier livers were observed at 0.1% and higher levels. Heavier kidneys were noticed from 0.025%. In the 400-day group at 0.2 and 0.4% EQ, females showed no distinct lesions, but clear lesions were observed in the kidneys, livers, and thyroid glands in males. Kidneys showed tubular atrophy, fibrosis, focal tubular dilatation, and lymphocytic infiltration characteristic of chemical pylonephrites. Renal calcification and necrosis was also observed. The effects were dose dependent. In the thyroid glands a decrease in stored colloid and a diffuse increase in the height of follicular epithelium was observed, indicating mild hyperplasia. In the 700-day group, in males at the

0.2% level the lesions were comparable to those of the 400-day group. But in females some patchy changes were observed in the kidneys. Occasional mammary, uterine, and adrenal tumors were also observed. At lower dosage levels of 0.0062%, there were mild changes in males and none in females (Wilson and DeEds, 1959). In a recent study in rats, Manson et al. (1992) have also observed that the degree of nephrosis was dependent on age, sex, and duration of treatment. In another study on the nephrotoxicity of EQ in Fischer 344 rats, Hard and Neal (1992) have reported that EQ increased the cellular accumulation of lipofuscin-related pigments involving proximal tubules in female rats. They also observed that in female rats papillary changes developed at a later stage than males and the lesions never progressed beyond interstitial degeneration.

The modifying effects of EQ on various chemical carcinogens have been studied in rats. EQ administered by gavage or in drinking water significantly enhanced the hepatotoxic effect of N-nitrosodimethylamine (Skaare et al., 1977). EQ significantly enhanced the colon carcinogenesis initiated by 1,2-dimethyl hydrazine (Shirai et al., 1985) and liver carcinogenesis initiated by diethyl nitrosamine (Ito et al., 1987). EQ enhanced the preneoplastic and neoplastic lesions in the kidneys and inhibited liver carcinogenesis initiated by N-ethyl-N-hydroxyethylnitrosamine (Tsuda et al., 1984). EQ enhanced the urinary bladder carcinogenesis induced by N-butyl-N-(4 hydroxybutyl) nitrosamine (Fukushima et al., 1984). In a recent study Hasegawa et al. (1990) observed that EQ inhibited lung carcinogenesis and significantly enhanced the thyroid carcinogenesis initiated by N-bis-(2-hydroxypropyl) nitrosamine in male rats.

Skin Toxicity. In rabbits and guinea pigs, repeated application of EQ produced a slight erythema followed by a papular eruption and in some instances scab formation. When treatment was stopped the lesions disappeared, leaving a normal-appearing skin after a few weeks (Wilson and DeEds, 1959). EQ is also reported to cause allergic contact dermatitis in apple packers and animal feed mill workers (Burrows, 1975; Van Hecke, 1977; Savini et al., 1989).

Reproduction. Reproduction studies have been conducted in rats (Wilson and DeEds, 1959) and rabbits (Isensein, 1970). In rats fed EQ at levels of 0.025–0.1% and in rabbits at 0.0025–0.01%, no reproductive or teratogenic effects were observed following administration of EQ before mating, throughout pregnancy, or during organogenesis. EQ was also reported to prevent the occurrence of congenital malformities associated with vitamin E deficiency (King, 1964).

Anoxomer

Anoxomer (Poly AO™ 79) is a synthetic phenolic polymer developed by Weinshenker et al. (1976). Anoxomer is a condensation product of divinyl benzene, hydroxyanisole, TBHQ, and *tert*-butyl phenol. Anoxomer is not a single molecular weight compound, but is a distribution of molecular weights centered about a "peak" at 4000 daltons (Weinshenker, 1980). Anoxomer is a off-white powder highly soluble in fats and oils and organic solvents, is thermostable, and does not undergo depolymerization at frying temperatures of 190°C over a period of 6 hours (Weinshenker, 1980). Anoxomer is highly effective in frying fats and oils and provides carry-through protection to the fried product. Anoxomer was accepted as a food-grade antioxidant in 1982. The JECFA has allocated an ADI of 0–8 mg/kg bw (FAO/WHO, 1984).

Biochemical Studies

Anoxomer was very poorly absorbed and metabolized because of the large molecular size. Absorption studies indicated that the compound was minimally absorbed (0.1–0.6% of the dose) in rats and mice, in guinea pigs, rabbits, and also in humans (Parkinson et al., 1978a,b). Anoxomer had no adverse effects on liver weight, hepatic cytochrome P-450 level, and hepatic mixed-function oxygenase systems in rats at levels of 250 and 2500 mg/kg bw for 60 days (Halladay et al., 1980).

Toxicological Studies

Anoxomer was found to be nontoxic in acute studies in rats, mice, and dogs at single doses of up to 10 g/kg bw and in subchronic feeding studies in rats at doses of up to 5% in the diet (unpublished data, cited in Walson et al., 1979) and dogs (Weinshenker, 1980). In in vitro mammalian and microbial mutagenicity studies, Anoxomer was negative (Brown et al., 1977). Anoxomer had no adverse effects on reproduction data in rats or rabbits and was not teratogenic (Weinshenker, 1980).

Trolox-C

Trolox-C (6-hydroxy-2,5,7,8-tetramethyl chroman-2-carboxylic acid), a synthetic derivative of α-tocopherol, was developed by Scott et al. (1974). Trolox-C resembles α-tocopherol structurally, except for the replacement of the hydrocarbon chain by a COOH group at the 2-position (Fig. 15). In thin layer tests in vegetable oils and animal fats, Trolox C was found to have two to four times the antioxidant activity of BHA and BHT and was more active than tocopherols, propyl gallate, and ascorbyl palmitate. In vegetable oils, a combination of Trolox-C with certain amino acids was found to be highly effective. Trolox-C is a colorless, tasteless solid, is sparingly soluble in oils, and is 95–100% stable for 2 months at room temperature (22°C) and 45°C (Cort et al., 1975a,b). However, Trolox-C is not being used commercially at present.

Trolox-C was found to have a low order of toxicity. In mice the acute oral, i.p., and s.c. LD_{50} in mg/kg bw was 1630, 1700, and 1930, respectively. In adult rats the acute oral and i.p. LD_{50} in mg/kg bw was 4300 and 1800, respectively. In neonatal rats acute oral LD_{50} was 1120 mg/kg bw and in rabbits it was >2000 mg/kg bw. In a short-term study in dogs fed Trolox-C in doses pyramiding daily up to 320 mg/kg bw for over 14 days, no adverse effects were observed on hematocrit, hemoglobin levels, differential leukocyte counts, blood chemistry, plasma glucose levels, activities of serum glutamic oxaloacetic transaminase, glutamic pyruvic transaminase, and alkaline phosphatase (Cort el al., 1975a).

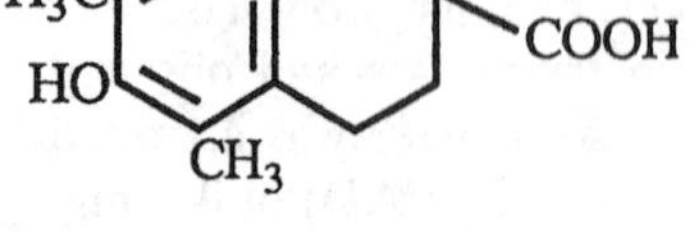

Fig. 15   Trolox-C.

V. BIOCHEMICAL AND TOXICOLOGICAL ASPECTS OF FOOD ANTIOXIDANTS: Synergistic/Secondary Antioxidants

A. Oxygen Scavengers

Sulfites

Sulfites represent a group of compounds comprising sulfur dioxide (SO_2), sodium sulfite (Na_2SO_3), sodium metabisulfite ($Na_2S_2O_5$), and sodium bisulfite ($NaHSO_3$). Sulfites are widely used as antimicrobials in wine making and corn wet-milling and as antioxidants, especially in raw packaged or unpackaged fruits and vegetables, to prevent enzymatic browning and preserve freshness. Sulfites are also added to dehydrated fruits, vegetables, soups, fruit juices, and beer. Sulfites have been GRAS substances since 1959. However, in 1986 the use of sulfiting agents in raw packaged or unpackaged fruits and vegetables was banned by the FDA due to some adverse reactions in sulfite-sensitive individuals. Most of the adverse reactions were associated with the use of sulfites in salad bars in restaurants. Sulfites precipitate attacks of asthma in some individuals, and up to 17 possible fatalities have been attributed to sulfite ingestion in sulfite-sensitive asthamatics. The patients most likely to have sulfite sensitivity seem to be more severely ill with asthma and dependent on corticosteroid medication for control of the disease (Bush, 1986). An ADI of 0–0.7 mg/kg bw has been allocated to sulfites by the JECFA (as SO_2) (FAO/WHO, 1974).

Biochemical Studies

Absorption, Metabolism, and Excretion. Sulfites were readily absorbed and quickly metabolized either by oxidation or by the formation of S-sulfonates (Gunnison and Palmes, 1978; Oshino and Chance, 1975). In rats given single oral doses of sodium metabisulfite in a 0.2% solution, 55% of the sulfur was eliminated as sulfates in the urine within the first 4 hours (Bhagat and Lockett, 1960). In rats, mice, and monkeys following an oral administration of 10 or 50 mg SO_2 (as sodium bisulfite)/kg, 70–95% was absorbed and eliminated in the urine within 24 hours. Most of the remaining dose was eliminated in the feces and only 2% or less remained in the body after one week (Gibson and Strong, 1973).

In mammals, the primary route of sulfite metabolism was via enzymatic oxidation to sulfates by the mitochondrial enzyme sulfite:cytochrome *c* reductase (sulfite oxidase), which occurs predominantly in the liver and also in lower concentrations in almost all other tissues of the body. Sulfite oxidase had a very high capacity for sulfite oxidation with a first-order rate constant of the order of 0.7–1/min, equivalent to a half-life of approximately 1 minute for sulfite (Gunnison et al., 1977). Gunnison et al. (1977) also reported that rats exhibit approximately three to five times greater activity of sulfite oxidase than do rabbits and monkeys. A small but significant amount of sulfites was also metabolized to S-sulfonate compounds in rats, monkeys, and rabbits (Gunnison and Palmes 1978; Wever, 1985). At higher concentrations, sulfites reacted with β-mercaptopyruvate, an intermediate in sulfur-amino acid catabolism, forming inorganic thiosulfate, which has been detected in the urine of normal humans and rats (Gunnison, 1981). Gunnison and Palmes (1973, 1978) also detected free sulfites in the plasma of rats, rabbits, and monkeys both prior to and after administration of sulfites.

Reactions of Sulfites in Vitro.   In vitro, sulfites react reversibly with open-chain aldehydes and ketones to form hydroxysulfonate compounds (Schroeter, 1966; Petering and Shih, 1975) and also with pyridine and flavin nucleotides to form sulfonic acid compounds (Shih and Petering, 1973). Sodium bisulfite adds reversibly to uracil, cytosine, and their derivatives (Hayatsu et al., 1970; Shapiro et al., 1973; Hayatsu, 1976) forming a sulfonate adduct. Sulfites induced sulfitolysis of thiamine, an irreversible reaction resulting in the cleavage of thiamine (Williams et al., 1935) and also irreversible cleaving of disulfide bonds in free cystine, forming cysteine S-sulfonate (Cecil, 1963). The aerobic oxidation of sulfites involves a free radical mechanism resulting in the formation of free radicals, which have potential biological significance (Hayatsu, 1976). Significant cleavage of the glycosidic linkage of uridine and cytidine (Kitamura and Hayatsu, 1974), oxidation of methionine and certain other diallyl sulfides (Yang, 1970), destruction of tryptophan (Yang, 1973), and oxidation of lipids (Kaplan et al., 1975) are some of the effects of the free radicals arising from sulfite autoxidation.

In vitro, sulfites inhibit a number of enzymes associated with NAD or flavin nucleotide cofactors. Ciaccio (1966) observed a 50% inhibition of a number of NAD-dependent dehydrogenases (lactate dehydrogenase, malate dehydrogenase, alcohol dehydrogenase, and glutamate dehydrogenase) in the presence of 0.03–0.5 mM sulfite. Massey et al. (1969) observed that a series of flavin-dependent enzymes like D and L amino acid oxidases, lactate oxidase react reversibly with sulfites forming flavin sulfite adducts, which were unstable in the absence of sulfites. Sulfites also inhibited cytochrome oxidase (Cooperstein, 1963), α-glucan phosphorylase (Kamogawa and Fukui, 1973), and most of the sulfatase enzymes (Roy, 1960).

Toxicological Studies

Acute Toxicity.   The acute i.p. LD_{50} of sodium bisulfite in mg/kg bw in rats was 498, in rabbits 300, in dogs 244, and in mice 675 (Wilkins et al., 1968). Acute i.v. LD_{50} in mg/kg bw in rats was 115, in mice 130, in hamsters 95, and in rabbits 65 (Hoppe and Goble, 1951).

Short-Term/Long-Term Studies.   Short-term studies have been conducted in rats and pigs. In rats fed 0.6% sodium metabisulfite for 6 weeks, a reduction in growth rate was observed in rats fed a fresh diet, which was attributed to lack of thiamine. Rats fed the same diet after 75 days showed signs of thiamine deficiency and additional toxic effects like diarrhea and reduced growth rate, which could not be completely corrected by the administration of thiamine (Bhagat and Lockett, 1964). Thiamine deficiency was not observed when sulfite was administered in drinking water (Lhuissier et al., 1967). In rats fed 0–8% sodium metabisulfite for 10–56 days in a thiamine–enriched diet, levels of 6% or above depressed food intake and growth accompanied by glandular hyperplasia, hemorrhage, ulceration, necrosis, and inflammation of the stomach. Anemia occurred in all animals receiving 2% or above. Leukocytosis and splenic hematopoiesis were also observed. The effects were found to be reversible (Til et al., 1972a). Gunnison (1981) has observed that the anemia results from the interaction of sulfite with dietary constituents, possibly cyanocobalamine.

In long-term and multigeneration feeding studies, rats were fed 0.125, 0.25, 0.5, 1, or 2% sodium metabisulfite in a thiamine-enriched diet for 2 years. A significant reduction of thiamine levels in the urine and the liver was observed, and addition of thiamine prevented the symptoms at lower levels of sulfite. At 1 and 2% occult blood was present in the feces. At the 2% level a slight growth retardation in the F_1 and F_2 generations was observed. Increase in the relative weight of the kidneys not accompanied by any functional or histological changes was observed in females of the F_2 generation. Pathological examination revealed hyperplastic changes in both fore and glandular stomach at 1 and 2% levels in all three generations. There was no indication that sulfite had any carcinogenic effect. Sulfites had no effect on reproduction data or early development (Til et al., 1972a).

In short-term and long-term feeding studies, pigs were fed sodium metabisulfite in thiamine-enriched diets at levels of 0.125, 0.25, 0.5, 1, or 2% for 15 weeks and up to 48 weeks. Thiamine levels were markedly reduced in urine and liver in animals fed 0.16% or more, and added thiamine prevented the deficiency with sulfite levels up to 0.83%. No adverse effects on health, mortality, or the blood picture were observed. A reduction in body weight and food conversion was observed at 1.72%. An increase in the weight of liver, kidneys, heart and spleen and mild inflammatory, hyperplastic changes were observed in the gastric mucosa at 0.83 and 1.72% levels. In paired feeding studies, esophageal intraepithelial micro abscesses, epithelial hyperplasia, and accumulation of neutrophilic leukocytes in the papillae tips were observed (Til et al., 1972b).

Mutagenicity. The genotoxic effect of sulfites have been studied in a number of test systems and reviewed by Gunnison (1981) and Shapiro (1976). Sulfites were mutagenic in a number of in vitro systems like *Escherichia coli* (Mukai et al., 1970), yeasts (Shapiro, 1976), Chinese hamster ovary cells (MacRae and Stich, 1979), and also enhanced the UV mutagenicity in Chinese hamster cell lines by the inhibition of excision repair of DNA (Mallon and Rossman, 1981). The mutagenic effects of sulfites have been attributed to their reaction with cytosine and uracil and also to the free radicals formed during the autoxidation of sulfites. Sulfites were negative in a dominant lethal test in mice (Generoso et al., 1978) and did not induce chromosomal aberrations in mouse oocytes in vitro following a single i.v. injection of up to 2 mmol/kg (Jagiello et al., 1975).

Ascorbic Acid and Sodium Ascorbate

L-Ascorbic acid or vitamin C (3-keto-L-glucofuranolactone) (Fig. 16) (ASA) occurs widely in nature. ASA and sodium ascorbate (SA) are used as oxygen scavengers and also as synergists in a wide variety of food products, including canned or bottled products with a headspace, vegetable oils, beverages, fruits, vegetables, butter, cured meat, and fish products. ASA is a white, odorless solid highly soluble in

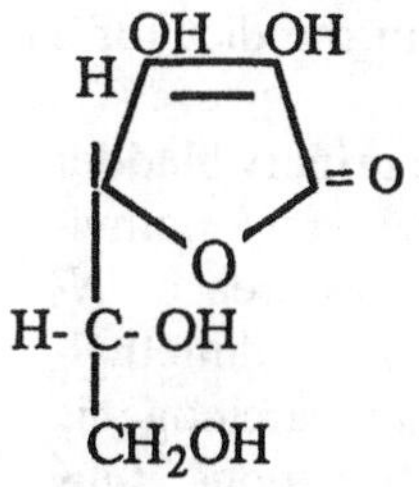

Fig. 16 Ascorbic acid.

water and insoluble in fats and oils. In the presence of oxygen and metal ions in aqueous solutions, ASA readily undergoes oxidation to form dehydroascorbic acid. ASA and SA have been allocated an ADI "not limited" by the JECFA (FAO/ WHO, 1981).

Biochemical Studies: Absorption, Metabolism, and Excretion

Absorption studies have been carried out in rats and humans. In rats after an i.p. injection of 1.5–5.9 mg of ^{14}C ASA, 19–29% was converted to CO_2 and only 0.4% was excreted as oxalic acid within 24 hours (Curtin and King, 1955). In humans, the average absorption of ASA has been estimated to be 84% (Kallner et al., 1981). Kuebler and Gehler (1970) observed that increasing oral intakes from 1.5 to 12 g decreased the relative absorption of ASA from about 50% to only 16%. In humans oxalic acid was the major urinary metabolite. Other metabolites observed were dehydroascorbic acid, 2,3-keto-gluconic acid, and ascorbic acid sulfate (Wilson, 1974). ASA was excreted by glomerular filtration and active tubular reabsorption. High doses of ASA (4 g or more) increased the urinary excretion of oxalate. About 40% of the urinary oxalate was derived from ASA, but the mechanism of its formation is not clear (Wilson, 1974). Briggs et al. (1973) observed that at daily intakes of 4 g ASA, the urinary oxalate level increased 10-fold, which may lead to the formation of kidney stones. However, Hornig and Moser (1981), in an evaluation of safety of high vitamin C intakes, observed that even with large daily intakes, the amount of oxalic acid formed was far too little to contribute significantly to oxalate formation.

Toxicological Studies

Acute Toxicity.   In mice and rats, the acute oral and i.v. LD_{50} of ASA in mg/ kg bw was >5000 and >1000, respectively, and in guinea pigs it was >5000 and >500, respectively (Demole, 1934).

Short-Term Studies.   Administration of ASA orally, subcutaneously, and intravenously in daily doses of 500–1000 mg/kg bw to mice and 400–2500 mg/kg bw to guinea pigs for 6–7 days showed no adverse effects on weight gain, general behavior, or histopathological examination of the various organs (Demole, 1934). Ohno and Myoga (1981) observed that in guinea pigs vitamin C at 10–100 times the normal daily requirement (600 mg/kg bw/day) daily for 112 days resulted in fat deposition and congestion in the liver, resulting in death.

Long-Term/Carcinogenicity Studies.   In rats given daily doses of 1000, 1500, or 2000 mg/kg bw of ASA for 2 years, no adverse effects were observed in hematological examination, urine analysis, liver, and renal function tests. Pathological examination revealed no toxic lesions attributable to ASA (Surber and Cerioli, 1971, unpublished report, cited in FAO/WHO, 1974). In a carcinogenic bioassay, ASA was not carcinogenic in rats and mice fed 2.5 or 5% ASA in the diet for 2 years (National Institutes of Health, 1983).

In rats, SA at a 5% level in the diet has been shown to promote urinary bladder carcinogenesis initiated by N-butyl-N-(4 hydroxybutyl)nitrosamine or N-methylnitrosourea, forestomach carcinogenesis initiated by N-methylnitrosourea or N-methyl-N'-nitro-N-nitrosoguanidine, and colon cancer initiated by 1,2-dimethylhydrazine (Ito et al., 1986). However, ASA was shown to have anticarcinogenic and antimutagenic properties, and it also prevented nitrosation reactions, thus inhibiting the formation of carcinogenic nitroso compounds (Mirvish, 1975). ASA suppressed UV-induced skin cancer (Black and Chan, 1975) and inhibited mutagenicity of a number of compounds (Guttenplan, 1977, 1978; Shamberger et al., 1979).

Reproduction. Information on reproduction is conflicting. In some studies, it has been observed that large daily doses of ASA increased abortion in guinea pigs and rats (Samborskaya, 1964; Samborskaya and Ferdman, 1966). In later studies, Alleva et al. (1976) and Frohberg et al. (1973) reported no adverse effects in rats, mice, hamsters, and guinea pigs at dosages comparable to the earlier studies. The reason for the discrepancy is not known.

Mutagenicity. ASA was reported to be mutagenic in a number of in vitro systems (Stich et al., 1976; Omura et al., 1978; Speit et al., 1980; Rosin et al., 1980). However, in in vivo systems ASA was negative in Chinese hamster bone marrow tests, rat dominant lethal assay, and guinea pig intrahepatic host-mediated test (Chauhan et al., 1978; Speit et al., 1980; Norkus et al., 1983). In in vitro systems, ASA was mutagenic only in the presence of oxygen and metal ions in the incubation medium. Under these conditions ASA completely oxidizes to form hydrogen peroxide, which is a known mutagen (Hornig and Moser, 1981). These observations indicate that ASA is not mutagenic.

Studies in Humans. Studies in humans indicate that ASA has a diuretic effect at 5 mg/kg bw, and glycosuria was observed with doses of 30–100 mg/kg bw. With very high doses of 6000 mg/day, adverse effects observed were nausea, vomiting, diarrhea, flushing of the face, headache, fatigue, and disturbed sleep. In children the main reaction observed was skin rashes (Widenbauer, 1936).

Ascorbyl Palmitate

Ascorbyl palmitate (Fig. 17), the ester of ascorbic acid and palmitic acid, is highly effective in frying fats, oils, and fried products. Alone, ascorbyl palmitate is better than BHA and BHT, and in combination with other antioxidants it improves the shelf life of all vegetable oils (Cort, 1974a). Ascorbyl palmitate is a white or yellowish white solid insoluble in cold water and sparingly soluble in fats and oils. In 1940s food-grade ascorbyl palmitate normally contained a significant amount of ascorbyl stearate, and toxicological studies have been done in samples containing 5–20% stearate and 80–90% palmitate. An ADI of 0–1.25 mg/kg bw has been allocated by the JECFA (FAO/WHO, 1974) for ascorbyl palmitate or ascorbyl stearate or the sum of both.

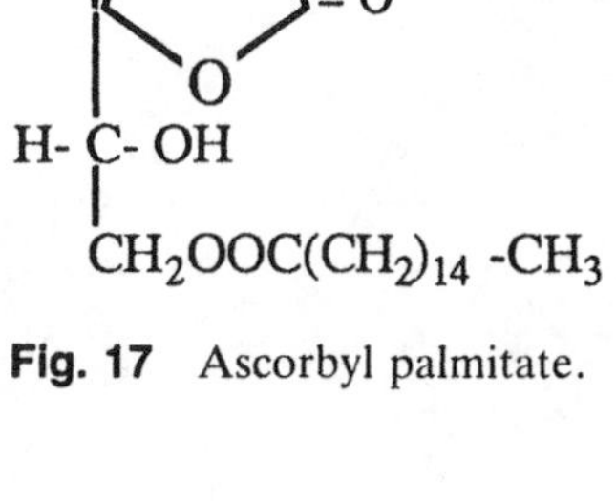

Fig. 17 Ascorbyl palmitate.

Biochemical Studies

No information is available on the metabolism of ascorbyl palmitate, but it is assumed that ascorbyl palmitate is hydrolyzed to ascorbic acid and palmitic acid (Gwo et al., 1985).

Toxicological Studies

In mice the acute oral LD_{50} was 25 g/kg bw (FAO/WHO, 1974). In short-term studies in rats fed 2 and 5% ascorbyl palmitate for 9 months, at the 5% level a significant retardation in growth rate, bladder stones, and hyperplasia of the bladder epithelium was observed. At the 2% level only a slight retardation in growth was observed. In long-term studies in rats fed 1 or 5% ascorbyl palmitate for 2 years, no adverse effects on growth rate, mortality, and pathological studies were observed (Fitzhugh and Nelson, 1946).

Erythorbic Acid and Sodium Erythorbate

Erythorbic acid (3-keto-D-glucofuranolactone) (Fig. 18) is the D-isomer of ascorbic acid. Erythorbic acid has no vitamin C activity and does not occur naturally in food products. Erythorbic acid and its sodium salt are effective in the stabilization of nitrate- and nitrite-cured meat products, in dehydrated fruit and vegetable products, and as synergists for tocopherols in fats and oils (Nakao, et al., 1972; Kanematsu et al., 1984; Movaghar, 1990). Erythorbic acid in combination with citric acid can be an effective alternative to the use of sulfites in frozen seafood, salad vegetables, and apples. In model solutions erythorbic acid was more rapidly oxidized as compared to ascorbic acid (Yourga et al., 1944). Erythorbic acid is highly soluble in water and soluble in ethanol. Erythorbic acid is not permitted for food use in European Economic Countries. In a 1974 reevaluation, the JECFA allocated an ADI of 0–5 mg/kg bw (FAO/WHO, 1974).

Biochemical Studies: Absorption, Metabolism, and Excretion

Erythorbic acid was readily absorbed and rapidly metabolized. In guinea pigs erythorbic acid decreased the tissue uptake of ascorbic acid, thereby lowering its level in different organs like spleen, adrenal glands, and kidneys (Hornig et al., 1974; Hornig and Weiser, 1976; Arakawa et al., 1986).

Toxicological Studies

No information is available on the acute toxicity of erythorbic acid. In short-term studies in rats fed 1% erythorbic acid for 36 weeks, no adverse effects were observed on growth rate and mortality. Gross and histopathological studies of various organs

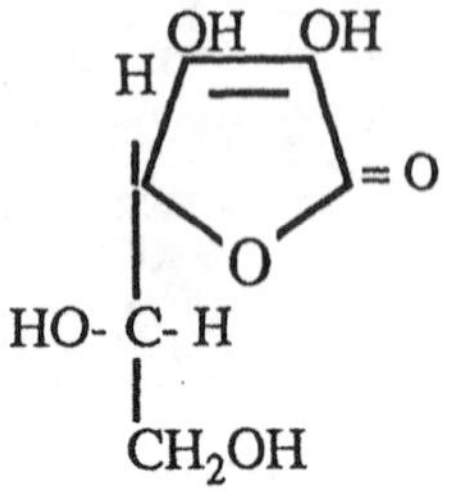

Fig. 18 Erythorbic acid.

revealed no changes (Fitzhugh and Nelson, 1946). In long-term studies in rats fed 1% erythorbic acid, no adverse effects on growth rate or mortality and no histopathological changes were observed (Lehman et al., 1951). In a carcinogenicity test in F344 rats, sodium erythorbate given at levels of 1.25 or 2.5% in drinking water for 104 weeks was not carcinogenic (Abe et al., 1984).

Sodium erythorbate at a 5% level was found to have a promoting effect on the N-butyl-N-4-hydroxy butyl nitrosamine–initiated urinary bladder carcinogenesis in rats. However, when tested alone it was without any effect (Fukushima et al., 1984). Erythorbic acid was weakly positive in the Ames *S. typhimurium* reverse mutation assays with and without metabolic activation. In in vitro assay for chromosomal aberrations in Chinese hamster fibroblast cell lines, erythorbic acid was negative (Ishidate et al., 1984).

B. Chelating Agents

Polyphosphates

Phosphoric acid and its salts are widely used in the food industry as chelating agents, emulsion stabilizers, anticaking agents, and antimicrobial agents. Some of the food products in which phosphates are used include meat products, poultry, cheese, and soft drinks. Phosphoric acid is an essential biological constituent of bone and teeth and also plays an important role in carbohydrate, fat, and protein metabolism. Phosphates used as chelators include sodium and potassium orthophosphates (Na_2HPO_4, NaH_2PO_4, K_2HPO_4, KH_2PO_4), sodium pyrophosphates ($Na_4P_2O_7$, $Na_2P_2H_2O_7$), sodium tripolyphosphate ($Na_5P_3O_{10}$), and sodium hexametaphosphate ($NaPO_3)_n$, of which sodium pyrophosphate and sodium tripolyphosphate are the most effective chelators. Phosphoric acid also functions as a synergist with other antioxidants in vegetable shortenings. The JECFA has allocated an ADI of 0–70 mg/kg bw, which applies to the sum of added phosphate and food phosphate (FAO/WHO, 1974).

Biochemical Studies

The orthophosphates were readily absorbed through the intestinal wall. The pyrophosphates and polyphosphates were converted to monophosphate by an inorganic diphosphatase enzyme before absorption. The hexametaphosphates were more slowly degraded than tripolyphosphates. The degree of hydrolysis and absorption decreased with increase in molecular weight (Gosselin et al., 1952; Ebel, 1958; Grossman and Lang, 1962). The level of inorganic phosphate in the blood was found to be regulated by the action of the parathyroid hormone. This hormone also inhibited the tubular reabsorption of phosphates by the kidneys. Excretion of phosphates was mainly in the feces as calcium phosphate. Hence excessive intake of phosphates may result in a depletion of calcium and bone mass (Ellinger, 1972; FAO/WHO, 1974).

Toxicological Studies

Phosphates in general were without any adverse effects at low dosages. At high levels adverse effects observed were retarded growth, increase in kidney weight, hypertrophy of the parathyroid glands, and metastatic calcification in the soft tissues, especially the kidneys, stomach, and aorta.

Phosphoric Acid. In rats in a 44-day study, phosphoric acid levels of 2.94% caused extensive kidney damage (McKay and Oliver, 1935). At lower levels of 0.75%, phosphoric acid had no adverse effects (Bonting, 1952). Feeding studies in dogs showed that phosphoric acid was well tolerated up to 13 g/day before signs of enterites appeared. In humans, phosphoric acid had no adverse effects up to 26 g/day (Nazario, 1952).

Monosodium Phosphate. In a 42-day study in rats, monosodium phosphate at 3.4 g/kg bw level caused kidney damage (McFarlane, 1941). In guinea pigs, the levels of magnesium and potassium also had a significant effect on the physiological damage by phosphates. Diets containing 0.9% calcium, 1.7% phosphorus, 0.04% magnesium, and 0.41% potassium resulted in a severe reduction in weight gain, stiffness in leg joints, and numerous deposits of calcium phosphates in the footpads. The symptoms were significantly reduced or eliminated when the diet contained 0.35% magnesium and 1.5% potassium with the same levels of phosphorus and calcium.

Disodium and Dipotassium Phosphates. Hahn et al. (1958) reported that in rats disodium phosphate at levels of 1.8, 3, and 5% for 6 months caused extensive physiological damage only at the 3 and 5% levels. Dipotassium phosphate at 0.87 and 5% levels for 150 days had no adverse effects in rats (Dysmsza et al., 1959). In both studies no adverse effects on the levels of iron, calcium, and copper in the blood were observed. In a three-generation study in rats fed diets containing 0.5–5% of a mixture of mono- and disodium phosphates at levels of 1% or more, renal damage and a reduction in growth rate and fertility was observed. A reduction in the life span in the 5% group was also observed (Van Esch et al., 1957).

Pyrophosphates. In rats fed 0.5–5% pyrophosphate for 6 months (Hahn and Seifen, 1959), 4 months (Datta et al., 1962), and in a multigeneration study (Van Esch et al., 1957), 1% or more of the pyrophosphate produced kidney damage and calcification.

Polyphosphates. In rats sodium tripolyphosphate or sodium hexametaphosphate at 3 and 5% for 6 months caused severe kidney damage equivalent to that found when similar amounts of disodium phosphate were fed in the diet, indicating the hydrolysis of polyphosphates to orthophosphates before absorption (Hahn et al., 1958; Hahn and Seifen, 1959). Hodge (unpublished report cited in Ellinger, 1972) found that in dogs 0.1 g/kg bw/day of sodium tripolyphosphate or sodium hexametaphosphate produced no adverse effects. On increasing the dosage to 4 g/kg bw/day over a 5-month feeding period, a reduction in body weight was observed.

Human Studies. Phosphoric acid at levels of 2000–4000 mg for 10 days or 3900 mg for 14 days had no adverse effects on urine composition (Lauersen, 1953). Long-term administration of 5–7000 mg of monosodium phosphate was also without any adverse effects (Lang, 1959). Phosphate-enriched diets (700 mg calcium and 1 g phosphorus/day for 4 weeks followed by 700 mg calcium and 2.1 g phosphorus/day for 4 weeks) resulted in mild diarrhea, soft stools, increase in serum and urinary phosphorus, and a decrease in serum and urinary calcium. An increase in hydroxypyroline and cyclic AMP excretion was also observed (Raines Bell et al., 1977).

Ethylenediaminetetraacetic Acid

Ethylenediaminetetraacetic acid (EDTA) (Fig. 19) and its disodium (Na_2 EDTA) and calcium disodium salts ($CaNa_2$ EDTA) are used as chelating agents in the food

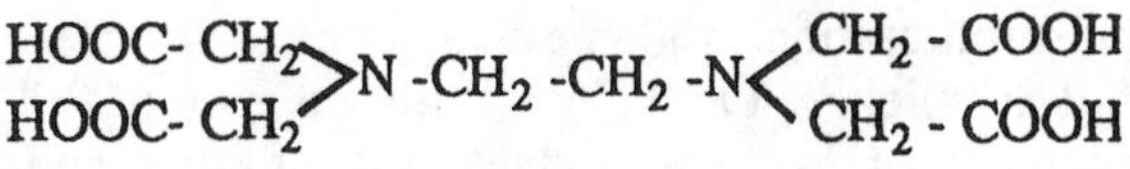

$$\begin{array}{l} \text{HOOC- CH}_2 \\ \text{HOOC- CH}_2 \end{array} \!\!\! >\!\! \text{N -CH}_2\text{ -CH}_2\text{ -N} \!\! <\!\! \begin{array}{l} \text{CH}_2\text{ - COOH} \\ \text{CH}_2\text{ - COOH} \end{array}$$

Fig. 19 Ethylenediaminetetraacetic acid.

industry. They are highly effective in a wide variety of products like fats and oils, salad dressings, sauces, dairy products, meat, processed fruits and vegetables, and fruit juices for the stabilization of vitamin C. EDTA forms stable water-soluble complexes with many di- or polyvalent metal ions. Maximum chelating efficiency occurs at higher pH values where the carboxyl groups are dissociated. EDTA is a white crystalline powder sparingly soluble in water (0.2 g/100 g at 20°C) and insoluble inorganic solvents. The CaNa$_2$ salt is considered as the compound with lowest toxicity, and the JECFA has allocated an ADI of 2.5 mg/kg bw (FAO/WHO, 1974).

Biochemical Studies

Absorption, Metabolism, and Excretion. Absorption studies have been carried out in rats and humans. EDTA was poorly absorbed and rapidly excreted from the body. In rats fed ^{14}C CaNa$_2$ EDTA at doses of 50 mg/kg bw, only 2–4% of the dose was absorbed and 80–90% was excreted in feces within 24 hours (Foreman et al., 1953). In rats given a single oral dose of 95 mg Na$_2$ EDTA, 93% was eliminated in 32 hours. The amount of EDTA recovered was also found to be directly proportional to the dose level, suggesting that EDTA was absorbed from the gastrointestinal tract by passive diffusion (Chan, 1956). The elimination of EDTA from the kidneys was mainly by tubular excretion and glomerular filtration (Foreman et al., 1953). In normal healthy humans given a dose of 1.5 mg of ^{14}C CaNa$_2$ EDTA in a gelatin capsule, only 5% absorption was observed (Foreman and Trujillo, 1954). After an i.v. injection of 3000 mg of ^{14}C CaNa$_2$ EDTA, the compound was almost completely eliminated in 12–16 hours, and only 2.5% of the dose was recovered in the urine (Srbova and Teisinger, 1957).

Reactions of EDTA. EDTA chelates with a number of physiologically important metal ions like calcium, zinc, and iron and may induce essential mineral deficiency. CaNa$_2$ EDTA enhanced the excretion of Zn (Perry and Perry, 1959). EDTA was found to inhibit the activity of a number of heavy metal–containing enzymes because of its metal-chelating capacity. At concentrations of 10^{-3} M, EDTA inhibited aldehyde oxidase and homogentisinase (Westerfield, 1961). Na$_2$EDTA at 5.5×10^{-6} M was a strong inhibitor of γ-amino levulinic acid dehydrogenase (Gibson et al., 1955). At 1722 mg/kg bw, CaNa$_2$ EDTA inhibited alkaline phosphatase in the liver, prostrate, and serum in rats (Nigrovic, 1964).

Toxicological Studies

Acute Toxicity. The acute oral LD$_{50}$ of Na$_2$ EDTA in rats was 2000–2200 mg/kg bw (Yang, 1952) and in rabbits was 2300 mg/kg bw (Shibata, 1956). The acute oral LD$_{50}$ in rats was 10,000 mg/kg bw, in rabbits 7000 mg/kg bw, and in dogs 12,000 mg/kg bw (Oser et al., 1963).

Short-Term Studies. Short-term studies have been conducted in rats, rabbits, and dogs. In rats given 250 or 500 mg/kg bw of CaNa$_2$ EDTA i.p. daily for 21 days, no deleterious changes were observed in weight gain, histology of the liver, lung, spleen, adrenals, small gut, and heart. A moderate renal hydropic change with focal subcapsular swelling and proliferation in glomerular loops at the 500-mg level was observed (Reuber and Schmieller, 1962). In rats i.v. infusion of 0.1 M $CaNa_2$ EDTA at the rate of 6 mmol/kg for 24 hours produced vacuolization and increased lysosomal activity in the kidneys (Braide, 1976). On dietary administration of 0.5 and 1% $CaNa_2$ EDTA for 205 days in rats, no significant effects were observed in weight gain, mortality, and histopathology of the liver, kidney, and spleen. No change in blood coagulation time, total bone ash, and blood calcium levels was observed (Chan, 1956). In rats fed 0.5 and 1% Na_2 EDTA for 6 months with a low-mineral diet, at the 1% level a reduced growth rate in males, lowered blood cell counts, a prolonged blood coagulation time, a slight but significant increase in blood calcium level, lower bone ash levels, considerable erosion of the molars, and diarrhea were observed. Rats fed the same dose of Na_2 EDTA in normal mineral diet showed no dental erosion (Chan, 1956). In another study in rats given i.p. 250, 400, or 500 mg/kg bw of Na_2EDTA for 3–31 days, at the 400- and 500-mg levels all the rats became lethargic and 100% mortality was observed in 9–14 days. Moderate dilatation of the bowel, subserosal hemorrhages, and swollen kidneys were observed. At the 250-mg level one rat showed hemorrhage of the thymus. All the groups showed hydropic necrosis of the renal proximal convoluted tubules with epithelial sloughing. The effects were found to be reversible on cessation of the treatment (Reuber and Schmieller, 1962). The nephrotoxic effects of EDTA were caused mainly by the chelation of metal ions, leading to an alteration of their distribution in the tissue.

In rabbits given 0.1, 1, 10, or 20 mg/kg bw Na_2 EDTA i.v. or orally at 50, 100, 500, and 1000 mg/kg bw for 1 month, all the animals at the highest oral level had severe diarrhea and died. Histopathological studies showed degenerative changes in the liver, kidney, parathyroid, and endocrine glands, and edema in muscles, brain, and heart at all treatment levels (Shibata, 1956). In dogs fed 50, 100, and 250 mg/kg bw of $CaNa_2$ EDTA for 12 months, no adverse effects were observed in survival rate, blood chemistry, and histology of the various organs (Oser et al., 1963).

Long-Term Studies. In rats fed 0.5, 1, and 5% Na_2 EDTA for 2 years, no significant effects on weight gain, blood coagulation time, red blood cell counts, or bone ash was observed. At the 5% level severe diarrhea was observed. No significant changes were observed in gross and microscopic examination of the various organs due to Na_2EDTA (Yang, 1952). In a four-generation study over a period of 2 years in rats fed 50, 125, and 250 mg/kg bw of $CaNa_2$ EDTA, no adverse effects were observed in weight gain, feed efficiency, hemopoiesis, organ weights, and histopathology of various organs. Fertility, lactation, and weaning were not affected (Oser et al., 1963).

Skin Toxicity. EDTA caused acute allergic conjunctivitis and periorbital dermatitis in some cases following the use of eyedrops containing EDTA at a 0.1% level. However, with a 10% aqueous solution of $CaNa_2$ EDTA, no adverse effects were observed (Raymond and Gross, 1969).

Mutagenicity. The genotoxic effect of EDTA has been studied with various test systems, and the subject has been reviewed by Heindorff et al. (1983). EDTA was nonmutagenic in bacterial systems such as *E. coli* and *S. typhimurium* (McCann et al., 1975). EDTA induced inhibition of DNA synthesis in kidney cortex cells (Lieberman and Ove, 1962), in regenerating rat liver cells (Fujioka and Lieberman,

1964), and in phytohemagglutinin-stimulated lymphocytes (Alford, 1970). EDTA also induced dominant lethal mutations in insects such as wasps (LaChance, 1959) and in *Drosophila* (Ondrej, 1965; Baranauskajte et al., 1972). EDTA was positive in tests for chromosomal aberrations in bone marrow cells and splenic cells in mice (Das and Manna, 1972) and also in human leukocytes (Basrur and Baker, 1963). In a bone marrow micronucleus assay, Muralidhara and Narasimhamurthy (1991) reported that oral administration of acute doses of Na_2 EDTA at 5–20 mg/kg bw in mice induced a dose-dependent increase in the incidence of micronucleated polychromatic erythrocytes. EDTA interferes with the DNA repair process that takes place after exposure to mutagens. In Chinese hamster cells and human cell lines, the fast repair component detectable after treatment with ionizing radiation of bleomycin was inhibited by EDTA (Kleijer et al., 1973; Leontjiva et al., 1976; Sognier and Hittelman, 1979). EDTA also had a modulating effect on the mutagenic response of a variety of chemical and physical mutagens in plant and insect systems (Heindorff et al., 1983).

Reproduction. In a reproduction study in rats fed 0.5, 1, and 5% Na_2 EDTA for 12 weeks, rats at the 5% level failed to produce a litter (Yang, 1952). In a teratogenic study rats were injected i.m. 20–40 mg EDTA/day during pregnancy on days 6–8, 10–15, and 16 to the end of pregnancy. At the 40-mg level injected during days 6–8 or 10–15, some dead or malformed fetuses with polydactyly, double tail, generalized edema, or circumscribed edema were observed (Tuchmann-Duplessis and Mercier-Parot, 1956). The adverse effects could be due to the binding of Zn by EDTA, resulting in maternal Zn deficiency, which is known to cause gross congenital malformations in rats. Swernerton and Hurley (1971) reported that when Na_2 EDTA was administered with Zn supplementation, no teratogenic effects were observed in rats.

Tartaric Acid

L-Tartaric acid (2,3-dihydrosuccinic acid) (HOOC—CHOH—CHOH—COOH) occurs naturally in many fruits and is a byproduct of wine making. Tartaric acid and its salts are used as synergists and acidulants in a number of products such as confectionary, bakery products, and soft drinks. Tartaric acid is a colorless, odorless, crystalline solid highly soluble in water. An ADI of 0–30 mg/kg bw (calculated as L-tartaric acid) has been allocated by the JECFA (FAO/WHO, 1974).

Biochemical Studies: Absorption, Metabolism, and Excretion

L-Tartaric acid was almost completely absorbed in the gastrointestinal tract, and significant amounts were metabolized to CO_2 in body tissues. Studies in rats and humans have indicated a species difference in the metabolism. Also, L-tartaric acid, the naturally occurring form of tartaric acid, was eliminated more rapidly compared to the synthetic racemate DL-tartaric acid (Lewis, 1977). Following an oral administration of L-tartaric acid, rats excreted 73% of the dose unchanged in the urine. In humans, 17% of an oral dose was recovered in the urine whereas after a parenteral administration, recovery was almost quantitative. The difference in excretion indicated metabolism of tartaric acid in the intestine, presumably by bacterial action (Finkle, 1933; Gry and Larsen, 1978).

In rats administered single oral doses of ^{14}C monosodium L-tartarate (400 mg/kg bw), excretion in the urine, feces, and expired air within 48 hours was 70, 13.6, and 15.6%, respectively. In i.v. administration the corresponding figures were 81.8, 0.9, and 7.5%, respectively (Chasseaud et al., 1977). In another study in rats ^{14}C monosodium DL-tartarate was administered orally, intraperitoneally, and by direct injection to the cecum. With oral administration, 51% was excreted in the urine and 21% was observed in the expired air. Following i.p. administration 63% of the dose was excreted unchanged in the urine within 24 hours and 9% was excreted as CO_2 in 6 hours. However, after cecal injection less than 2% was excreted in the urine and 67% in the expired air. In humans the major portion of the oral dose was excreted as CO_2 (46%), and only 12% was found in the urine. In i.v. administration 64% was excreted in the urine in 22 hours and 18% was excreted as CO_2 in 8 hours (Chadwick et al., 1978).

Toxicological Studies

Acute Toxicity. In mice the acute oral LD_{50} was 4360 mg/kg bw and in rabbits was approximately 5290 mg/kg bw (Locke et al., 1942).

Short-Term Studies. In short-term studies in dogs fed daily oral doses of 900 mg/kg bw for 90–114 days, blood chemistry remained normal except in one dog in which azotaemia developed resulting in death in 90 days. Weight changes were equivocal. In some cases casts appeared in the urine (Krop and Gold, 1945). In rats fed 7.7% of sodium L-tartarate, no adverse effects were observed (Packman et al., 1963). Renal damage was observed in rabbits and rats only after i.v. administration of L-tartaric acid in doses of 0.2–0.3 g (Bodansky et al., 1942; Gold and Zahm, 1943).

Long-Term Studies. In long-term studies in rats fed 0.1, 0.5, 0.8, and 1% L-tartaric acid for 2 years, no significant effects on growth rate, mortality, gross, and pathological studies of the organs were observed (Fitzhugh and Nelson, 1947). In another long-term study, 21-day-old weanling rats were fed L-tartaric acid at levels of up to 1.2% without any adverse effects (Packman et al., 1963). L-Tartaric acid was not teratogenic in mice, rats, hamsters, or rabbits at levels of 274, 181, 225, and 215 mg/kg bw, respectively (FDA, 1973c).

Citric Acid

Citric acid and its salts are widely used as chelators and acidulants in food industry. Citric acid is used as a synergist both with primary antioxidants and oxygen scavengers at levels of 0.1–0.3% (Fig. 20). In fats and oils, citric acid chelates metal ions at levels of 0.005–0.2% (Dziezak, 1986). Citric acid is widely distributed in plant and animal tissue and is an intermediate in the Krebs cycle. Citric acid is a white, odorless solid highly soluble in water. The potassium and sodium salts have been extensively used in medicine for many years without any adverse effects. The JECFA has allocated an ADI "not limited" for citric acid (FAO/WHO, 1974).

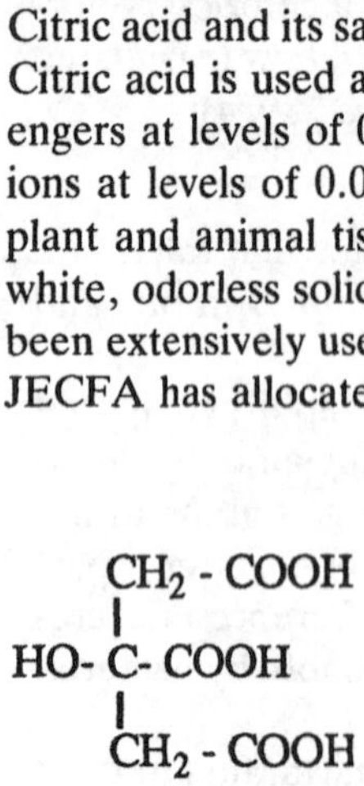

$$CH_2 - COOH$$
$$|$$
$$HO- C- COOH$$
$$|$$
$$CH_2 - COOH$$

Fig. 20 Citric acid.

Citric acid and its salts have been found to have a low order of toxicity. The acute i.p. LD_{50} in mice was 96 mg/kg bw and in rats was 884 mg/kg bw. The acute i.v. (rapid infusion) LD_{50} in mice was 42 mg/kg bw (Gruber and Halbeisen, 1948).

In short-term studies in dogs given daily doses of 1380 mg/kg bw for 112–120 days, no adverse effects were observed (Krop and Gold, 1945). In a two-generation study in rats fed 1.2% citric acid for 90 weeks, no adverse effects in growth rate, blood picture, histopathological studies, and reproduction were observed. In rabbits fed 7.7% sodium citrate for 60 days, no adverse effects were observed in blood or urine chemistry or histological studies (Packman et al., 1963). In humans, both potassium and sodium salts have been used in daily doses of up to 10 g as mild diuretics without any adverse effects (Martindale's Extra Pharmacopoeia, 1972).

Citric acid at high levels was found to have an adverse effect on calcium absorption. Cramer et al. (1956) observed that in rats fed sodium citrate or citric acid in a vitamin D–free diet with low levels of phosphorus, citric acid completely prevented the absorption of calcium. Gomori and Gulyas (1944) observed that in dogs fed 520–1200 mg/kg bw of sodium citrate, urinary calcium levels increased. Gruber and Halbeisen (1948) suggested that the effects of high levels of citric acid resembled symptoms of calcium deficiency. In rats a dose level of 50% resulted in lowered food intake and slight abnormalities in blood chemistry (Horn et al., 1957; Yokotani et al., 1971)

Citrate Esters

Esters of citric acid like isopropyl citrate mixture and stearyl citrate are also used as synergists in food products. Citrate esters are readily soluble in fats and oils from propylene glycol solution concentrates. Formulations containing various mixtures of antioxidants and citrates in propylene glycol are commercially available.

Isopropyl Citrate Mixture

Isopropyl citrate mixture consists of monoisopropyl citrate 27%, diisopropyl citrate 9%, triisopropyl citrate 2%, and mono- and diglycerides 62%. In rats isopropyl citrate mixture is readily absorbed when incorporated in the diet at a 10% level (Calbert et al., 1951). The acute oral LD_{50} in rats was 2800–2250 mg/kg bw and in dogs was 2250 mg/kg bw (Deuel et al., 1951). No deleterious effects were observed in short-term studies in rats (1500–2000 mg/rat/day for 6 weeks), rabbits (3600 mg/rabbit/day for 6 weeks), dogs (0.06% for 6 weeks), and in long-term studies in rats at levels of 0.28, 0.56, and 2.8% for 2 years. Multigeneration studies at levels of 2.8% in the diet in rats also showed no adverse effects (Deuel et al., 1951). However, because of the known toxicity of isopropyl alcohol, and ADI of 0–14 mg/kg bw (calculated as monoisopropyl citrate) has been allocated by the JECFA (FAO/WHO, 1974).

Stearyl Citrate

Stearyl citrate was hydrolyzed readily to stearyl alcohol and citric acid in dogs and to a lesser extent in rats (Calbert et al., 1951). In rats the oral LD_{50} was >5400 mg/kg bw and in dogs was >5600 mg/kg bw (Deuel et al., 1951). In short-term studies in rats at levels of 1.3, 2.5, 5, and 10% for 10 weeks, in rabbits at 2 and 10% for 6 weeks, and in dogs at levels of 3% for 12 weeks, no adverse effects were observed on body weight, growth rate, or histological studies. In a five-generation study in rats at levels of 1.9 and 9.5%, no adverse effects were observed on litter size, fertility, lactation, and growth rate of the progeny (Deuel et al., 1951). Stearyl citrate at levels of 2.5 and 10% reduced the digestibility of fat to 77 and 71%, respectively, in rats. In dogs at a 3% level fat digestibility was reduced to 80% (Calbert et al., 1951). An ADI of 0–50 mg/kg bw has been allocated by the JECFA (FAO/WHO, 1974).

Phytic Acid

Phytic acid (myoinositol hexaphosphoric acid) (Fig. 21) is a major component of all seeds constituting 1–5% by weight of many cereals, nuts, oilseeds, and edible legumes and occurs as a mixture of calcium, magnesium, and potassium salts. Some of the important physiological functions of phytic acid include storage of phosphorus, high-energy phosphate groups, cations, and a cell wall precursor (Graf, 1983). Phytic acid is a potential chelating agent. At low pH it precipitates Fe^{3+} quantitatively. At intermediate and high pH it forms insoluble complexes with all other polyvalent cations. Phytic acid is a potential inhibitor of iron mediated hydroxy radical formation. Hydroxy radical formation requires at least one coordination site that is free or occupied by an easily dissociable group in the iron atom. Iron phytate chelates lack the coordination site and do not support free radical formation (Graf et al., 1984). Phytic acid also prevents browning and putrifaction of fruits and vegetables by inhibiting polyphenol oxidase activity (Graf et al., 1987). Phytic acid is effective in preventing both autoxidation and hydrolysis of soybean oil and stabilizes a number of food products like fish products, lipid containing foods, natural and artificial coloring agents etc. Phytic acid is also effective in removing iron from diluted molasses, wine, and other beverages (Graf, 1983). Phytic acid is used widely in medicine. In countries like Japan it is also used as a food additive. In the United States phytic acid has not been considered for inclusion in the food additive list because of lack of information of its use in food manufacture (*Federal Register*, 1982).

Biochemical Studies

Phytic acid undergoes hydrolysis in the gastrointestinal tract to form inositol and orthophosphate mainly by the action of the enzyme phytase. Phytases are widely distributed in plants, animals, and fungi (Cosgrove, 1966). Phytases have been isolated and characterized in rats, calves, and humans (Bitar and Reinhold, 1972). In humans the hydrolysis of phytates occurs most probably by microbial phytases or by nonenzymatic cleavage (Hegsted et al., 1954; Subrahmanyan et al., 1955). Nearly 61 and 39% of the ingested phytate was hydrolyzed in weanling and mature

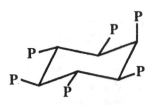

$P : H_2PO_4$

Fig. 21   Phytic acid.

rats, respectively (Nelson and Kirby, 1979). In humans nearly 85% of the ingested phytic acid was hydrolyzed (Subrahmanyan et al., 1955).

Phytic acid forms insoluble complexes with a number of essential minerals like calcium, iron, and zinc, decreasing their bioavailability and resulting in mineral deficiency in humans (Graf, 1983). Phytic acid also precipitates most proteins at low pH in the absence of cations and at high pH in the presence of cations forming a ternary protein, metal, and phytate complex (Okubo et al., 1976). Phytic acid inhibits trypsin (Singh and Krikorian, 1982) and binds to hemoglobin, thereby reducing its affinity for O_2 or CO (Benesch and Benesch, 1974; Isaacks et al., 1977). The nutritional implications of phytic acid have been exhaustively reviewed (Erdman, 1979; Cheryan, 1980; Reddy et al., 1982).

Toxicological Studies

Toxicological studies have been done in recent years, with just one-long term study and a subacute study in rats. The LD_{50} in rats calculated by the moving average method was 450–500 mg/kg bw for males and 480 mg/kg bw for females (Ichikawa et al., 1987).

In a subacute study in F344 rats, phytic acid administered at levels of 0.6, 1.25, 2.5, 5, or 10% in drinking water for 12 weeks resulted in high mortality at 5 and 10% levels. In the 1.25 and 2.5% groups, the reduction in body weight was less than 10% compared to the control. In a 100- to 108-week study at dose levels of 1.25 and 2.5%, a 50% mortality was observed in females at the 2.5 level. Mean final body weights were significantly lower at both dose levels, the effect being more marked in females. No significant differences in hematology or clinical chemistry values or relative organ weights were observed. Necrosis and calcification of the renal papillae were observed in both dose levels, the incidence being higher in females. In males hyperplasia of the renal pelvis at higher doses was significantly higher than that in controls (Hiasa et al., 1992).

In a teratogenicity study in mice, pregnant mice were given orally 1.6, 3.1, and 6.3% phytic acid in aqueous solution on day 7 through day 15 of gestation. Although no clear teratogenic effects were observed with external or skeletal malformations, the incidence of late resorbed fetuses increased in the 6.3% group (Ogata et al., 1987).

Lecithin

Lecithin (Phosphatidyl choline) is a naturally occurring phospholipid and makes up 1–2% of many crude vegetable oils and animal fats. The commercial source of lecithin is predominantly soybeans. Commercial lecithin is a mixture of phospholipids and contains phosphatidyl ethanolamine and phosphatidyl inositol in addition to lecithin. Structurally lecithin is a mixture of the diglycerides of the stearic, palmitic, and oleic acids combined with the choline ester of phosphoric acid (Fig. 22). Lecithin functions as a potent synergist in fats and oils with a range of primary antioxidants and oxygen scavengers at elevated temperatures above 80°C. Lecithin is more effective at lower concentrations of the antioxidant. Lecithin was found to be highly effective in ternary mixtures with vitamin E and vitamin C, to such an extent that the induction times in oils were extended about 25-fold for 500 ppm of vitamin E and 1000 ppm of vitamin C (Loliger, 1991). Similar effects have been observed in mixtures comprising of ascorbyl palmitate, α-tocopherol, and lecithin

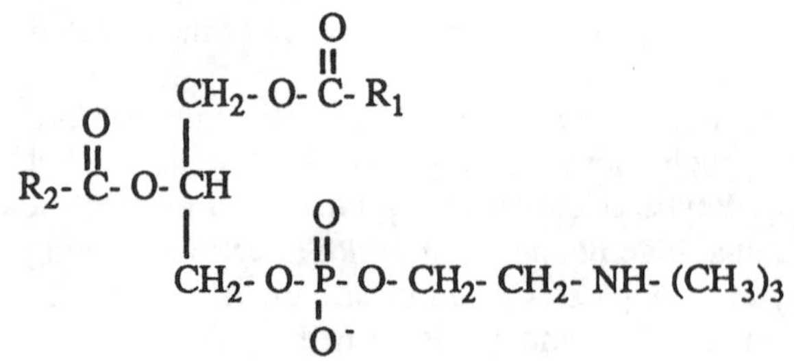

$$
\begin{array}{c}
\text{O} \\
\parallel \\
R_2\text{-}\overset{\text{O}}{\overset{\parallel}{\text{C}}}\text{-O-}\,\underset{\displaystyle |}{\overset{\displaystyle \text{CH}_2\text{-O-}\overset{\text{O}}{\overset{\parallel}{\text{C}}}\text{-R}_1}{\text{CH}}}
\end{array}
$$

CH$_2$-O- P- O- CH$_2$- CH$_2$- NH- (CH$_3$)$_3$

R1, R2 : Hydrocarbon side chains.

Fig. 22 Lecithin.

(Hudson and Ghavami, 1984). However, the mechanism of action of lecithin is not clear. It is postulated that in ternary mixtures the regeneration of vitamin E by ascorbic acid or ascorbyl palmitate is mediated by lecithin (Tappel, 1968; Loliger, 1991). Phosphatidyl ethanolamine is also highly effective as a synergist. Phosphatidyl serine is less effective, and phosphatidyl inositol has no synergistic effect (Dziedzic and Hudson, 1984). An ADI of "not limited" has been allocated by the JECFA (FAO/WHO, 1974).

No information on the acute toxicity of lecithin is available in literature. In cats rapid infusion of a 1.2% egg yolk phosphatide emulsion containing 5% glucose had no adverse effects. A rapid infusion of soybean phosphatides caused a fall in blood pressure with apnea (Schuberth and Wretlind, 1961). In humans, administration of large doses of 25–40 g/day for some months resulted in a lowering of serum cholesterol (Merrill, 1959). Although no conventional toxicological studies have been carried out, lecithin is considered as a nontoxic substance based on extensive nutritional and clinical experience in humans.

C. Secondary Antioxidants

Thiodipropionic Acid and Dilauryl, Distearyl Esters

Thiodipropionic acid (TDPA), dilauryl thiodipropionate (DLTDP), and distearyl thiodipropionate (DSTDP) (Fig. 23) are generally regarded as secondary antioxidants or synergists. Free TDPA has the ability to chelate metal ions (Schwab et al., 1953) and also functions as a sulfide, decomposing alkyl hydroperoxides into more stable compounds. In model systems containing performic acid, nonanal, ethyl oleate, or cholesterol, Karahadian and Lindsay (1988) observed that DLTDP was preferentially oxidized to sulfoxide and prevented the formation of nonanoic acid, 9-epoxy oleate, and 5-6-epoxy cholesterol, respectively. Though TDPA and its salts have been approved for food use, they are not being used as direct additives in food products. The JECFA has allocated an ADI of 0–3 mg/kg bw. This evaluation is largely based on the toxicological studies of Lehman et al. (1951).

Biochemical Studies: Absorption, Metabolism, and Excretion

In rats, single oral doses of ^{14}C TDPA in the range 241–650 mg/kg bw were almost completely absorbed from the gastrointestinal tract and rapidly eliminated. During

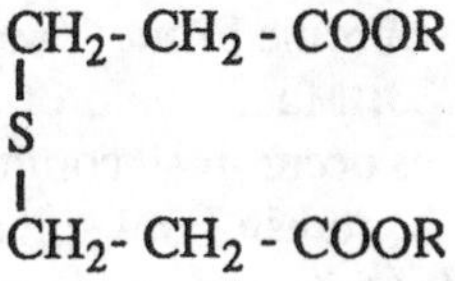

$$CH_2\text{-}CH_2\text{-}COOR$$
$$|$$
$$S$$
$$|$$
$$CH_2\text{-}CH_2\text{-}COOR$$

R : - H   thiodipropionic acid

  - $(CH_2)_{11}$ -CH_3 dilauryl ester

  - $(CH_2)_{17}$ -CH_3 distearyl ester

Fig. 23 Thiodipropionic acid and esters.

a period of 4 days 87–95% of the total dose was recovered, 78–88% in the urine, 0.1–0.9% in the feces, and 3–8% as CO_2. TDPA was excreted in urine either largely unchanged or as an acid-labile conjugate, which was not a glucuronide. Single oral doses of ^{14}C DLTDP (107–208 mg/kg bw) were completely absorbed and rapidly eliminated, mostly in the urine (85–88%), with just 1.8–3.5% in the feces and 3–4% as CO_2. TDPA and a acid-labile conjugate were the metabolites in the urine indicating the hydrolysis of DLTDP (Reynolds et al., 1974).

Toxicological Studies

Acute Toxicity.   The acute oral, i.p., and i.v. LD_{50} of TDPA in mg/kg bw in mice was 2000, 250, and 175, respectively, and in rats it was 3000, 500, and >300, respectively. The acute oral and i.p. LD_{50} of DLTDP in mice was >2000 mg/kg bw, and in rats acute oral LD_{50} was >2500 mg/kg bw. The acute oral and i.p. LD_{50} of DSTDP in mice was >2000 mg/kg bw, and in rats acute oral LD_{50} was >2500 mg/kg bw (Lehman et al., 1951).

Short-Term/Long-Term Studies.   In short-term studies in rats (3% for 120 days), guinea pigs (0.5% for 120 days), and dogs (0.1 and 3% for 100 days), no adverse effects were observed with TDPA and DLTDP. In long-term studies in rats fed TDPA or its esters at levels of 0.5, 1, and 3% for 2 years, no discernable adverse effects were observed as determined by growth rate, mortality, and pathological examination (Lehman et al., 1951).

D. Miscellaneous Antioxidants

Nitrates and Nitrites

Sodium nitrate ($NaNO_3$) and sodium nitrite ($NaNO_2$) are widely used in meat curing and fish products. Some of the important functions of these compounds include formation of a stable color pigment nitrosylmyoglobin by reacting with myoglobin, texture improvement, cured meat flavor formation, and antimicrobial and antioxidant activities. It is postulated that nitrites and nitrates probably function as antioxidants by converting heme proteins to inactive nitric oxide forms and by chelating metal ions, especially nonheme iron, copper, and cobalt present in meat. Both heme proteins and metal ions have been implicated as major prooxidants in meat system. Nitrosylmyoglobin also reacts with peroxy radicals terminating the oxidative chain reaction. On heating, the stable nitrosylhemochrome formed blocks the release of heme iron (Waters, 1971; Kanner et al., 1980; MacDonald et al., 1980; Morrissey and Tichivangana, 1985). Nitrates and nitrites occur in all common food products. Certain vegetables like beets, celery, lettuce, radish, and spinach tend to accumulate more nitrates. The use of nitrates and nitrites has become a controversial issue because of their involvement in the formation of nitrosamines in situ in the food or in the body. Nitrosamines are powerful carcinogens, mutagens, and also have embryopathic and teratogenic properties (Magee, 1971). The JECFA has allocated an ADI of 0–5 mg/kg bw for sodium nitrate and a temporary ADI of 0–0.2 mg/kg bw for sodium nitrite (FAO/WHO, 1974).

Biochemical Studies: Absorption, Metabolism, and Excretion

Nitrates were readily absorbed and almost completely eliminated unchanged. A small amount of the nitrates was converted to nitrite by bacterial action in the gastrointestinal tract (Bradley et al., 1939; Kuebler, 1958). In humans, approximately 20% of the salivary nitrate was reduced by bacterial action to nitrite (Spiegelhalder et al., 1976; Mirvish, 1983). Nitrates inhibit the uptake of iodine by the thyroid gland in rats and sheep (Wyngaarden et al., 1953; Reid et al., 1969), which results in an interference in vitamin A formation from β-carotene, vitamin A deficiency, and lower liver stores (Emerick and Olson, 1962).

Nitrites were also readily absorbed from the gastrointestinal tract. Of the absorbed nitrite, 30–40% was excreted unchanged in the urine, but the fate of 60–70% was not clear. Some of the important reactions of nitrites include conversion of myoglobin to nitrosomyoglobin and hemoglobin to methemoglobin, degradation of β-carotene under acidic conditions, and formation of dialkyl, acylalkyl nitrosamines, and nitrosoguanidines with secondary amines (Lehman, 1958; Emerick and Olson, 1962; Sander and Seif, 1969; Sen et al., 1969).

Toxicological Studies

Acute Toxicity. The acute oral LD_{50} of sodium nitrate in rats was 3236 mg/kg bw (FAO/WHO, 1974). The acute oral LD_{50} of sodium nitrite in mice was 220 mg/kg bw and in rats was 85 mg/kg bw (Greenberg et al., 1945).

Short-Term Studies. In short-term studies in dogs fed 2% sodium nitrate for 105 and 125 days, no adverse effects were observed (Lehman, 1958). In cattle a level of 1.5% potassium nitrate in the forage caused all symptoms of nitrate poisoning (Bradley et al., 1939).

In rats given 100, 300, and 2000 mg/L of sodium nitrite in drinking water for 60 days, abnormalities in EEG was observed at all dose levels (Gruener and Shuval, 1973). At levels of 170 and 340 mg/kg bw/day for 200 days, methemoglobinemia, raised hematocrit, increased spleen weights in females, increased heart weight in males, and increase in kidney weights in both sexes were observed (Musil, 1966). In mice given sodium nitrite in drinking water at levels of 100, 1000, 1500, and 2000 mg/L drinking water, a reduction in motor activity was observed at higher dose levels (Gruener and Shuval, 1973).

Long-Term/Carcinogenicity Studies. In rats fed sodium nitrate at levels of 0.1, 1, 5, and 10% for 2 years, no adverse effects were observed except for a slight reduction in growth rate at the 5 and 10% levels (Rosenfield and Huston, 1950). Sodium nitrite at low levels was without any adverse effects. In a long-term study with canned meat (40% of the diet) treated with 0.5 or 0.02% sodium nitrite and glucono-δ-lactone, no adverse effects were observed in hematology, histopathology, and clinical biochemistry. No evidence of any preneoplastic change or tumor formation was observed (Van Logten et al., 1972). In a three-generation study with 100 mg/kg bw in rats, no adverse effects were observed (Lehman, 1958). At high doses sodium nitrite has been reported to cause stomach and esophageal cancer. Newberne (1979) reported an increased incidence of lymphoma in rats fed 250–2000 ppm of nitrite in food or water. In another study Shank and Newberne (1976) reported that in rats and hamsters, nitrites in combination with N-nitrosomorpholine, a cyclic amine, induced a dose-related hepatocellular carcinoma and angiosarcoma. N-Nitrosomorpholine is an anticorrosive agent and an unintentional additive to foods such as canned ham. Nitrite alone caused lymphoreticular tumors. Incidence of lung adenomas by morpholine and high levels of sodium nitrite in mice has also been reported (Greenblatt et al., 1971).

Reproduction. Sodium nitrite was found to have an adverse effect on reproduction. In a reproduction study in rats sodium nitrite at levels of 2000 or 3000 mg/L resulted in mortality of the newborn and also maternal anemia (Gruener and Shuval, 1973). In guinea pigs fed 0.03–1% sodium nitrite, no live births were observed at or above the 0.5% level. Maternal deaths, abortions, fetal resorptions, mummification, placental lesions, and inflammation of the uterus were observed (Sleight and Atallah, 1968). In cattle, sodium nitrite at levels to produce 40–50% methemoglobinemia caused no adverse effects (Winter and Hokanson, 1964). Sodium nitrate had no adverse effects on reproduction in guinea pigs (Sleight and Atallah, 1968) and in cattle (Winter and Hokanson, 1964).

Amino Acids

Amino acids are effective both as primary antioxidants and as synergists (Bishov and Henick, 1975). At lower concentrations most of the amino acids have antioxidant properties, but at higher concentrations they function as prooxidants (Marcuse, 1962). Also, at low pH most of the amino acids are prooxidants, while higher pH favors antioxidant activity. Glycine, tryptophan, methionine, histidine, proline, and lysine have been found to be effective in fats and oils. Glycine has been listed as a GRAS substance for addition to fats and oils up to 0.01%. Covalent attachment of tryptophan, cystine, methionine, and histidine significantly enhanced the antioxidant action of Trolox-C, a synthetic analog of α-tocophero (Taylor et al., 1981).

Excessive intake of amino acids has been reported to cause a reduction in growth rate, feed intake, and survival rate in rats. In a 3-week study in weanling rats at diet levels of 1–10% of 17 different amino acids, Daniel and Waisman (1968) found methionine, cystine, phenylalanine, and tryptophan to be highly toxic, histidine, tyrosine, and lysine to be toxic, glycine, proline, valine, and arginine to be slightly toxic, and serine, aspartic acid, glutamic acid, isoleucine, leucine, and alanine to be nontoxic at all levels tested. Similar results were obtained when the amino acids were given i.p. in three daily doses of 25–350 mg/55 g rat. In studies in rats fed 5% glycine, reduced weight gain and the ability to use food, reduction in the activity of certain enzymes (e.g., transaminase), and increased plasma cholesterol level were observed (Anonymous, 1971).

Spice Extracts

Spice extracts form a potential source of naturally occurring antioxidants. Spice extracts are effective in fats, meat products, and baked goods. The subject has been reviewed by Pruthi (1980). Chipault et al. (1952) examined 78 samples representing 36 spices for their antioxidant properties and observed that rosemary and sage exhibited pronounced antioxidant properties in lard. Vanillin, used extensively as a food-flavoring agent, has potent antioxidant properties even in dry mixes like rice flakes (Burri et al., 1989). Eugenol, the major flavor compound in cloves, and curcumin, the major pigment in turmeric, also have antioxidant properties (Cort, 1974b). Spice extracts find limited use as antioxidants only in products compatible with the specific spice flavor because of their color, odor, and taste.

Rosemary (*Rosmarinus officinalis* L. family Labiatae) is generally recognized as the most potent antioxidant spice. Industrial processes have been developed to produce a purified antioxidant that is bland, odorless, and tasteless (Chang et al., 1977; Bracco et al., 1981). Rosemary antioxidant is available commercially as a fine powder soluble in fats and oils and insoluble in water. Rosemary antioxidant is recommended for use at 200–1000 mg/kg of the food product to be stabilized. Approximately 90% of the antioxidant activity in rosemary extract has been attributed to carnosol, a phenolic diteprene. Other active molecules so far identified are rosmarinic acid, carnosic acid, and rosmaridiphenol (Houlihan et al., 1985; Loliger, 1991). No toxicological or biochemical information is available on rosemary antioxidant.

Flavonoids

Flavonoids form a group of naturally occurring phenolics widespread in common edible plants. The estimated daily intake of flavonoids is nearly 1 g/day in western diets (Kuhnau, 1976). Quercetin and rutin were found to be very effective as antioxidants in fats and oils (Whittern et al., 1984). Flavonoids function both as primary antioxidants and as chelators. Flavonoids are effective in milk, lard, and butter in combination with synergists such as citric acid and ascorbic acid. At present, flavonoids are not being used commercially due to insufficient or in some instances adverse toxicological information.

Flavonoids in general were poorly absorbed in the gastrointestinal tract in mammalian systems (Gugler et al., 1975), efficiently metabolized, and eliminated (Ueno et al., 1983). They also undergo extensive microbial degradation to form inactive derivatives in the large bowel (Simpson et al., 1969; Griffiths and Smith, 1972). In a carcinogenicity bioassay in mice, rats, and hamsters, quercetin was negative even at high doses of 10% in the diet (Saito et al., 1980; Hirono et al., 1981; Hosaka and Hirono, 1981; Morino et al., 1982). However, in another study in rats, quercetin at a 0.1% level for 1 year caused intestinal and bladder cancer (Pamukçu et al., 1980). Quercetin was found to be a potent mutagen in a number of in vitro systems and a weak mutagen in in vivo systems (Sahu et al., 1981; MacGregor et al., 1983). Ahmed et al. (1992) in a recent report observed that several flavonoids including quercetin and rutin caused DNA strand scission in the presence of copper.

Vitamin A

Vitamin A or all-*trans*-retinol (Fig. 24) has very limited use as an antioxidant because of its high susceptibility to oxidation on exposure to air and light, conditions under which vitamin A becomes prooxidant. However, retinol was found to be effective in fats and oils when kept in the dark. Retinol also inhibited the formation of free acids in vegetable oils. Structurally retinol consists of a β-ionine ring and a 8 carbon polyene side chain. Retinol occurs widely in all animal tissues, mainly in the liver and also in eggs and milk. In nature, retinol occurs as the ester of acetate or palmitate. In the liver, palmitate is the primary storage form of vitamin A. Retinol is soluble in fats and oils and insoluble in water. The recommended daily intake is 750 mg/kg bw (FAO/WHO, 1967).

Biochemical Studies

In the intestinal mucosa, dietary retinol was esterified with long-chain fatty acids, incorporated into chylomicra and transported via the lymphatic system to the liver (Goodman et al., 1965, 1966). Retinol was mobilized from the liver and delivered to various organs in bound form to a specific retinol-binding protein. The major metabolite of retinol was retinoic acid. Retinoic acid was excreted in the urine either as free acid or as a glucuronide conjugate. Other metabolites have not been characterized (Frolik, 1984).

Toxicological Studies

The preclinical and clinical toxicity of vitamin A has been reviewed by Kamm et al. (1984). The acute oral LD_{50} in mice was 1510–2570 mg/kg bw (Kamm, 1982). In rodents in general, signs of hypervitaminosis A have been associated with anorexia, weight loss, hair loss, emaciation, anemia, spontaneous fractures due to the destruction of bone matrix, and extensive hemorrhages. Some of the effects on internal organs include fatty infiltration of the liver, testicular hypertrophy, and fatty changes in the heart and kidney (Kamm et al., 1984). Bone toxicity of vitamin A has also been reported in dogs (Maddock et al., 1949), cats (Seawright et al., 1967), calves (Grey et al., 1965), and hogs (Wolke et al., 1968). Retinol was nonmutagenic in the Ames test (Kamm, 1982) and also did not induce sister chromatid exchanges in Chinese hamster ovary cells (Huang et al., 1982).

High intakes of retinol have also been associated with adverse effects on reproduction like testicular changes and inhibition of ovulating activity in rats (Gellert, 1977; Lamano-Carvalho et al., 1978). High doses of retinol has been reported to be teratogenic in a number of species including mice, hamsters, dogs, pigs, monkeys, and humans. More than 70 types of abnormalities affecting almost every organ or tissue system have been reported. The teratogenic effects of retinol were

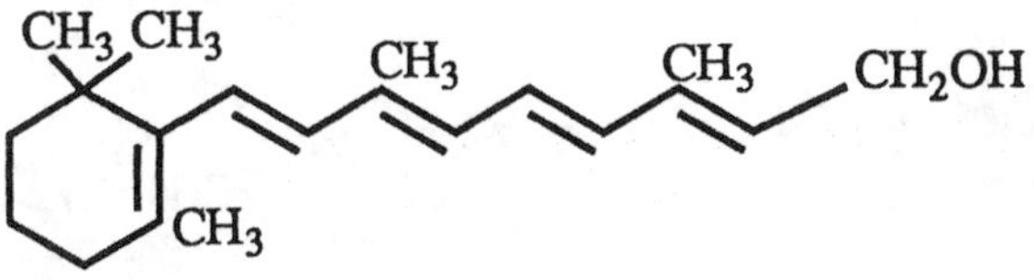

Fig. 24 Vitamin A.

mainly due to the major metabolite retinoic acid, a potent teratogen (Shenefelt, 1972; Geelen, 1979; Rosa et al., 1986).

In humans, the symptoms of hypervitaminosis A include skin scaling, tenderness of bones, headache, anorexia, weight loss, general fatigue, edema, and hemorrhage. Most of the symptoms disappeared on discontinuing vitamin A except for the changes in bones, which took a longer time for reversal (Toomey and Morissette, 1947; Pease, 1962; Koerner and Voellm, 1975).

β-*Carotene*

β-Carotene (provitamin A) (Fig. 25) is mainly used as a food colorant. β-Carotene and related carotenoids are effective quenchers of singlet oxygen (Foote and Denny, 1968; Terao, 1989) and can act as antioxidants by preventing the formation of hydroperoxides (Gordon, 1990). Structurally, β-carotene consists of two β-ionine rings and a 18-carbon polyene side chain. The antioxidant action is limited to low oxygen partial pressures less than 150 mm Hg, and at higher oxygen pressures β-carotene may become prooxidant. β-Carotene occurs widely as a lipoprotein complex in all green parts of plants. It is found in abundance in carrots, some tropical fruits like papayas and mangoes, and all dark green leafy vegetables. β-Carotene and related carotenoids have also been chemically synthesized. β-Carotene has the highest provitamin A activity of all carotenoids. β-Carotene is insoluble in water and slightly soluble in vegetable oils. It is very sensitive to oxidative decomposition when exposed to air or light. An ADI of 0–5 mg/kg bw has been allocated by the JECFA (FAO/WHO, 1975).

Biochemical Studies

In humans, 10–41% of an ingested dose of β-carotene was absorbed and 30–90% was excreted in the feces (Kuebler, 1963). β-Carotene was cleaved by β-carotene-15,15'-oxygenase in the intestine and liver to two molecules of retinaldehyde in the presence of oxygen (Goodman and Huang, 1965). In the intestinal mucosa, liver, and eye, retinaldehyde was reduced to retinol by retinaldehyde reductase (Olson, 1961; Zachman and Olson, 1961; Huang and Goodman, 1965; Blaner and Churchich, 1980).

Toxicological Studies

β-Carotene was not toxic to rats, dogs, and humans. The acute oral LD_{50} in dogs was >8000 mg/kg bw (Nieman and Klein Obbink, 1954) and in rats was >1000 mg/bw (Zbinden and Studer, 1958). Doses of 100 mg β-carotene/kg bw 5 days a week for 13 weeks had no significant effect on growth rate and also no evidence for toxicity was observed in dogs. In a four-generation study in rats fed 0.1% β-carotene for 110 weeks, no adverse effects were observed (Zbinden and Studer,

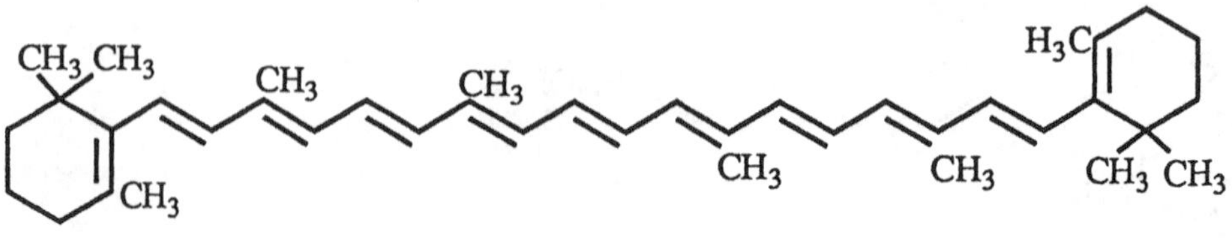

Fig. 25 β-Carotene.

1958; Bagdon et al., 1960). In humans administered 100,000 units of β-carotene/day for 3 months, no signs of vitamin A toxicity were observed (Greenberg et al., 1959).

Tea Extracts

Tea extracts form a potential source of natural antioxidants for food products. Extracts of black tea and green tea were found to be highly effective in fats and oils (Lee and Sher, 1984; Mai et al., 1985). The polyphenols present in tea have antioxidant properties.

The acute oral and i.p. LD_{50} in mice was 10g and 0.7g respectively. In subchronic tests in rats at levels as high as 1000 mg/kg bw, growth rate, feed efficiency, and protein efficiency ratio were not affected. No adverse effects were observed in hematological analysis, gross and microscopic examination of the organs, and litter size (Lee et al., 1984).

VI. TOXICOLOGICAL IMPLICATIONS ASSOCIATED WITH LEACHING OF ANTIOXIDANTS FROM PLASTICS USED IN FOOD PACKAGING

In recent years the possible health hazards associated with the migration of additives from food-packaging materials have attracted a lot of attention. Efforts are being made to assess the significance of migration of various additives and their decomposition products into food system. Plastics are extensively used as films, containers, and coating materials for packaging food products. Some of the commonly used plastics include high density, low density polyethylenes, polypropylenes, polyvinyl chloride, polystyrenes, and copolymers of ethylene and vinyl acetate. Apart from high molecular weight polymers, plastics also contain a number of low molecular weight additives like antioxidants, heat stabilizers, UV absorbers, and plasticizers. The additives are added either during the processing and fabrication stages as processing aids or as end product use additives after molding. Most of the additives have a high mobility in the polymer materials and are readily leached from the polymer into the food product.

Polymers undergo oxidative degradation at all stages of fabrication in the presence of oxygen and also during long-term storage. The process of oxidation involves the formation of polymer hydroperoxides, which decompose to form reactive hydroxy radicals, thus initiating a chain reaction in the polymer. Antioxidants are used to remove the hydroperoxides formed or retard their decomposition (preventive antioxidants) and also to remove the reactive radicals formed (chain-breaking antioxidants). Preventive antioxidants include phosphite esters, sulfides, and dithiophosphates. Chain-breaking antioxidants include aromatic amines, hindered phenols, quinones, and nitro compounds. Antioxidants are usually incorporated in the range of 0.1–0.5% by weight of the polymer (Al-Malaika, 1991). Phenolic antioxidants like BHA and BHT are also commonly added by spray or roll coat application to films or dissolved in paraffin wax used for coating containers. High-fat candies, bakery products, and dry breakfast cereals are some applications in which antioxidant-treated packaging material is used.

Al-Malaika (1991) has reviewed the effect of some of the parameters on the leaching of antioxidants in the human environment. Migration of antioxidants from the packaging material to food product is determined by the interaction of a number of physical and chemical parameters like the nature of the polymer and the food product, molecular weight, volatility, and solubility of the antioxidant, temperature, light, irradiation, and time of contact with the food product. Migration studies have been conducted in food systems and also in food-simulating model systems. In a study on the migration of Irganox-1010, a complex high molecular weight antioxidant, Schwope et al. (1987a) observed that the antioxidant migrated rapidly from ethylene vinyl acetate films into n-heptane, 100% ethanol, and corn oil as compared to low-density polyethylene films. In aqueous media, little migration of the antioxidant was observed from ethylene vinyl acetate films, whereas the migration from low-density polyethylene films was relatively high. Chang et al. (1982) reported similar findings with BHT, a low molecular weight volatile compound compared to Irganox-1010. In another study comparing the migration of BHT and Irganox-1010 from low-density polyethylene films, Schwope et al. (1987b) observed that BHT migrated more rapidly compared to Irganox-1010. Figge (1972) observed that higher temperatures increased the migration of Ionox-330 from high-density polyethylenes, polyvinyl chloride, or polystyrene films. γ-Irradiation resulted in a 30% loss of Irganox-1010 and Irgafos-168, an arylphosphite antioxidant, in a range of polymers like polyvinyl chloride, polyethylenes, and polypropylenes. Little of Irgafos-168 remained after a dose of 10 kGy, but its triarylphosphate oxidation product was found in the extracts of the irradiated polymer. With increasing irradiation Irganox-1010 showed no increase in migration into aqueous-based food simulants and a decrease in migration into a fatty food simulant (Allen et al., 1988). Antioxidants used in plastics are extensively tested for toxicity like other food additives before being accepted for incorporation into food-packaging materials. However, very little attention has been paid to the assessment of health risks presented by the chemical transformation products formed during processing (Al-Malaika, 1991). Further work is required to elucidate the biotransformation, metabolism, and toxicity of these indirect food additives.

ACKNOWLEDGMENTS

The senior author wishes to thank Dr. Charles E. Carpenter, Assistant Professor, Department of Nutrition and Food Sciences, Utah State University, and Dr. Vishwasrao M. Ghorpade, Research Associate, Industrial Agricultural Products Center, University of Nebraska, for their constant encouragement and support during the preparation of this manuscript.

REFERENCES

Abdo, K. M., Huff, J. E., Haseman, J. K., and Alden, C. J. (1968a). No evidence of carcinogenicity of D-mannitol and propyl gallate in F344 rats or B6C3F1 mice. *Food Chem. Toxicol. 24*:1091–1097.

Abdo, K. M., Rao, G., Montgomery, C. A., Dinowitz, M., and Kanagalingam, K. (1986b). Thirteen-week toxicity study of a d-α-tocopheryl acetate (vitamin E) in Fischer 344 rats. *Food Chem. Toxicol. 24*:1043–1050.

Abe, I., Saito, S., Hori, K., Suzuki, M., and Sato, H. (1984). Sodium erythorbate is not carcinogenic in F344 rats. *Exp. Mol. Pathol. 41*:35–43.

Abe, S., and Sasaki, M. (1977). Chromosome aberrations and sister chromatid exchanges in Chinese hamster cells exposed to various chemicals. *J. Natl. Cancer Inst. 58*:1635–1640.

Adamson, I. Y. R., Bowden, D. H., Cote, M. G., and Witschi, H. P. (1977). Lung injury induced by butylated hydroxytoluene. Cytodynamic and biochemical studies in mice. *Lab. Invest. 36*:26–32.

Addis, P. B. (1986). Occurrence of lipid oxidation products in foods. *Food Chem. Toxicol. 24*:1021–1030.

Addis, P. B., and Warner, G. J. (1991). The potential health aspects of lipid oxidation products in foods. In *Free Radicals and Food Additives*, Arouma, O. I. and Halliwell, B. (eds.). Taylor and Francis, London, pp. 77–120.

Addis, P. B., Csallany, A. S., and Kindom, S. E. (1983). Some lipid oxidation products as xenobiotics. In *Xenobiotics in Foods and Feeds*, Finley, J. W. and Schwass, D. E. (eds.). ACS Symposium Series 234, American Chemical Society, Washington, D.C. pp. 85–98.

Aeling, J. L., Panagotacos, P. J., and Andreozzi, R. J. (1973). Allergic contact dermatitis to vitamin E aerosol deodorant. *Arch. Dermatol. 108*:579–580.

Ahmad, S. M., Fazal, F., Rahman, A., Hadi, S. M., and Parish, J. H. (1992). Activities of flavonoids for the cleavage of DNA in the presence of Cu (II): correlation with generation of active oxygen species. *Carcinogenesis 13*:605–608.

Akagi, M., and Aoki, I. (1962a). Studies on food additives. VI. Metabolism of 2,6-di-tert-butyl phenol (BHT) in a rabbit. (1) Determination and paper chromatography of a metabolite. *Chem. Pharm. Bull. 10*:101–105.

Akagi, M., and Aoki, I. (1962b). Studies on food additives. VIII. Metabolism of α-hydroxy 2,6-di-tert-butyl-*p*-cresol. Isolation of metabolites. *Chem. Pharm. Bull. 10*:200–204.

Al-Malaika, S. (1991). Toxicological implications associated with loss of antioxidants from plastics for use in food packaging applications. In *Free Radicals and Food Additives*, Arouma, O. I. and Halliwell, B. (eds.). Taylor and Francis, London, pp. 151–172.

Alford, R. H. (1970). Metal cation requirements for phytohemagglutinin induced transformation of human peripheral blood lymphocytes. *J. Immunol. 104*:698–703.

Allen, D. W., Leathard, D. A., Smith, C., and McGuinness, J. D. (1988). The effects of gamma irradiation on the fate of polymer additives and the implications for migration from plastic food contact materials. *Food Addit. Contam. 5*:433–435.

Allen, J. R. (1976). Long-term antioxidant exposure effects on female primates. *Arch. Environ. Health 31*:47–50.

Allen, J. R., and Engblom, J. F. (1972). Ultrastructural and biochemical changes in the liver of monkey given butylated hydroxyanisole and butylated hydroxytoluene. *Food Cosmet. Toxicol. 10*:769–779.

Allen, S. C., and DeEds, F. D. (1951). The chronic toxicity of lauryl gallate. *J. Am. Oil Chem. Soc. 28*:304–306.

Alleva, F. R., Alleva, J. J., and Balazs, T. (1976). Effect of large daily doses of ascorbic acid on pregnancy in guinea pigs, rats, and hamsters. *Toxicol. Appl. Pharmacol. 35*:393–395.

Altmann, H. J., Grunov, W., Mohr, U., Richter-Reichhelm, H. B., and Wester, P. W. (1986). Effects of BHA and related phenols on the forestomach of rats. *Food Chem. Toxicol. 24*:1183–1188.

Amo, H., Kubota, H., Lu, J., and Matsuyuma, M. (1990). Adenomatous hyperplasia and adenomas in the lung induced by chronic feeding of butylated hydoxyanisole of Japanese house musk shrew (*Sancus murinus*). *Carcinogenesis 11*:151–154.

Anonymous. (1971). Use of glycine and its salts as food additives will be banned by FDA in 6 months. *Chem. Eng. News 48* (22):27.

Aoki, I. (1962). Studies on food additives in a rabbit. VII. Metabolism of 2,6-di-tert-butyl phenol (BHT) in a rabbit. (2) Isolation of a metabolite. *Chem. Pharm. Bull.* *10*:105–112.

Arakawa, N., Suzuki, E., Kurata, T., Otsuka, M., and Inagaki, C. (1986). Effect of erythorbic acid administration on ascorbic acid content in guinea pig tissues. *J. Nutr. Sci. Vit.* *32*:171–181.

Armstrong, K. E., and Wattenberg, L. W. (1985). Metabolism of 3-tert-butyl-4-hydroxyanisole to 3-tert-butyl-4,5-dihydroxyanisole by rat liver microsomes. *Cancer Res.* *45*:1507–1510.

Astill, B. D., Fassett, D. W., and Roudabush, R. L. (1959). The metabolism of 2:4:5-trihydroxy butyrophenone in the rat and dog. *Biochem. J.* *72*:451–459.

Astill, B. D., Fassett, D. W., and Roudabush, R. L. (1960). The metabolism of phenolic antioxidants. 2. The metabolism of butylated hydroxyanisole in the rat. *Biochem. J.* *75*:543–551.

Astill, B. D., Mills, J., Fasset, D. W., Roudabush, R. L., and Terhaar, C. J. (1962). Food additive metabolism: fate of butylated hydroxyanisole in man and rat. *J. Agric. Food Chem.* *10*:315–321.

Astill, B. D., Terhaar, C. J., Krasavage, W. J., Wolf, G. L., Roudabush, R. L., Fassett, D. W., and Morgareidge, K. (1975). Safety evaluation and biochemical behavior of 2-tert-butyl hydroquinone. *J. Am. Oil Chem. Soc.* *52*:53–58.

Atkinson, A., Van der Merwe, R. P., and Swart, L. G. (1972). Effect of high levels of different fish meals, of several antioxidants, and poultry byproduct meal on the flavor and fatty acid composition of the broilers. *Agroanimalia* *4*:63–68.

Bagdon, R. E., Zbinden, G., and Studer, A. (1960). Chronic toxicity studies of β-carotene. *Toxicol. Appl. Pharmacol.* *2*:225–236.

Baranauskatje, A. P., Vasiljauskajte, O. I., and Ranchyalis, V. P. (1972). Specific induction of mutations and modification of mutagenic effect of ethylenimine in *Drosophila* under the influence of ethylenediaminetetraacetate (in Russian). *Lietuvos. TSR Mokslu. Akad. Darb. Ser. B.* *2*:107–113.

Bascoul, J., Domerue, N., Olle, M., and Crastes De Paulet, A. (1986). Autoxidation of cholesterol in tallows heated under deep frying conditions: evaluation of oxysterols by GLC and TLC. *Lipids* *21*:383–387.

Basrur, V. R., and Baker, D.G. (1963). Human chromosome breakage in low-calcium cultures. *Lancet* *1*:1106–1107.

Basu, A. K., and Marnett, L. J. (1983). Unequivocal demonstration that malonaldehyde is a mutagen. *Carcinogenesis* *4*:331–333.

Basu, A. K., O'Hara, S. M., Valladier, P., Stone, K., Mols, O. and Marnett, L. J. (1988). Identification of adducts formed by the reaction of guanine nucleosides with malonaldehyde and structurally related aldehydes. *Chem. Res. Toxicol.* *1*:53–59.

Beckman, C., Roy, R. M., and Sproule, A. (1982). Modification of radiation induced sex linked recessive lethal mutation frequency by tocopherol. *Mut. Res.* *105*:73–77.

Benesch, R. E., and Benesch, R. (1974). Mechanism of interaction of red cell organic phosphates with hemoglobin. *Adv. Prot. Chem.* *28*:211–237.

Benson, A. M., Batzinger, R. P., Ou S-Y L., Beuding, E., Cha Y-N., and Talalay, P. (1978). Elevation of hepatic gluthathione-S-transferase activities and protection against mutagenic metabolities of benzo(a)pyrene by dietary antioxidants. *Cancer Res.* *38*:4486–4495.

Bettger, W. J., and Olson, R. E. (1982). Effect of α-tocopherolquinone on vitamin K dependent carboxylation in the rat. *Fed. Proc.* *41*:344 (abst.).

Bhagat, B., and Lockett, M. F. (1960). The absorption and elimination of metabisulfite and thiosulfate by rats. *J. Pharm. Pharmacol.* *12*:690–694.

Bhagat, B., and Lockett, M. F. (1964). The effect of sulfite in solid diets on the growth of rats. *Food Cosmet. Toxicol. 2*:1–13.

Bickel, A. F., Kooijman, E. C., La Lau, C., Roest, W., and Piet, P. (1953). Alkylperoxy radicals. I. Reactions with 2,4,6-trialkylphenols. *J. Chem. Soc. Part III*, 3211–3218.

Bickoff, E. M., Livingston, A. L., Guggolz, J., and Thompson, C. R. (1954). Quinone derivatives as antioxidants for carotene. *J. Agric. Food Chem. 2*:1229–1231.

Bieri, J. G. (1972). Aspects of vitamin E metabolism relating to the dietary requirement. *Ann. NY Acad. Sci. 203*:181–191.

Bird, R. P., and Draper, H. H. (1980). Effect of malonaldehyde and acetaldehyde on cultured mammalian cells: growth, morphology, and synthesis of macromolecules. *J. Toxicol. Environ. Health 6*:811–823.

Bird, R. P., Draper, H. H., and Basrur, P. K. (1982). Effect of malonaldehyde and acetaldehyde on cultured mammalian cells. *Mut. Res. 101*:237–246.

Bishov, S. J., and Henick. A. S. (1975). Antioxidant effect of protein hydrolysates in freeze dried model systems. *J. Food Sci. 40*:345–348.

Bitar, D. J., and Reinhold, J. G. (1972). Phytase and alkaline phosphatase activities in intestinal mucosa of rat, chicken, calf, and man. *Biochim. Biophys. Acta 268*:442–452.

Black, H. S., and Chan, J. T. (1975). Suppression of ultraviolet light induced tumor formation by dietary antioxidants. *J. Invest. Derm. 65*:412–414.

Blackburn, G. M., Rashid, A., and Thompson, M. H. (1979). Interactions of 5 α, 6 α cholesterol oxide with DNA and other nucleophiles. *J. Chem. Soc. Chem. Commun. 9*:421.

Blaner, W. S., and Churchich, J. E. (1980). The membrane bound retinol dehydrogenase from bovine rod outer segments. *Biochim. Biophys. Res. Commun. 94*:820–826.

Bodansky, O., Gold, H., Zahm, W., Civin, H., and Salzman, C. (1942). The toxicity and laxative action of sodium fumarate. *J. Am. Pharm. Assoc. 31*:1–8.

Bonting, S. L. (1952). *The Effect of a Prolonged Intake of Phosphoric Acid and Citric Acid in Rats*. PhD thesis, University of Amsterdam, Amsterdam.

Booth, A., Masri, M., Robbins, D. J., Emerson, O. H., Jones, F. T., and DeEds, F. (1959). The metabolic fate of gallic acid and related compounds. *J. Biol. Chem. 234*:3014–3016.

Botham, C. M., Conning, D. M., Hayes, J., Litchfield, M. H., and McElligott, T. F. (1970). Effects of butylated hydroxytoluene on the enzyme activity and ultrastructure of rat hepatocytes. *Food Cosmet. Toxicol. 8*:1–8.

Bracco, U., Loliger, J., and Viret, J. L. (1981). Production and use of natural antioxidants. *J. Am. Oil Chem. Soc. 58*:686–690.

Bradley, W. B., Eppson, H. T., and Beath, O. A. (1939). Nitrites as the cause of oat hay poisoning. *J. Am. Vet. Med. Assoc. 47*:541–543.

Braide, V. B. (1976). Renal ultrastructural changes induced by calcium EDTA in rats. *Res. Vet. Sci. 20*:295–301.

Branen, A. L. (1975). Toxicology and biochemistry of butylated hydroxyanisole and butylated hydroxytoluene. *J. Am. Oil Chem. Soc. 52*:59–63.

Briggs, M. (1974). Vitamin E supplements and fatigue. *N. Engl. J. Med. 290*:579–580.

Briggs, M. H., Garcia-Webb, P., and Davies, P. (1973). Urinary oxalate and vitamin C supplements. *Lancet 2*:201.

Brodkin, R. H., and Bleiberg, J. (1965). Sensitivity to topically applied vitamin E. *Arch. Dermatol. 92*:76–77.

Brooks, T. M., Hunt, P. F., Thorpe, E., and Walker, A. T. (1974). Unpublished data, cited in *Federal Register 42*:27603 (1974).

Brown, J. P., Brown, R. J., and Roehm, G. W. (1977). The application of short-term microbial mutagenicity tests in the identification and development of non-toxic, nonabsorbable food additives. In *Progress in Genetic Toxicology*, Scott, D., Bridges, B. A., and Sobels, F. H. (eds). Elsevier/North-Holland Biomedical Press, Amsterdam.

Brown, W. D., Johnson, A. R., and Halloran, M. W. (1959). The effect of the level of dietary fat on the toxicity of phenolic antioxidants. *Aust. J. Exp. Biol. Med.* 37:533–548.

Bruce, W. R., and Heddle, J. A. (1979). The mutagenic activity of 61 agents as determined by the micronucleus, *Salmonella*, and sperm abnormality test. *Can. J. Genet. Cytol.* 21:319–334.

Brun, R. (1964). Kontaktekzem auf Laurylgallat und *p*-Hydroxybenzoesaure ester. *Berufsderm.* 12:281–284.

Brun, R. (1970). Eczema de contact a une antioxydant de la margarine. *Dermatologica* 140:390–394.

Buck, D. F. (1984). Food antioxidants: applications and uses in snack food. *Cereal Foods World* 29(5):301–303.

Buck, D. F. (1985). Antioxidant applications. *Manuf. Confect.* 65:45–49.

Burkhardt, W., and Fierz, U. (1964). Antioxidantien in der Margarine als Ursache von Gewerbeekzemen. *Dermatologica* 129:431–432.

Burri, J., Graf, M., Lambelet, P., and Loliger, J. (1989). Vanillin more than a flavoring agent—a potent antioxidant. *J. Sci. Food Agric.* 48:49–56.

Burrows, D. (1975). Contact dermatitis in animal feed mill workers. *Br. J. Dermatol.* 92:167–170.

Bush, R. (1986). Sulfites in food: health risk. *Food Technol.* 40:49.

Calbert, C. E., Greenberg, S. M., Kryder, G., and Deuel, H. J., Jr. (1951). The digestibility of stearyl alcohol, ispropyl citrates, and stearyl citrate and the effect of these materials on the rate and degree of absorption of margarine in rats. *Food Res.* 16:294–305.

Carlson, A. J., and Brewer, N. R. (1953). Toxicity studies on hydroquinone. *Proc. Soc. Exp. Biol.* 84:684–688.

Cawthorne, M. A., Bunyan, J., Sennit, M. V., Green, J., and Grasso, P. (1970). Vit.E and hepatotoxic agents. 3. Vit.E, synthetic antioxidants, and carbon tetrachloride toxicity in the rat. *Br. J. Nutr.* 24:357–384.

Cecil, R. (1963). Intramolecular bonds in proteins. I. The role of sulfur in proteins. In *The Proteins*. Vol. 1, Neurath, H. (ed). Academic Press, New York, pp. 379–476.

Cha, Y. N., and Heine, H. S. (1982). Comparative effects of dietary administration of 2(3) tert-butyl-4-hydroxyanisole and 3,5-di-tert butyl-4-hydroxytoluene on several hepatic enzyme activities in mice and rats. *Cancer Res.* 42:2609–2615.

Cha, Y. N., and Beuding, E. (1979). Effect of 2(3) tert-butyl-4-hydroxyanisole administration on the activities of several hepatic microsomal and cytoplasmic enzymes in mice. *Biochem. Pharm.* 28:1917–1921.

Chadwick, V. S., Vince, A., Killngley, M., and Wrong, O. M. (1978). The metabolism of tartarate in man and the rat. *Clin. Sci. Mol. Med.* 54:273–281.

Chan, M. S. (1956). *Some Toxicological and Physiological Studies of Ethylenediaminetetraacetic Acid in the Albino Rat.* PhD thesis, University of Massachusetts, Amherst, MA.

Chang, S. S., Ostric-Matijaseric, B., Hsieh, O. A. L., and Huang, C. (1977). Natural antioxidants from rosemarry and sage. *J. Food Sci.* 42:1102–1106.

Chang, S. S., Senich, G. A., and Smith, L. E. (1982). *Migration of Low Molecular Weight Additives in Polyolefins and Copolymers.* Final report, National Bureau of Standards, NBSIR 82-2472.

Chasseaud, L. F., Down, W. H., and Kirkpatric, D. (1977). Absorption and biotransformation of L(+)-tartaric acid in rats. *Experientia* 33:998–999.

Chauhan, P. S., Aravindakshan, M., and Sundaram, K. (1978). Evaluation of ascorbic acid for mutagenicity by dominant lethal test in male wistar rats. *Mut. Res.* 53:166–167.

Cheryan, M. (1980). Phytic acid interactions in food systems. *CRC Crit. Rev. Food Sci. Nutr. 13*:297–335.

Chipault, J. R., Mizuna, G. R., Hawkins, J. M., and Lundberg, W. O. (1952). The antioxidant properties of natural spices. *Food Res. 17*:46–55.

Ciaccio, E. I. (1966). The inhibition of lactate dehydrogenase by 3-acetylpyridine adenine dinucleotide and bisulfite. *J. Biol. Chem. 241*:1581–1586.

Cillard, J., Cillard, P., and Cormier, M. (1980). Effects of experimental factors on the prooxidant behavior of tocopherol. *J. Am. Oil Chem. Soc. 57*:255–261.

Clapp, N. K., Tyndall, R. L., and Cumming, R. B. (1973). Hyperplasia of hepatic bileducts in mice following long-term administrationse of butylated hydroxytoluene. *Food Cosmet. Toxicol. 11*:847–849.

Clapp, N. K., Tyndall, R. L., Cumming, R. B., and Otten, J. A. (1974). Effects of butylated hydroxytoluene alone or with diethyl nitrosamine in mice. *Food Chem. Toxicol. 12*:367–371.

Clegg, D. J. (1965). Absence of teratogenic effect of butylated hydroxyanisole and butylated hydroxytoluene in rats and mice. *Food Cosmet. Toxicol. 3*:387–430.

Cook, M. G., and McNamara, P. (1980). Effect of dietary vitamin E on dimethylhydrazine induced colonic tumors in mice. *Cancer Res. 40*:1329–1331.

Cooperstein, S.J. (1963). Reversible inactivation of cytochrome oxidase by disulfide bond reagents. *J. Biol. Chem. 238*:3606–3610.

Cort, W. M. (1974a). Antioxidant activity in tocopherols, ascorbyl palmitate, and ascorbic acid and their mode of action. *J. Am. Oil Chem. Soc. 51*:321–325.

Cort, W. M. (1974b). Hemoglobin peroxidation test screens antioxidants. *Food Technol. 28*(10):60–66.

Cort, W. M., Scott, J. W., Araujo, M., Mergens, W. J., Cannalinga, M. A., Osadca, M., Harley, H., Parrish, D. R., and Pool, W. R. (1975a). Antioxidant activity and stability of 6-hydroxy-2,5,7,8-tetramethylchroman-2-carboxylic acid. *J. Am. Oil Chem. Soc. 52*:174–178.

Cort, W. M., Scott, J. W., and Harley, J. H. (1975b). Proposed antioxidant exhibits useful properties. *Food Technol. 29*(11):46–50.

Cosgrove, D. J. (1966). The chemistry and biochemistry of inositol phosphates. *Rev. Pure Appl. Chem. 16*:209–224.

Cramer, J. W., Porrata-Doria, E. I., and Steenbock, H. (1956). A rachitogenic and growth promoting effect of citrate. *Arch. Biochim. Biophys. 60*:58–63.

Cranston, E. M., Jensen, M. J., Moren, A., Brey, T., Bell, E. T., and Bieter, R. N. (1947). The acute and chronic toxicity of nordihydroguairetic acid. *Fed. Proc. 6*:318–319.

Creaven, P. J., Davies, W. H., and Williams, R. T. (1966). The effect of butylated hydroxyanisole, butylated hydroxytoluene, and octyl gallate upon liver weight and biphenyl-4-hydroxylase activity. *J. Pharm. Pharmacol. 18*:485–489.

Csallany, A. S., Draper, H. H., and Shah, S. N. (1962). Conversion of d-α-tocopherol-^{14}C to tocopheryl-*p*-quinone in vivo. *Arch. Biochim. Biophys. 98*:142–145.

Curtin, C. O. H., and King, C. G. (1955). The metabolism of ascorbic acid-1-C^{14} and oxalic acid C^{14} in the rat. *J. Biol. Chem. 216*:539–548.

Cutler, M. G., and Schneider, R. (1973a). Sensitivity of feeding tests in detecting carcinogenic properties in chemicals: examination of 7,12-dimethyl benz(a)anthracene and oxidized linoleate. *Food Chem. Toxicol. 11*:443–457.

Cutler, M. G., and Schneider, R. (1973b). Malformations produced in mice by oxidized linoleate. *Food Chem. Toxicol. 11*:935–942.

Czyba, J. C. (1966). Effects de l'hypervitaminse E sur le testicule du hamster dore. *C. R. Soc. Biol. 160*:765–768.

Dacre, J. C. (1960). Metabolic pathways of the phenolic antioxidants. *J. NZ Inst. Chem. 24*:161–171.

Dacre, J. C. (1961). The metabolism of 3,5-di-tert-butyl-4- hydroxytoluene and 3,5-di-tert-butyl-4- hydroxybenzoic acid in the rabbit. *Biochem. J. 78*:758–766.

Dacre, J. C. (1970). Toxicologic studies with 2,6-di-tert-butyl-4-hydroxymethyl phenol in the rat. *Toxicol. Appl. Pharmacol. 17*:669–678.

Dacre, J. C. (1974). Long-term toxicity study of *n*-propyl gallate in mice. *Food Cosmet. Toxicol. 12*:125–129.

Dacre, J. C., Denz, F. A., and Kennedy, T. H. (1956). Metabolism of butylated hydroxyanisole in the rabbit. *Biochem. J. 64*:777–782.

Dahl, S. (1974). Vitamin E in clinical medicine. *Lancet 1*:465.

Daniel, J. W., and Gage, J. C. (1965). The absorption and excretion of butylated hydroxytoluene in the rat. *Food Cosmet. Toxicol. 3*:405–415.

Daniel, J. W., Gage, J. C., Jones, D. I., and Stevens, M. A. (1967). Excretion of butylated hydroxyanisole and butylated hydroxytoluene by man. *Food Cosmet. Toxicol. 5*:475–479.

Daniel, J. W., Gage, J. I., and Jones, D. I. (1968). The metabolism of 3,5-di-tert-butyl-4-hydroxytoluene in the rat and in man. *Biochem. J. 106*:783–790.

Daniel, R. G., and Waisman, H. A. (1968). The effect of excess amino acids on growth of the young rat. *Growth 32*:255–265.

Das, R. K., and Manna, G. K. (1972). Differential chromosomal abberations produced in the bone marrow and spleen cells of mice treated with two chemicals. *Proc. Indian Sci. Congress 59*:413–414.

Datta, P. K., Frazer, A. C., Sharrat, M., and Sammons, H. G. (1962). Biological effects of food additives. II. Na pyrophosphate. *J. Sci. Food Agric. 13*:556–566.

Deichmann, W. B., Clemmer, J. J., Prakoczy, R., and Biachine, J. (1955). Toxicity of dietary butyl methyl phenol. *A.M.A. Arch. Ind. Health 11*:93–101.

Demole, V. (1934). The physiological action of ascorbic acid and some related compounds. *Biochem. J. 28*:770–773.

Demole, V. (1939). Pharmakologisches über vitamin E (Verträglichkeit des synthetischen dl-α-Tocopherols und seines Acetats). *Int. Z. Vitaminforsch. 8*:338–341.

Denz, F. A., and Llaurado, J. G. (1957). Some of the effects of phenolic antioxidants on sodium and potassium balance in the rabbit. *Br. J. Nutr. 38*:515–524.

DeSesso, J. M. (1981). Amelioration of teratogenesis. I. Modification of hyroxyurea induced teratogenesis by the antioxidant propyl gallate. *Teratology 24*:19–35.

DeStafney, C. M., Prabhu, U. D. G., Sparnius, V. L., and Wattenberg, L. W. (1986). Studies related to the mechanism of 3-BHA induced neoplasia of the rat forestomach. *Food Chem. Toxicol. 24*:1149–1157.

Deuel, H. J., Jr., Greenberg, S. M., Calbert, C. E., Baker, R., and Fisher, H. R. (1951). Toxicological studies on isopropyl citrate and stearyl citrate. *Food Res. 16*:258–280.

Dysmsza, H. A., and Park, J. (1975). Excess dietary vitamin E in rats. *Fed. Am. Soc. Exp. Biol. 34*:912 abst.

Dysmsza, H. A., Reussner, G., and Thiessen, R. (1959). Effect of normal and high intakes of orthophosphate and metaphosphate in rats. *J. Nutr. 69*:419–428.

Dziedzic, S. Z. and Hudson, B. J. F. (1984). Phosphatidyl ethanolamine as a synergist for primary antioxidants in edible oils. *J. Am. Oil Chem. Soc. 61*:1042–1045.

Dziezak, J. D. (1986). Antioxidants, the ultimate answer to oxidation. *Food Technol. 40*(9):94–102.

Ebel, J. P. (1958). Physiological and toxicological effects of condensed phosphates. *Ann. Nutr. Alim. 12*:57–97.

EEC Commission Documents. (1982). *Report of the Scientific Committee for Food on Tertiary Butyl Hydroquinone*. EEC Commission Document III/26/82, Brussels.

Ellinger, R. H. (1972). Phosphates in food processing. In *CRC Handbook of Food Additives*, Vol. 1, Furia, T. E. (ed). CRC Press, Boca Raton, FL, pp 617–780.

El-Rashidy, R., and Niazi, S. (1980). Comparative pharmacokinetics of butylated hydroxyanisole and butylated hydroxytoluene in rabbits. *J. Pharm. Sci.* *69*:1455–1457.

El-Rashidy, R., and Niazi, S. (1983). A new metabolite of butylated hydroxyanisole in man. *Biopharm. Drug Dispos.* *4*:389–396.

Emerick, R. J., and Olson, O. E. (1962). Effect of nitrate and nitrite on vitamin A storage in the rat. *J. Nutr.* *78*:73–77.

Erdman, J. W. (1979). Oilseed phytates: nutritional implications. *J. Am. Oil Chem. Soc.* *56*:736–741.

FAO/WHO. (1967). *Requirement of Vitamin A, Thiamin, Riboflavin, and Niacin.* WHO Tech Rep. Series No. 362, World Health Organization, Geneva, Switzerland.

FAO/WHO. (1969). *Joint FAO/WHO Meeting on Pesticide Residues in Food.* WHO Technical Report Series No. 458./FAO Agricultural Studies No. 84, World Health Organization, Geneva, Switzerland.

FAO/WHO. (1974). *Toxicological Evaluation of Some Food Additives Including Anticaking Agents, Antimicrobials, Antioxidants, Emulsifiers, and Thickening Agents.* WHO Food Additive Series No. 5, World Health Organization, Geneva, Switzerland.

FAO/WHO. (1975). *Toxicological Evaluation of Some Food Colors, Enzymes, Flavor Enhancers, Thickening Agents, and Certain Other Food Additives.* WHO Food Additive Series No. 6, World Health Organization, Geneva, Switzerland.

FAO/WHO. (1981). 25th Report of the Joint FAO/WHO Expert Committee on Food Additives. WHO Tech. Rep. Series No. 669, World Health Organization, Geneva, Switzerland.

FAO/WHO. (1984). *28th Report of the Joint FAO/WHO Expert Committee on Food Additives.* WHO Technical Report Series No. 710, World Health Organization, Geneva, Switzerland.

FAO/WHO. (1987). *Toxicological Evaluation of Certain Food Additives and Contaminants.* WHO Tech. Rep. Series No. 21, World Health Organization, Geneva, Switzerland.

FAO/WHO. (1989). *Evaluation of Certain Food Additives and Contaminants.* WHO Tech. Rep. Series No. 776, World Health Organization, Geneva, Switzerland.

FDA. (1972a). *Teratologic Evaluation of FDA 71-24 (Butylated Hydroxyanisole) in Mice, Rats, and Hamsters.* NTIS PB-221783. Maspeth, N.Y.

FDA. (1972b). *Teratologic Evaluation of FDA 71-25 (Butylated Hydroxytoluene-Ionol).* NTIS PB-221782. Maspeth, N.Y.

FDA. (1973a). *Teratologic Evaluation of 71-39 (Propyl gallate).* NTIS PB-223816. Maspeth, N.Y.

FDA. (1973b). *Teratologic Evaluation of FDA 71-58 (dl-α-Tocopheryl Acetate) in Mice, Rats, Hamsters, and Rabbits.* NTIS PB-233809. Maspeth, N.Y.

FDA. (1973c). *NAS/NRC Questionnaire on Tartaric Acid.* Contract 71-75, Food and Drug Administration, Rockville, MD.

FDA. (1974a). *Teratologic Evaluation of FDA 71-24 (Butylated Hydroxyanisole) in Rabbits.* NTIS PB-267200. Maspeth, N.Y.

FDA. (1974b). *Teratologic Evaluation of FDA 71-24 (Butylated Hydroxytoluene) in Rabbits.* NTIS PB-267201. Maspeth, N.Y.

Fassett, D. W., Terhaar, C. J., and Astill, B. D. (1968). *Summary of the Safety Evaluation of monotertiary butyl hydroquinone.* Unpublished report cited in FAO/WHO, WHO Food Additive Series No. 8, 1975.

Federal Register. (1974). *39* (185, Sept. 23):34172–34173.

Federal Register. (1982). *47*:27806.

Feurer, G., Gaunt, I. F., Goldberg, L., and Fairweather, F. A. (1965). Liver response tests. VI. Application to a comparative study of food antioxidants and hepatotoxic agents. *Food Cosmet. Toxicol.* *3*:457–469.

Figge, K. (1972). Migration of additives from plastic films into edible oils and fat simulants. *Food Cosmet. Toxicol. 10*:815–828.

Finkle, P. (1933). The fate of tartaric acid in the human body. *J. Biol. Chem. 100*:349–351.

Fitzhugh, O. G., and Nelson, A. A. (1946). Subacute and chronic toxicities of ascorbyl palmitates. *Proc. Soc. Exp. Biol. 61*:195–198.

Fitzhugh, O. G., and Nelson, A. A. (1947). The comparative chronic toxicities of fumaric, tartaric, oxalic, and malic acids. *J. Am. Pharm. Assoc. 36*:217–219.

Foote, C. S. and Denny, R. W. (1968). Chemistry of singlet oxygen. VII. Quenching by β-carotene. *J. Am. Oil Chem. Soc. 90*:6233–6235.

Foreman, H., Vier, M., and Magee, M. (1953). The metabolism of ^{14}C labelled ethylene-diaminetetraacetic acid in the rat. *J. Biol. Chem. 203*:1045–1053.

Foreman, H., and Trujillo, T. T. (1954). The metabolism of ^{14}C labeled ethylenediamine-tetraacetic acid in human beings. *J. Lab. Clin. Med. 43*:566–571.

Frankel, E. N. (1984). Lipid oxidation: mechanisms, products, and biological significance. *J. Am. Oil Chem. Soc. 61*:1908–1917.

Frawley, J. P., Kohn, F. E., Kay, J. H., and Calendra, J. C. (1965). Progress report on the multigeneration reproduction studies in rats fed butylated hydroxytoluene (BHT). *Food Chem. Toxicol. 3*:377–386.

Frohberg, H., Gleich, J., and Kieser, H. (1973). Reproduktions toxikologische Studien mit Ascorbinsäure an Mausen and Ratten. *Arzneim. Forsch. 23*:1081–1082.

Frolik, C. A. (1984). Metabolism of retinoids. In *The Retinoids*, Vol. 2, Sporn, B. M., Roberts, A. B. and Goodman, D. S. (eds). Academic Press Inc., London, pp. 177–208.

Fujimoto, K., Neff, W. E., and Frankel, E. N. (1984). The reaction of DNA with lipid oxidation products, metals, and reducing agents. *Biochim. Biophys. Acta 795*:100–107.

Fujioka, M., and Lieberman, J. (1964). A Zn^{++} requirement for synthesis of deoxyribo-nucleic acid by rat liver. *J. Biol. Chem. 239*:1164–1167.

Fukuhara, Y., Yoshida, D., and Goto, F. (1981). Reduction of mutagenic products in the presence of polyphenols during pyrolysis of protein. *Agric. Biol. Chem. 45*:1061–1066.

Fukushima, S., Kurata, Y., Shibata, M., Ikawa, E., and Ito, N. (1984). Promotion by ascorbic acid, sodium erythorbate, and ethoxyquin of neoplastic lesions in rats initiated with N-butyl-N-(4-hydroxybutyl)nitrosamine. *Cancer Lett. 23*:29–37.

Gallo-Torres, H. E. (1980a). Absorption. In *Vitamin E: A Comprehensive Treatise*, Vol. I., Machlin, L. J. (ed). Marcel Dekker, Inc., New York, pp. 170–192.

Gallo-Torres, H. E. (1980b). Transport and metabolism. In *Vitamin E: A Comprehensive Treatise*, Vol. I., Machlin, L. J. (ed). Marcel Dekker, Inc., New York, pp. 193–267.

Garton, G. A., and Williams, R. T. (1949). Studies on detoxification. 21. The fates of quinol and resorcinol in the rabbit in relation to the metabolism of benzene. *Biochem. J. 44*:234–238.

Gaunt, I. F., Feuer, G., Fairweather, F. A., and Gilbert, D. (1965). Liver response tests. IV. Application to short-term feeding studies of butylated hydroxytoluene and butylated hydroxyanisole. *Food Cosmet. Toxicol. 3*:433–443.

Gebhart, E., Wagner, H., Grziwok, K., and Behnsen, H. (1985). The actions of anticlas-togens in human lymphocyte cultures and their modification by rat liver S9 mix. II. Studies with vitamins C and E. *Mut. Res. 149*:83–94.

Gellen, J. A. (1979). Hypervitaminosis A induced teratogenesis. *Crit. Rev. Toxicol. 6*:351–375.

Gellert, R. J. (1977). Inhibition of cyclic ovarian activity in rats treated chronically with vit.A. *J. Reprod. Fertil. 50*:223–229.

Generoso, W. M., Huff, S. W., and Cain, K. T. (1978). Tests on induction of chromosome aberrations in mouse germ cells with sodium bisulfite. *Mut. Res. 56*:363–365.

Gibson, K. D., Neuberger, A., and Scott, J. C. (1955). Purification and properties of γ-aminolevulinic acid dehydrase. *Biochem. J. 61*:618–629.

Gibson, W. B., and Strong, F. M. (1973). Metabolism and elimination of sulfite by rats, mice, and monkeys. *Food Cosmet. Toxicol. 11*:185–198.

Gilbert, D., and Goldberg, L. (1965). Liver response tests. III. Liver enlargement and stimulation of microsomal processing enzyme activity. *Food Cosmet. Toxicol. 3*:417–432.

Giri, A. K., Sen, S., Talukder, G., and Sharma, A. (1984). Mutachromosomal effects of tert-butyl hydroquinone in bone marrow cells of mice. *Food Chem. Toxicol. 22*:459–460.

Glavind, J., Christensen, F., and Sylven, C. (1971). Intestinal absorption and in vivo formation of lipoperoxides in vit.E deficient rats. *Acta Chem. Scand. 25*:3220–3226.

Gold, H., and Zahm, W. (1943). Method for the evaluation of laxative agents in constipated human subjects with a study of the comparative laxative potencies of fumarates, sodium tartarate, and magnesium acid citrate. *J. Am. Pharm. Assoc. 32*:173–178.

Golder, W. S., Ryan, A. J., and Wright, S. E. (1962). The urinary excretion of tritiated butylated hydroxyanisole in the rat. *J. Pharm. Pharmacol. 14*:268–271.

Gomori, G., and Gulyas, E. (1944). Effect of parenterally administered citrate on the renal excretion of calcium. *Proc. Soc. Exp. Biol. Med. 56*:226–228.

Goodman, D. S., and Huang, H. S. (1965). Biosynthesis of vit.A with rat intestinal enzymes. *Science 149*:879–880.

Goodman, D. S., Huang, H. S., and Shiratori, T. (1965). Tissue distribution of newly absorbed vit.A in the rat. *J. Lipid Res. 6*:390–396.

Goodman, D. S., Blomstrand, R, Werner, B., Huang, H. S., and Shiratori, T. (1966). Intestinal absorption and metabolism of vit.A and β-carotene in man. *J. Clin. Invest. 45*:1615–1623.

Goodman, T., Grice, H., Becking, G. C., and Salem, F. A. (1970). Cystic nephropathy induced by nordihydroguairetic acid in the rat: light and electron microscopic investigations. *Lab. Invest. 23*:93–107.

Gordon, M. H. (1990). The mechanism of antioxidant action in vitro. In *Food Antioxidants*, Hudson, B. J. F. (ed). Elsevier, London, pp. 1–18.

Gosselin, R. E., Rothstein, A., Miller, G. J., and Berke, H. L. (1952). Hydrolysis and excretion of polymeric phosphate. *J. Pharmacol. Exp. Ther. 106*:180–192.

Graf, E. (1983). Applications of phytic acid. *J. Am. Oil Chem. Soc. 60*:1861–1867.

Graf, E., Mahoney, J. R., Bryant, R. G., and Eaton, J. W. (1984). Iron catalysed hydroxyl radical formation: stringent requirement for free iron coordination site. *J. Biol. Chem. 259*:3620–3624.

Graf, E., Empson, K. L., and Eaton, J. W. (1987). Phytic acid—a natural antioxidant. *J. Biol. Chem. 262*:11647–11650.

Greenberg, M., Birnkrant, W. B., and Schiftner, J. J. (1945). Outbreak of sodium nitrite poisoning. *J. Am. Public Health 35*:1217–1220.

Greenberg, R., Cornbleet, T., and Jeffny, A. I. (1959). Accumulation and excretion of vit.A like fluorescent material by sebaceous glands after oral feeding of various carotenoids. *J. Invest. Dermatol. 32*:599–604.

Greenblatt, M., Mirvish, S., and So, B. T. (1971). Nitrosamine studies: induction of lung adenomas by concurrent administration of sodium nitrite and secondary amines in Swiss mice. *J. Natl. Cancer Inst. 46*:1029–1034.

Grey, R. M., Nielsen, S. W., Rousseau, J. E. Jr., Calhoun, M. C., and Eaton, H. D. (1965). Pathology of skull, radius, and rib in hypervitaminosis A of young calves. *Pathol. Vet. 2*:446–467.

Grice, H. C., Becking, G., and Goodman, T. (1968). Toxic properties of nordihydroguairetic acid. *Food Cosmet. Toxicol. 6*:155–161.

Griepentrog, F. (1961). Allergy studies with simple chemical compounds. VII. Nordihy-droguairetic acid. *Arzneimittel forsch. 11*:920–922.

Griffiths, L. A., and Smith, G. E. (1972). Metabolism of apigenin and related compounds in the rat: metabolite formation in vivo and by intestinal microflora in vitro. *Biochem. J. 128*:901–911.

Grossman, D., and Lang, K. (1962). Inorganic poly- and metaphosphatases and polyphosphate in animal cell nuclei. *Biochem. Z. 336*:351–370.

Gruber, C. M., and Halbeisen, W. A. (1948). A study of the comparative toxic effects of citric acid and its sodium salts. *J. Pharmacol. Exp. Ther. 94*:65–67.

Gruener, N., and Shuval, H. I. (1973). Toxicology of nitrites. *Environ. Qual. Safety 2*:219–229.

Gry, J., and Larsen, J. C. (1978). Metabolism of L(+)- and D(−)- tartaric acids in different animal species. *Arch. Toxicol. 36*:351.

Gugler, R., Leschik, M., and Dengler, H. J. (1975). Disposition of quercetin in man after single intravenous doses. *Eur. J. Clin. Pharmacol. 9*:229–234.

Gunnison, A. F. (1981). Sulfite toxicity: a critical review of in vitro and in vivo data. *Food Chem Toxicol. 19*:667–682.

Gunnison, A. F., and Palmes, E. D. (1973). Persistance of plasma S-sulfonates following exposure of rabbits to sulfite and sulfur dioxide. *Toxicol. Appl. Pharmacol. 24*:266–278.

Gunnison, A. F., and Palmes, E. D. (1978). Species variability in plasma S-sulfonate levels during and following sulfite administration. *Chemico-Biol. Interact. 21*:315–329.

Gunnison, A. F., Bresnahan, C. A., and Palmes, E. D. (1977). Comparative sulfite metabolism in the rat, rabbit, and rhesus monkey. *Toxicol. Appl. Pharmacol. 42*:99–109.

Guttenplan, J. B. (1977). Inhibition by L-ascorbate of bacterial mutagenesis induced by two N-nitroso compounds. *Nature 268*:368–370.

Guttenplan, J. B. (1978). Mechanisms of inhibition by ascorbate of microbial mutagenesis induced by N-nitroso compounds. *Cancer Res. 38*:2018–2022.

Gwo, Y. Y., Flick, J. R., and Dupuy, H. P. (1985). Effect of ascorbyl palmitate on the quality of frying fats for deep frying operations. *J. Am. Oil Chem. Soc. 62*:1666–1671.

Hageman, G. J., Verhagen, H., and Kleinjans, J. C. S. (1988). Butylated hydroxyanisole and butylated hydroxytoluene and tert-butyl-quinone are not mutagenic in the *Salmonella*/microsome assay using new tester strains. *Mut. Res. 208*:207–211.

Hahn, F., and Seifen, E. (1959). Further studies on the effect of chronic feeding of phosphates. *Arzneimittel forsch. 9*:501–503.

Hahn, F., Jacobi, H., and Seifen, E. (1958). Do ortho- and polyphosphates show variable compatibilities on chronic feeding? *Arzneimittel forsch. 8*:286–289.

Hallady, S. C., Ryerson, B. A., Smith, C. R., Brown, J. P., and Parkinson, T. M. (1980). Comparison of effects of dietary administration of butylated hydroxytoluene or a polymeric antioxidant on the hepatic and intestinal cytochrome P-450 mixed function oxygenase system in the rat. *Food Cosmet. Toxicol. 18*:569–574.

Hanck, A. (1986). Spektrum Vitamine, Vitamin E. In *Arzneimitteltherapie Heute*, Vol. 42. Aesopus-Verlag, pp. 36–42.

Hard, G. C., and Neal, G. E. (1992). Sequential study of the chronic nephrotoxicity induced by dietary administration of ethoxyquin in Fischer 344 rats. *Fundam. Appl. Toxicol. 18*:278–287.

Harman, D., Curtis, H. J., and Tilley, J. (1970). Chromosomal aberrations in liver cells of mice fed free radical reaction inhibitors. *J. Gerontol. 25*:17–19.

Hasegawa, R., Furukawa, F., Toyoda, K., Takahashi, Y., Hirose, M., and Ito, N. (1990). Inhibitory effects of antioxidants on N-bis (2-hydroxypropyl) nitrosamine induced lung carcinogenesis in rats. *Jpn. J. Cancer Res. 81*:871–877.

Hathway, D. E. (1966). Metabolic fate in animals of hindered phenolic antioxidants in relation to their safety evaluation and antioxidant function. *Adv. Food Res. 15*:1–56.

Hausen, B. M., and Beyer, W. (1992). The sensitizing capacity of the antioxidants propyl, octyl, and dodecyl gallates and some related gallic acid esters. *Contact Dermatitis 26*:253–258.

Hansen, E. and Meyer, O. (1978). A study of the teratogenicity of butylated hydroxyanisole in the rabbit. *Toxicology 10*:195–201.

Hayatsu, H. (1976). Bisulfite modification of nucleic acids and their constituents. *Prog. Nucl. Acid Res. Mol. Biol. 16*:75–124.

Hayatsu, H., Wataya, Y., Kai, K., and Iida, S. (1970). Reaction of sodium bisulfite with uracil, cytosine, and their derivatives. *Biochemistry 9*:2858–2865.

Hegsted, D. M., Trulson, M. F., and Stare, F. J. (1954). Role of wheat and wheat products in human nutrition. *Physiol. Rev. 34*:221–258.

Heindorff, K., Aurich, O., Michaelis, A., and Rieger, R. (1983). Genetic toxicology of ethylenediaminetetraacetic acid (EDTA). *Mut. Res. 115*:149–173.

Hiasa, Y., Konishi, N., Kitahori, Y., and Shimoyama, T. (1985). Carcinogenicity study of a commercial sodium oleate in Fischer rats. *Food Chem. Toxicol. 23*:619–623.

Hiasa, Y., Kitahori, Y., Morimoto, J., Konishi, N., Nakakoa, S., and Nishioka, H. (1992). Carcinogenicity study in rats of phytic acid 'Daichi', a natural food additive. *Food Chem. Toxicol. 30*:117–125.

Hillman, R. W. (1957). Tocopherol excess in man. Creatinuria associated with prolonged ingestion. *Am. J. Clin. Nutr. 5*:597–600.

Hirai, K. I., Witschi, H. P., and Cote, M. G. (1977). Electron microscopy of butylated hydroxytoluene induced lung damage in mice. *Exp. Mol. Pathol. 27*:295–308.

Hirono, I., Ueno, I., Hosaka, S., Takanashi, H., Matsushima, T., Sugimura, T., and Natori, S. (1981). Carcinogenicity examination of quercetin and rutin in ACI rats. *Cancer Lett. 13*:15–21.

Hirose, M., Shibata, M., Hagiwara, A., Imaida, K., and Ito, N. (1981). Chronic toxicity of butylated hydroxytoluene in wistar rats. *Food Chem. Toxicol. 19*:147–151.

Hodge, H. C., Fassett, D. W., Maynard, E. A., Downs, W. L., and Coye, R. D. Jr. (1964). Chronic feeding studies of butylated hydroxyanisole in dogs. *Toxicol. Appl. Pharmacol. 6*:512–519.

Holmes, R. P., and Yoss, N. L. (1984). 25-Hydroxysterols increase the permeability of liposomes to Ca^{2+} and other cations. *Biochim. Biophys. Acta 770*:285–332.

Hoppe, J. O., and Goble, F. C. (1951). The intravenous toxicity of sodium bisulfite. *J. Pharmacol. Exp. Ther. 101*:101–106.

Horn, H. J., Holland, E. G., and Hazelton, L. W. (1957). Safety of adipic acid as compared with citric acid and tartaric acid. *J. Agric. Food Chem. 5*:759–761.

Hornig, D., and Weiser, H. (1976). Interaction of erythorbic acid with ascorbic acid catabolism. *Int. J. Vit. Nutr. Res. 46*:40–47.

Hornig, D., Weber, F., and Wiss, O. (1974). Influence of erythorbic acid on vitamin C in guinea pigs. *Experientia 30*:173–174.

Hornig, D. H., and Moser, U. (1981). The safety of high vitamin C intakes in man. In *Vitamin C (Ascorbic Acid)*, Counsell, J. N. and Hornig, D. H.(eds). Applied Science Publishers, London, pp. 225–248.

Hosaka, S., and Hirono, I. (1981). Carcinogenicity test of quercetin by pulmonary-adenoma assay in strain A mice. *Gann 72*:327–328.

Houlihan, M. C., Ho, C. H., and Chang, S. S. (1985). The structure of rosmariquinone—a new antioxidant isolated from *R. officinalis* L. *J. Am. Oil Chem. Soc. 62*:96–98.

Huang, C. C., Huseh, J. L., Chen, H. H., and Batt, T. R. (1982). Retinol inhibits sister chromatid exchanges and cell cycle delay induced by cyclophosphamide and aflatoxin B1 in Chinese hamster V79 cells. *Carcinogenesis 3*:1–5.

Huang, H. S., and Goodman, D. S. (1965). Vitamin A and carotenoids. I. intestinal absorption and metabolism of ^{14}C labeled vit.A alcohol and β-carotene in the rat. *J. Biol. Chem. 240*:2839–2844.

Hudson, B. J. F., and Ghavami, M. (1984). Phospholipids as antioxidant synergists for tocopherols in the autoxidation of edible oils. *Leben. Wiss. Technol. 17*:191–194.

Ichihara, I. (1967). The fine structure of testicular interstitial cells in the mouse administered with vit.E. *Okajimas Folia Anat 43*:203–217.

Ichikawa, H., Ohishi, S., Takahashi, O, Kobayashi, H., Yuzawa, K., Hoshokawa, N., and Hashimoto, T. (1987). *Studies on the Acute Oral Toxicities of Phytic Acid and Sodium Phytate in Rats.* Annual Report of the Tokyo Metropolitan Research Laboratory of Public Health, Tokyo, pp. 371–376.

Ikeda, G. J., Stewart, J. E., Sapienza, P. P., Peggins, J. O., Michel, T. C., Olivito, V, Alam, H. Z., and O'Donnell, M. W., Jr. (1986). Effect of subchronic dietary administration of butylated hydroxyanisole on canine stomach and hepatic tissue. *Food Chem. Toxicol. 24*:1201–1221.

Imai, H., Werthessen, N. J., Subrahmanyam, V., Lequesne, P. W., Soloway, A. H., and Kanasawa, M. (1980). Angiotoxicity of oxygenated sterols and possible precursors. *Science 207*:651–653.

Inai, K., Kobuke, T., Nambu, S., Takemoto, T., Kou, E., Nishina, H., Fujihara, M., Yonehara, S., Suehiro, S., Tsuya, T., Horiuchi, K., and Tokuoka, S. (1988). Hepatocellular tumorigenicity of butylated hydroxytoluene administered orally to B6C3F1 mice. *Gann 79*:49–58.

Isaacks, R. E., Harkness, D. R., Goldman, P. H., Adler, J. L., and Kim, C. Y. (1977). Studies on avian erythrocyte metabolism. VII. Effects of inositol pentaphosphate and other organic phosphates on oxygen affinity of the embryonic and adult type hemoglobins of the turkey embryo. *Hemoglobin 1*:577–593.

Isensein, R. S. (1970). Ethoxyquin in rabbit feed: study of relationship to abortion and early neonatal death. *Am. J. Vet. Res. 31*:907–909.

Ishidate, M., Jr., and Odashima, S. (1977). Chromosome tests with 134 compounds on Chinese hamster cells in vitro. A screening of 14 carcinogens. *Mut. Res. 48*:337–354.

Ishidate, M. Jr., Sofumi, T., Yoshikawa, K., Hayashi, M., Nohmi, T., Sawada, M., and Matsuoka, A. (1984). Primary mutagenicity screening of food additives currently used in Japan. *Food Chem. Toxicol. 22*:623–636.

Ito, N., Hagiwara, A., Shibata, M., Ogiso, T., and Fukushima, S. (1982). Induction of squamous cell carcinoma in the forestomach of F344 rats treated with BHA. *Gann 73*:332–334.

Ito, N., Fukushima, S., Hagiwara, A., Shibata, M., and Ogiso, T. (1983a). Carcinogenicity of butylated hydroxyanisole in F344 rats. *J. Natl. Cancer Inst. 70*:343–352.

Ito, N., Fukushima, S., Imaida, K., Sakata, T., and Masui, T. (1983b). Induction of papilloma in the forestomach of hamsters by butylated hydroxyanisole. *Gann 74*:459–461.

Ito, N., Hirose, M., Kurata, Y.M., Ikawa, E., Nera, Y., and Fukushima, S. (1984). Induction of forestomach hyperplasia by crude BHA, a mixture of 3-tert and 2-tert isomers in Syrian golden hamsters is due to 3-tert BHA. *Gann 75*:471–474.

Ito, N., Hirose, M., Fukushima, S., Tsuda, H., Shirai, T., and Tatematsu, M. (1986). Studies on antioxidants: their carcinogenic and modifying effects on chemical carcinogenesis. *Food Chem. Toxicol. 24*:1071–1082.

Ito, N., Fukushima, S., and Hirose, M. (1987). Modification of the carcinogenic response by antioxidants. In *Toxicological Aspects of Food*, Miller, K. (ed). Elsevier Applied Sci., New York, pp. 253–293.

Iverson, F., Truelove, J., Nera, E., Lok, E., Clayson, D.B., and Wong, J. (1986). A 12 week study of butylated hydroxyanisole in the cyanomalgus monkey. *Food Chem. Toxicol. 24*:1197–1200.

Jagiello, G. M., Lin, J. S., and Ducayen, M. B. (1975). SO$_2$ and its metabolites: effects on mammalian egg chromosomes. *Environ. Res. 9*:84–93.

Johnson, A. R. (1965). A re-examination of the possible teratogenic effect of butylated hydroxytoluene (BHT) and its effect on the reproductive capacity of the mouse. *Food. Cosmet. Toxicol. 3*:371–375.

Johnson, A. R., and Hewgill, F. R. (1961). The effect of antioxidants, butylated hydroxyanisole, butylated hydroxytoluene, and propyl gallate on growth, liver, and serum lipids and serum sodium levels of the rat. *Aust. J. Exp. Biol. Med. Sci. 39*:353–360.

Johnson, F. C. (1971). A critical review of the safety of phenolic antioxidants in foods. *CRC Crit. Rev. Food Technol 2*:267–304.

Johnson, V., Carlson, A. J., Kleitman, N., and Bergstrom, P. (1938). Action of gum guaiacum upon the animal organism. *Food Res. 3*:555–574.

Jurgens, G., Lang, J., and Esterbauer, H. (1986). Modification of the human low density lipoproteins by the lipid peroxidation product 4-hydroxynonenal. *Biochim. Biophys. Acta 875*:103–114.

Kallner, A. B., Hartman, D, and Hornig, D. H. (1981). On the requirements of ascorbic acid in man: steady state turnover and bodypool in smokers. *Am. J. Clin. Nutr. 34*:1347–1355.

Kamm, J. J. (1982). Toxicology, carcinogenicity, and teratogenicity of some orally administered retinoids. *J. Am. Acad. Dermatol. 6*:652–659.

Kamm, J. J., Ashenfelter, K. O., and Ehmann, C. W. (1984). Preclinical and clinical toxicology of selected retinoids. In *The Retinoids*, Vol. 2, Sporn, B. M., Roberts, A. B. and Goodman, D. S. (eds). Academic Press Inc., London, pp. 287–326.

Kamogawa, A., and Fukui, T. (1973). Inhibition of α-glucan phosphorylase by bisulfite competition at the phosphate binding site. *Biochim. Biophys. Acta 302*:158–166.

Kanazawa, K., and Ashida, H. (1991). Target enzymes on hepatic dysfunction caused by dietary products of lipid peroxidation. *Arch. Biochim. Biophys. 288*:71–78.

Kanazawa, K., Kanazawa, E., and Natake, M. (1985). Uptake of secondary autoxidation products of linoleic acid by the rat. *Lipids 20*:412–419.

Kanazawa, K., Ashida, H., Minamoto, S., Danno, G., and Natake, M. (1988). The effects of orally administered secondary autoxidation products of linoleic acid in the rat. *J. Nutr. Sci. Vit. 34*:363–373.

Kanematsu, H., Aoyama, M., Maruyama, T., Niiya, I., Tsukamoto, M., Tokairin, S., and Matsumoto, T. (1984). Studies on the improvement of antioxidant effect of tocopherols. IV. Synergistic effect of ascorbic and erythorbic acids (in Japanese). *Yukagaku 33*:361–365.

Kanner, J., Ben-Gera, I., and Berman, S. (1980). Nitric oxide myoglobin as an inhibitor of lipid oxidation. *Lipids 15*:944–948.

Kaplan, D., McJilton, C., and Luchtel, D. (1975). Bisulfite induced lipid oxidation. *Arch. Environ. Health 30*:507–509.

Kappus, H. (1991). Lipid peroxidation: mechanisms and biological significance. In *Free Radicals and Food Additives*, Arouma, O. I., and Halliwell, B. (eds.). Taylor and Francis, London, pp. 59–75.

Kappus, H., and Diplock, A. T. (1992). Tolerance and safety of vitamin E: a toxicological position report. *Free Rad. Biol. Med. 13*:55–74.

Karahadian, C., and Lindsay, R. C. (1988). Evaluation of the mechanism of dilauryl thiodipropionate antioxidant activity. *J. Am. Oil Chem. Soc. 65*:1159–1165.

Karplyuk, I. A. (1959). Toxicological characteristics of phenolic antioxidants of edible fats. *Voprosy Pitaniya 18*:24–29.

Karplyuk, I. A. (1962). Effects of phenolic antioxidants of nutritive fats on the animal organism. *Trudy 2-oi (vtor) Nauchn. Konf. Po Vopr. Probl. Zhira. V Pitanii Leningrad*: 318–325.

Kawachi, T., Yahagi, T., Kada, T., Tazyma, Y., Ishidate, M., Sasaki, M., and Sugiyama, T. (1980). Cooperative program on short-term assays for carcinogenicity in Japan. In *Molecular and Cellular Aspects of Carcinogen Screening Tests*, Montesano, R., Bartsch, H., and Tomatis, L. (eds). International Agency for Research on Cancer, IARC Scientific Publication No. 27. Lyon.

Kawano, S., Nakao, T., and Hiraga, K. (1980). Species strain differences in the butylated hydroxytoluene produced induction of hepatic drug oxidation enzymes. *Jpn. J. Pharmac. 30*:861–870.

Kim, H. L. (1991). Accumulation of ethoxyquin in the tissue. *J. Toxicol. Environ. Health 33*:229–236.

King, D. W. (1964). Comparative effects of certain antioxidants on gestational performance and teratogenicity in vitamin E deficient rats. *J. Nutr. 83*:123–132.

King, M. M., and McCay, P. B. (1980). DMBA-induced mammary tumor incidence: effect of propyl gallate supplementation in purified diets containing different types and amounts of fat. *Proc. Am. Assoc. Cancer Res. 21*:113 abst.

King, M. M., and McCay, P. B. (1983). Modulation of tumor incidence and possible mechanisms of inhibition of mammary carcinogenesis by dietary antioxidants. *Cancer Res. 43*:2485S–2490S.

Kitamura, N., and Hayatsu, H. (1974). Cleavage of the glycosidic linkage of pyramidine ribonucleosides by bisulfite-oxygen system. *Nucleic Acids Res. 1*:75–86.

Kleijer, W. J., Hoeksema, J. L., Sluyter, M. L., and Bootsma, D. (1973). Effects of inhibitors on repair of DNA in normal human and xeroderma pigmentosum cells after exposure to X-rays and ultraviolet irradiation. *Mut. Res. 17*:385–394.

Koerner, W. F., and Voellm, J. (1975). New aspects of the tolerance of retinols in humans. *Int. J. Vit. Nutr. Res. 45*:363–372.

Krasavage, W. J. (1977). Evaluation of the teratogenic potential of teritary butyl hydroquinone (TBHQ) in the rat. *Teratology 16*:31–33.

Krasavage, W. J., and Terhaar, C. J. (1977). d-α-Tocopheryl poly(ethylene glycol) 1000 succinate. Acute toxicity, subchronic feeding, reproduction, and teratologic studies in the rat. *J. Agric. Food Chem. 25*:273–278.

Krop, S., and Gold, H. (1945). Toxicity of hydroxyacetic acid after prolonged administration: comparison with its sodium salt and citric and tartaric acids. *J. Am. Pharm. Assoc. 34*:86–89.

Kuebler, W. (1958). Importance of nitrate content of vegetables in the nutrition of infants. *Z. Kinderheilkd. 81*:405–416.

Kuebler, W. (1963). Carotene in the nutrition of infants. *Wiss. veroeffentl. Dtsch. Ges. Ernahr. 9*:222–234.

Kuebler, W., and Gehler, J. (1970). Kinetics of enteral ascorbic acid absorption. Calculation of dose-nonproportional absorption processes. *Int. J. Vit. Res. 40*:442–453.

Kuhnau, J. (1976). The flavonoids, a class of semi-essential food components: their role in human nutrition. *World Rev. Nutr. Diet. 24*:117–191.

Kwon, T. W., and Brown, W. D. (1965). Complex formation between malonaldehyde and bovine serum albumin. *Fed. Proc. Fed. Am. Soc. Exp. Biol. 24*:592 (Abst.).

Labuza, T. P. (1971). Kinetics of lipid oxidation in foods. *CRC Crit. Rev. Food Technol. 2*:355–405.

LaChance, L. E. (1959). The effect of chelation and X-rays on fecundity and induced dominant lethals in *Habrobracon*. *Radiation Res. 11*:218–228.

Ladomery, L. G., Ryan, A. J., and Wright, S. E. (1967). The excretion of ^{14}C butylated hydroxytoluene in the rat. *J. Pharm. Pharmacol. 19*:383–387.

Lamano-Carvalho, T. L., Lopes, R. A., Azoubel, R., and Ferreira, A. L. (1978). Morphometric study of testicle alterations in rats submitted to hypervitaminosis A. *Int. J. Vit. Nutr. Res. 48*:307–315.

Lang, K. (1959). Comprehensive review. Phosphate requirements and injury with high phosphate feeding. *Z. Lebensmitt. Untersuch. 110*:450–456.

Lauersen, F. (1953). Comprehensive review. The health considerations on the use of phosphoric acid and primary phosphates in refreshment drinks. *Z. Lebensmitt. Untersuch. 96*:418–440.

Lee, M. H. and Sher, R. L. (1984). Extraction of green tea antioxidants and their antioxidant activities in various edible oils and fats (in Chinese). *J. Chin. Agric. Chem. Soc. 22*:226–231.

Lee, M. H., Sher, R. L., Sheu, C. H., and Tsai, Y. C. (1984). Safety evaluation of natural antioxidant from tea (in Chinese). *J. Chin. Agric. Chem. Soc., 22*:128–135.

Lehman, A. J. (1958). Quarterly report to the editor on topics of current interest-nitrites and nitrates in meat products. *Quart. Bull. Ass. Food Drug Off. 22*:136–138.

Lehman, A. J., Fitzhugh, O. G., Nelson, A. A., and Woodard, G. (1951). The pharmacological evaluation of antioxidants. *Adv. Food Res. 3*:197–208.

Leontjiva, G. A., Mantzighin, Y. A., and Gaziev, A. I. (976). The ultrafast repair of single strand breaks in DNA of gamma irradiated Chinese hamster cells. *Int. J. Radiat. Biol. 30*:577–580.

Lewis, J. D. (1977). Comparison of the distribution of L+ and DL forms of tartaric acid in the rat. *Acta Pharmacol. Toxicol. 41*:144–145.

Lhuissier, M., Hugot, D., Leclerc, J., and Causeret, J. (1967). Physiological and nutritional effects of sulfite ingestion. *Cah. Nutr. Diet. 2*:23–28.

Lieberman, J., and Ove, P. (1962). Deoxyribonucleic acid synthesis and its inhibition in mammalian cells cultured from the animal. *J. Biol. Chem. 237*:1634–1642.

Lin, J. S., and Olcott, H. S. (1975). Ethoxyquin nitroxide. *J. Agric. Food Chem. 23*:798–800.

Lindenschmidt, R. C., Tryka, A. F., Goad, M. E., and Witschi, H. P. (1986). The effect of dietary butylated hydroxytoluene on liver and colon tumor development in mice. *Toxicology 38*:151–160.

Litton Bionetics Inc. (1974a). *Mutagenic Evaluation of the Compound FDA 71-39, Propyl Gallate.* NTIS PB-245 441. Kensington, MD.

Litton Bionetics, Inc. (1974b). *Mutagenic Evaluation of the Compound FDA 71-24 (Butylated Hydroxyanisole).* NTIS PB-245 460. Kensington, MD.

Lo, L. W., and Stich, H. F. (1978). The use of short-term tests to measure the preventive action of carcinogenic nitroso compounds. *Mut. Res. 57*:57–67.

Locke, A., Locke, R. B., Schlesinger, H., and Carr, H. (1942). The comparative toxicity and cathartic efficiency of disodium tartarate and fumarate and magnesium fumarate for the mouse and rabbit. *J. Am. Pharm. Assoc. 31*:12–14.

Loliger, J. (1991). The use of antioxidants in foods. In *Free Radicals and Food Additives*, Arouma, O. I., and Halliwell, B. (eds). Taylor and Francis, London, pp. 121–150.

Lundberg, W. O., Dockstader, W. B., and Halvorson, H. O. (1947). The kinetics of oxidation of several antioxidants in oxidizing fats. *J. Am. Oil Chem. Soc. 24*:89–92.

MacDonald, D. S., Gray, J. I., and Gibbins, L. N. (1980). Role of nitrite in cured meat flavor: antioxidant role of nitrite. *J. Food Sci. 45*:893–897.

MacGregor, J. T., Wehr, C. M., Manners, G. D., Jurd, L., Minkler, J. K., and Carrano, A. V. (1983). In vivo exposure to plant flavonols: influence of frequencies of micronuclei in mouse erythrocytes and sister chromatid exchange in rabbit lymphocytes. *Mut. Res. 124*:255–270.

MacRae, W. D., and Stich, H. F. (1979). Induction of sister chromatid exchanges in Chinese hamster cells by the reducing agents bisulfite and ascorbic acid. *Toxicology 13*:167–174.

Maddock, C. L., Wolbach, S. B., and Maddock, S. (1949). Hypervitaminosis A in the dog. *J. Nutr. 39*:117–137.

Magee, P. N. (1971). Toxicity of nitrosamines: their possible human health hazards. *Food Cosmet. Toxicol. 9*:207–218.

Mai, J., Chambers, L. J., and McDonald, R. E. (1985). *Tea Extract Used for Food Preservation*. U.K. Patent GB 2151123A.

Mallon, R. G., and Rossman, T. B. (1981). Bisulfite is a comutagen in *E. coli* and in Chinese hamster cells. *Mut. Res. 88*:125–133.

Manson, M. M., Green, J. A., Wright, B. J., and Carthrew, P. (1992). Degree of ethoxyquin induced nephrotoxicity in rat is dependent on age and sex. *Arch. Toxicol. 66*:51–56.

March, B. E., Wong, E., Seier, L., Sim, J., and Biely, J. (1973). Hypervitaminosis E in the chick. *J. Nutr. 103*:371–377.

Marcuse, R. J. (1962). The effect of some amino acids on the oxidation of linoleic acid and its methyl ester. *J. Am. Oil Chem. Soc. 39*:97–103.

Marino, A. A., and Mitchell, J. T. (1972). Lung damage in mice following intraperitoneal injection of butylated hydroxytoluene. *Proc. Soc. Exp. Biol. Med. 140*:122–125.

Martin, A. D., and Gilbert, D. (1968). Enzyme changes accompanying liver enlargement in rats treated with 3-tert-butyl-4-hydroxyanisole. *Biochem. J. 106*:22p (Abst.).

Martindale's Extra Pharmacopoeia. (1972). 26th ed. The Pharmaceutical Press, London.

Massey, V., Muller, F., Feldberg, R., Schuman, M., Sullivan, P., Howell, L. G., Mayhew, S. G., Matthews, R. G., and Foust, G. P. (1969). The reactivity of flavoproteins with sulfite. Possible relevance to the problem of oxygen reactivity. *J. Biol. Chem. 244*:3999–4006.

Masui, T., Hirose, M., Imaida, K., Fukushima, S., Tamano, S., and Ito, N. (1986). Sequential changes of the forestomach of F344 rats, Syrian golden hamsters, and B6C3F1 mice treated with butylated hydroxyanisole. *Gann. 77*:1083–1090.

Matsuo, M., Mihara, K., Okuno, M., Ohkawa, H., and Miyamoto, J. (1984). Comparative metabolism of 3,5 di-tert-butyl-4-hydroxytoluene (BHT) in mice and rats. *Food Chem. Toxicol. 22*:345–354.

Matsuoka, K., Matsui, M., Miyata, N., Sofuni, T., and Ishidate, M., Jr. (1990). Mutagenicity of 3-tert-butyl-4-hydroxyanisole and its metabolites in short term tests in vitro. *Mut. Res. 241*:125–132.

Matsushita, S. (1975). Specific interactions of linoleic acid hydroperoxides and their secondary degradation products with enzyme proteins. *J. Agric. Food Chem. 23*:150–154.

McCann, J. E., Chio, E., Yamasaki, E., and Ames, B. N. (1975). Detection of carcinogens as mutagens in the *Salmonella/* microsome test: assay of 300 chemicals. *Proc. Nat. Acad. Sci. 72*:5135–5139.

McFarlane, D. (1941). Experimental phosphate nephritis in the rat. *J. Path. Bacteriol. 52*:17–24.

McKay, E. M., and Oliver, J. (1935). Renal damage following the ingestion of a diet containing an excess of inorganic phosphate. *J. Exp. Med. 61*:319–333.

Menzel, D. B. (1967). Reaction of oxidizing lipids with ribonuclease. *Lipids 2*:83–84.

Merrill, J. M. (1959). Symposium on significance of lowered cholesterol levels. *J. Am. Med. Assoc. 170*:2202–2203.

Meyer, O., Blom, L., and Olsen, P. (1978). Influence of diet and strain of rat on kidney damage observed in toxicity studies. *Arch. Toxicol.* (Suppl. 1): 355–358.

Mikhailova, Z., Vachkova, R., Vasileva, L., Stavreva, T., Donchev, N. Goranov, I., and Tyagunenko, E. (1985). Toxicological study of the long-term effect of the antioxidant dodecyl gallate on white rats (in Russian). *Voprosy-Pitaniya 2*:49–52.

Minkin, W., Cohen, H. J., and Frank, S. B. (1973). Contact dermatitis from deodorants. *Arch. Dermatol. 107*:774–775.

Mirvish, S. S. (1975). Blocking the formation of N-nitroso compounds with ascorbic acid in vitro and in vivo. *Ann. NY Acad Sci. 258*:175–180.

Mirvish, S. S. (1983). The etiology of gastric cancer: intragastric nitrosamine formation and other theories. *J. Natl. Cancer. Inst. 71*:630–647.

Moore, M. A., Tsuda, H., Thamvit, W., Masui, T., and Ito, N. (1987). Differential modification of development of preneoplastic lesions in the Syrian golden hamsters initiated with a single dose of 2,2'-dioxo-N-nitrosodipropylamine: influence of subsequent butylated hydroxyanisole, α-tocopherol or carbazole. *J. Natl. Cancer Inst. 78*:289–293.

Morino, K., Matsukura, N., Kawachi, T., Ohgaki, H., Sugimura, T., and Hirono, I. (1982). Carcinogenicity test of quercetin and rutin in golden hamster by oral administration. *Carcinogenesis 3*:93–97.

Morrissey, P. A., and Tichivangana, J. Z. (1985). The antioxidant activities of nitrite and nitrosylmyoglobin in cooked meats. *Meat Sci. 14*:175–190.

Movaghar, K. N. (1990). *Fruit and Vegetable Dried Products*. U.S. Patent No. 4,948,609.

Mukai, F. H., and Goldstein, B. D. (1976). Mutagenicity of malonaldehyde, a decomposition product of polyunsaturated fatty acids. *Science 191*:868–869.

Mukai, F., Hawryluk, I., and Shapiro, R. (1970). The mutagenic specificity of sodium bisulfite. *Biochim. Biophys. Res. Commun. 39*:983–988.

Mukherjee, A., Talukder, G., and Sharma, A. (1989). Sister chromatid exchanges induced by tertiary butyl hydroquinone in bone marrow cells of mice. *Environ. Mol. Mutagen 13*:234–237.

Muralidhara, and Narasimhamurthy, K. (1991). Assessment of in vivo mutagenic potency of ethylenediaminetetraacetic acid in albino mice. *Food Cosmet. Toxicol. 29*:845–849.

Musil, J. (1966). Effect of chronic sodium nitrite intoxication in rats. *Acta Biol. Med. Ger. 16*:380–386.

Nafstad, I., and Skaare, J. U. (1978). Ultrastructural hepatic changes in rats after oral administration of ethoxyquin. *Toxicol. Lett. 1*:295–299.

Nakagawa, Y., and Tayama, K. (1988). Nephrotoxicity of butylated hydroxytoluene in phenobarbital-pretreated male rats. *Arch. Toxicol. 61*:359–365.

Nakao, Y., Takagi, S., and Nakatani, H. (1972). *Meat Color Stabilization*. U.S. Patent No. 3,666,488.

Naruszewicz, M., Wozny, E., Mirkiewicz, E., Nowioka, G., and Szostak, W. B. (1987). The effect of thermally oxidized soybean oil on metabolism of chylomicrons: increased uptake and degradation of oxidized chylomicrons in cultured mouse macrophages. *Atherosclerosis 66*:45–33.

National Institutes of Health (1983). *Carcinogenesis Bioassay of L-Ascorbic Acid in F344 Rats and B6C3F1 Mice (Feed Study)*. NIH Publication No. 83-2503. Research Triangle Park, NC.

Nazario, G. (1952). Use of acids in foods. *Rev. Inst. Adolfo. Lutz. 2*:141–158.

Nelson, T. S., and Kirby, L. K. (1979). Effect of age and diet composition on the hydrolysis of phytate phosphorus by rats. *Nutr. Rep. Int. 20*:729–734.

Nera, E. A., Lok, E., Iverson, F., Ormsby, E., Karpinski, K. F., and Clayson, D. B. (1984). Short-time pathological and proliferative effects of butylated hydroxyanisole and other phenolic antioxidants in the forestomach of Fischer 344 rats. *Toxicology 32*:197–213.

Newberne, P. M. (1979). Nitrite promotes lymphoma incidence in rats. *Science 204*:1079–1081.

Neyes, L., Stimpel, M., Locher, R., Vetter, W., and Streuli, R. (1985). Oxidized derivatives of cholesterol and its interference with the calcium channel. *J. Am. Oil Chem. Soc. 62*:634 (Abst.).

Nieman, C., and Klein Obbink, H. J. (1954). The biochemistry and pathology of hypervitaminosis A. *Vit. Horm. 12*:69–99.

Nigrovic, V. (1964). The in vivo inactivation of alkaline phosphatase by DTPA and EDTA. *Arch. Exp. Pathol. Pharmacol. 249*:206–214.

Nishigaki, I., Hagihara, M., Maseki, M., Tomoda, Y., Nagayama, K., Nakashima, T., and Yagi, K. (1984). Effect of linoleic acid hydroperoxide on uptake of low density lipo-protein by cultured smooth muscle cells from rabbit aorta. *Biochem. Int.* 8:501–506.

Norkus, E. P., Kuenzig, W., and Conney, A. H. (1983). Studies on the mutagenic activity of ascorbic acid in vitro and in vivo. *Mut. Res.* 117:183–191.

Ogata, A., Ando, H., Kubo, Y., Sasaki, M., and Hosokawa, N. (1987). *Teratological Studies of Phytic Acid in ICR Mice.* Annual Report of the Tokyo Metropolitan Research Laboratory of Public Health. Tokyo, pp. 377–381.

Ohno, T., and Myoga, K. (1981). The possible toxicity of vit.C in the guinea pigs. *Nutr. Rep. Int.* 24:291–294.

Okubo, K., Myers, D., and Iacobucci, G. A. (1976). Binding of phytic acid to glycinin. *Cereal Chem.* 53:513–524.

Olcott, H. S. (1958). The roles of free fatty acids on nutritional effectiveness of unsaturated fats. *J. Am. Oil Chem. Soc.* 35:597–599.

Olsen, P., Meyer, O., Billie, N., and Wurtzen, G. (1986). Carcinogenicity study on butylated hydroxytoluene in wistar rats exposed in utero. *Food Chem. Toxicol.* 24:1–12.

Olson, J. A. (1961). The conversion of radioactive β-carotene into vitamin A by the rat intestine in vitro. *J. Biol. Chem.* 236:349–356.

Olson, R. E. Jones, J. P. (1979). The inhibition of vitamin K action by d-α-tocopherol and its derivatives. *Fed. Proc.* 38:710 abst.

Omura, H., Shinohara, K., Maeda, H., Nonaka, M., and Murakami, H. (1978). Mutagenic action of triose reductone and ascorbic acid on *Salmonella typhimurium* TA 100 strain. *J. Nutr. Sci. Vitaminol* 24:185–194.

Ondrej, M. (1965). *Influence of Interaction Between EDTA and X-rays on Mutation and Crossover Frequencies in Drosophila melanogaster.* Induction Mut. Mutation Process Proc. Symp., pp. 26–29. Prague.

Orten, J. M., Kuyper, A. C., and Smith, A. H. (1948). Studies on the toxicity of propyl gallate and of antioxidant mixtures containing propyl gallate. *Food Technol.* 2:308–316.

Oser, B. L., Oser, M., and Spencer, H. C. (1963). Safety evaluation studies of calcium EDTA. *Toxicol. Appl. Pharmacol.* 5:142–162.

Oshino, N. and Chance, B. (1975). The properties of sulfite oxidation in perfused rat liver: Interaction of sulfite oxidase with the mitochondrial respiratory chain. *Arch. Biochim. Biophys.* 170:514–528.

Packman, E. W., Abbot, D. D., and Harrison, J. W. E. (1963). Comparative subacute toxicity for rabbits of citric, fumaric, and tartaric acids. *Toxicol. Appl. Pharmacol.* 5:163–167.

Pamukçu, A. M., Yalciner, S., Hatcher, J. F., and Bryan, G. T. (1980). Quercetin, a rat intestinal and bladder carcinogen present in bracken fern (*Pteridium aquilinum*). *Cancer Res.* 40:3468–3472.

Parke, D. V., Rahim, A., and Walker, R. (1972). Effects of ethoxyquin on hepatic micro-somal enzymes. *Biochem. J.* 130:84p (Abst.).

Parke, D. V., Rahim, A., and Walker, R. (1974). Reversibility of hepatic changes caused by ethoxyquin. *Biochem. Pharmacol.* 23:1871–1876.

Parkinson, T. M., Halladay, S. C., and Enderlin, F. E. (1978a). Metabolic fate of orally administered poly AO®-79 in experimental animals. *J. Am. Oil Chem. Soc.* 55:242A.

Parkinson, T. M., Honohan, T., Enderlin, F. E., Halladay, S. C., Hale, R. L., de Keczer, S. A., Dubin, P. L., Ryerson, B. A., and Read, A. R. (1978b). Intestinal absorption, distribution, and excretion of an orally administered polymeric antioxidant in rats and mice. *Food Cosmet. Toxicol.* 16:321–330.

Paschin, Yu. V., and Bahitova, L. M. (1984). Inhibition of the mutagenicity of benzo(a)pyrene in the V79/HGPRT system by bioantioxidants. *Mut. Res.* 137:57–59.

Patterson, R. M., Keith, L. A., and Stewart, J. (1987). Increase in chromosomal abnormalities in Chinese hamster ovary cells treated with butylated hydroxytoluene in vitro. *Toxicol. In Vitro 1*:55–57.

Pearson, A. M., Gray, J. I., Wolzak, A. M., and Horenstein, N. A. (1983). Safety implications of oxidized lipids in muscle foods. *Food Technol. 37*:121–129.

Pearson, C. K., and MacBarnes, M. (1970). Absorption of tocopherols by small intestinal loops of the rat in vivo. *Int. Z. Vitaminforsch. 40*:19–22.

Pease, G. M. (1962). Focal retardation and arrestment of growth of bones due to vitamin A intoxication. *J. Am. Med. Assoc. 182*:980–985.

Peng, S. K., and Morin, R. J. (1987). Effects on membrane function by cholesterol oxidation derivatives in cultured smooth muscle aortic cells. *Artery 14*:85–99.

Peng, S. K., Taylor, C. B., Tham, P., Werthessen, N. J., and Mikkelson, B. (1978). Effects of autoxidation products from cholesterol on aortic smooth muscle cells. *Arch. Path. Lab. Med. 102*:57–61.

Peng, S. K., Morin, R. J., Tham, P., and Taylor, C. B. (1985a). Effects of oxygenated derivatives of cholesterol on cholesterol uptake by cultured aortic smooth muscle cells. *Artery 13*:144–164.

Peng, S. K., Morin, R. J., and Sentovich, S. (1985b). Effects of cholesterol oxidation products on membrane functions. *J. Am. Oil Chem. Soc. 62*:634 (Abst.).

Perry, H. M., Jr., and Perry, E. F. (1959). Normal concentration of some trace metals in human urine: changes produced by ethylenediaminetetraacetate (EDTA). *J. Clin. Invest. 38*:1452–1463.

Petering, D. H., and Shih, N. T. (1975). Biochemistry of bisulfite-sulfur dioxide. *Environ. Res. 9*:55–65.

Peters, J. M., and Boyd, E. M. (1969). Toxic effects from a rancid diet containing large amounts of raw egg white powder. *Food Cosmet. Toxicol. 7*:197–207.

Piche, L. A., Draper, H. H., and Cole, P. D. (1988). Malonaldehyde excretion by subjects consuming codliver oil vs a concentrate of n-3 fatty acids. *Lipids 23*:370–371.

Placer, Z., Veselkova, Z., and Petrasek, R. (1964). Hemmung von Esterasen-systemem durch Felt-antioxydanten. *Nahrung 8*:707–708.

Powell, C. J., Connelly, S. M., Jones, S. M., Grasso, P., and Bridges, J. W. (1986). Hepatic responses to the administration of high doses of BHT to the rat: their relevance to hepatocarcinogenicity. *Food Chem. Toxicol. 24*:1131–1143.

Pruthi, J. S. (1980). *Spices and condiments: chemistry, microbiology, and technology*. Academic Press, London.

Raines Bell, R., Draper, H. H., Tzeng, D. Y. M., Shin, H. K., and Schmidt, G. R. (1977). Physiological responses of human adults to foods containing phosphate additives. *J. Nutr. 107*:42–50.

Raj, A. S., and Katz, M. (1984). Corn oil and its minor constituents as inhibitors of DMBA induced chromosomal breaks in vivo. *Mut. Res. 136*:247–253.

Raymond, J. Z., and Gross, P. R. (1969). EDTA: preservative dermatitis. *Arch. Dermatol. 100*:436–440.

Reddy, N. R., Sathe, S. K., and Salunkhe, D. K. (1982). Phytates in legumes and cereals. *Adv. Food Res. 28*:1–92.

Reid, R. L., Jung, G. A., Weiss, R., Post, A. J., Horn, F. P., Kahle, E. B., and Carlson, C. E. (1969). Performance of ewes on nitrogen fertilized orchard grass pasture. *J. Animal Sci. 29*:181–186.

Reuber, M. D., and Schmieller, G. C. (1962). Edetate kidney lesions in rats. *Arch. Environ. Health 5*:430–436.

Reynolds, R. C., Astill, B. D., and Fassett, D. W. (1974). The fate of thiodipropionates in rats. *Toxicol. Appl. Pharmacol. 28*:133–141.

Rogers, C. G., Nayak, B. N., and Heroux-Metcalf, C. (1985). Lack of induction of sister chromatid exchanges and of mutation to 6-thioguanine resistance in V79 cells by butylated hydroxyanisole with and without activation by rat or hamster hepatocytes. *Cancer Lett. 27*:61–69.

Rogers, C. G., Boyes, B. G., Matula, T. I., and Stapley, R. (1992). Evaluation of genotoxicity of tert-butyl hydroquinone in an hepatocyte mediated assay with V79 Chinese hamster lung cells and in strain D7 of *Saccharomyces cerevisiae. Mut. Res. 280*:17–27.

Rosa, F. W., Wilk, A. L., and Kelsey, F. O. (1986). Teratogen update: vitamin A congeners. *Teratology 33*:355–364.

Rosenfield, A. B., and Huston, R. (1950). Infant methemoglobinemia in Minnesota due to nitrites in well water. *Minn. Med. 33*:787–796.

Rosin, M. P., and Stich, H. F. (1980). Enhancing and inhibiting effect of propyl gallate on carcinogen induced mutagenesis. *J. Environ. Path. Toxicol. 4*:159–167.

Rosin, M. P., San, R. H. C., and Stich, H. F. (1980). Mutagenic activity of ascorbate in mammalian cell cultures. *Cancer Lett. 8*:299–305.

Roy, A. B. (1960). The synthesis and hydrolysis of sulfate esters. *Adv. Enzymol. 22*: 205–235.

Ryan, A. J., and Wright, S. E. (1964). Food additives project report. *Food Technol. Aust. 16*:626–629.

Saheb, W., and Witschi, H. P. (1975). Lung growth in mice after a single dose of butylated hydroxytoluene. *Toxicol. Appl. Pharmacol. 33*:309–319.

Sahu, R. K., Basu, R., and Sharma, A. (1981). Genetic toxicological testing of some plant flavonoids by the micronucleus test. *Mut. Res. 89*:69–74.

Saito, D., Shirai, A., Matsushima, T., Sugimura, T., and Hirono, I. (1980). Test of carcinogenicity of quercetin, a widely distributed mutagen in food. *Teratogen Carcinogen Mutagen 1*:213–221.

Samborskaya, E. P. (1964). The effect of high ascorbic acid doses on the course of pregnancy on the guinea pig and on the progeny (translation). *Byull. Eksp. Biol. Med. 57*:105–108.

Samborskaya, E. P., and Ferdman, T. D. (1966). The mechanism of termination of pregnancy by ascorbic acid (translation). *Byull. Eksp. Biol. Med. 62*:96–98.

Sander, J., and Seif, F. (1969). Bakteriele Reduktion von Nitrat im Magen des Menschen als Ursache einer Nitrosaminbildung. *Arzneimittel forsch 19*:1091–1093.

Sasaguri, Y., Nakashima, T., Morimatsu, M., and Yagi, K. (1984). Injury to cultured endothelial cells from human umbilical cord vein by linoleic acid hydroperoxides. *J. Appl. Biochem. 6*:144–150.

Sasaguri, Y., Morimatsu, M., Nakashima, T., Tokunaga, O., and Yagi, K. (1985). Difference in the inhibitory effect of linoleic acid hydroperoxide on prostacyclin biosynthesis between cultured endothelial cells from human umbilical cord vein and cultured smooth muscle cells from rabbit aorta. *Biochem. Int. 11*:517–521.

Savini, C., Morelli, R., Piancastelli, E., and Restani, S. (1989). Contact dermatitis due to ethoxyquin. *Contact Dermatitis 21*:342–343.

Schmandke, H., and Schmidt, G. (1968). Degradation of α-tocopherol in man. *Int. Z. Vitaminforsch. 38*:75–78.

Schmandke, H., Sima, C., and Maune, R. (1969). α-Tocopherol absorption in man. *Int. Z. Vitaminforsch. 39*:296–298.

Schroeter, L. C. (1966). *Sulfur Dioxide. Applications in Foods, Beverages, and Pharmaceuticals.* Pergamon Press, Oxford, England.

Schuberth, O., and Wretlind, A. (1961). Intravenous infusion of fat emulsions, phosphatides, and emulsifying agents. *Acta. Chir. Scand. 278*(Suppl.):1–21.

Schwab, A. W., Moser, H. A., Curley, R. S., and Evans, C. D. (1953). The flavor problem of soybean oil. XIII. Sulfur coordination compounds effective in edible oil stabilization. *J. Am. Oil Chem. Soc. 30*:413–417.

Schwope, A. D., Till, D. E., Ehntholt, D. J., Sidman, K. R., Whelan, R. H., Schwartz, P. S., and Reid, R. C. (1987a). Migration of Irganox-1010 from ethylene-vinyl acetate films to foods and food simulating liquids. *Food Chem. Toxicol. 25*:327–330.

Schwope, A. D., Till, D. E., Ehntholt, D. J., Sidman, K. R., Whelan, R. H., Schwartz, P. S., and Reid, R. C. (1987b). Migration of BHT and Irganox-1010 from low density polyethylene to foods and food simulating liquids. *Food Chem. Toxicol. 25*:317–326.

Sciorra, L. J., Kaufman, B. N., and Maier, R. (1974). The effects of butylated hydroxytoluene on the cell cycle and chromosome morphology of phytohemagglutinin stimulated leukocyte cultures. *Food Cosmet. Toxicol. 12*:33–44.

Scott, J. W., Cort, W. M., Harley, J. H., Parrish, D. R., and Saucy, G. (1974). 6-Hydroxychroma-2-carboxylic acids: novel antioxidants. *J. Am. Oil Chem. Soc. 51*:200–203.

Seawright, A. A., English, P. B., and Gartner, R. J. W. (1967). Hypervitaminosis A and deforming spondylosis of the cat. *J. Comp. Pathol. 77*:29–39.

Sen, N. P., Smith, D. C., and Schwinghamer, L. (1969). Formation of N-nitrosamines from secondary amines and nitrite in human and animal gastric juice. *Food Cosmet. Toxicol 7*:301–307.

Sevanian, A., and Peterson, A. R. (1986). The cytotoxic and mutagenic properties of cholesterol oxidation products. *Food Chem. Toxicol. 24*:1103–1110.

Shamberger, R. J., Baughman, F. F., Kalchert, S. L., Willis, C. E., and Hoffman, G. C. (1973). Carcinogen induced chromosomal breakage decreased by antioxidants. *Proc. Natl. Acad. Sci. 70*:1461–1463.

Shamberger, R. J., Andrione, T. L., and Wills, C. E. (1974). Antioxidants and cancer. IV. Malonaldehyde has initiating activity as a carcinogen. *J. Natl. Cancer Inst. 53*:1771–1773.

Shamberger, R. J., Corlett, C. L., Beaman, K. D., and Kasten, B. L. (1979). Antioxidants reduce the mutagenic effect of malonaldehyde and β-propiolactone. IX. Antioxidants and cancer. *Mut. Res. 66*:349–355.

Shank, R. C., and Newberne, P. M. (1976). Dose-response study of the carcinogenicity of dietary sodium nitrite and morpholine in rats and hamsters. *Food Chem. Toxicol. 14*:1–8.

Shapiro, R. (1976). Genetic effects of bisulfite (sulfur dioxide). *Mut. Res. 39*:149–176.

Shapiro, R., Braverman, B., Louis, J. B., and Servis, R. E. (1973). Nucleic acid reactivity and conformation. II. Reaction of cytosine and uracil with sodium bisulfite. *J. Biol. Chem. 248*:4060–4064.

Shelef, L. A., and Chin, B. (1980). Effect of phenolic antioxidants on the mutagenicity of aflatoxin B_1. *Appl. Environ. Microbiol. 40*:1039–1043.

Shenefelt, R. E. (1972). Animal model for human disease: treatment of various species with a large dose of vit.A at known stages of pregnancy. *Am. J. Pathol. 66*:589–592.

Sherwin, E. R. (1976). Antioxidants for vegetable oils. *J. Am. Oil Chem. Soc. 53*:430–438.

Shibata, S. (1956). Toxicological studies of EDTA salt (disodium ethylenediaminetetracetate). *Nippon Yakurigaku Zasshi 52*:113–119.

Shih, N. T., and Petering, D. H. (1973). Model reactions for the study of the interaction of sulfur dioxide with mammalian organisms. *Biochim. Biophys. Res. Commun. 55*:1319–1325.

Shirai, T., Hagiwara, A., Kurata, Y., Shibata, M., Fukushima, S., and Ito, N. (1982). Lack of carcinogenicity of butylated hydroxytoluene on long-term administration to B6C3F1 mice. *Food Chem. Toxicol. 20*:861–865.

Shirai, T., Ikawa, E., Hirose, M., Thamvit, W., and Ito, N. (1985). Modification by five antioxidants of 1,2-dimethylhydrazine initiated colon carcinogenesis in F344 rats. *Carcinogenesis 6*:637–639.

Shklar, G. (1982). Oral mucosal carcinogenesis in hamsters: inhibition by vitamin E. *J. Natl. Cancer Inst. 68*:791–797.

Simon, E. J., Gross, C. S., and Milhorat, A. T. (1956). The metabolism of vitamin E. I. The absorption and excretion of d-α-tocopheryl-5-methyl-^{14}C-succinate. *J. Biol. Chem. 221*:797–805.

Simpson, F. J., Jones, J. A., Wolin, E. A. (1969). Anaerobic degradation of some bioflavonoids by microflora of the rumen. *Can. J. Microbiol. 15*:972–974.

Singh, M., and Krikorian, A. D. (1982). Inhibition of trypsin activity in vitro by phytate. *J. Agric. Food Chem. 30*:799–800.

Skaare, J. U. (1979). Studies on the biliary excretion and metabolites of the antioxidant ethyoxyquin in the rat. *Xenobiotica 9*:659–668.

Skaare, J. U., and Solheim, E. (1979). Studies on the metabolism of the antioxidant ethoxyquin in the rat. *Xenobiotica 9*:649–657.

Skaare, J. U., Nafstad, I., and Dahle, H. K. (1977). Enhanced hepatotoxicity of dimethylnitrosamine by pretreatment of rats with antioxidant ethoxyquin. *Toxicol. Appl. Pharmacol. 42*:19–31.

Sleight, S. D., and Atallah, O. A. (1968). Reproduction in the guinea pig as affected by chronic administration of potassium nitrate and potassium nitrite. *Toxicol. Appl. Pharmacol. 12*:179–185.

Sluis, K. J. H. (1951). The higher alkyl gallates as antioxidants. *Food Manuf. 26*:99–101.

Smith, L. L. (1981). *Cholesterol Autoxidation*. Plenum Press, New York.

Smith, L. L., and Johnson, B.H. (1989). Biological activities of oxysterols. *Free Radicals Biol. Med. 7*:285–332.

Smith, L. L., Matthews, W. S., Price, V. C., Bachmann, R. C., and Reynolds, B. (1967). Thin layer chromatographic examination of cholesterol oxidation products. *J. Chromat. 27*:187–205.

Sognier, M. A., and Hittelman, W. N. (1979). Repair of bleomycin-induced DNA damage and its relationship to chromosome aberration repair. *Mut. Res. 62*:517–527.

Solomon, D., Strummer, D., and Nair, P. P. (1972). Relationship between vitamin E and urinary excretion of ketosteroid fractions in cystic mastitis. *Ann. NY Acad. Sci. 203*:103–110.

Speit, G., Wolf, M., and Vogel, W. (1980). The SCE-inducing capacity of vitamin C: investigations in vitro and in vivo. *Mut. Res. 78*:273–278.

Spiegelhalder, B., Eisenbrand, G., and Preussmann, R. (1976). Influence of dietary nitrate on nitrite content of human saliva: possible relevance to in vivo formation of N-nitroso compounds. *Food Cosmet. Toxicol. 14*:545–548.

Srbova, J. and Teisinger, J. (1957). Resorption of the calcium salt of EDTA administered per os. *Pracovni lekarstui 9*:385–390.

Stanford Research Institute. (1972). *Study of the Mutagenic Effects of Ionol C.P. (Butylated Hydroxytoluene)*. NTIS PB-221 827. Menlo Park, CA.

Stanford Research Institute. (1977). *Study of the Mutagenic Effects of Butylated Hydroxytoluene (71-25) by a Dominant Lethal Test*. NTIS PB- 279 026. Menlo Park, CA.

Stevenson, D. E., Chambers, P. L., and Hunter, C. G. (1965). Toxicological studies with 2,4,6-tri(3′,5′-di-tert-butyl-4′-hydroxybenzyl)mesitylene in the rat. *Food Chem. Toxicol. 3*:281–288.

Stich, H. F., Karim, J., Koropatnick, J., and Lo, L. (1976). Mutagenic action of ascorbic acid. *Nature 260*:722–724.

Stokes, J. D., and Scudder, C. R. (1974). The effect of butylated hydroxyanisole and butylated hydroxytoluene on behavioral development in mice. *Dev. Psychobiol.* 7:343–350.

Stokes, J. D., Scudder, C. R., and Karczmar, A. G. (1972). Effects of chronic treatment with established food preservatives on brain chemistry and behavior of mice. *Fed. Proc.* 31:596 (abst.).

Stuckey, B. N. (1972). Antioxidants as food stabilizers. In *CRC Handbook of Food Additives*, Vol. I., Furia, T. E. (ed). CRC Press, Boca Raton, FL, pp. 185–223.

Stuckey, B. N., and Gearhart, W. M. (1957). Trihydroxy butyrophenone. A food grade antioxidant. *Food Technol.* 11:676–679.

Subrahmanyan, V., Narayana Rao., M., Rama Rao, G., and Swaminathan, M. (1955). The metabolism of nitrogen, calcium, and phosphorus in human adults on a poor vegetarian diet containing Ragi (*Eleusine Coracana*). *Bull. Central Food Technol. Res. Inst.* 4:87–88.

Suzuki, K., Bruce, W. R., Baptista, J., Furrer, R., Vaughan, D. J., and Krepinsky, J. J. (1986). Characteristics of cytotoxic steroids in human feces and their putative role in the etiology of human colonic cancer. *Cancer Lett.* 33:307–316.

Swernerton, H., and Hurley, L. S. (1971). Teratogenic effects of a chelating agent and their prevention by zinc. *Science 173*:62–63.

Tajima, K., Yamamoto, K., and Mitzutani, T. (1981). Biotransformation of butylated hydroxytoluene (BHT) to BHT quinone methide in rats. *Chem. Pharm. Bull.* 29:3738–3741.

Takahashi, O. (1988). Inhibition of phylloquinone epoxide reductase by BHT quinone methide, salicyclic acid, and α-tocopherolquinone. *Biochem. Pharmacol.* 37:2857–2895.

Takahashi, O. (1992). Hemorrhages due to defective blood coagulation do not occur in mice and guinea pigs fed butylated hydroxytoluene, but nephrotoxicity is found in mice. *Food Chem. Toxicol.* 30:89–97.

Takahashi, O. and Hiraga, K. (1978). Dose-response study of hemorrhagic death by dietary butylated hydroxytoluene (BHT) in male rats. *Toxicol. Appl. Pharmacol.* 43:399–406.

Takahashi, O., and Hiraga, K. (1979). Preventive effects of phylloquinone on hemorrhagic death induced by butylated hydroxytoluene in male rats. *J. Nutr.* 109:453–457.

Takahashi, O., and Hiraga, K. (1984). Effects of dietary butylated hydroxytoluene on functional and biochemical properties of platelets and plasma preceding the occurrence of hemorrhage in rats. *Food Chem. Toxicol.* 22:97–103.

Takahashi, O., Hayashida, S., and Hiraga, K. (1980). Species differences in the hemorrhagic response to butylated hydroxytoluene. *Food Chem. Toxicol.* 18:229–235.

Takahashi, O., Ichikawa, H., and Sasaki, M. (1990). Hemorrhagic toxicity of d-α-tocopherol in the rat. *Toxicology 63*:157–165.

Tamano, S., Fukushima, S., Shirai, T., Hirose, M., and Ito, N. (1987). Modification by α-tocopherol, propyl gallate, and tert-butyl hydroquinone of urinary bladder carcinogenesis in Fischer 344 rats pretreated with N-butyl-N-(4-hydroxybutyl)nitrosamine. *Cancer Lett.* 35:39–46.

Tanaka, S., Kawashima, K., Nakaura, S., Nagao, S., and Omori, Y. (1979). Effect of dietary administration of propyl gallate during pregnancy and postnatal development of rats. *Shokuhin Eiseigaku Zasshi 20*:378–384.

Tappel, A. L. (1968). Will antioxidant nutrients slow aging processes? *Geriatrics 23*(10):97–105.

Tappel, A. L. (1980). Measurement and protection from in vivo lipid peroxidation. *Free Radicals Biol.* 4:1–47.

Tappel, A. L., and Marr, A. G. (1954). Effect of α-tocopherol, propyl gallate, and nordihydroguairetic acid on enzyme reactions. *J. Agric. Food Chem.* 2:554–558.

Taylor, C. B., Peng, S. K., Werthessen, N. T., Tham, P., and Lee, K. T. (1979). Spontaneously occurring angiotoxic derivatives of cholesterol. *Am. J. Clin. Nutr. 32*:40–57.

Taylor, M. J., Richardson, T., and Jasensky, R. D. (1981). Antioxidant activities of amino acids bound to Trolox-C. *J. Am. Oil Chem. Soc. 58*:622–626.

Terao, J. (1989). Antioxidant activity of β-carotene related carotenoids in solution. *Lipids 24*:659–661.

Terhaar, C. J., Vis, E. A., and Kesel, H. J. (1968). *Acute Oral Toxicity of Monotertiary Butyl Hydroquinone.* Unpublished report cited in FAO/WHO, WHO Food Additive Series No. 8, 1975.

Theunissen, J. J. H., Jackson, R. L., Kempen, H. J. M., and Daniel, R. A. (1986). Membrane properties of oxysterols: interfacial orientation influence on membrane permeability and redistribution between membranes. *Biochim. Biophys. Acta 860*:66–74.

Til, H. P., Feron, V. J., and De Groot, A. P. (1972a). The toxicity of sulfite. I. Long-term feeding and multigeneration studies in rats. *Food Cosmet. Toxicol. 10*:291–310.

Til, H. P., Feron, V. J., and De Groot, A. P. (1972b). The toxicity of sulfite. II. Short- and long-term feeding studies in pigs. *Food Cosmet. Toxicol. 10*:463–473.

Tobe, M., Furuya, T., Kawasaki, Y., Naito, K., Sekita, K., Matsumoto, K., Ochai, T., Usui, A., Kokubo, T., Kanno, J., and Hayashi, Y. (1986). Six month toxicity study of butylated hydroxyanisole in beagle dogs. *Food Chem. Toxicol. 24*:1223–1228.

Tollenar, F. D. (1957). Prevention of rancidity in edible fats with special reference to the use of antioxidants. *Proc. Pacific Sci. Congr. 5*:92.

Tomassi, G., and Silano, V. (1986). An assessment of the safety of tocopherols as food additives. *Food Chem. Toxicol. 24*:1051–1061.

Tong, C., and Williams, G. M. (1980). Definition of conditions for the detection of genotoxic chemicals in the adult rat liver hypoxanthine-guanine phosphoribosyl transferase (ARL/ HGPRT) mutagenesis assay. *Mut. Res. 74*:1–9.

Toomey, J. A., and Morissette, R. A. (1947). Hypervitaminosis A. *Am. J. Dis. Child. 73*:473–480.

Tsai, A. C., Kelley, J. J., Peng. B., and Cook, N. (1978). Study on the effect of megavitamin E supplementation in man. *Am. J. Clin. Nutr. 31*:831–837.

Tsuda, H., Sakata, T., Masui, T., Imaida, K., and Ito, N. (1984). Modifying effects of butylated hydroxyanisole, ethoxyquin, and acetaminophen on induction of neoplastic lesions in rat liver and kidney initiated by N-ethyl-N-hydroxyethyl-nitrosamine. *Carcinogenesis 5*:525–531.

Tuchmann-Duplessis, H., and Mercier-Parot, L. (1956). The influence of a chelation agent ethylenediaminetetraacetate on gestation and fetal development of rats. *Compt. Rend. 243*:1064–1066.

Tye, R., Engel, J. D., Rapien, I., and Moore, J. (1965). Summary of toxicological data. Disposition of butylated hydroxytoluene in the rat. *Food Cosmet. Toxicol. 3*:547–551.

Ueno, I., Nakano, N., and Hirono, I. (1983). Metabolic fate of ^{14}C quercetin in the ACI rat. *Jpn. J. Exp. Med. 53*:41–50.

Vaca, C. E., Wilhelm, J., and Harms- Ringdahl, M. (1988). Interaction of lipid peroxidation products with DNA. A review. *Mut. Res. 195*:137–149.

Van Der Heijden, C. A., Janssen, P. J. C. M., and Strik, J. J. T. W. A. (1986). Toxicology of gallates: a review and evaluation. *Food Chem. Toxicol. 24*:1067–1070.

Van Duuren, B. L., Nelson, N., Orris, L., Palmes, E. D., and Schmitt, F. L. (1963). Carcinogenicity of epoxides, lactones, and peroxy compounds. *J. Natl. Cancer Inst. 31*:41–55.

Van Duuren, B. L., Langseth, L., Orris, L., Baden, M, and Kuschner, M. (1967). Carcinogenicity of epoxides, lactones, and peroxy compounds. V. Subcutaneous injection in rats. *J. Natl. Cancer Inst. 39*:1213–1216.

Van Esch, G. J. (1955). The toxicity of the antioxidants propyl, octyl, and dodecyl gallate. *Voeding 16*:683–686.

Van Esch, G. J., and Van Gendersen, H. (1954). Netherland Inst. Public Hlth. Report No. 481.

Van Esch, G. J., Vink, H. H., Wit, S. J., and Van Gendersen, H. (1957). The physiologic action of polyphosphates. *Arzneimittel Forsch. 7*:172–175.

Van Hecke, E. (1977). Contact dermatitis to ethoxyquin in animal feeds. *Contact Dermatitis 3*:341–342.

Van Ketel, W. G. (1978). Dermatitis from octyl gallate in peanut butter. *Contact Dermatitis 4*:60–61.

Van Logten, M. J., den Tonkelaar, E. M., Kroes, R., Berkvens, J. M., and Van Esch, G. J. (1972). Long-term experiment with canned meat treated with sodium nitrite and glucono-δ-lactone. *Food Cosmet. Toxicol. 10*:475–488.

Verhagen, H., Thijssen, H. H. W., ten Hoor, F., and Kleinjans, J. C. S. (1989a). Disposition of single oral doses of butylated hydroxyanisole in man and rat. *Food Chem. Toxicol. 27*:151–158.

Verhagen, H., Beckers, H. H. G., Comuth, P. A. W. V., Mass, L. M., ten Hoor, F., Henderson, P.Th., and Kleinjans, J. C. S. (1989b). Disposition of single oral doses of butylated hydroxytoluene in man and rat. *Food Chem. Toxicol. 27*:765–772.

Verhagen, H., Furhee, C., Schutte, B., Bosman, F. T., Blijham, G. H., Henderson, P.Th., ten Hoor, F., and Kleinjans, J. C. S. (1990). Dose dependent effects of short-term dietary administration of the food additive butylated hydroxyanisole on cell kinetic parameters in rat gastrointestinal tract. *Carcinogenesis 11*:1461–1468.

Vorhees, C. V., Butcher, R. E., Brunner, R. L., and Sobotka, T. J. (1981). Developmental neurobehavioral toxicity of butylated hydroxytoluene in rats. *Food Chem. Toxicol. 19*:153–162.

Walson, P. D., Carter, D. E., Iverson, B. A., and Halladay, S. C. (1979). Intestinal absorption of two potential polymeric food additives in man. *Food Cosmet. Toxicol. 17*:201–203.

Waters, W. A. (1971). The kinetics and mechanism of metal catalysed autoxidation. *J. Am. Oil Chem. Soc. 48*:427–433.

Weil, J. T., Van der Veen, J., and Olcott, H. S. (1968). Stable nitroxides as lipid antioxidants. *Nature 219*:168–169.

Weinshenker, N. M. (1980). Anoxomer: a new non absorbable antioxidant. *Food Technol. 34*:40–49.

Weinshenker, N. M., Bunes, L. A., and Davis, R. (1976). Oil soluble antioxidant prepared by condensation of divinylbenzene, hydroxyanisole, tertiary butyl hydroquinone, tertiary butyl phenol, and bisphenol A under ortho alkylation conditions. U.S. Patent 3,996,199.

Weissberger, L. H., and Harris, P. L. (1943). Effect of tocopherols on phosphorus metabolism. *J. Biol. Chem. 151*:543–551.

Westerfield, W. W. (1961). Effect of metal binding agents on metalloproteins. *Fed. Proc. 20*:158–176.

Wever, J. (1985). Appearance of sulfite and S-sulfonates in the plasma of rats after intra-duodenal sulfite application. *Food Chem Toxicol. 23*:895–898.

Wheldon, G. H., Bhatt, A., Keller, P., and Hummler, H. (1983). dl-α-Tocopheryl acetate: a long-term toxicity and carcinogenicity study in rats. *Int. J. Vit. Nutr. Res. 53*:287–296.

Whittern, C. C., Miller, E. E., and Pratt, D. E. (1984). Cottonseed flavonoids as lipid antioxidants. *J. Am. Oil Chem. Soc. 61*:1072–1078.

Widenbauer, F. (1936). Toxic secondary effects of ascorbic acid-C-hypervitaminosis. *Klin. Wschr. 15*:1158.

Wiebe, L. I., Mercer, J. R., and Ryan, A. J. (1978). Urinary metabolites of 3,5- di (1-^{13}C methyl-1-methyl ethyl) 4-hydroxytoluene (BHT-^{13}C) in man. *Drug Metab. Dispos.* 6:296–299.

Wilder, O. H. M., and Kraybill, H. R. (1948). *Summary of Toxicity Studies on Butylated Hydroxyanisole.* American Meat Institute Foundation, University of Chicago, Chicago.

Wilder, O. H. M., Ostby, P. C., and Gregory, B. R. (1960). Effect of feeding butylated hydroxyanisole to dogs. *J. Agric Food Chem.* 8:504–506.

Wilkins, J. W., Jr., Greene, J. A., Jr., and Weller, J. M. (1968). Toxicity of intraperitoneal bisulfite. *Clin. Pharmac. Ther.* 9:328–332.

Williams, G. M. (1977). The detection of chemical carcinogens by unscheduled DNA synthesis in rat liver primary cell cultures. *Cancer Res.* 37:1845–1851.

Williams, G. M. (1986). Epigenetic promoting effects of BHA. *Food Chem. Toxicol.* 24:1163–1166.

Williams, R. R., Waterman, R. E., Keresztesy, J. C., and Buchman, E. R. (1935). Studies on crystalline vitamin B1. III. Cleavage of vitamin with sulfite. *J. Am. Chem. Soc.* 57:536–537.

Williamson, D., Esterez, P., and Witschi, H. P. (1978). Studies on the pathogenesis of butylated hydroxytoluene induced lung damage in mice. *Toxicol. Appl. Pharmacol.* 43:577–587.

Wilson, C. W. M. (1974). Vitamin C: tissue metabolism, oversaturation, desaturation, and compensation. In *Vitamin C: Recent Aspects of Its Physiological and Technological Importance*, Birch, G. G. and Parker, K. H. (eds). John Wiley and Sons, New York, pp. 203–220.

Wilson, R. H., and DeEds, F. (1959). Toxicity studies of the antioxidant 6-ethoxy-1,2-dihydro-2,2,4-trimethylquinoline. *J. Agric. Food Chem.* 3:203–206.

Wilson, R. H., Thomas, J. O., Thompson, R. A., Launer, H. F., and Kohler, G. O. (1959). Absorption, metabolism, and excretion of the antioxidant 6-ethoxy-1,2-dihydro-2,2,4-trimethylquinoline. *J. Agric. Food Chem.* 3:206–209.

Winkler, H. (1943). What is the optimal dose of vitamin E in man? The effect of overdosage of vitamin E upon the ovary and hypophysis. *Zentr. Gynakol.* 67:32–41.

Winter, A. J., and Hokanson, J. F. (1964). Effects of long-term feeding of nitrate, nitrite, or hydroxylamine in pregnant dairy heifers. *Am. J. Vet. Res.* 25:353–361.

Wiss, O., Bunnel, H. R., and Gloor, U. (1962). Absorption and distribution of vit E in the tissues. *Vit. Horm.* 20:441–455.

Witschi, H. P., and Saheb, W. (1974). Stimulation of DNA synthesis in mouse lung following intraperitoneal injection of butylated hydroxytoluene. *Proc. Soc. Exp. Biol. Med.* 147:690–693.

Witschi, H. P., Hascheck, W. M., Liein-Szanto, A. J. P., and Hakkinen, P. J. (1981). Alteration of diffuse lung damage by oxygen: determining variables. *Am. Rev. Respir. Dis.* 123:98–103.

Wolke, R. E., Nielsen, S. W., and Rousseau, J. E. Jr. (1968). Bone lesins of hypervitaminosis A in the pig. *Am. J. Vet. Res.* 29:1009–1024.

Woodard, G., Hagan, E. C., and Radomski, J. L. (1949). The toxicity of hydroquinone for laboratory animals. *Fed. Proc.* 8:348.

Wright, A. S., Crowne, R. S., and Hathway, D. E. (1965a). The fate of 2,4,6-tri-(3′,5′-ditert-butyl-4′-hydroxybenzyl)mesitylene (Ionox-330) in the dog and rat. *Biochem. J.* 95:98–103.

Wright, A. S., Akintonwa, D. A. A., Crowne, R. S., and Hathway, D. E. (1965b). The metabolism of 2,6-di-tert-butyl-4-hydroxymethyl phenol (Ionox-100) in the dog and the rat. *Biochem. J.* 97:303–310.

Wright, A. S., Crowne, R. S., and Hathway, D. E. (1966). The fate of di(3,5-di-tert-butyl-4-hydroxyphenyl) methane (Ionox-220) in the rat. *Biochem. J.* 99:146–154.

Wright, A. S., Crowne, R. S., and Hathway, D. E. (1967). The metabolism of di(3,5-di-tert-butyl-4-hydroxybenzyl) ether (Ionox-201) in the rat. *Biochem. J. 102*:351–361.

Wurtzen, G., and Olsen, P. (1986a). BHA study in pigs. *Food Chem. Toxicol. 24*:1229–1233.

Wurtzen, G., and Olsen, P. (1986b). Chronic study on BHT in rats. *Food Chem. Toxicol. 24*:1121–1125.

Wyngaarden, J. B., Stanbury, J. B., and Rapp, B. (1953). The effects of iodide, perchlorate, thiocyanate, and nitrate administration upon the iodide concentrating mechanism of the rat thyroid. *Endocrinology 52*:568–574.

Yagi, K., Ohkawa, H., Ohishi, N., Yamashita, M., and Nakashima, T. (1981). Lesion of aortic intima caused by intravenous administration of linoleic acid hydroperoxide. *J. Appl. Biochem. 3*:58–65.

Yagi, K., Inagaki, T., Sasaguri, Y., Nakano, R., and Narasimha, T. (1987). Formation of lipid laden cells from cultured aortic smooth muscle cells and macrophages by linoleic acid hydroperoxide and low density lipo-protein. *J. Clin. Biochem. Nutr. 3*:87–94.

Yamamoto, K., Tajima, K., and Mitzutani, T. (1979). Identification of new metabolites of butylated hydroxytoluene (BHT) in rats. *J. Pharm. Dyn. 2*:164–168.

Yang, N. Y., and Desai, I. D. (1977). Effect of high levels of dietary vitamin E on hematological indices and biochemical parameters in rats. *J. Nutr. 107*:1410–1417.

Yang, S. F. (1970). Sulfoxide formation from methionine or its sulfide analogs during aerobic oxidation of sulfite. *Biochemistry 9*:5008–5014.

Yang, S. F. (1973). Destruction of tryptophan during aerobic oxidation of sulfite ions. *Environ. Res. 6*:395–402.

Yang, S. S. (1952). *Toxicological Investigations of Ethylenediaminetetraacetic Acid in the Rat.* Ph.D. thesis, University of Massachusetts, Amherst, MA.

Yokotani, H., Usui, T., Nakaguchi, T., Kanabayashi, T., Tanda, M., and Aramaki, Y. (1971). Acute and subacute toxicological studies of TAKEDA citric acid in mice and rats. *J. Takeda Res. Lab. 30*:25–31.

Yourga, F. J., Esselen, W. B., and Fellers, C. R. (1944). Some antioxidant properties of D-isoascorbic acid and its sodium salt. *Food Res. 9*:188–196.

Zachman, R. D., and Olson, J. A. (1961). A comparison of retinene reductase and alcohol dehydrogenase of the rat liver. *J. Biol. Chem. 236*:2309–2313.

Zbinden, J., and Studer, A. (1958). Tierexperimentelle Untersuchungen über die chronische Verträglichkeit von β-Carotin, Lycopin, 7,7' Dihydro β-carotin, und Bixin. *Z. Lebensm. Unters. Forsch. 108*:113–134.

4
Food Colors

V. M. Ghorpade,* S. S. Deshpande,† and D. K. Salunkhe
Utah State University
Logan, Utah

I. INTRODUCTION

Although our entire sensory system (olfactory, visual, gustatory, auditory, and tactile) is involved in the recognition and identification of objects in the surrounding environment, the single most important sense is undoubtedly the visual pathway. The visual stimulus is provided by the transmitted or reflected light from objects illuminated by a light source. It is interpreted generally in terms of morphological characteristics, size, shape, organization, and specific light-modifying properties, which provide the basis for perception of such appearance characteristics as color, opacity, translucency, glossiness, and texture.

Color is often the first sensory quality by which foods are judged. Similarly, both food quality and flavor are associated with color. Our senses are trained to expect foods of certain colors and reject any deviations from our expectations. Foods that are aesthetically pleasing are more likely to be consumed, thereby contributing to a varied diet and, hence, better nutrition.

The natural pigments associated with most fresh foods, especially fruits and vegetables, are vivid and brilliant. However, these pigments are subjected to adverse physical and chemical conditions during processing that cause their partial degradation. Processing therefore often results in undesirable changes in color and thus diminishes the visual perception of foods. In the developed countries, as much as 75% of the food is processed in some form before it reaches the consumer. Food manufacturers and processors therefore must replace the lost color if the

---

*Current affiliation: Industrial Agricultural Products Center, University of Nebraska, Lincoln, Nebraska.
†Current affiliation: Idetek, Inc. Sunnyvale, California.

acceptable attractive appearance is to be restored. Colors are primarily used in foods for the following reasons (NAS, 1971):

1. To restore the original appearance of the food where the natural colors have been destroyed by heat processing and subsequent storage.
2. To ensure uniformity of color due to natural variations in color intensity.
3. To intensify colors naturally occurring in foods to meet consumer expectations—Examples include fruit yogurts, sauces, and soft drinks.
4. To help protect flavor and light-sensitive vitamins during shelf storage.
5. To give an attractive appearance to foods, such as colorless gelatin-based desserts, which would otherwise look unappetizing.
6. To help preserve the identity or character by which foods are recognized and thus aid in product identification.
7. To serve as visual indication of food quality.

Both synthetic and natural food colors, therefore, play a significant role in enhancing the aesthetic appeal of processed foods as well as in food manufacture, storage, and quality control. They are also important ingredients in many convenience foods such as confectionery, instant desserts, ice creams, snacks, and beverages, since many of these are naturally colorless. Colors are also used to supplement the natural appearance of a given food system and to ensure batch-to-batch uniformity where raw materials have varying color intensities.

Prior to 1900, there was no regulation in the United States on the usage of food colors in processed foods. Many of the colors used were toxic, and their overuse often resulted in food poisoning. They were often used to make foods of poor quality acceptable. The National Academy of Sciences (NAS, 1971) cites the following cases in which colors were deliberately used in foods to defraud the consumer or to disguise adulteration.

1. In 1920, Frederick Accum mentioned the fate of a woman who, while at her hairdressers, habitually ate pickles colored green with copper sulfate. She later became ill and died.
2. Cheese colored with vermillion (HgS) and red lead (Pb_3O_4) also caused several cases of food poisoning.
3. In a Manchester tea shop, stocks of copper arsenite, lead chromate, and indigo were found on hand to color used tea leaves for resale.
4. Because of the lack of synthetic dyes, candies were generally colored with mineral pigments. An analysis of 100 samples of candy revealed that 59 contained lead chromate, 12 red lead, 6 vermillion, and 4 white lead (basic lead carbonate).
5. In Boston, 46% of the candy sampled in the year 1880 contained one or more mineral pigments. The primary pigment was found to be lead chromate.
6. In 1860, a caterer wishing to have a green pudding at a public dinner asked a druggist to provide a color. The copper arsenite he received and used caused two deaths.
7. In London around 1900, the addition of yellow coloring to milk was so common that housewives refused to buy uncolored milk, thinking it had been adulterated. The yellow tint was commonly added to prevent detection of skimmed

or watered milk. It was not until 1925 that British law prohibited the coloring of milk.

During the course of this century, food colors have been evaluated rigorously for their technical suitability and toxicological properties. The stricter government guidelines have greatly reduced the range of colors available for food use. However, these guidelines and a stricter government policy have greatly helped to eliminate dishonest practices and protect consumer health and safety. This chapter summarizes the uses of natural and synthetic colorants in our food supply, their chemical properties, and their toxicology.

II. HISTORY

Colors have been used to make food more attractive and appetizing for centuries. Spices and condiments played an important role as coloring ingredients in the early Indian and Chinese civilizations. Similarly, paintings in Egyptian tombs dating as far back as 1500 B.C. depict the making of colored candy (Marmion, 1984). Wine was probably first colored around 400 B.C. Colorants derived from naturally occurring minerals, plants, and animals were prepared along with the spices that played a prominent role in the development of early civilizations (Tannahill, 1973).

The discovery of the first synthetic dye—mauve—in 1856 is credited to Sir William Henry Perkins. This was followed soon by the synthesis of a host of new and different synthetic dyes. These colors, as compared with natural extracts from animals, vegetables, and minerals, were superior in tinctorial strengths, hues, and stability. They were also readily available in many different shades and hues. Some of these synthetic dyes were used almost immediately in Europe. The United States first legalized the use of synthetic organic dyes in foods by an act of Congress that authorized the addition of coloring matter to butter in 1886. The second such act was passed in 1896 to add synthetic colors to cheese. However, by the year 1900, some 80 different food colors were being used in a wide variety of products including ketchup, jellies, cordials, butter, cheese, ice cream, candy, sausage, noodles, and wine. Colors were also increasingly being used in several drug and cosmetic products.

The U.S. Congress soon recognized the proliferation in the use of color additives as a threat to public health. Of particular concern was the fact that substances known to be poisonous were often incorporated into foods and that dyes were frequently used to hide poor quality and to add weight or bulk to certain items. Moreover, the synthetic colors, also known as aniline dyes, were manufactured from coal tar derivatives. Although sold in highly purified forms, the negative connotation of their association with coal tar resulted in much unfavorable publicity. This also prompted the development of synthetic dyes from petrochemicals.

The increasing public concern over the misuse of colors in foods prompted the U.S. government to initiate a comprehensive testing program to investigate the relationship of coloring matters to public health and to establish principles that should be followed to govern their use. By 1904, the U.S. Department of Agriculture issued a series of Food Inspection Decisions. Under the guidance of Dr. Bernard C. Hesse, a German dye expert, the department also undertook the arduous task of studying the chemistry and physiology of the then nearly 700 extant coal tar dyes as well as the laws of various countries and states regarding their use in food products. Until then, very few colorants were ever tested for their effects on health. Of the 80 colorants used widely in foods in the United States by the turn of the century, 30 were never tested, and their safety was simply unknown. Of the remaining colorants, 26 had been tested but the results were contradictory: 8 were considered by most experts to be unsafe, and the remaining 16 were deemed more or less harmless. These 16 colors were then tested physiologically by determining their acute short-range effects in dogs, rabbits, and human beings. Based on these studies and Hesse's recommendations, the first comprehensive legislation, the Food and Drug Act of 1906, listed seven dyes for use in foods. These were amaranth, Ponceau 3R, erythrosine, indigotine, Light Green SF, Naphthol Yellow S, and Orange 1. These new regulations also established a system for voluntary certification of synthetic organic food colors by the Department of Agriculture.

The original list of seven dyes, however, could not fulfill the industry's need for additional colors. Hence, during the following three decades, several new colorants were added to the system after rigorous physiological testing. A chronological history of synthetic, certifiable food colors is presented in Table 1. In 1938, the Federal Food, Drug and Cosmetic Act that superseded the Act of 1906 established mandatory certification, requiring submission of samples from each batch of col-

Table 1 A Chronological History of Synthetic Food Colors in the United States

Year listed for food use	Common name	FDA name	Color Index Number	Year delisted	Current status for food use
1907	Ponceau 3R	FD&C Red No. 1	16155	1961	Not allowed
1907	Amaranth	FD&C Red No. 2	16185	1976	Not allowed
1907	Erythrosine	FD&C Red No. 3	45430	—	Allowed
1907	Orange 1	FD&C Orange No. 1	14600	1956	Not allowed
1907	Naphthol Yellow S	FD&C Yellow No. 1	10316	1959	Not allowed
1907	Light Green SD Yellowish	FD&C Green No. 2	42095	1966	Not allowed
1907	Indigotine	FD&C Blue No. 2	73015	—	Allowed
1916	Tartrazine	FD&C Yellow No. 5	19140	—	Allowed
1918	Sudan 1	—	12055	1918	Not allowed
1918	Butter Yellow	—		1918	Not allowed
1918	Yellow AB	FD&C Yellow No. 3	11380	1959	Not allowed
1918	Yellow OB	FD&C Yellow No. 4	11390	1959	Not allowed
1922	Guinea Green B	FD&C Green No. 1	42085	1966	Not allowed
1927	Fast Green FCF	FD&C Green No. 3	42053	—	Not allowed
1929	Ponceau SX	FD&C Red No. 4	14700	1976	Not allowed
1929	Sunset Yellow FCF	FD&C Yellow No. 6	15985	—	Allowed
1929	Brilliant Blue FCF	FD&C Blue No. 1	42090	—	Allowed
1939	Naphthol Yellow S	FD&C Yellow No. 2	10316	1959	Not allowed
1939	Orange SS	FD&C Orange No. 2	12100	1956	Not allowed
1939	Oil Red XO	FD&C Red No. 32	12140	1956	Not allowed
1950	Benzyl Violet 4B	Fd&C Violet No. 1	42640	1973	Not allowed
1959	Citrus Red No. 2	Citrus Red No. 2	12156	—	Allowed
1966	Orange B	Orange B	19235	—	Allowed
1971	Allura® Red AC	FD&C Red No. 40	16035	—	Allowed

orant for evaluation of purity. The Act also created three new categories of synthetic coal tar dyes for various applications as follows:

1. FD&C colors: those certifiable for use in coloring foods, drugs and cosmetics.
2. D&C colors: dyes and pigments considered safe in drugs and cosmetics when in contact with mucous membranes or when ingested.
3. External D&C colors: those colorants that, because of their oral toxicity, were not certifiable for use in products intended for ingestion, but were considered safe for use in products externally applied.

Under this new law, all common names of dyes and colors were also changed to color prefix and numbers. Thus certified amaranth became FD&C Red No. 2. During the following two decades, the situation with regard to color additives appeared to be finally under control. In the early 1950s, several cases of sickness in children who had eaten candy and popcorn colored with excessive amounts of dyes were reported. The Food and Drug Administration (FDA) also initiated a new round of pharmacological testing of food colors. These studies were conducted at higher levels and for longer test periods than any of the earlier studies, and hence contradicted the assumption of safety of such widely used colors as FD&C Orange No. 1, FD&C Orange No. 2, and FD&C Red No. 32. Following a series of legal battles in which the validity of the 1938 Act to set quantity limitation was questioned, and through the efforts of the Certified Color Industry and the FDA, a new law was passed. This Color Additives Amendments of 1960 defines the term *color additive* as "any dye, pigment or other substance made or obtained from a vegetable, animal or mineral or other source capable of coloring a food, drug or cosmetic or any part of the human body." The law consists of two parts or titles. Title I of the Delaney-type clause prohibited addition to food of any colorant found to induce cancer in humans or animals. Title II of the clause allowed the use of existing color additives under a provisional listing pending the completion of scientific investigations needed to ascertain their safety for permanent listing. Synthetic colorants were thus required to undergo premarketing safety clearance, and previously authorized colorants were reevaluated. Natural colorants were also required to undergo similar testing, but were not required to undergo certification for purity specification. The law also eliminated any distinction between "coal tar" colors and other color additives and empowered the Secretary of Health, Education and Welfare to decide which colors must be certified and which could be exempted from certification based on their relationship to public health. The law also allowed the Secretary to list color additives for specific uses and also to set conditions and tolerances on the use of color additives. Under the provisions of this law, both producers and consumers of the color additives were required to provide the necessary scientific data to obtain "permanent" listing of a color additive. The economic considerations dictated testing of only those colors of commercial importance, and consequently many previously certifiable colors were eventually delisted by default. Most colorants are now "permanently" listed; those that are not continue to be listed provisionally.

With the passage of the Medical Device Amendments of 1976, the Congress created a new category of color additive by mandating the separate listing of colorants for use in medical devices if the color additive in them comes in direct contact with the body for a significant period of time. Food colors that are currently allowed for use in foods in the United States and their current status are summarized in Table 2. To add any new colors to this list, the FDA (U.S. FDA, 1982) now requires results from the following toxicological studies.

1. One subchronic feeding study, of 90 days duration, in a nonrodent species, usually dog
2. Acute toxicity studies in rats
3. Chronic feeding studies in at least two animal species, e.g., rats and mice (one with in utero exposure), lasting at least 24–30 months
4. One teratology study
5. One multigeneration reproduction study using mice
6. One mutagenicity test

The development and use of food colors in European countries have been somewhat different than in the United States. For example, the United Kingdom did not establish any legislation for food colorants until the mid-1950s (Haveland-Smith and Combes, 1980). Some countries still permit the use of any colorants, while others prohibit the use of all synthetic colorants for food applications. A major difficulty involved in the lack of a universal regulatory policy appears to be controversies regarding the physiological and pharmacological testing of synthetic colorants. Nevertheless, several synthetic colorants approved for use in foods by the FDA are also commonly used in Europe. The United Kingdom at present monitors food colors based on a Color Index System. Hence, for the benefit of the readers, wherever applicable, the Color Index Numbers are also provided for the synthetic colorants approved for use in foods in both Europe and the United States.

III. CLASSIFICATION

The color additives permitted for use in foods can be broadly classified into two categories: colorants subject to certification and those exempt from certification. A schematic diagram for the classification of various food colors is shown in Figure 1.

A. Colorants Subject to Certification

The synthetic food colors subject to certification are normally very pure chemicals with standardized color strengths. Because of the starting materials used in their manufacture in the past, certified colors have also been known as "coal tar" dyes. However, at present they are manufactured as a byproduct of the petroleum industry.

Compared to colorants exempt from certification, certified colors are cheaper, brighter, more uniform, and better characterized with higher tinctorial strengths and a wider range of hues. They are available as is ("primary colors") or as admixtures with other certified colors ("secondary mixes"). A nearly infinite number of shades can be prepared by properly blending the available primary colors. Some examples are summarized in Table 3.

Certified colors are available as water-soluble dyes or as insoluble pigments or "lakes." The soluble dyes readily dissolve in water and certain polyhydric solvents such as propylene glycol. Their coloring power is directly dependent on their chemical dye content. FD&C dyes must contain a minimum of 85% pure dye; however, they are commercially available with 90–93% pure dye content. By law, each batch of colorant must be certified for purity prior to approval for use in foods. The dyes are available as powders, pastes, granules, and solutions. In addition, the blends are also available in jelly or fat-based sticks for convenience of use. The powders or granules are used for beverages, pastes, or dispersions for baked goods and confectionery, and liquid colors for dairy products (Meggos, 1984). Glycerin or propylene glycol carriers may be used as solvents for nonaqueous forms. Although specific concentration limits are not set for certified dyes, good manufacturing practices suggest that they should be used at less than 300 ppm (IFT, 1986).

Several certified colors are also available as the aluminum lake of the dye. The aluminum lakes are produced by reacting solutions of the water-soluble colors with freshly prepared alumina (aluminum hydroxide). Alumina is the only base approved for manufacturing FD&C lakes. The lakes are essentially insoluble in water and organic solvents (Rayner, 1991). They are produced as extremely fine powders with the dye content ranging from 10 to 40%. Unlike dyes, a minimum dye content is not specified for lakes. Similarly, the tinctorial strength of the lakes is not proportional to their dye content. Unlike dyes that color foods through their adsorption or attachment from solution to the material being colored, lakes, like other pigments, impart color by dispersing them in the medium to be colored. As a consequence of this pigmentlike character, both the shade and tinctorial strength of lakes are highly dependent on the conditions used in their manufacture as well as their physical properties, such as particle size and crystal structure.

Lakes are marketed as is or mixed with other lakes or approved diluents, as dispersed in various edible carriers such as hydrogenated vegetable oil, coconut oil, propylene glycol, glycerin, or sucrose syrup. Lakes generally have enhanced light stability as compared to the soluble dyes. They are used to color dry powder products, snack products, chewing gums, sugar confectionery, and compressed tablets.

Although more expensive than the FD&C dyes, FD&C lakes have proven especially useful because of their opacity, their ability to be incorporated into the products in the dry state, and their superior stability toward heat and light (Marmion, 1984). FD&C lakes are often used to color water-repelling foods such as fats, gums, and oils and for coloring food-packaging materials including lacquers, plastic films, and inks from which soluble dyes would be quickly leached.

The FDA considers lakes toxicologically equivalent to their corresponding dyes. The agency, however, has not yet established regulations for their use in foods. Except for the lake of FD&C Red No. 40, all lakes are provisionally listed by the FDA (Table 4).

Chemically, FD&C dyes and lakes belong to one of four classes: azo dyes (FD&C Yellow No. 5, FD&C Yellow No. 6, FD&C Red No. 40, Citrus Red No. 2, and Orange B), triphenylmethane dyes (FD&C Blue No. 1 and FD&C Green No. 3), xanthene dyes (FD&C Red No. 3), and sulfonated indigo dyes (FD&C Blue No. 2) (Fig. 1).

Azo dyes comprise the largest group of certified colorants. They are characterized by the presence of one or more azo bonds ($-N=N-$). They are synthesized

Table 2 A Summary of Colorants Permitted and Their Current Status for Use in Foods

Food and Drug Administration official name	Color Index Number	Limitations[a]	Current status
		Subject to Certification	
FD&C Blue No. 1	42090		Listed
FD&C Blue No. 2	73015		Provisional
FD&C Green No. 3	42053		Listed
FD&C Red No. 3	45430		Listed
FD&C Red No. 40	16035		Listed
FD&C Yellow No. 5	19140		Listed
FD&C Yellow No. 6	15985		Provisional
Citrus Red No. 2	12156	Orange skins only, 2.0 ppm max., based on the weight of the whole fruit	Listed
Orange B	19235	Sausage and frankfurter casings or surfaces only, 150 ppm max., based on the weight of finished products	Listed
		Exempt from Certification	
Annatto extract	75120		Listed
β-Apo-8'-carotenol[b]	40820	Maximum 15 mg/lb of solid or semisolid food, or pint of liquid food	Listed
Canthaxanthin[b]	40850	Maximum 30 mg/lb of solid or semisolid food, or pint of liquid	Listed
Caramel	75130 (natural) 40800 (synthetic)		Listed
Carrot oil			Listed
Cochineal extract and carmine	75470		Listed
Corn endosperm oil		Chicken feed only	Listed

Name	CI number	Restriction	Status
Dehydrated beets and beet powder			Listed
Dried algae meal		Chicken feed only	Listed
Ferrous gluconate[b]		Ripe olives only	Listed
Fruit juice			Listed
Grape color extract		Nonbeverage food only	Listed
Grape skin extract		Beverages only	Listed
Paprika			Listed
Paprika oleoresin			Listed
Riboflavin[b]			Listed
Saffron	75100		Listed
Synthetic iron oxide[b]	77491 77492 77499	Dog and cat food only, 0.25% (w/w) max.	Listed
Tagetes meal and extract	75125	Chicken feed only	Listed
Titanium dioxide	77891	1% (w/w) maximum in finished food	Listed
Toasted, partially defatted, and cooked cottonseed flour			Listed
Turmeric	75300		Listed
Turmeric Oleoresin	75300		Listed
Ultramarine blue[b]	77007	Salt for animal feed only, 0.5% (w/w) max.	Listed
Vegetable juice			Listed

[a]No color additive or product containing one can be used in the area of the eye, in surgical sutures, or in injections, unless so stated. Also, no colorant can be used to color foods for which standards of identity have been promulgated under Section 401 of the Federal Food, Drug and Cosmetic Act, unless the use of added color is authorized by the standard.

[b]Synthetic but nature identical.

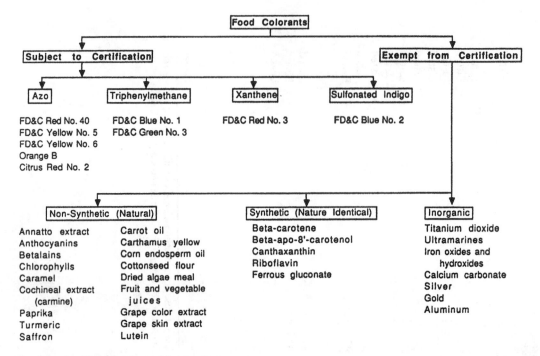

Fig. 1 Classification of food colorants.

by the coupling of a diazotized primary aromatic amine to a component capable of coupling, usually a naphthol. The azo dyes are easily reduced by metallic ions or strong reducing agents such as sulfur dioxide, and thus are liable to fade with time. They are also susceptible to ultraviolet light oxidation. Certified dyes belonging to the other three classes are more resistant to chemical reduction. However, FD&C Blue No. 2 and FD&C Red No. 3 are easily oxidized by ultraviolet light and fade rapidly (Newsome, 1990).

B. Colorants Exempt from Certification

This class of color additives is comprised of the so-called "natural" colors. Although according to the Color Additives Amendment Act of 1960 the exempt colorants need not be certified prior to their sale, they are still subject to surveillance by FDA to ensure that they meet the government regulations and are used in accordance with the law. All exempt colorants in use prior to the 1960 amendment continue to be provisionally listed, pending the completion of testing to obtain their permanent listing.

Colorants exempt from certification could be broadly classified as nonsynthetic (natural), nature-identical, and inorganic colorants (Fig. 1). The nonsynthetic colorants, comprised of a wide variety of organic and inorganic compounds, are extracted from animal, plant, and mineral sources. The nature-identical colorants are the synthetic counterparts of the naturally occurring pigments.

Several inorganic pigments as well as extracts from natural foods are also used as colorants in many parts of the world. In the United States, several of these

Table 3 Some Representative Examples of Secondary Mixes and the Shades Obtained by Combining Different Ratios of Primary Colors[a]

Shade[b]	FD&C Blue No. 1	FD&C Blue No. 2	FD&C Red No. 3	FD&C Red No. 40	FD&C Yellow No. 5	FD&C Yellow No. 6
Strawberry			5	95		
Black (licorice)	36			22		42
Egg yellow					85	15
Cinnamon	5			35	60	
Lime green	3				97	
Mint green	25				75	
Orange						100
				25	20	55
					84	16
Grape	20			80		
		8.2		91.8		
Black cherry	5			95		
Chocolate	10			45	45	
	8			52	40	
Tea, root beer, or cola	8			52	40	
	5			25	70	
Butterscotch	3			22	57	18
	2			24	74	
	1.5		8.5		90	
Caramel	6		21		64	9
Peach				60		40
Raspberry	5		75			20
Cheddar cheese					55	45

[a]Values represent parts by weight.
[b]More than one combination of colorants can be used to produce a particular shade. The mixture depends on the effect desired and the product to be colored.
Source: Marmion, 1984.

Table 4 Lakes Listed for Use in Foods and Their Current Status[a]

Lake	Current status
FD&C Red No. 40	Permanent
FD&C Yellow No. 6	Provisional
FD&C Red No. 3	Provisional
FD&C Blue No. 1	Provisional
FD&C No. 2	Provisional
FD&C Green No. 3	Provisional
FD&C Yellow No. 5	Provisional

[a]As of January 1986, pending the release of FDA's Color Additives Scientific Review Panel Report.

colorants are exempt from certification. However, they have been defined in the Code of Federal Regulations.

Compared to synthetic colorants subject to certification, the exempt colors generally have poor tinctorial power, and thus need to be used at higher concentrations. Those from plants also tend to be chemically unstable and more variable in shade and are likely to impart undesirable flavors and odors to food products. The composition of exempt colorants also varies with the source from which they are obtained, geographical location, and season, thus resulting in a very high batch-to-batch variation. They are also likely to be contaminated with undesirable toxic trace metals, insecticides, herbicides, and potentially harmful microorganisms (Marmion, 1984; Newsome, 1990). They are also difficult to obtain in a steady supply. Many of the colorants exempt from certification, therefore, have found only limited applications in foods. They are classified and regulated as such only because of the broad definition of a color additive given in the 1960 amendments.

IV. COLORANTS SUBJECT TO CERTIFICATION

Colorants subject to certification in the United States include the FD&C dyes and the FD&C lakes. These colors and their toxicological properties are briefly described below. Although only nine FD&C colors are permitted for use in food, several others that have been delisted in the United States are still used in many parts of the world. Hence, information is also provided on some of these delisted colorants.

A. FD&C Red No. 1

FD&C Red No. 1 (Ponceau 3R, Color Index No. 16155) was one of the seven synthetic colorants approved for food use by the Food and Drug Act of 1906. This disodium salt of 1-pseudocumylazo-2-naphthol-3,6-disulfonic acid belongs to the monoazo group of synthetic dyes (Fig. 2). FD&C Red No. 1 is a dark red powder. It dissolves readily in water to yield a poppy red solution.

FD&C Red No. 1 has proven to be a liver carcinogen when fed to both sexes of Osborne-Mendel rats at 0.5, 1.0, 2.0, and 5.0% levels (Hansen et al., 1963; Mannell, 1964). Grice et al. (1961) have also reported a dose-related incidence of

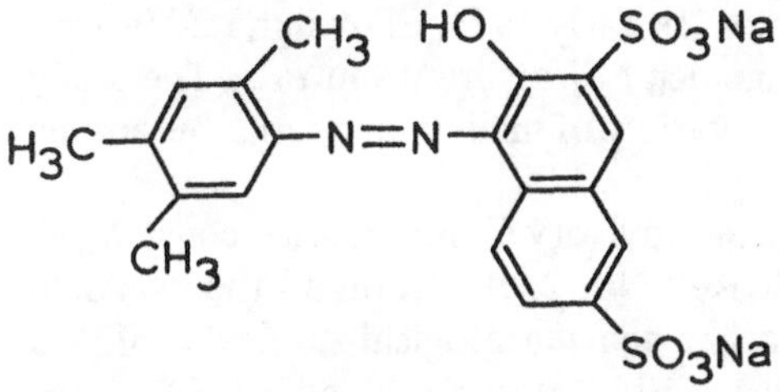

Fig. 2 FD&C Red No. 1.

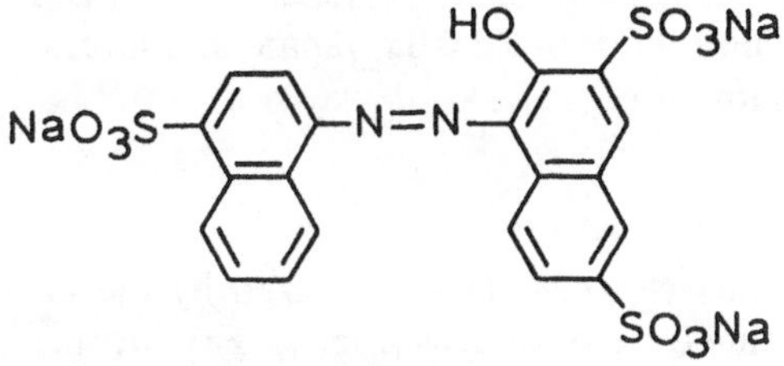

Fig. 3 FD&C Red No. 2.

trabecular cell carcinoma of the liver. Its hepatocarcinogenicity was also observed in mice and dogs.

The toxicity of FD&C Red No. 1 appears to be due to its two trimethylaniline derivatives, mesidine and pseudocumidine, since xylidines were also shown to be hepatotoxic to rats and dogs (Magnusson et al., 1971). The hepatocarcinogenic nature of FD&C Red No. 1 led to its delisting in 1961.

B. FD&C Red No. 2

FD&C Red No. 2 (amaranth, Color Index No. 16185) belongs to the monoazo group of synthetic dyes. It was also one of the seven original dyes certified for use by the Food and Drug Act of 1906. It is synthesized by coupling one mole of diazotized naphthionic acid with one mole of 2-naphthol-3,6-disulfonic acid (Fig. 3). Amaranth is a reddish-brown powder that dissolves rapidly in water to yield a magenta-red or bluish-red solution.

Early physiological studies with amaranth accounting for up to 5% of the total diet produced no pathological damage, mutagenicity, or increase in tumor incidence in rats (Cook et al., 1940; Willheim and Ivy, 1953; Mannell et al., 1958). Long-term, 7-year duration studies conducted by the FDA also showed no evidence of pathological damage in dogs when the dye was fed at 2% level (U.S. FDA, 1974). Similarly, several studies in mice, rats, rabbits, hamsters, cats, and dogs have also shown no significant teratogenic, reproductive, or other harmful effects (WHO, 1975). Amaranth, therefore, was being considered for permanent listing. However, two studies from the former Soviet Union reported carcinogenic and embryotoxic responses in rats fed 0.8–1.6% amaranth in the diet (Baigusheva, 1968; Andrianova, 1970). Based on the overwhelming data supporting the nontoxic nature of amaranth, FDA discredited these two studies. In early 1971, FDA initiated its own in-house study to confirm the embryotoxigenicity of amaranth in rats. The study found a "statistically significant increase in a variety of malignant neoplasms among aged Osborne-Mendel female rats."

In 1975, FDA appointed a Toxicological Advisory Committee to consider all aspects of controversy surrounding FD&C Red No. 2. Based on all the available data, the committee concluded that the earlier pharmacological studies of FD&C Red No. 2 did not meet the then newly established rigorous standards of testing with respect to the number of animals and the extent of histopathological examination. Based on the committee's recommendations, FDA terminated the provisional listing of amaranth in 1976. A subsequent petition for permanent listing of amaranth was denied in 1980, based again on insufficient evidence (U.S. FDA 1980). However, amaranth is still used to color foods in Canada, Japan, and several countries of the European Economic Community.

C. FD&C Red No. 3

FD&C Red No. 3 (erythrosine, Color Index No. 45430), synthesized by the iodination of fluorescein, belongs to the xanthene group of dyes (Fig. 4). Erythrosine is a brown-colored powder that yields a red solution with a slight fluorescence in 95% alcohol.

In the United States, FD&C Red No. 3 has been approved for use in foods since 1907. Its use in foods, drugs, and cosmetics is widespread. With the exception of an International Research and Development Corporation (IRDC) study, most chronic and subchronic studies in rats, mice, gerbils, hamsters, dogs, and swine have shown it to be noncarcinogenic. The IRDC study (1982), requested by the FDA prior to permanent listing of this dye, found adverse in utero effects and development of thyroid tumors in rats fed diets containing 4% erythrosine. No adverse effects, however, were observed at lower levels of 0.1, 0.5, and 1% dye in the diet.

Subchronic feeding studies indicated that erythrosine inhibits conversion of thyroxine to triiodothyronine, thus resulting in an increased secretion of thyrotropin by the pituitary gland. This in turn results in an increased stimulation of the thyroid and, hence, the tumor formation. No effect levels for the tumor formation process in male rats have been established at 0.5% (302 mg/kg body weight/d). Human studies, however, have failed to identify any adverse effects following the ingestion of FD&C Red No. 3 (Anderson et al., 1964; Bora et al., 1969).

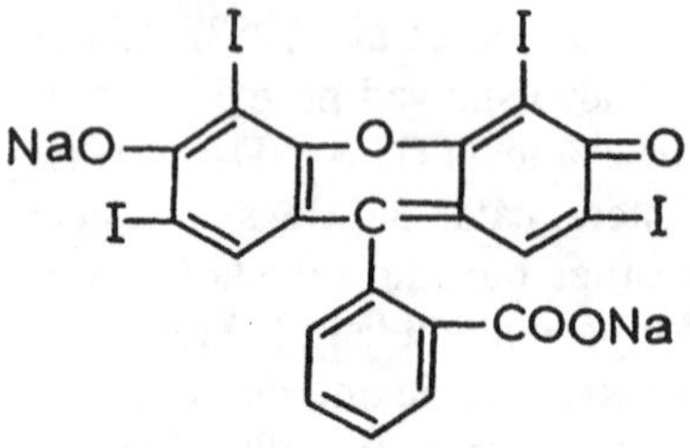

Fig. 4 FD&C Red No. 3.

Erythrosine was also implicated in behavior modification (neurotoxicity) processes. Several researchers have studied the effects of this dye on neurotransmitter release and iron transfer across cell membranes (Swanson and Logan, 1980; Augustine and Levitan, 1983; Sibergeld et al., 1983; Vorhees et al., 1983; Kantor et al., 1984). However, no conclusive evidence was found that linked this color to possible adverse behavioral effects.

D. FD&C Red No. 4

FD&C Red No. 4 (Ponceau SX, Color Index No. 14700) was approved for food use in 1929. This monoazo dye (Fig. 5) is synthesized by coupling one mole each of diazotized 1-amino-2,4-dimethylbenzene-5-sulfonic acid and 1-naphthol-4-sulfonic acid. A red-colored powder, it is readily soluble in water, yielding orange-red solution.

FD&C Red No. 4 was originally approved to color butter and margarine. It was found to be noncarcinogenic to rats when fed at a 5% level in the diet for up to 2 years (Davis, 1966). These researchers, however, found the dye to be toxic to dogs. When fed at a 1% level in the diet for a period of 7 years, FD&C Red No. 4 produced chronic folicular cystitis with hematomatous projections into the urinary bladder, hemosiderotic focal lesions in the liver, and atrophy of the zona glomerulosa of the adrenals. In one study, three of the five dogs fed a diet containing 2% dye died prematurely within 6 months. Thus, its provisional listing as a permissible food color was terminated in 1976 (U.S. FDA, 1983b).

E. FD&C Red No. 32

FD&C Red No. 32 (Oil Red XO, Color Index No. 12140) was approved for food use in 1939. This monoazo dye (Fig. 6) is synthesized by diazotizing one mole of

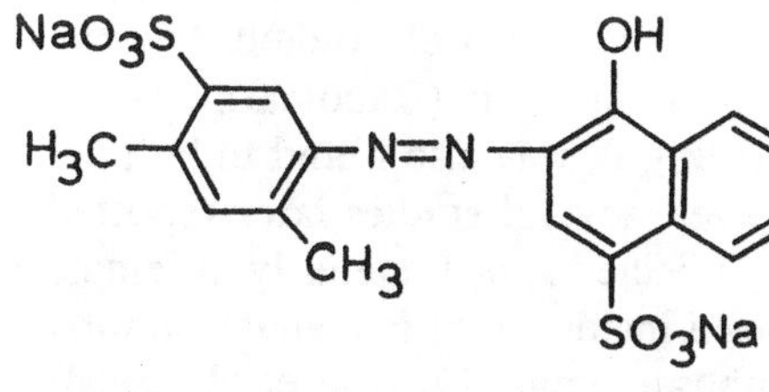

Fig. 5 FD&C Red No. 4.

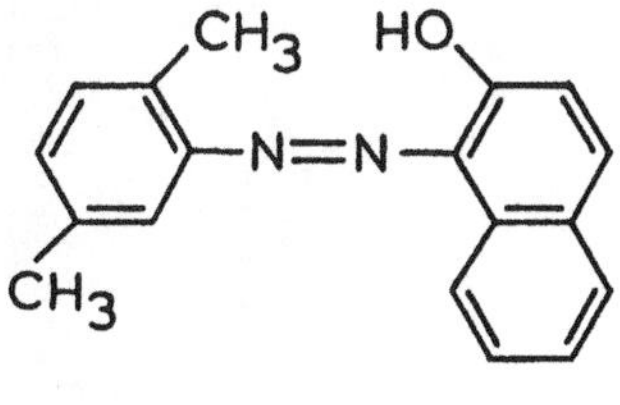

Fig. 6 FD&C Red No. 32.

xylidine mixture from which the *meta* components are partially removed with one mole of 2-naphthol. It is a brownish-red powder soluble in oil.

FD&C Red No. 32 was found to be a strong cathartic in dogs and rats (Radomaski, 1961). It is also highly toxic to rats (Fitzhugh et al., 1956). Rats fed the dye at 0.1% level in the diet for 2 years showed growth retardation, damage to liver and heart tissue, and higher mortality rates compared to those on control diets. Dogs thus treated also showed similar toxic effects (Fitzhugh et al., 1956). The dye was banned in 1956 for food use in the United States.

F. FD&C Red No. 40

FD&C Red No. 40 (Allura® Red AC, Color Index No. 16035) is a monoazo dye (Fig. 7). Developed in the mid-1960s, it is manufactured by coupling diazotized 5-amino-4-methoxy-2-toluenesulfonic acid with 6-hydroxy-2-naphthalenesulfonic acid.

In the United States, FD&C Red No. 40 was approved for food use in 1971. However, it was refused similar legal status in Canada after the Health and Protection Branch (HPB) of Health and Welfare Canada concluded that the data submitted by the manufacturers to support its safety were inadequate (IFT, 1986). These toxicological studies were terminated after 21 months, when pneumonia swept the rat colony, instead of after the required 24-month period. While the Canadian HPB deemed these studies inadequate, FDA accepted the test results as being adequate proof of safety. Later studies proved its safety for food use, thus allowing its use in Canada. The dye, however, is not permitted for food use in the United Kingdom, Switzerland, Sweden, The Netherlands, and other countries of the European Economic Community.

G. Citrus Red No. 2

Citrus Red No. 2 (Solvent Red 80, Color Index No. 12156) is principally 1-(2,5-dimethoxy-phenylazo)-2-naphthol (Fig. 8). It belongs to the monoazo group of dyes. Its use is limited to coloring skins of oranges not intended for processing.

Toxicological properties of Citrus Red No. 2 have been well studied. Feeding studies in rats and dogs have shown it to be noncarcinogenic (Radomaski, 1962). In the same study, its metabolite, 1-amino-2-naphthol, was also found to be noncarcinogenic when fed to rats and dogs. However, several studies later reported this dye to be a carcinogen. When the dye was injected subcutaneously in female mice, Sharratt et al. (1966) observed an increased incidence of malignant tumors, such as adenocarcinomas of the lungs of lymphosarcomas. Clayson et al. (1968)

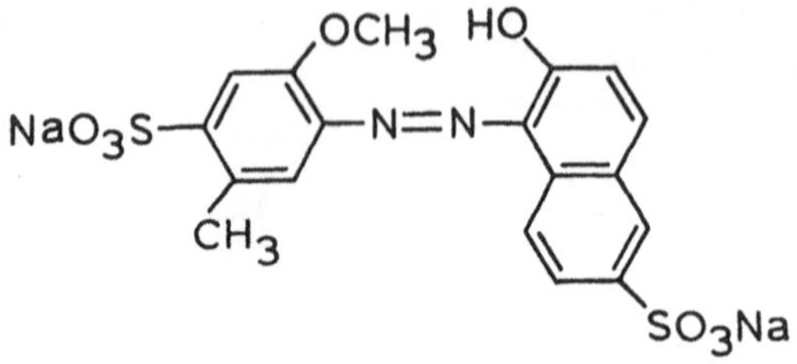

Fig. 7 FD&C Red No. 40.

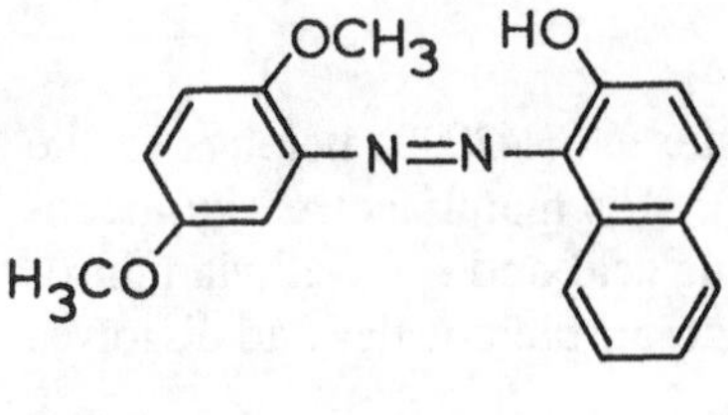

Fig. 8 Citrus Red No. 2.

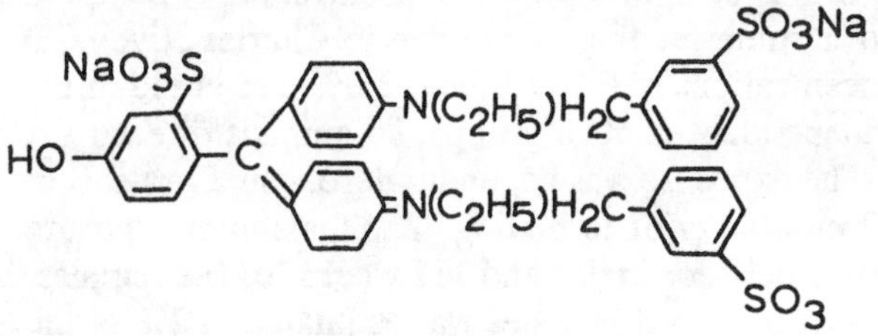

Fig. 9 FD&C Green No. 3.

also observed a similar, statistically significant increase in bladder cancer in mice following implantation of a pellet containing the dye into the lumen of the bladder. Dacre (1965) reported hyperplasia and benign tumors of the bladder in rats and mice fed diets containing Citrus Red No. 2. While all these studies reported the carcinogenic nature of the dye, FDA still would not remove its listing as a permitted dye for coloring orange skins (U.S. FDA, 1983a). This decision was based on the opinions of Grasso (1970) and the joint WHO/FAO Expert Committee (1969), who suggested that only those tests involving the oral route are relevant to the question of carcinogenicity of the ingested product. Similarly, a number of 2-*N*-hydroxy metabolites that are known carcinogens from compounds of these types have not been detected for Citrus Red No. 2 or any other permissible azo dyes. Furthermore, even if Citrus Red No. 2 is unequivocally shown to be carcinogenic by the oral route, it still would pose negligible hazards to humans, unless, of course, the dyed skins of oranges are ingested in products such as orange marmalade.

H. FD&C Green No. 3

FD&C Green No. 3 (Fast Green FCF, Color Index No. 42053) belongs to the triphenylmethane group of dyes (Fig. 9). It is synthesized by a condensation reaction of *p*-hydroxybenzaldehyde-*o*-sulfonic acid with α-(*N*-ethylanilino)-*m*-toluenesulfonic acid, followed by oxidation and conversion to a disodium salt. The dye is a reddish or brownish-violet powder. It is readily soluble in water, yielding bluish-green solutions.

Recent toxicological studies have shown both Indigo Carmine and FD&C Green No. 3 to induce sister chromatid exchanges in bone marrow cells, when the dyes were injected intraperitonially into mice at doses exceeding 25 and 10 mg/kg body weight, respectively. FD&C Green No. 3 was introduced in 1929 and is currently a permanently listed dye for food use in the United States.

I. FD&C Blue No. 1

FD&C Blue No. 1 (Brilliant Blue FCF, Color Index No. 42090) belongs to the triphenylmethane group of synthetic dyes (Fig. 10). It is manufactured by a condensation reaction involving benzaldehyde-*o*-sulfonic acid and α-(*N*-ethylanilino)-*m*-toluenesulfonic acid. FD&C Blue No. 1 is a bronze-purple powder and dissolves readily in water, giving a greenish-blue solution.

FD&C Blue No. 1 was introduced for food use in 1929. After being tested for chronic toxicity and having undergone teratology and reproduction studies, it was listed permanently for food use in the United States. Recent studies have shown the toxicological effects of FD&C Blue No. 1 to be concentration dependent. Borzelleca et al. (1990) studied lifetime feeding of the dye in Charles River CD rats and CD1 mice. Dietary concentrations of 0.1, 1.0, and 2.0% were used in the rat study. In addition to two independent control groups, 70 animals of each sex were used at each dosage level. The exposure was begun in utero. The F_0 rats were fed the dye for approximately 2 months prior to mating. The maximum exposure times for the F_1 animals were 116 weeks for males and 111 weeks for the females. Whereas the no-observed-adverse-effect level in males was estimated at 2% of the dye level, it was found to be only 1% for the female rats. The latter was based on a 15% decrease in the body weight and a significant decrease in survival when the dye was fed at 2% level in the diet.

In the above study (Borzelleca et al., 1990), groups of mice (60 of each sex) were also fed the dye at 0.5, 1.5, and 5% levels. The maximum exposure time was 104 weeks for both sexes, and the no-observed-effect level was estimated to be 0.5% of the dye in the diet.

J. FD&C Blue No. 2

FD&C Blue No. 2 (Indigotine, Indigo Carmine, Color Index No. 73015) was one of the seven original dyes allowed for food use by the Food and Drug Act of 1906. It belongs to the indigoid family of synthetic dyes (Fig. 11) and is manufactured by the sulfonation of indigo dye. It is a blue, brown-to-reddish powder and is readily soluble in water, yielding blue solutions.

When tested for at a concentration of 0.5 g/100 mL in cultures of *E. coli*, FD&C Blue No. 2 showed no significant mutagenic effects (Luck and Rickerl, 1960). Similar observations were made in an FDA study with rats. The dye also did not show any carcinogenic potential in both short-term and long-term feeding studies conducted at several different concentrations with beagles, pigs, and mice. The

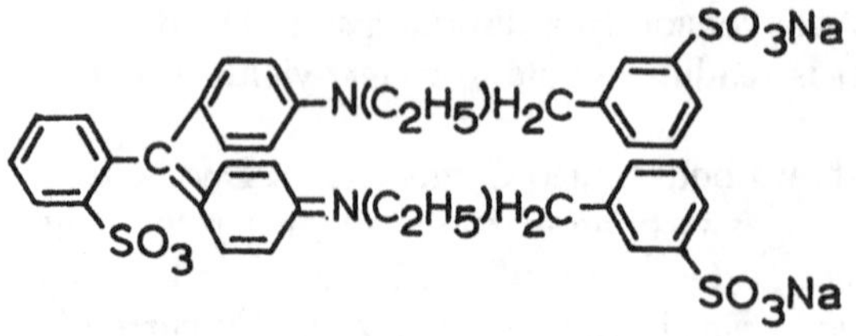

Fig. 10   FD&C Blue No. 1.

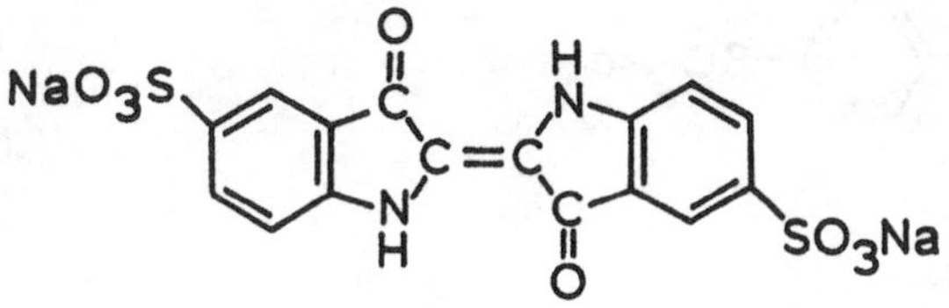

Fig. 11   FD&C Blue No. 2.

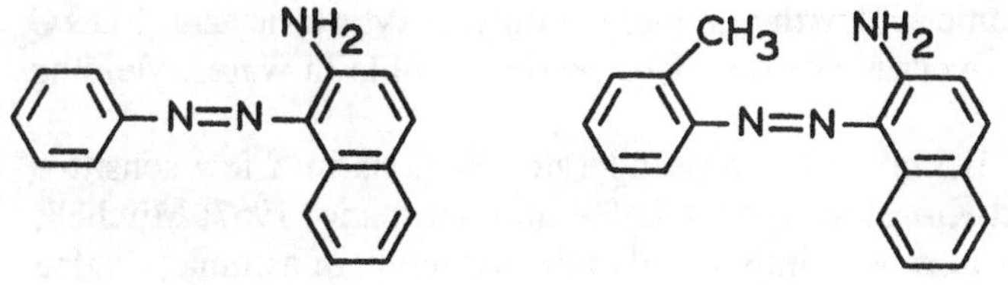

(a)   (b)

Fig. 12   (a) FD&C Yellow No. 3. (b) FD&C Yellow No. 4.

metabolic studies on this color are fairly complete and do not suggest any potential toxicity problems concerning its use in foods.

K. FD&C Yellow No. 3 and FD&C Yellow No. 4

Both these dyes belong to monoazo group of dyes (Fig. 12). FD&C Yellow No. 3 (Yellow AB, Color Index No. 11380) is prepared by coupling diazotized aniline and 2-naphthylamine in equimolar ratios. FD&C Yellow No. 4 (Yellow OB, Color Index No. 11390), in contrast, is synthesized by reacting diazotized *o*-toluidine with 2-naphthylamine. Both are orange-colored powders and are oil-soluble dyes.

FD&C Yellow No. 3 and FD&C Yellow No. 4 were introduced in the United States for food use in 1918 for coloring oleomargarine. Allamark et al. (1955) showed both these dyes to be hepatotoxic to rats and dogs. Even at 0.05% dietary levels, both these dyes induced significant weight loss in experimental animals (Hansen et al., 1963). Right-side cardiac atrophy and hypertrophy were observed in rats fed diets containing greater than 0.05% dyes for a period of up to 2 years. These two dyes are metabolized under the acid conditions of stomach to byproducts of 2-naphthylamine (Harrow and Jones, 1954; Radomaski and Harrow, 1966). 2-Naphthylamine is a known liver carcinogen in mice and a bladder carcinogen in dogs (Clayson and Gardner, 1976). In the United States, both of these dyes were delisted from the category of certified colors in 1959.

L. FD&C Yellow No. 5

FD&C Yellow No. 5 (Tartrazine, Color Index No. 19140) is a monoazo dye having pyrazoline ring structure (Fig. 13). It is synthesized by condensing phenylhydrazine-*p*-sulfonic acid with oxalacetic ester. The reaction product is then coupled with diazotized sulfanilic acid. The resulting ester is then hydrolyzed with sodium hydroxide. Alternatively, tartrazine can also be synthesized by condensing two moles

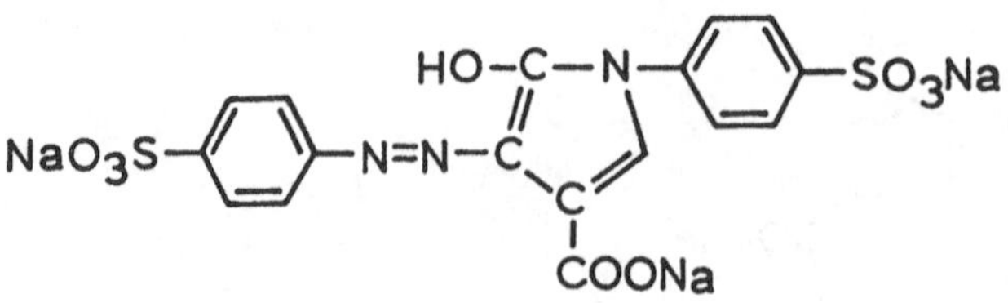

Fig. 13 FD&C Yellow No. 5.

of phenylhydrazine-*p*-sulfonic acid with one mole of dihydroxytartaric acid. FD&C Yellow No. 5 is an orange-yellow powder. It is readily soluble in water, yielding golden yellow solutions.

FD&C Yellow No. 5 is known to cause allergic reactions in a few sensitive individuals (Kevansky and Kingsley, 1964; Chafee and Settipane, 1967; Mitchell, 1971; Lockey, 1972). It has also been implicated in the induction of asthma (Chafee and Settipane, 1967). Azo dyes, particularly tartrazine, have been implicated in adverse food reactions involving immune mechanisms such as urticaria (Chafee and Settipane, 1967; Weber et al., 1979). Gerber et al. (1979) also noted nonimmunological reactions such as bronchospasm in asthmatic aspirin-intolerant individuals and those with chronic urticaria. Symptoms in sensitive individuals include itching hives, tissue swelling, asthma, and rhinitis. Miller (1982) also noted that such symptoms appear more often in asthmatic allergic and aspirin-intolerant individuals than in the general public. Zlotlow and Settipane (1977) reported a clinical case of tartrazine-induced chronic urticaria in a 16-year-old white male patient. Population studies have indicated that of about one million aspirin-sensitive individuals in the United States, about 15% are also sensitive to tartrazine (Chafee and Settipane, 1974; Settipane et al., 1974).

Recent studies by Loblay and Swain (1985) suggested that the reactions to tartrazine represented individual idiosyncrasy and that the propensity to react to tartrazine and other natural as well as artificial food colorants is probably genetically determined. Tartrazine does not inhibit the action of cyclooxygenase and has no effect on prostaglandin formation. This led Morales et al. (1985) to conclude that the tartrazine sensitivity in aspirin-intolerant individuals is not surprising. Although not well documented and established yet, the impurities in the colorant, rather than the dye itself, may also be involved in such adverse reaction mechanisms. In a recent study, tartrazine was also found to be nonmutagenic (Brown and Dietrich, 1983). After an extensive review of all the scientific evidence from tests conducted prior to tartrazine's approval for food use, FDA concluded that the colorant is neither carcinogenic nor genotoxic.

Listed for food use in the United States since 1916, tartrazine is used in some 60 countries around the world for coloring foods. However, its association with allergic-type reactions in sensitive individuals has resulted in regulations that either limit its use or require declaration of its name in the list of ingredients (44FR 3721226, June 1976).

M. FD&C Yellow No. 6

FD&C Yellow No. 6 (Sunset Yellow FCF, Color Index No. 15985) is a monoazo dye (Fig. 14). It is synthesized by coupling diazotized sulfanilic acid with 2-naphthol-

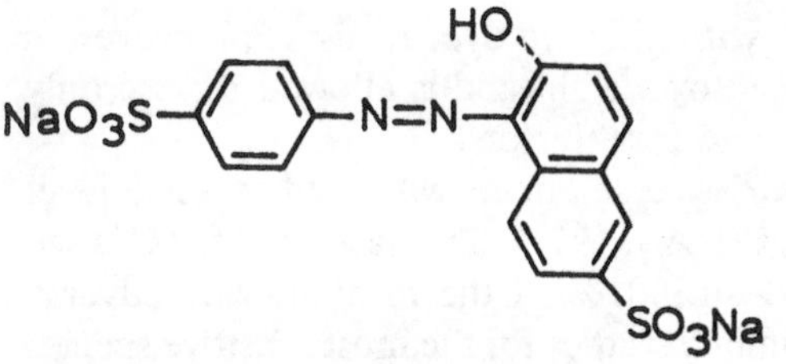

Fig. 14 FD&C Yellow No. 6.

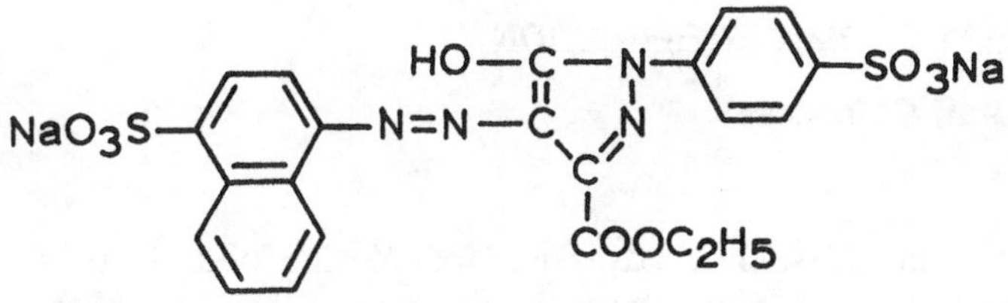

Fig. 15 Orange B.

6-sulfonic acid. The dye is an orange-red powder and is readily soluble in water, giving an orange-yellow solution.

Similar to amaranth and tartrazine, FD&C Yellow No. 6 also causes allergic reactions and induces urticaria in sensitive individuals. The controversies surrounding the dye are primarily due to the results obtained in an FDA lifetime feeding study of rats. In this study, a number of female rats developed proliferative renal lesions when the dye was fed at 5% level in the diet. Such a high concentration would result in an average daily consumption of 3926 mg/kg/d, while the normal consumption in humans for this dye is only about 0.15 mg/kg/d (Newsome, 1990). FDA has submitted the data to the National Toxicology Program (NTP) for a peer review (50FR 51455, December 1985). An earlier NTP study in which the rats received a lower dietary concentration of the color (1.25 and 2.5%) for a period of 24 months did not show any harmful effects related to the consumption of this dye. A concurrent study in mice was also negative. The NTP Expert Committee, after reviewing the data provided by FDA, concluded that FD&C Yellow No. 6 is noncarcinogenic. Similar to tartrazine, its use in foods must be accompanied by specific listing of its name in the list of ingredients.

N. Orange B

Orange B is principally the disodium salt of 1-(4-sulfophenyl)-3-ethylcarboxy-4-(4-sulfonaphthylazo)-5-hydroxypyrazole (Fig. 15). It belongs to the pyrazolone group of azo dyes.

Orange B is manufactured by reacting phenylhydrazine *p*-sulfonic acid with the sodium derivative of diethyl hydroxymaleate. It is then partially hydrolyzed to remove one ethyl group, followed by coupling with diazotized naphthionic acid (Marmion, 1984).

Orange B is permanently listed as a synthetic food dye. Its usage, however, is restricted at a level not to exceed 150 ppm by weight and is allowed for use only in casings or on the surfaces of sausages and frankfurters.

Orange B has been shown to have no adverse effects when fed at a 5% level to rats and mice and at a 1% level to dogs (NAS, 1971). The safe level for Orange B for human ingestion, calculated based on 0.01% of the maximum no adverse effect level established by the long-term animal studies for the most sensitive species and assuming a daily dietary intake of 1814 g for humans, was tentatively established at 181 mg/person/d. Based on the CCIC (1968) survey, the estimated maximum ingestion of Orange B in human nutrition was found to be only 0.31 mg/person/d.

V. COLORANTS EXEMPT FROM CERTIFICATION

A. Nonsynthetic (Natural) Colorants

Annatto Extracts

Annatto extracts are some of the oldest known dyes used for coloring foods, textiles, and cosmetics. These pigments are extracted from the pericarp of the seeds of the annatto tree (*Bixa orellana* L.). It is a large, fast-growing shrub native to the tropical climates of India, South America, East Africa, and the Caribbean. The tree produces large clusters of brown or crimson capsular fruits. Their seeds are coated with a thin, highly colored resinous coating that serves as a raw material for the colorant (Marmion, 1984).

Annatto extracts are prepared by leaching the seeds with one or more of approved food-grade solvents such as edible vegetable oils and fats and alkaline and alcoholic solutions. Depending on the end use, the pigments from the alkaline extracts are precipitated with food-grade acids. They may also be further purified by recrystallization from approved solvents.

The major coloring compound of the oil-soluble extract is the carotenoid bixin (Color Index No. 75120) (Fig. 16a). This orange-yellow–colored compound exhibits

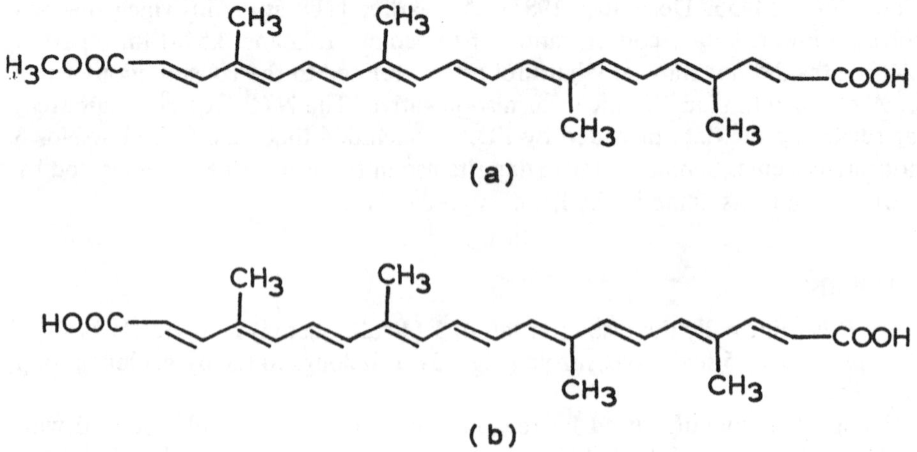

(a)

(b)

Fig. 16 Annatto extracts: (a) bixin, (b) norbixin.

fairly good light and heat stability. It is, however, susceptible to oxidation, which is accelerated by heat and light. Bixin is primarily used in dairy and fat-based products such as processed cheese, butter, margarine, cooking oils, salad dressings, desserts, baked goods, and snack foods (Noonan, 1972; Marmion, 1984; Rayner, 1991).

Bixin can be hydrolyzed by alkaline treatment during or after extraction to produce the water-soluble diacid norbixin (Fig. 16b). Norbixin precipitates in an acidic environment. It also reacts with metallic salts in water to produce hazy solutions. Upon complexation with proteins, its light stability is greatly enhanced (Rayner, 1991). Norbixin is widely used for coloring cheese, smoked fish, sausage casings, flour confectionery, cereal products, ice creams, ice cream cones, and desserts in North American, European Economic Community, and Scandinavian countries.

Annatto extracts are available commercially in several physical forms, including dry powders, propylene glycol/monoglyceride emulsions, oil solutions and suspensions, and alkaline and aqueous solutions (Marmion, 1984). The active colorant in these preparations, expressed as bixin, may range from 1 to 15%. It is generally used in products at 0.5–10 ppm as pure color. This results in hues ranging from butter yellow to peach, depending on the type of color preparation employed and the product colored. Annatto extracts can be blended also with turmeric to produce a more yellow shade or with paprika for a redder shade.

The mutagenic action of annatto extracts was tested at 0.5 g/100 mL in cultures of *E. coli*. No adverse effects were found (Luck and Rickerl, 1960). The administration of aqueous extracts of bixa roots depresses the spontaneity of motor activity in mice, the intraperitoneal effective dose ED_{50} being 21 mg/kg body weight. The extract also affects the volume of gastric secretion but not its pH when injected intraduodenally at a 400 mg/kg level. Annatto extracts are also antispasmodic (1 mg/mL, isolated guinea pig ileum) and hypotensive (intravenous at 50 mg/kg body weight in rats) (Durham and Allard, 1960). Several long-term tests in mice and rats performed on well-defined types of extracts containing 0.1–2.6% bixin, however, have not shown any carcinogenic potential associated with their use.

Anthocyanins

Anthocyanins are one of the most important and widely distributed groups of water-soluble natural pigments. They are responsible for the attractive red, purple, and blue colors of the many flowers, fruits, and vegetables. Their distinctive color is normally not produced by a single pigment. It is rather more often a combination or system of pigments (IFT, 1986). For example, blackberries contain one of the simpler systems consisting of only one primary pigment (cyanidin-3-glucoside), while the color of others such as blueberries may be due to as many as 10–15 different pigments. Generally, most fruits and vegetables contain four to six pigments.

More than 200 individual anthocyanins have been identified thus far, of which 20 have been shown to be present naturally in black grapes, the major commercial source of anthocyanin pigments for food coloration (Rayner, 1991).

Anthocyanins are the glycosides of anthocyanidins consisting of 2-phenyl benzopyrilium (flavylium) structure (Fig. 17). The anthocyanidin aglycone may be esterified to one or more sugars, which may or may not be acylated. Glucose,

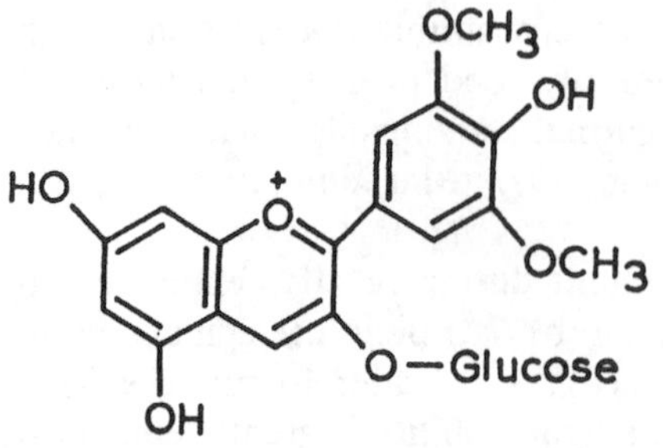

Fig. 17   General structure of anthocyanin pigments.

Table 5   Commercial Sources of Major Anthocyanin Pigments

Source	Scientific name	Major anthocyanins present
Grape skins	*Vitis vinifera*	Cy, Dp, Pt, Mv monoglycosides, free and acylated
Grape lees	*Vitis labrusca*	Cy, Dp, Pt, Mv monoglycosides, free and acylated
Cranberry	*Vaccinium macrocarpon*	Cy and Pn monoglycosides
Roselle calyces	*Hibiscus sabdariffa*	Cy and Dp mono- and diglycosides
Red cabbage	*Brassica oleracea*	Cy glycosides
Elderberry	*Sambucus nigra*	Cy glycosides
Black currant	*Ribes nigrum*	Cy and Dp mono- and diglycosides free and acylated
Purple corn	*Maize morado*	Pg, Cy, and Pn monoglycosides

Cy = Cyanidin; Dp = delphinidin; Mv = malvidin; Pg = pelargonidin; Pn = peonidin; Pt = petunidin.
Source: Rayner, 1991.

rhamnose, galactose, xylose, and arabinose are the principal sugars associated with different anthocyanins. When acylated, the sugar molecules may be associated with one or more molecules of *p*-coumaric, ferulic, caffeic, or acetic acid. The six most common anthocyanins are pelargonidin, cyanidin, delphinidin, petunidin, peonidin, and malvidin (Rayner, 1991). Extracts from different sources (Table 5) exhibit different stabilities.

Anthocyanin pigments are obtained by extraction with acidified water or alcohol, followed by concentration under vacuum and/or reverse osmosis. The extracts can also be spray or vacuum dried to give powders.

Anthocyanins are natural indicators of pH. In acidic media, they appear red, while as the pH is progressively increased, they become more blue. The anthocyanin double-ring benzopyrilium structure is cationic and thus is very reactive. Anthocyanins exhibit their most intense colors below pH 3.5 (Newsome, 1990). These pigments are therefore suitable for coloring acidic foods only. Anthocyanins easily undergo discoloration in the presence of amino acids and phenolic sugar derivatives due to condensation reactions (Sankaranarayanan, 1981). They are also oxidized in the presence of ascorbic acid. The stabilities of these pigments can be greatly enhanced by substitution at the C-4 position with a methyl or phenyl group.

Anthocyanin pigments are widely used for coloring soft drinks, alcoholic beverages, sugar confectionery and preserves, fruit toppings and sauces, pickles, dry mixes, canned and frozen foods, and dairy products.

Dehydrated Beets (Beet Powder, Betalains)

Betalains are found in the members of the Centrospermae family of plants such as red beets, chards, cactus fruits, pokeberries, bougainvillea, and amaranthus flowers. The color additive beet powder is defined as "a dark red powder prepared by dehydrating sound, mature, good quality, edible beets" (Marmion, 1984).

Beet roots contain both red pigments (betacyanins) and yellow pigments (betaxanthins). Collectively, they are known as betalains. The betacyanin content generally far exceeds that of betaxanthins. Betanin (Fig. 18) is the principal pigment in beet colorant, accounting for 75–95% of the total betacyanins.

The color extract is prepared by crushing mature, sound, clean beet roots. The juice can then be concentrated under vacuum to a total solids content of 40–60%. The powders are prepared by spray drying the concentrates. Ascorbic or citric acid is used as a stabilizer in both the concentrate and the dry powder. On a dry weight basis, beet colorant typically contains between 0.4–1.0% betanin, 80% sugar, 8% ash, and 10% crude protein (Marmion, 1984). The actual quantity of the pigment varies with the raw material and the processing conditions employed.

Betalains are sensitive to light, pH, and heat (Marmion, 1984; Newsome, 1990; Rayner, 1991). Beet colorants readily dissolve in water and water-based products. The carbohydrates associated with the colorant impart it with the natural flavor of beets. Its solutions produce hues resembling raspberry or cherry. When used in combination with water-soluble annatto, it produces strawberry shades.

Beet colorants are used primarily in foods of short shelf life that do not require high or prolonged heat treatment. In the latter instance, it may be added to the product after the heat treatment is over or as near the end of the heating cycle as possible (Marmion, 1984). Betalains are used at 0.1–1% levels to color foods such as hard candies, yogurts, ice creams, salad dressings, ready-made frostings, cake mixes, meat substitutes, powdered drink mixes, gravy mixes, marshmallow candies, soft drinks, and gelatin desserts.

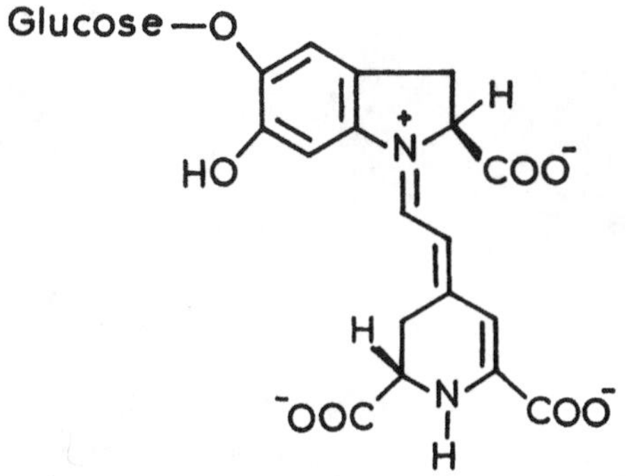

Fig. 18 Batanin.

Chlorophylls

Chlorophylls, the most abundant of naturally occurring plant pigments, are the green and olive-green pigments in green plants. Although they exist in four different forms—chlorophyll *a*, *b*, *c*, and *d*—chlorophyll *a* and chlorophyll *b* are the two predominant forms (Francis, 1985).

Because of the light and acid sensitivity of their magnesium-chelated porphyrin structures (Fig. 19), chlorophylls are the least useful food colors (Sankaranarayanan, 1981). The green color is easily destroyed under even the mildest processing conditions. The resulting pheophytinization, in which the magnesium is replaced by hydrogen, destroys the porphyrin ring structure, yielding a dull olive-brown color (Francis, 1985). Chlorophylls are generally stabilized by replacing the magnesium with copper ions.

Chlorophyll extracts are not permitted for food use in the United States. However, they may be added to foods in the form of green vegetables. In such cases, they are classified as food ingredients. Chlorophylls marketed as chlorophyll-copper complexes are permitted food colorants in Canada and Europe (Newsome, 1990).

Caramel

Caramel belongs to the group of melanoidin pigments. This group of compounds is responsible for the attractive red-brown color of cooked foods. When carbohydrates are heated at high temperatures, they caramelize to produce a characteristic flavor and color. Melanoidin pigments are responsible for the color of caramels, malt extracts, and toasted carob flour (Rayner, 1991).

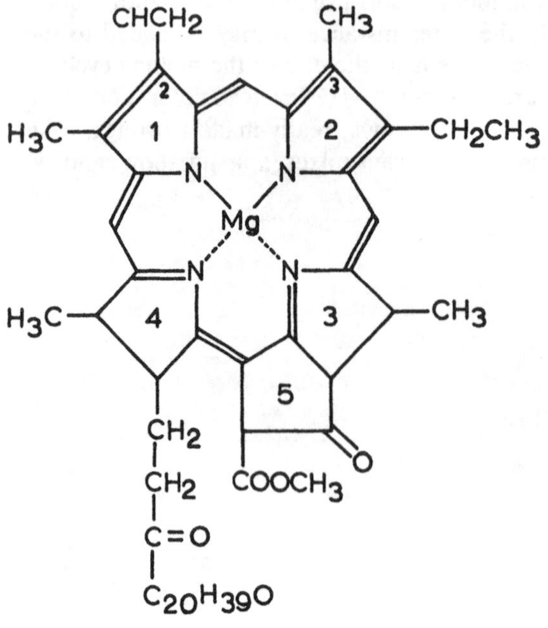

Fig. 19 Chlorophyll *a* (chlorophyll *b* differs in having a formyl group at carbon 3).

Caramel colors are probably the most widely used food colors in foods and drinks. The FDA defines caramel as "the dark brown liquid or solid material resulting from the carefully controlled heat treatment of the following food-grade carbohydrates: dextrose, invert sugar, lactose, malt syrup, molasses, starch hydrolysates and fractions thereof, or sucrose" (Marmion, 1984).

Liquid corn syrup of 60° Brix or higher reducing sugar content is the most widely used raw material for the manufacture of caramel. Because of its high cost and processing difficulties, sucrose is seldom used. Liquid corn sugars are heated at about 250°F (121°C) in the presence of accelerators for several hours or until the proper tinctorial strength is obtained. The product is then rapidly cooled, filtered, blended, and standardized. It can also be spray-dried to produce a powdered colorant.

Several different grades of caramel are available commercially. The positively charged caramel is manufactured using ammonia as an accelerator. Electropositive caramels with an isoelectric point of about pH 6.0 are especially useful in the brewing industry, where stability in the presence of positively charged fining colloids is required. This is essential to avoid problems related to flocculation and hazing of beers.

The negatively charged caramel is manufactured under acidic conditions using ammonium bisulfite as a catalyst. Electronegative caramels have isoelectric points below pH 3.0 and, hence, are prized by the soft drink industry where stability at low pH is desired. In contrast, the spirit caramel is manufactured using sodium hydroxide as a catalyst. These caramels possess only a weak ionic charge and are therefore stable in high-alcohol products such as whiskey and rum.

The exact chemical composition of caramel is difficult to define. The color is freely soluble in water and insoluble in most organic solvents. The specific gravity of caramel syrups containing 50–75% total solids ranges from 1.25 to 1.38 (Marmion, 1984). The color is used to produce shades such as delicate yellow to red to the darkest brown. Typically used at 0.1–30% levels, caramel color is relatively inexpensive and exhibits good stability in most food products.

Approximately 75–85% of the caramel produced in the United States is used in soft drinks, especially root beers and colas. They are also used extensively to standardize the hue of blended whiskey, liqueurs, wines, and beers. Other food uses of caramel include coloring of baked goods, syrups, preserves, candies, pet foods, gravies, canned meat products, soups, condiments, vinegars, and dark sugars.

In toxicological studies, no abnormalities were detected after observation of the animals for 14 days following administration of 12 different caramel color products (Foote et al., 1958; Chacharonis, 1960, 1963). These products were prepared using either ammonia or ammonium sulfate catalysts. Sharratt (1971) showed that a single dose of caramels, prepared by either ammonia-catalyzed closed pan process or the sodium hydroxide process up to 10 g/kg body weight in mice and 15 g/kg body weight in rabbits did not cause convulsions or others signs of distress. Several short-term toxicological studies in rats at levels of 10–15 g caramel/kg body weight or 10–20% caramel/kg body weight did not show any abnormalities or significant differences in histochemical and hematological studies (Prier, 1960; Haldi and Calandra, 1962; Key and Calandra, 1962). Similarly, many long-term toxicological and reproduction studies (WHO, 1975) also showed no adverse effects in up to three generations.

Cochineal Extract (Carmine, Carminic, Acid)

Cochineal extract (Color Index No. 75470) is the concentrated solution obtained after the removal of alcohol from an aqueous, alcoholic extract of cochineal. Cochineal is obtained from the dried bodies of the female insect *Coccus cacti* (*Dactylopius coccus costa*). These insects grow on a specific variety of cactus that is native to the Canary Islands and parts of South America.

Cochineal extracts consist mainly of carminic acid (Fig. 20). This anthraquinone pigment constitutes approximately 10% of cochineal and 2% of its extract (Marmion, 1984). In the traditional purification process, the aqueous extract is precipitated as the insoluble aluminum lake. The lake is known as cochineal carmine. Carmine is normally 50% or more carminic acid.

Cochineal extract is typically acid (pH 5.0–5.3) and has a total solids content of about 6%. It varies in shade from orange to red to violet as the pH is increased. It is insoluble in typical solvents, including water, glycerine, and propylene glycol, but can be dispersed easily in water. The aluminum lake, carmine, can be solubilized by strong acids and bases that cause degradation of the substratum and release of the color. Cochineal exhibits good stability toward light and oxidation but has poor stability toward pH and microbiological attack (Marmion, 1984). Sodium benzoate, therefore, is often used as a preservative in cochineal extracts.

Carmine is widely used in producing pink shades in retorted protein products, candy, confections, alcoholic and soft drinks, jams, jellies, rouge, eye shadow, and pill coatings at 0.04–0.2% levels.

Short-term toxicological studies on cochineal extracts were conducted in mice and rabbits. When 1–2% aqueous solutions of the lithium salt of carminic acid were injected intraperitoneally for a period of 60 days, the only abnormality observed in mice was a proliferation of spleen tissue (WHO, 1975). Similar effects were also observed in rabbits given intravenous injections of 3–10 ml of 2–4% aqueous solution of the lithium salt of carminic acid every 5–6 days. In another study, groups of 40 rats received cochineal carmine in 0.4% aqueous gum tragacanth at 0, 2.5, 5.0, and 10 mg/kg body weight, by intubation. The process was carried out 5 days per week for a period of 13 weeks. No adverse hematological effects were noted (WHO, 1975).

Paprika and Paprika Oleoresin

Paprika is the deep red, sweet, pungent powder prepared from the ground dried pods of mild capsicum (*Capsicum annum*). Paprika is one of two principal kinds of red pepper, the other being cayenne pepper or cayenne. Paprika is largely

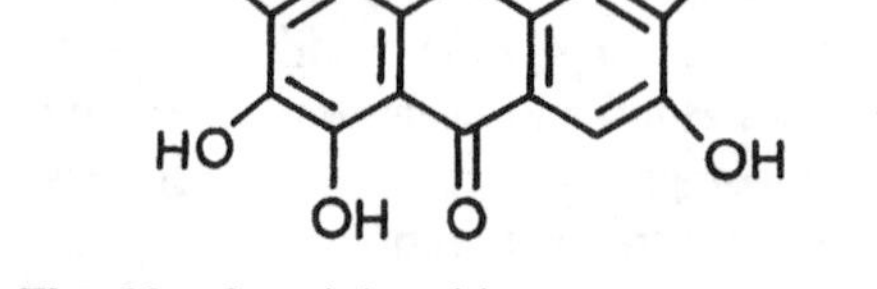

Fig. 20 Carminic acid.

produced in the warm climate areas of Africa, Spain, Hungary, and the American tropics (Marmion, 1984).

Paprika oleoresins are the combination of flavor and color principles obtained by extracting paprika with any one or a combination of approved solvents. These include acetone, ethyl alcohol, ethylene dichloride, hexane, isopropyl alcohol, methyl alcohol, methylene chloride, and trichloroethylene. Depending on their source, paprika oleoresins are brown-red, slightly viscous, homogeneous liquids, pourable at room temperature, and containing 2–5% sediment (Marmion, 1984). Paprika oleoresins are available in various standardized forms in which 1 lb of the oleoresin is equivalent to 10–30 lb of the natural colorant.

Paprika extracts normally have a spicy flavor that tends to restrict their use to savory or highly flavored products. Paprika oleoresin is used in meat products, such as sausages, for flavor and color. It is also used at levels of 0.2–100 ppm to produce orange to bright red shades in seasonings, snack products, soups, relishes, sugar confectionery, cheese, fruit sauces, and toppings.

Turmeric and Turmeric Oleoresin

Turmeric (Color Index No. 75300) is the fluorescent yellow extract of the dried, ground rhizome of *Curcuma longa*. It is a perennial herb of the Zingiberaceae family native to south Asia. It is cultivated widely in China, India, South America, and the East Indies.

Turmeric oleoresin is the combination of flavor and color principles obtained from turmeric by extracting the roots with one or a combination of the following solvents: acetone, ethyl alcohol, ethylene dichloride, hexane, isopropyl alcohol, methyl alcohol, methylene chloride, and trichloroethylene.

The major pigment in turmeric, and its oleoresin is curcumin (1,6-heptadiene-3,5-dione-1,7-bis[4-hydroxy-3-methoxyphenyl]). Curcumin (Fig. 21) is an orange-yellow crystalline powder, insoluble in water and ether but soluble in ethanol and glacial acetic acid (Marmion, 1984). Turmeric extracts are oil soluble. The pigment is relatively stable to heat but fades rapidly in light in the presence of oxygen. Both turmeric and its oleoresin exhibit good tinctorial strength. While the basic turmeric extracts have a spicy flavor and aroma, the curcumin pigment has very little of both.

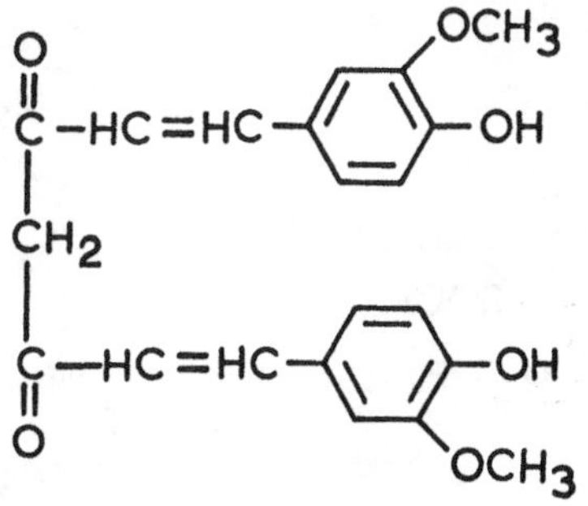

Fig. 21 Curcumin.

Turmeric is available commercially as a powder and as a suspension in a variety of carriers, including edible vegetable oils and fats and mono- and diglycerides. Turmeric oleoresin is most often sold as solutions in propylene glycol with or without added emulsifying agents. The dry powder is typically used at 0.2–60 ppm and the oleoresin at 2–640 ppm to produce bright yellow to greenish-yellow shades in foods. They can be used alone or in combination with other colorants such as annatto to shade pickles, mustard, spices, margarine, ice creams, cheeses, pies, cakes, candies, soups, cooking oils, salad dressings, and canned and dry mix foods. Turmeric and its oleoresin are often used to replace FD&C Yellow No. 5.

Saffron (Crocin and Crocetine)

Saffron is the dried stigma of *Crocus sativus*. It is indigenous to the Orient, but is also grown in North Africa, Spain, Switzerland, Greece, Austria, and France. Saffron is a reddish-brown or golden yellow odoriferous powder with a slight bitter taste (Marmion, 1984). Saffron is an expensive color, since stigmas of approximately 165,000 flowers are required to produce 1 kg of saffron containing about 50 g of the pigment.

The principal coloring pigments of saffron are crocin (Fig. 22a) and crocetin (Fig. 22b). Crocin is a yellow-orange glycoside that is freely soluble in hot water, slightly soluble in absolute alcohol, glycerine, and propylene glycol, and insoluble in vegetable oils. Crocetin is a dicarboxylic acid that forms brick red rhombs from acetic anhyride (Marmion, 1984; Rayner, 1991). It is very sparingly soluble in water and most organic solvents, but soluble in pyridine and similar organic bases as well as in dilute sodium hydroxide.

Saffron and saffron extracts are normally used as much for flavor as for their color. As a food colorant, it is generally stable toward light, oxidation, pH, and microbial attack and has a high tinctorial strength. Saffron is typically used at levels of 1–260 ppm in baked goods, rice dishes, soups, meat dishes, and sugar confectionery.

Crocin is extracted commercially from the less expensive, dried fruit of the *Gardenia jasminoides* bush, which grows in the Far East. The color extract does

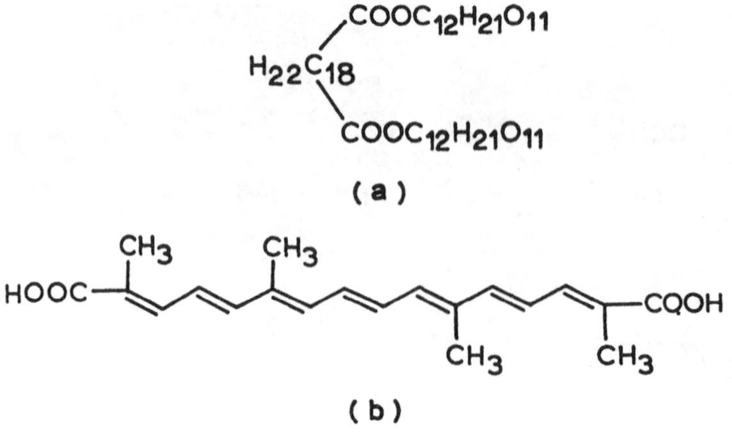

Fig. 22 Saffron pigments: (a) crocin, (b) crocetin.

not have the flavor of saffron but is ideal for coloring smoked white fish such as cod and haddock, where it binds to the flesh (Rayner, 1991). Other applications of crocin from this source include dairy products, sugar and flour confectionery, jams and preserves, rice, and pasta dishes.

Gardenia fruits also yield other pigments of the iridoid and flavonoid groups. These extracts can give red, green, and blue colors. They are used in Japan and the Far East to color confectionery, ices, cakes, noodles, beans, and other dishes.

Carrot Oil

Carrot oil is available as a liquid or the solid portion of a mixture prepared by hexane extraction of edible carrots (*Daucas carota* L.). After removal of hexane by vacuum distillation, the resultant mixture of solid and liquid extractives consists mainly of oils, fats, waxes, and carotenoids occurring naturally in carrots. Its use in foods is consistent with good manufacturing practices.

Carthamus Yellow

Carthamus yellow is the water-soluble extract of the dried petals of flowers of safflower (*Carthamus tinctorius*). The extract imparts a lemon yellow color and a mild flavor to various food products (Rayner, 1991). The color is stable between pH 3 and 9 and exhibits good heat and light stability. It is used for coloring soft drinks and alcoholic beverages in some countries.

Corn Endosperm Oil

Corn endosperm oil is obtained by isopropyl alcohol and hexane extraction of the gluten fraction from yellow corn grain. This reddish-brown liquid contains primarily glycosides, fatty acids, sitosterols, and carotenoid pigments. Its use in the United States is restricted to chicken feed only.

Cottonseed Flour

Cottonseed flour is prepared by delinting and decorticating food-quality glandless (gossypol-free) cottonseeds. The meats are screened, aspirated, and rolled. After tempering and oil extraction, the cooked meats are cooled, ground, and selected to obtain a product varying in shade from light to dark brown. It is a listed food colorant in the United States and used according to good manufacturing practices in baked cereal products.

Dried Algae Meal

The algae biliproteins or phycobiliproteins are a group of pigments occurring naturally in the red algae (Rhodophyta), the blue-green algae (Cyanobacteria), and the cryptomonad (Cryptophyta). It is produced as a dried mixture of algae cells separated from their culture broth, molasses, cornsteep liquor, and a maximum of 0.3% ethoxyquin. The algae cells are produced by fermentation under controlled conditions from a pure culture of the genus *Spongiococcum*.

The red phycoerythrins and the blue phycocyanins are prepared as water- or alcohol-soluble extracts. They are sometimes used in some countries as colorants in sugar confectionery, sherbets, frozen confections, ices, and chewing gum. In the United States, the use of dried algae meal is restricted to chicken feed only.

Fruit and Vegetable Juices

Fruit juices are the concentrated or unconcentrated liquids expressed from mature varieties of fresh, edible fruits. Sometimes they are also prepared by water infusion of dried fruits. Vegetable juices are similarly prepared from a variety of fresh, edible vegetables. Both are listed food colorants in the United States subject to use according to good manufacturing practices.

Grape Color Extract

This is an aqueous solution of anthocyanin grape pigments made from Concord grapes or a dehydrated water-soluble powder prepared by the spray-drying of its aqueous extract (Marmion, 1984). The aqueous solution is prepared by extracting the pigments from the precipitated lees produced during the storage of Concord grape juice. It is composed of anthocyanins, tartarates, malates, sugars, and minerals. Its purple color is primarily due to the 3-mono- and 3,5-diglucosides of malvidins, delphinidins, and cyanidins and their acylated derivatives.

Grape color extract is widely used to color jams and nonstandard jellies and to preserve the color of sherbets, icepops, raspberry, grape, and strawberry yogurts, gelatin desserts, canned fruits, fruit sauces, candy, confections, and bakery fillings and toppings. It is used at 0.05–0.8% levels based on the weight of the finished products. In the United States, its use is restricted to nonbeverage foods only.

Grape Skin Extract (Enocianina)

Grape skin extract is a purplish-red liquid prepared by the aqueous extraction (steeping) of the fresh, deseeded marc remaining after grapes have been pressed to produce grape juice or wine (Marmion, 1984). Its composition is similar to that of grape color extract. In the United States, grape skin extract is restricted to colored beverages and soft drinks only.

Lutein (Tagetes Meal and Extract)

This xanthophyll type of carotenoid is found in all green leaves, green vegetables, eggs, and some flowers. Commercially, it is obtained as an oil-soluble yellow extract of Aztec marigold (*Tagetes erecta*). The color exhibits good stability to heat, light, and sulfur dioxide and is less sensitive to oxidation than most other carotenoid pigments (Rayner, 1991).

Lutein extracts are used as colorants primarily in salad dressings, ice creams, dairy products, emulsified fats, and other food products containing high levels of fats. They are also used in soft drinks and flour and sugar confectionery. In the United States, its use is restricted to chicken feed only.

B. Nature-Identical Colorants

β-Carotene (Provitamin A)

β-Carotene (Color Index No. 75310) is a normal constituent of the human diet. It is an isomer of the naturally occurring carotenoid pigment carotene. Carotene or provitamin A occurs naturally in products such as butter, cheese, carrots, alfalfa, and yellow-colored cereal grains. β-Carotene was one of the first "natural" colorants synthetically produced on a commercial scale. The original process for the synthesis of this optically inactive all-*trans* isomer from acetone was developed in the 1950s by Hoffman-La Roche. Its use in food as a permitted colorant eventually led to the creation of the category of colorants called "colorants exempt from certification" (Marmion, 1984).

β-Carotene (Fig. 23) is sensitive to alkali and very sensitive to air and light, especially at high temperatures. It is insoluble in water, ethanol, glycerine, and propylene glycol, but is slightly soluble in edible oils at room temperature. β-Carotene is one of the rare color additives having nutritional value, since it is converted biologically by humans into provitamin A. One gram of β-carotene is equivalent to 1.6×10^6 USP (1.6 IU/mg) units of vitamin A.

β-Carotene is marketed commercially as dry crystals packed under nitrogen, as a dry water-dispersible powder containing 1% β-carotene, dextrin, gum arabic, partially hydrogenated vegetable oil, sucrose, sodium ascorbate and dl-α-tocopherol, as liquid and semisolid suspensions in edible oils including vegetable, peanut, and butter oil, as water-dispersible beadlets composed of colorant, vegetable oil, sugar, gelatin, and carbohydrates, and as emulsions (Marmion, 1984).

Unlike other nature-identical carotenoid colorants allowed for food use, the FDA permits the addition of β-carotene to color foods at any levels consistent with good manufacturing practices. It imparts a yellow-to-orange color when used at 2–50 ppm levels in foods. β-Carotene is used to shade or color a wide range of foods, including butter, margarine, hydrogenated fats, oils, cheese, soft drinks, ice creams, eggnogs, yogurts, desserts, flour and sugar confectionery, macaroni products, soups, jellies, preserves, dressings, and meat products.

In humans, about 30–90% of the ingested β-carotene is normally excreted in the feces. A concomitant intake of fat does not improve its absorption. Excessive doses of β-carotene depress the vitamin A activity of the absorbed fraction; only a small fraction appears in the serum. When dissolved in oil, as much as 10–41% and 50–80% of β-carotene is absorbed in adults and children, respectively (Fraps and Meinke, 1945). Although hypercarotenemia associated with excessive intakes of β-carotene is harmless and produces no adverse symptoms, it usually disappears when the vitamin intake is discontinued (Abrahamson and Abrahamson, 1962; Nieman et al., 1954). Bagdon et al. (1960) also noted the absence of hypervitaminosis in human volunteers given β-carotene over an extended period of time. Similarly, Greenberg et al. (1959) failed to see symptoms of hypervitaminosis in 15 individuals who received daily doses of 60 mg of β-carotene over a 3-month period. Serum carotene levels rose from 120 to a maximum of 308 µg/100 ml after one month, while the vitamin A levels remained essentially unchanged. Long-term

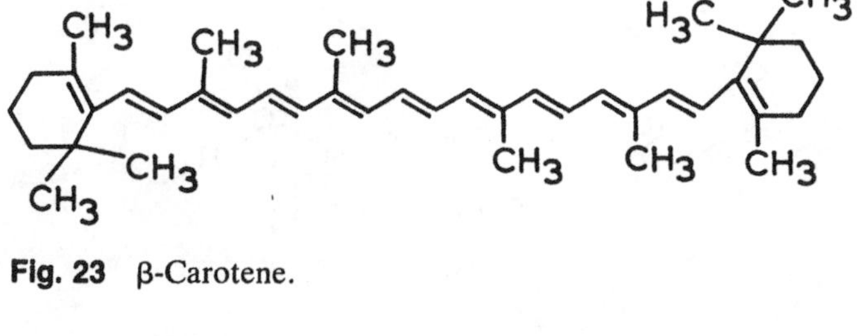

Fig. 23 β-Carotene.

studies of up to four generations in rats fed 0 to 1000 ppm of β-carotene daily for 110 weeks also failed to show adverse effects in any of the generations (Bagdon et al., 1960).

β-Apo-8'-Carotenal (Apocarotenal)

β-Apo-8'-carotenal (Color Index No. 40820) is an aldehydic carotenoid occurring naturally in oranges, spinach, grass, tangerines, and marigolds. It is available commercially as a synthetic color.

Apocarotenal (Fig. 24) is synthetically produced as a crystalline, all-*trans* stereoisomer. Its physicochemical properties are similar to those of β-carotene. However, it is more sensitive to oxidation than β-carotene and less stable to light. It also has provitamin A activity, with 1 g colorant being equivalent to 1.2×10^6 USP (1.2 IU/mg) units of vitamin A.

Apocarotenal is marketed commercially as a dry powder, as 1–1.5% vegetable oil solutions, as 20% suspension in vegetable oils, as 2–4% solutions in a mixture of monoglycerides and dl-α-tocopherol, and as 10% dry beadlets (Marmion, 1984).

Apocarotenal is used at 1–20 ppm levels to impart orange-red colors to cheese, sauces, spreads, oils, fats, ice creams, cake mixes, cake toppings, snack foods, and soft drinks. Because of its reddish shade, it is often blended with β-carotene to produce a rich orange shade. In the United States, FDA restricts its use as a colorant to a maximum of 15 mg/lb of solid or semisolid food or pint of liquid food.

In toxicological studies, no adverse effects were observed in dogs of both sexes when apocarotenol was fed at daily levels of 0.1 or 1 g per animal during a 14-week period. In other studies, three- to fivefold higher vitamin A levels were found in test animals as compared to the respective controls. Histopathological examination also showed pigmentation of the kidney, adipose tissue and of the adrenal cortex (Bagdon et al., 1962).

Canthaxanthin

The carotenoid pigment canthaxanthin (Color Index No. 40850) occurs naturally in an edible mushroom (*Cantharellus cinnabarinus*), sea trout, algae, daphnia, salmon, brine shrimp, and several species of flamingo. It has been available commercially as a synthetic food color since 1969.

Canthaxanthin (Fig. 25) is synthesized from acetone or β-ionone using procedures similar to those used for β-carotene and β-apo-8'-carotenal (Marmion, 1984). It is crystallized from various solvents as brownish-violet, shiny leaves. It is stable at pH 2–8 and is unaffected by heat in systems with a minimal oxygen content. Similar to other carotenoid pigments, canthaxanthin is sensitive to both

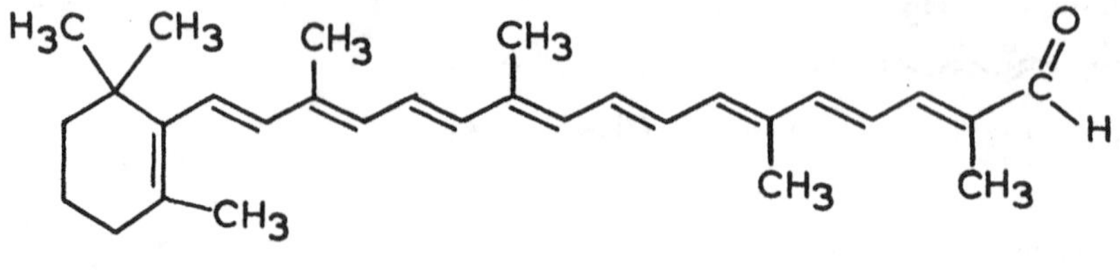

Fig. 24   β-Apo-8'-carotenal.

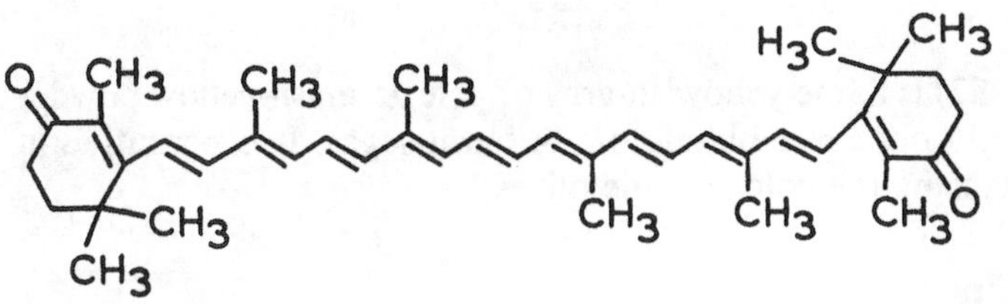

Fig. 25 Canthaxanthin.

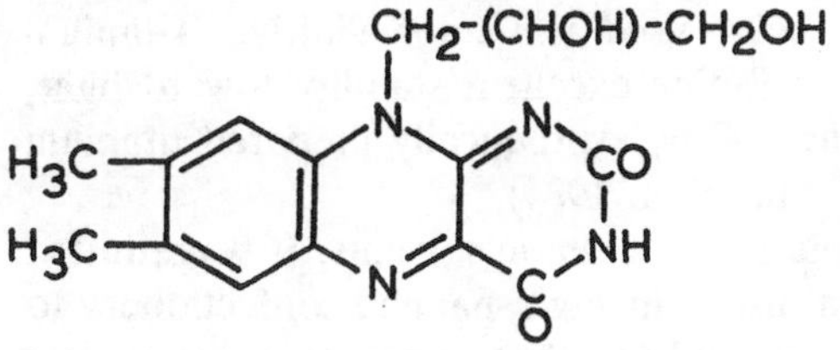

Fig. 26 Riboflavin.

light and oxygen and, hence, needs to be stored under nitrogen at low temperatures. Unlike β-carotene, canthaxanthin does not exhibit any provitamin A activity.

Compared with other carotenoid pigments, canthaxanthin is poorly soluble in oil and is insoluble in water. It is available commercially as a dry powder and as a water-dispersible, dry beadlet composed of 10% colorant, gelatin, vegetable oil, sugar, starch, antioxidant, and preservatives (Marmion, 1984).

Canthaxanthin is used at 5–60 ppm levels to impart red color to a wide range of foods, including tomato products such as soups, spaghetti sauce, and pizza sauce. Russian and French dressings, fruit drinks, sausage products, sugar confectionery, meat and fish products, ice cream, biscuits, and breadcrumbs. It also blends well with β-carotene to produce orange shades. Its use in the United States is restricted to a maximum of 30 mg per pound of solid or semisolid food or pint of liquid food.

Toxicological studies conducted with three dogs of each sex fed 100 and 400 mg/kg body weight canthaxanthin for one week have shown no adverse effects on body weight or the general health of the animals as compared to the control dogs (WHO, 1975). Similarly, when tested at 1000 ppm levels, canthaxanthin did not produce any adverse teratological effects in three generations of rats.

Riboflavin (Vitamin B$_2$)

Riboflavin is a yellow to orangish-yellow pigment (Fig. 26) naturally occurring in plant and animal cells such as milk and yeast. Most of the product commercially sold, however, is synthesized. Riboflavin is sparingly soluble in water and ethanol, yielding greenish-yellow fluorescent solutions. It is soluble in alkali, but decomposes rather rapidly.

Riboflavin is responsible for the natural yellow color of milk, butter, and cheese. Primarily used as a source of vitamin, riboflavin is sometimes used to color cereal products, sugar-coated confectionery, sherbets, ice creams, and tablets.

Ferrous Gluconate

Ferrous gluconate (Fig. 27) is a fine yellowish-gray or pale greenish-yellow powder or granules having a slight odor resembling that of burnt sugar. It is permitted in some countries for enhancing the color of ripe olives.

C. Inorganic Colorants

Titanium Dioxide (TiO_2)

Titanium dioxide (Color Index No. 77891) is obtained from the natural mineral ilmenite ($FeTiO_3$). It exists in nature in three crystalline forms—anatase, brookite, and rutile—with only the anatase form being used as a color additive. Titanium dioxide is an intensely white pigment exhibiting excellent stability toward light, oxidation, pH, and microbiological attack. Only synthetically prepared titanium dioxide can be used as a food colorant (Marmion, 1984).

Titanium dioxide is virtually insoluble in all common solvents. It is permitted in foods at levels up to 1%. Its principal use is in sugar-panned confectionery to give an opaque white finish or as a background to other colors. It is also widely used in tableted drug products and in numerous cosmetics in amounts consistent with good manufacturing practices.

Ultramarines (Ultramarine Blue)

Ultramarines are synthetic, inorganic pigments of somewhat indefinite composition. They are principally sodium aluminosulfosilicates and are intended to mimic the colors produced from the naturally occurring semiprecious gem lazurite. Their color is believed to be due to polysulfide linkages being in a highly resonant state.

Ultramarines are manufactured by heat treating and then very slow cooling of various combinations of kaolin (China clay), silica, sulfur, soda ash, and sodium sulfate with a carbonaceous reducing agent such as rosin or charcoal pitch (Marmion, 1984). The resulting color of the end product is determined by the formulation of ingredients, temperature, time, cooling rate, subsequent treatment, and other process variables.

Ultramarines are insoluble in water and organic solvents. They are used to impart a blue color to the product. They were once used to whiten sugar, although their use in foods is now severely restricted. They are, however, permitted for use in salt intended for animal feed at less than 0.5% color concentration. Ultramarines are widely used in cosmetics.

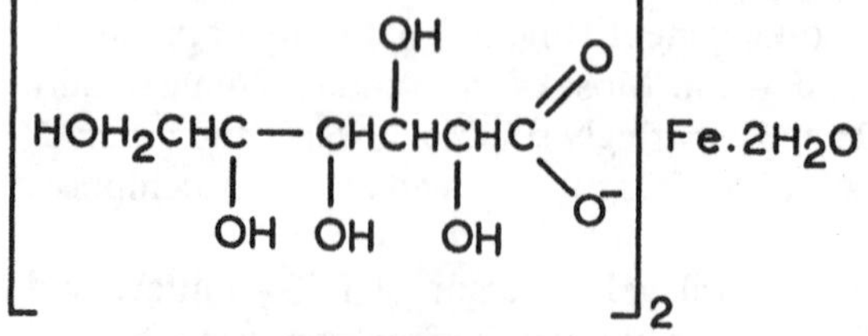

Fig. 27 Ferrous gluconate.

Iron Oxides and Hydroxides

Synthetic iron oxides and hydroxides provide a range of red, yellow, and black colors with excellent heat and light stability. Because of difficulties involved in their purification, the naturally occurring oxides are unacceptable as food colorants.

Iron oxides are insoluble in most solvents but are usually soluble in hydrochloric acid. They are primarily used at levels not exceeding 0.25% by weight in fish pastes and pet foods, where they withstand severe heat treatment during retorting and extruding.

Calcium Carbonate

Calcium carbonate occurs extensively in nature as chalk, limestone, marble, and feldspar. Only synthetically prepared calcium carbonate is allowed as a white colorant in certain foods to impart an opaque white appearance. Sometimes it is used in sugar confectionery instead of titanium dioxide.

Silver, Gold, and Aluminum

These are used as surface coloration in the form of finely divided powder or leaf (very thin sheets) for confectionery items and cake decorations in Middle and Far Eastern countries.

VI. PHYSICOCHEMICAL PROPERTIES

Because the potential areas and conditions of use for most food colors are so numerous, it is hard to define a perfect food colorant and even more difficult to produce it. Marmion (1984) suggested the following criteria for an ideal food colorant.

1. It must be safe at the levels used and under the conditions used.
2. It must not impart any offensive property to a product.
3. It must be stable to a wide variety of processing conditions.
4. It must be nonreactive with the products and containers in which it is used.
5. It must be easy to apply to products.
6. It should be inexpensive.
7. It should have a high tinctorial strength.

Data on several physicochemical properties of certified and exempt colorants are summarized in Tables 6 and 7. Solubility data for certified food colorants are presented in Table 8. Most colorants exempt from certification generally tend to be very poorly soluble in water, 25% ethanol, glycerin, propylene glycol, or vegetable oils. Detailed information on various physicochemical properties of different food colorants is available in several excellent reviews (Noonan, 1972; Noonan and Meggos, 1980; Sankaranarayanan, 1981; Santhanakrishnan, 1981; Marmion, 1984; Taylor, 1984; Newsome, 1990; Rayner, 1991).

VII. FOOD APPLICATIONS

The psychological basis for the importance of color in the perception of the quality, odor, flavor, and texture of food is well established. In a classic study showing how individuals react to sherbets of mismatched flavor and color, Hall (1985) observed

Table 6 Physicochemical Properties of Certified FD&C Food Colors

FD&C Name	Hue	Stability to			Compatability with other food components	Tinctorial strength	Overall rating
		Light	Oxidation	pH change			
Red No. 2	Bluish-pink	Fair	Fair	Poor	Poor	Very good	Poor-good
Red No. 40	Yellowish red	Very good	Fair	Good	Very good	Very good	Good
Citrus Red No. 2	Orangish red	—[a]	—	—	—	Good	—
Orange B	Orangish yellow	Moderate	Fair	—	—	Good	—
Yellow No. 6	Reddish	Moderate	Fair	Good	Moderate	Good	Moderate
Yellow No. 5	Lemon yellow	Good	Fair	Good	Moderate	Good	Good
Green No. 3	Bluish green	Fair	Poor	Good	Good	Excellent	Good
Blue No. 1	Greenish blue	Fair	Poor	Good[b]	Good	Excellent	Good
Blue No. 2	Deep blue	Very poor	Poor	Poor	Very poor	Poor	Very poor

[a]Data not available.
[b]Unstable in alkali.
Source: Marmion, 1984; Newsome, 1990; Rayner, 1991.

Physicochemical Properties of Colorants Exempt From Certification

FDA name	Hue range	Stability to				Compatibility with food components	Tinctorial strength[a]	Overall rating
		Light	Oxidation	pH change	Microbial attack			
Annatto extract	Yellow-peach	M	VG	VG	—	VG	G (0.5–10 ppm)	G
β-Apo-8'-carotenal[b]	Light to dark orange	F	P	G	P	G	G (1–20 ppm)	M
Dehydrated beets	Bluish red at pH <6, brown at pH >6	G	Ex	G	G	Ex	G (1000–5000 ppm)	G
Canthaxanthin[c]	Pink to red	M	F	G	—	G	G (5–60 ppm)	M
Caramel	Yellow tan to red brown	G	G	G	F	G	F (1000–5000 ppm)	G
β-Carotene	Yellow in oil, orange in water	F	P	G	P	G	G (2.5–50 ppm)	G
Cochineal extract	Orange to wine red in acid to base	G	G	P	P	G	M (25–1000 ppm)	G
Cottonseed flour[d]	Light to dark brown	G	G	G	G	—	P (1000–20,000 ppm)	—
Fruit and vegetable juices	Red to green to blue with increasing pH	P	P	VP to G	P	P to G	P (0.5–5%)	F
Grape skin extract[e]	Red to green to blue with increasing pH	P	P	P	M	G	P (0.5–5%)	—
Paprika extract and oleoresin	Orange to bright red	P	P	G	F	G	G (0.2–100 ppm)	F
Saffron	Yellow to orange with increasing pH	Ex	G	G	VG	VG	G (1.3–260 ppm)	G
Titanium dioxide[f]	White	Ex	Ex	Ex	Ex	Ex	Ex (50–5000 ppm)	G
Turmeric extract and oleoresin	Yellow	P	M	P	—	G	G (0.2–60 ppm extract, 2–640 ppm oleoresin)	F

VP = very poor; P = poor; F = fair; M = moderate; G = good; VG = very good; Ex = excellent.

[a] Effective concentration in food.
[b] Not to exceed 15 mg/lb or pint of food.
[c] Not to exceed 30 mg/lb or pint of food.
[d] Partially defatted, cooked, and toasted.
[e] Good dispersibility in water.
[f] Not to exceed 1% by weight of food.
Source: Marmion, 1984; Newsome, 1990; Rayner, 1991.

Table 8 Solubility (g/100 ml) Properties of Certified FD&C Colors

FD&C Name	Water	25% Ethanol	Glycerin	Propylene glycol	Vegetable oil
Red No. 3	9	8	20	20	Insoluble
Red No. 40	25	9.5	3	1.5	Insoluble
Citrus Red No. 2	Insoluble	Very slightly soluble	Very slightly soluble	Very slightly soluble	Insoluble
Yellow No. 6	19	10	20	2.2	Insoluble
Yellow No. 5	20	12	18	7	Insoluble
Green No. 3	20	20	20	20	Insoluble
Blue No. 1	20	20	20	20	Insoluble
Blue No. 2	1.6	0.5	1	0.1	Insoluble

Source: Marmion, 1984; Newsome, 1990; Rayner, 1991.

that white sherbets made with one of six test flavors (lemon, lime, orange, grape, pineapple, and almond) were confusing. The flavor was also difficult to identify. Similarly, most individuals failed to identify the right flavor when the sherbets were colored deceptively. Based on this and several other similar studies, the following two principles regarding the importance of colors in our foods are now firmly established.

1. Color far outweighs flavor in the impression it makes on the consumer, even when the flavors are pleasant and the food is a popular one.
2. Color powerfully influences not only one's ability to identify the flavor, but also the estimation of its strength and quality.

Synthetic colorants provide significant advantages in a variety of situations and varied food systems (NAS, 1971). They are especially advantageous in the following situations:

1. To help correct for natural variations and irregularities in color or changes during processing and storage, packaging and distribution, thereby assuring greater uniformity in appearance and, hence, acceptability.
2. To emphasize or identify flavors normally associated with various foods.
3. To help preserve the identity or character by which foods are recognized.

Each group of food products has its own technical requirements for certain colorants. These are based on the physicochemical properties of the food product as well as the colorants. Even within a given food category, several variables dictate the use of food colors. For example, colors that are light sensitive may be used in canned beverages, but not in glass-bottled beverages. Exposure to light in the latter case may result in fading if a light-sensitive colorant is used. The pH of the food product also affects the choice of colorants. Thus cola beverages require the use of colorants that are stable under acidic conditions. Similarly, heat-sensitive colors are better suited for use in frozen food products, whereas heat-insensitive colors find increasing applications in bakery products and hard-boiled sugar confections. Some of the common problems associated with the use of food colorants and their probable causes are listed in Table 9. Typical usages of certified and exempt colorants in various food systems are summarized in Tables 10 and 11. Data on the major categories of processed foods manufactured using certified colors and the levels of colorant used are presented in Table 12. These figures were obtained by the Certified Color Industry Committee from a survey of sales records of certified colorants used by the various segments of the color industries (CCIC, 1968).

Because of the public concern over the increasing use of food additives in processed foods, the National Academy of Sciences (NAS) and the National Research Council (NRC) conducted an extensive survey of more than 12,000 individuals and estimated their average daily intake of food additives, including certified and exempt food colorants (NAS/NRC, 1979). The results are summarized in Table 13. The average daily intake of the certified FD&C colorants by Americans over the age of 2 years ranged from 3.1 to 100 mg/kg/person, whereas that of colorants exempt from certification ranged from 0.43 to 250 mg/kg/person. Because the U.S. food supply is very complex and different food colorants can be used interchangeably in foods to achieve similar technical effects, the NAS estimated actual intakes to be approximately one fifth of the reported amount.

Table 9 Some Common Problems Associated With Food Colorants and Their Probable Causes

Problem	Probably cause
Precipitation from color solution or colored liquid food	Exceeded solubility limit
	Insufficient solvent
	Chemical reaction
Dulling effects instead of bright, pleasing shades	Low temperture, especially for concentrated colors
	Excessive color
	Exposure to high temperatures
Speckling and spotting during coloring of bakery and confectionery products	Color not completely dissolved while making a solution
	A liquid color containing sediment was used
	A dispersion in an aqueous color solution was attempted in products containing excessive fat
Fading due to light	Colored products not protected from sunlight
Fading due to metals	Colored solutions or colored products were in contact with certain metals (zinc, tin, aluminum, etc.) during dissolving, handling, or storage
Fading due to microorganisms	Color preparing facilities not thoroughly cleaned to avoid contaminating reducing organisms
Fading due to excessive heat	Processing temperatures were too high
Fading due to oxidizing and reducing agents	Contacted color with oxidizers such as ozone or hypochlorites or reducers such as sulfur dioxide and ascorbic acid
Fading due to retorting with protein material	Color is unstable under these conditions
Poor shelf life with colored canned carbonated beverages	Used an excessive amount of certified azo-type dyes

Source: Noonan, 1972.

Table 10 Food Applications of Synthetic Colors Regulated in the United Kingdom and the United States

Color	FD&C No.	Applications
Yellow/Orange Colors		
Tartrazine	Yellow No. 5	General purpose, powdered desserts, confectionery, ice cream, dairy products, soft drinks, pickles, sauces, fish, bakery products
Yellow 2G		General purpose
Quinoline yellow		General purpose, soft drinks, desserts, ice cream, dairy products, confectionery
Sunset Yellow FCF	Yellow No. 6	General purpose, soft drinks (not recommended if calcium ions are present), ice cream, canned foods, confectionery, baked goods, desserts
Orange RN		General purpose
Orange G		General purpose
Red Colors		
Carmoisine		Confectionery, soft drinks, ice cream, desserts, canned fruit
Ponceau 4R		Soft drinks, confectionery, jellies, canned goods, fish, lake to color cheese rind, and coated confections
Amaranth		Canned foods, soft drinks, jams, ice cream, powdered desserts
Red 2G		Meat products, sugar confectionery, jams
Erythrosine	Red No. 3	Only red color used with maraschino cherries and glacé, also used in meat products, confectionery, and canned foods
Allura Red	Red No. 40	General purpose
Citrus Red No. 2	Citrus Red No. 2	To color orange skins
Blue Colors		
Indigocarmine	Blue No. 2	Confectionery
Patent blue V		General purpose, confectionery, drinks, icings
Brilliant Blue FCF	Blue No. 1	General purpose, confectionery, drinks, icings
Green Colors		
Green S		General purpose, often blended with yellow to produce leafy green hues
Fast Green FCF	Green No. 3	General purpose, often blended to produce various shades
Brown Colors		
Brown FK		Coloring fish in brine without precipitation
Chocolate Brown FB		Baked cereal products, sugar confectionery, desserts
Chocolate Brown HT		General purpose, baked products, vinegar, confectionery
Black Colors		
Brilliant Black BN		General purpose color used in blends, also in fish roe products and confectionery
Black 7984		General purpose

Source: Marmion, 1984; Newsome, 1990; Rayner, 1991.

Table 11   Food Applications of Colorants Exempt From Certification[a]

Anthocyanins (blue-red shades)

Soft drinks, alcoholic drinks, sugar confectionery, preserves, fruit toppings and sauces, pickles, dry mixes, canned and frozen foods, dairy products

Annatto extracts (orange shades)

Oil-soluble bixin: dairy and fat-based products, processed cheeses, butter, margarine, creams, desserts, baked and snack foods

Water-soluble norbixin: sugar and flour confectionery, cheese, smoked fish, ice cream and dairy products, desserts, custard powders, cereal products, and bread crumbs

β-Carotene (yellow to orange)

Butter, margarine, fats, oils, processed cheeses, water-dispersible forms in soft drinks, fruit juices, sugar and flour confectionery, ice cream, yogurts, desserts, cheese, soups, and canned products

β-Apo-8'-carotenal (orange to orange-red)

Cheese, sauces, spreads, oils, fats, ice cream, cake mixes, cake toppings, snack foods, and soft drinks

Canthaxanthin (orange-red to red)

Sugar confectionery, sauces, soups, meat and fish dishes, ice cream, biscuits, bread crumbs, salad dressings

Paprika (orange to red)

Meat products, snack seasonings, soups, relishes, salad dressings, processed cheeses, sugar confectionery, fruit sauces and toppings

Saffron (yellow)

Baked goods, rice dishes, soups, meat dishes, sugar confectionery

Crocin (yellow)

Smoked white fish, dairy products, sugar and flour confectionery, jams and preserves, rice and pasta

Lutein (yellow)

Salad dressings, ice cream, dairy products, sugar and flour confectionery, soft drinks

Beet powder (bluish-red)

Frozen and short shelf-life foods, ice cream, flavored milks, yogurts, dry mix desserts, jelly crystals

Cochineal (orange)

Soft drinks and alcoholic drinks

Cochineal carmine (bluish-red)

Soft drinks, sugar and flour confectionery, flavored milks, desserts, sauces, canned and frozen products, pickles and relishes, preserves and soups

Sandalwood (orange to orange-red)

Fish processing, alcoholic drinks, seafood dressings, bread crumbs, snack seasonings, meat products

Table 11 (continued)

Alkannet (red)

Sugar confectionery, ice cream, alcoholic drinks

Chlorophyll (olive green)

Sugar confectionery, soups, sauces, fruit products, dairy products, pickles and relishes, jams and preserves, pet foods, drinks

Copper chlorophyll (green)

Flour and sugar confectionery, soups, sauces, pickles, relishes, fruit products, ice cream, yogurt, jelly, desserts, dry mix desserts, sauces and soups, soft drinks

Caramel (yellowish-tan to red-brown)

Alcoholic and soft drinks, sugar and flour confectionery, soups, sauces, desserts, dairy products, ice cream, dry mixes, pickles, and relishes

Malt extract (light brown)

Alcoholic and soft drinks, sugar and flour confectionery, soups, sauces, desserts, dairy products, ice cream, dry mixes, pickles, and relishes

Turmeric (bright yellow)

Ice cream, yogurt, frozen products, pickles and relishes, flour and some sugar confectionery, dry mixes, yellow fats

Riboflavin (yellow)

Cereal products, sugar-coated confectionery, sorbet, and ice cream

Vegetable carbon black (black)

Sugar confectionery, shading color

Orchil (red)

Soft drinks, alcoholic drinks, sugar confectionery

Safflower (yellow)

Soft drinks, alcoholic drinks

Titanium dioxide

Sugar-coated confectionery

Ferrous gluconate

Ripe olives

Iron oxides

Sugar-coated confectionery, pet foods, meat and fish pastes

Silver, gold, and aluminum

Surface coating of sugar confectionery, cake decorations

[a]Not all colors are permitted for food use in the United States.
Source: Marmion, 1984; Newsome, 1990; Rayner, 1991.

Table 12 Major Categories of Processed Foods Manufactured Using Certified Colors and Levels of Color Used

Category	Levels of color used (ppm)	
	Range	Average
Candy and confections	10–400	100
Beverages (liquid and powdered)	5–200	75
Dessert powders	5–600	140
Cereals	200–500	350
Maraschino cherries	100–400	200
Pet foods	100–400	200
Bakery goods	10–500	50
Ice cream and sherbets	10–200	30
Sausage (surface)	40–250	125
Snack foods	25–500	200
Miscellaneous[a]	5–400	—

[a]Includes nuts, salad dressings, gravy, spices, jams, jellies, food packaging, etc.
Source: CCIC, 1968.

Based on U.S. food-consumption patterns and the amount of FD&C colors certified by the FDA during the 1978–1981 period, Marmion (1984) estimated the consumption of certified color additives as 0.024 lb/day/person.

VIII. FOOD COLORANTS AND HYPERKINESIS

Food additive–induced hyperkinesis is characterized by several aberrant behaviors whereby the patients show one or more signs of the following: hyperactivity and fidgetiness, compulsive aggression, excitability, impulsiveness, impatience, short attention spans, poor sleep habits, and gross and fine muscle incoordination. Such behavior is generally accompanied by learning disabilities in the form of difficulty in reasoning, lack of auditory and visual memory, and difficulty in understanding ideas and concepts. Several clinical trials have confirmed that additive-free diets can indeed improve the behavior of hyperkinetic children (Brenner, 1977; Conners, 1980).

Such studies, however, should not be expected to provide definitive conclusions about the hyperkinetic effects of food additives, especially the synthetic food colors. Among other things, these studies are highly subject to the placebo effect (Spring and Sandoval, 1976; Harley and Matthews, 1977; Wender, 1977). Harley et al. (1978), while studying nine boys selected from a group of 46 hyperactive subjects, found only one subject responding with increased unfavorable behavior when challenged with cookies and candy bars containing 26 mg of a blend of eight approved food colors. In a similar study, Weiss et al. (1980) observed that, among 27 hyperactive children (22 males and 5 females aged 2.5–7 years) who previously responded favorably to additive-free diets, only two showed statistically significant, adverse responses when challenged daily with a mixture of about 35 mg of certified FD&C colors. One 3-year-old boy had a mild response based on several criteria. The food colors used in this study were FD&C Yellow No. 5, FD&C Yellow No.

Table 13 Consumption of Certified FD&C and Exempt Food Colorants

Category/Colorant	Average daily intake[a] (mg/kg/person)
Certified FD&C Colorants	
FD&C Red No. 3	24
FD&C Red No. 40	100
FD&C Blue No. 1	16
FD&C Blue No. 2	7.8
FD&C Yellow No. 5	43
FD&C Yellow No. 6	37
FD&C Green No. 3	4.3
Orange B	17.8
FD&C Red No. 3 Lake	15
FD&C Red No. 40 Lake	27
FD&C Blue No. 1 Lake	6.6
FD&C Blue No. 2 Lake	3.1
FD&C Yellow No. 5 Lake	22
FD&C Yellow No. 6 Lake	14
Colorants Exempt from Certification	
β-Apo-8′-carotenal	2.0
Annatto extract	3.2
Paprika	61
Paprika oleoresin	2.7
Turmeric	4.7
Turmeric oleoresin	0.44
Saffron	0.43
Cochineal extract (carmine)	7.1
Grape skin extract (enocianina)	46
Beet powder (dehydrated beets)	23
Carrot oil	250
Canthaxanthin	250

[a]Data represent the 99th percentile of persons over 2 years of age in the "eaters group" (those who consumed one or more foods containing the additive in question during the 14-day survey period). Ninety-nine percent of the population sampled was estimated to have intakes equal to or below the value shown. Total sample size was 12,000 persons.
Source: NAS/NRC, 1979.

6, FD&C Red No. 40, FD&C Red No. 3, FD&C Blue No. 1, FD&C Blue No. 2, and FD&C Green No. 3.

Yet another aspect of such double-blind studies was the fact that the food colors elicited hyperkinetic behavior rapidly and briefly. This is contrary to Feingold's (1975) initial claim that the effects persisted for several days. Thus if two different observers were to note behavioral changes several hours apart, they may report opposite effects. For example, Williams et al. (1978) have reported that the improvements or worsening of the hyperactive behavior of test children were noted only by the teachers who were in a better position to observe early behavioral changes than were their parents. Goytte et al. (1978) and Conners (1980) have observed the hyperkinetic effects within 3 hours after the food additive challenge. Levy et al., (1978) reported that significant effects in terms of deterioration in behavior could be detected only when measured within a few hours after a tartrazine challenge; the effect could not be observed after 24 hours.

The failure of some earlier studies (Harley et al., 1978; Levy et al., 1978; Swanson and Kinsbourne, 1979a,b) to detect effects of food-additive challenges may have been due to the low doses (1 to 26 mg of food colors) used in their experiments. Thus when much higher doses (up to 150 mg) of certified FD&C foods color blends were used, Swanson and Kinsbourne (1980) were able to document impaired behavior using a laboratory learning test based on the Conners scale in all 20 confirmed hyperactive children. Once again, the measurements were made within 3.5 hours after the challenge with a blend of nine dyes. The nonhyperactive children, in contrast, did not show any adverse effects. The amount of food color used in this study, according to an FDA estimate, was at the ninetieth percentile for the amount of artificial food colors consumed by 5- to 12-year-old children in the United States (Sobotka, 1976). Swanson and Kinsbourne (1980) have commented that the time course of the appearance of the effect, i.e., the initial appearance of 0.5 hour after administration, peaking at 1.5 hours and lasting up to at least 3.5 hours, suggested that the food additive effect was nonimmunological in nature.

This nonimmunological nature of the hyperkinetic effect of food colorants was also observed in animal studies. Mailman (1980) showed that the administration of 50–300 mg of FD&C Red No. 3 (erythrosine) per kg body weight to rats attenuates the suppressive effect of punishments monitored by the number of electric shocks received by the animals in an approach-and-avoidance test. This observed effect in rats is similar to that seen with barbiturate and benzodiazepin drugs, which also aggravate hyperkinesis in humans. In contrast, amphetamine reverses such effects (Cantwell, 1975). Levitan (1977) has reported membrane interactions with the FD&C Red No. 3 dye, whereas Logan and Swanson (1979) have observed that this dye also decreases the uptake of several neurotransmitters by homogenates prepared from rat brains. However, at least with dopamine, a major portion of the observed effects may have been an artifact resulting from its nonspecific interaction with brain membranes (Mailman, 1980). The dye also irreversibly increases acetylcholine release when applied to isolated neuromuscular synapses in the frog (Augustine and Levitan, 1980). The neurotransmitter release, which normally depends on the presence of calcium ions in the presynaptic terminals, was also independent of its concentration.

The studies cited above support essentially the basic premise of Feingold that food additives do induce certain behavioral changes in humans. However, at least with the artificial food colors, the hyperkinetic syndrome in humans may be induced or exacerbated in a subset of children. The evidence also shows that the basic mechanism may involve the central nervous system. Thus one important aspect of food toxicology, the behavioral toxicity of food components, is underscored by the experience encountered with artificial food colors. These studies perhaps will create a greater interest in this field and the unexplored aspects of behavioral food toxicology.

IX. FUTURE RESEARCH NEEDS

For centuries, colors have played a prominent role in three of the things most important to human beings: food, medicine, and physical appearance. With the exception of carotenoids and riboflavin, food colors do not contribute nutritionally, yet they are very important food ingredients.

No food colorant is completely suitable for use in all of the large variety of food applications and under the diverse processing conditions employed. Hence, research needs to be continued for the development of both synthetic and natural novel and better colorants. In this regard, nonabsorbable, nonmetabolizable polymeric colorants show considerable promise (Noonan and Meggos, 1980; Newsome, 1990). These colors can be produced by fixing a chromophore onto a polymer such that the molecular weight of the resulting colorant is high enough to prevent its migration across the gut mucosa from the gastrointestinal tract. The nonabsorbability, stability, blendability, tinctorial strength, and potential applications of such polymeric colorants have received considerable attention during the last decade (Santhanakrishnan, 1981; Newsome, 1990). Thus far, the long-term feeding studies for toxicological evaluation of these colors have also shown encouraging results.

The use of food colors is regulated by the Code of Federal Regulation (21 CFR Part 73) and is enforced by FDA. The document describes the color additives that are listed and defined and gives their uses, restrictions, and labeling requirements pertaining to the coloring of foods, drugs, and cosmetics. Today's food, pharmaceutical, and cosmetic manufacturers can draw from an array of dyes and pigments, either synthetic or naturally obtained, to color their products. Synthetic colors were favored until the hardline approach the FDA took towards them, a hostile antichemical press, increased consumer activism and hysteria, and the delisting of a number of important and widely used synthetic colors renewed the interest in natural food colors.

As the list of available synthetic colors shrank, it became obvious that manufacturers would turn to natural colors. The language of the CFR document also turns out to be useful in allowing new and much-needed natural colors to be accepted under the existing regulations.

Commercially available natural colors have been, and still are, viewed as mostly nonfunctional, expensive, and with low stability. Recent biotechnological developments in food colors that use plant tissue culture methods to overcome several of these drawbacks may further aid in the growing popularity and usage of this class of food colors. The production of colorants by plant tissue culture offers the advantages of a more reliable supply of color independent of weather and seasonal and plant variability, simplicity in chemical nature of the resultant color compounds, and elimination of strong, undesirable plant flavors from the end products (Ilker, 1987). In this context, anthocyanins and betalains are the most studied plant pigments; the feasibility of their commercial production by these methods, however, has not yet been determined.

Research on improving the stability of natural colorants should also be continued to make them more attractive to the end users. The stabilization of natural colors in foods is an extremely complex process. Each application must be considered individually and the optimum solution achieved largely by trial-and-error experiments. Stabilization by mimicking the local environment of colorants in vivo is appealing, but little is known about the subject (Taylor, 1984; Rayner, 1991). Further research on stabilization of natural colors will certainly help in increasing their applications in a wide variety of foods.

The users of food colors also need to be aware of the changes that are taking place in labeling requirements of food ingredients. The Nutrition Labeling and Education Act was passed by the U.S. Congress on October 24, 1990. This Act amends Section 403(1) of the Food, Drug and Cosmetic Act of 1938, with the aim of better informing consumers about the food they eat. The law will require FDA to implement the new changes. Certain sections with labeling in the new law appear to favor the users of natural colors. At present, it is interpreted to allow color additives that are "exempt from certification" to be declared in the ingredient statement generically as "color added" or "coloring." In contrast, the certified colors will need to be identified independently on the ingredient statement.

Research on the toxicological aspect of various colorants and their role in behavior modification will likely continue in the years ahead. Although absolute safety is unachievable, a high but realistic degree of relative safety, consistent with the benefits desired from every specific activity is still required. In the case of color additives, the degree of risk inherent in using any compound must be compared with the benefit it provides, whether cosmetic or psychological. The acceptable risk, however, will always remain minimal.

REFERENCES

Abrahamson, I. A., Sr., and Abrahamson, I. A., Jr. (1962). Hypercarotenemia. *Arch. Ophth. 68*:4–7.

Allamark, M. G., Grice, H. C., and Lu, F. C. (1955). Chronic toxicity studies on food colors. Part I. Observations on the toxicity of FD&C Yellow No. 3 (Oil Yellow AB) and FD&C Yellow No. 4 (Oil Yellow OB) in rats. *J. Pharm. Pharmacol. 7*:591–603.

Anderson, C. J., Keiding, N. R., and Brink Nielson, A. (1964). False elevation of serum protein-bound iodine caused by red colored drugs or foods. *Scand. J. Clin. Lab. Invest. 16*:249–259.

Andrianova, M. M. (1970). Carcinogenous properties of food pigments: amaranth, SX Purple and 4R Purple. *Vop. Pitan. 29*:61–65.

Augustine, G. J., and Levitan, H. (1980). Neurotransmitter release from a vertebrate neuromuscular synapse affected by a food dye. *Science 207*:1489–1490.

Augustine, G. J., and Levitan, H. (1983). Neurotransmitter release and nerve terminal morphology at the frog neuromuscular junction affected by the dye erythrosine. *Br. J. Physiol. 334*:47–63.

Bagdon, R. E., Impellizzeri, C., and Osadca, M. (1962). Studies on toxicity and metabolism of β-apo-8-carotenal in dog. *Toxicol. Appl. Pharm. 4*:444–456.

Bagdon, R. E., Zbinden, G., and Studer, A. (1960). Chronic toxicity of β-carotene. *Toxicol. Appl. Pharm. 2*:222–236.

Baigusheva, M. M. (1968). Carcinogenic properties of the amaranth paste. *Vop. Pitan. 27*:46–50.

Bora, S. S., Radichevich, I., and Werner, S. C. (1969). Artifactual elevation of PBI from and iodinated dyes used to stain medical capsules pink. *J. Clin. Endocrinol. Metab. 29*:1269–1271.

Borzelleca, J. F., Depukar, K., and Hallagan, J. B. (1990). Lifetime toxicity/carcinogenicity studies of FD&C Blue No. 1 (Brilliant Blue FCF) in rats and mice. *Food Chem. Toxicol. 28*:221–234.

Brenner, A. (1977). A study of the efficacy of the Feingold diet on hyperkinetic children. Some favorable personal observations. *Clin. Pediatr. 16*:652–656.

Brown, J. P., and Dietrich, P. S. (1983). Mutagenicity of selected sulfonated azo dyes in the salmonella microsome assay. Use of aerobic and anaerobic activation procedures. *Mutation Res. 116*:305–315.

Cantwell, D. P. (1975). *The Hyperactive Child*. Spectrum, New York.

CCIC. (1968). Guidelines for good manufacturing practices: use of certified FD&C colors in foods. Certified Color Industry Committee. *Food Technol. 22*:14.

Chacharonis, P. (1960). Unpublished report No. S.A. 54219 of Scientific Associates, Inc., submitted to WHO, 1975. *Toxicological Evaluation of Some Colors, Enzymes, Flavor Enhancers, Thickening Agents and Certain Other Food Additives*. Food Additives Series No. 6, World Health Organization, Geneva.

Chacharonis, P. (1963). Unpublished report No. S.A. 79105 of Scientific Associates, Inc., submitted to WHO, 1975. *Toxicological Evaluation of Some Colors, Enzymes, Flavor Enhancers, Thickening Agents and Certain Other Food Additives*. Food Additives Series No. 6, World Health Organization, Geneva.

Chafee, F. H., and Settipane, G. A. (1967). Asthma caused by FD&C approved dyes. *J. Allergy 40*:65–72.

Chafee, F. H., and Settipane, G. A. (1974). Aspirin intolerance. I. Frequency in an allergic population. *J. Allergy Clin. Immunol. 53*:193–199.

Clayson, D. B., and Gardner, R. K. (1976). Carcinogenic aromatic amine and related compounds. In *Chemical Carcinogens*, C. E. Searle (ed.). ACS Monograph 173, American Chemical Society, Washington, DC.

Clayson, D. B., Pringle, J. A. S., Bonser, G. M., and Wood, M. (1968). The technique of bladder implantation: further results and assessment. *Br. J. Cancer 22*:825–832.

Conners, C. K. (1980). *Food Additives and Hyperactive Children*. Plenum Press, New York.

Cook, H. W., Hewett, C. L., Kennaway, E. L., and Kennaway, N. M. (1940). Effects produced in the liver of mice by azo naphthalenes and related compounds. *Am. J. Cancer 40*:62–77.

Dacre, J. C. (1965). Chronic toxicity and carcinogenicity studies on Citrus Red No. 2. *Proc. Univ. Otago Med. Sch. 43*:31–33.

Davis, K. J. (1966). Chronic toxicity of Ponceau SX to rats, mice and dogs. *Toxicol. Appl. Pharmacol. 8*:306–317.

Durham, N. W., and Allard, R. K. (1960). A preliminary pharmacologic investigation of the *Bixa orellana. J. Am. Pharm. Assoc. 49*:218–228.

Feingold, B. F. (1975). Hyperkinesis and learning disabilities linked to artificial food flavors and colors. *Am. J. Nursing 75*:797–803.

Fitzhugh, O. G., Nelson, A. A., and Bourke, A. R. (1956). Chronic toxicities of two food colors, FD&C Red No. 32 and FD&C Orange No. 2. *Fed. Proc. 15*:422. (Abstract No. 1373).

Foote, W. L., Robinson, R. F., and Davidson, R. S. (1958). Unpublished reports of Battelle Memorial Institute, submitted to WHO, 1975. *Toxicological Evaluation of Some Colors, Enzymes, Flavor Enhancers, Thickening Agents and Certain Other Food Additives*. Food Additives Series No. 6, World Health Organization, Geneva.

Francis, F. J. (1985). Pigments and other contaminants. In *Food Chemistry*, O. R. Fennema (ed.). Marcel Dekker, New York.

Fraps, G. S., and Meinke, W. W. (1945). Digestibility by rats of α-, β- and neo-β-carotenes in vegetables. *Arch. Biochem. 6*:326–327.

Gerber, J. G., Payne, N. A., Olez, M. S., Nies, A. S., and Oates, J. A. (1979). Tartrazine and the prostaglandin system. *J. Allergy Clin. Immunol. 63*:289–294.

Goytte, C. H., Conners, C. K., Petti, T. A., and Curtis, L. E. (1978). Effects of artificial colors on hyperkinetic children. A double blind challenge study. *Psychopharmacol. Bull. 14*:39–40.

Grasso, P. (1970). Carcinogenicity testing and permitted lists. *Chem. Br. 6*:17–22.

Greenberg, R., Cornbleet, T., and Joffay, A. I. (1959). Accumulation and excretion of vitamin A-like fluorescent material by sebaceous glands after the oral feeding of various carotenoids *J. Invest. Dermatol.* 32:599–604.

Grice, H. C., Mannell, W. A., and Allmark, M. G. (1961). Liver tumors in rats fed Ponceau 3R. *Toxicol. Appl. Pharmacol.* 3:509–520.

Haldi, J., and Calandra, J. C. (1962). Unpublished reports of Emory University submitted to WHO, 1975. *Toxicological Evaluation of Some Colors, Enzymes, Flavor Enhancers, Thickening Agents and Certain Food Additives.* Food Additives Series No. 6, World Health Organization, 1975, Geneva.

Hall, R. L. (1958). Flavor study approach at McCormick & Co., Inc. In *Flavor Research and Food Acceptance.* Reinhold Publ. Corp., New York.

Hansen, W. H., Davis, K. J., Fitzhugh, O. G., and Nelson, A. A. (1963). Chronic oral toxicity of ponceau 3R. *Toxicol. Appl. Pharmacol.* 5:105–118.

Harley, J. P., and Matthews, G. C. (1977). *Hyperkinesis and Food Additives. A Challenge Experiment.* Presented at the Annual Meeting of the Nutrition Foundation, Food and Nutrition Liaison Committee, Palm Springs, CA.

Harley, J. P., Ray, R. S., Tomasi, L., and Eichman, P. L. (1978). Hyperkinesis and food additives. Testing the Feingold hypothesis. *Pediatrics 61*:818–828.

Harrow, L. S., and Jones, J. H. (1954). The decomposition of azo colors in acid solution. *J. Assoc. Off. Agric. Chem. 37*:1012–1020.

Haveland-smith, R. B., and Combes, R. D. (1980). Screening of food dyes for genotoxic activity. *Food Cosmet. Toxicol. 8*:215–221.

IFT. (1986). *Food Colors.* A scientific status summary by the Institute of Food Technologists Expert Panel on Food Safety and Nutrition. Institute of Food Technology, Chicago.

Ilker, A. (1987). In vitro pigment production: An alternative to color synthesis. *Food Technol. 41*(4):70–72.

IRDC. (1982). *Long-Term Dietary Toxicity/Carcinogenicity Study in Rats. Final Reports.* International Research and Development Corporation, Ottawa, Canada.

Kantor, M. A. Trout, J. R., and LaChance, P. A. (1984). Food dyes produce minimal effects on locomotor activity and vitamin B-6 levels in post-weanling rats. *J. Nutr. 114*:1402–1412.

Kevansky, H., and Kingsley, H. J. (1964). Fixed drug eruption caused by dyes. *S. Afr. Med. J. 88*:216.

Key, J. H., and Calandra, J. C. (1962). Unpublished reports of Industrial Bio-Test Laboratories Inc., submitted to WHO, 1975. *Toxicological Evaluation of Some Colors, Enzymes, Flavor Enhancers, Thickening Agents and Certain Other Food Additives.* Food Additives Series No. 6. World Health Organization, 1975, Geneva.

Levitan, H. (1977). Food, drug and cosmetic dyes: Biological effects related to lipid solubility. *Proc. Natl. Acad. Sci. USA 74*:2914–2918.

Levy, F., Dumbrell, S., Hobbes, G., Ryan, N., Wilton, N., and Woodhill, J. M. (1978). Hyperkinesis and Diet: A double-blind crossover trial with a tartrazine challenge. *Med. J. Aust. 1*:61–64.

Loblay, R. H., and Swain, A. R. (1985). Adverse reactions to tartrazine. *Food Technol. (Australia) 37*:508–510.

Lockey, S. D. (1972). Sensitizing properties of food additives and commercial products. *Ann. Allergy 30*:638–641.

Logan, W. J., and Swanson, J. M. (1979). Erythrosin B inhibition of neurotransmitter accumulation by rat brain homogenate. *Science 206*:363–364.

Luck, H., and Rickerl, E. (1960). Prüfung der in Westdeutschland zugelassenen und ursprunglich vor geschlagenen Lebensmittelfarbstoffe auf mutagene Wirkung an *Escherichia coli. Z. Lebensm.-Untersuch. 112*:157–174.

Magnusson, G., Bodin, N. D., and Hansson, E. (1971). Hepatic changes in dogs and rats induced by xylidine isomers. *Acta Pathol. Microbiol. Scand. 79A*:639–648.

Mailman, R. B. (1980). Erythrosine (Red No. 3) and its non-specific biochemical actions. What reactions to behavioral changes. *Science 207*:535–537.

Mannell, W. A. (1964). Further investigations on production of liver tumors in rats by Ponceau 3R. *Food Cosmet. Toxicol. 2*:169–174.

Mannell, W. A., Grice, H. C., Lu, F. C., and Allamark, M. G. (1958). Chronic toxicity studies on food colors. IV. Observations on the toxicity of tartrazine, amaranth, and sunset yellow in rats. *J. Pharmacol. 10*:625–634.

Marmion, D. M. (1984). *Handbook of U.S. Colorants for Foods, Drugs, Cosmetics*. John Wiley, New York.

Meggos, H. N. (1984). Colors: key food ingredients. *Food Technol. 38*(1):70.

Miller, K. (1982). Sensitivity to tartrazine. *Br. Med. J. 285*:1597–1598.

Mitchell, J. C. (1971). The skin and chemical additives in foods. *Arch. Dermatol. 104*:329–330.

Morales, M. C., Basomba, A., and Pelaez, A. (1985). Challenge tests with tartrazine in patients with asthma associated with intolerance to analgesics (ASA-Triad). *Clin. Allergy 15*:55–59.

NAS. (1971). *Food Colors*. National Academy of Sciences/National Research Council, Washington, DC.

NAS/NRC. (1979). *The 1977 Survey of Industry on the Use of Food Additives*. National Academy of Sciences/National Research Council, U.S. Dept. of Commerce, National Information Service, Washington, DC, Pub. No. 80-113418.

Newsome, R. L. (1990). Natural and synthetic coloring agents. In *Food Additives*, A. L. Branen, P. M. Davidson, and S. Salminen (eds.). Marcel Dekker, New York.

Nieman, C., Klein, S. P., and Obbink, H. J. (1954). The biochemistry and pathology of hypervitaminosis A. *Vit. Horm. 12*:69–99.

Noonan, J. (1972). Color additives in food. In *Handbook of Food Additives*, T. E. Furia (ed.). CRC Press, Boca Raton, FL.

Noonan, J. E., and Meggos, H. (1980). Synthetic food colors. In *Handbook of Food Additives*, Vol. 2, 2nd ed., T. E. Furia (ed.). CRC Press, Boca Raton, FL.

Prier, R. F. (1960). Unpublished reports No. 9070599 of Wisconsin Alumni Research Foundation, submitted to WHO, 1975. *Toxicological Evaluation of Some Colors, Enzymes, Flavor Enhancers, Thickening Agents and Certain Other Food Additives*. Food Additives Series No. 6. World Health Organization, 1975, Geneva.

Radomaski, J. L. (1961). The absorption fate and excretion of Citrus Red No. 2 (2,5-dimethoxyphenylazo-2-naphthol) and ext. D.C. Red No. 14 (1-xylylazo-2-naphthol). *J. Pharmacol. Exp. Ther. 134*:100–109.

Radomaski, J. L. (1962). 1-Amino-2-naphthylglucoronie, a metabolite of 2,5-dimethoxyphenylazo-2-naphthol and 1-xylylazo-2-naphthol. *J. Pharmacol. Exp. Ther. 136*:378–385.

Radomaski, J. L., and Harrow, L. S. (1966). The metabolism of 1-(o-talylazo)-2-naphthylamine (Yellow OB) in rats. *Ind. Med. Surg. 35*:882–888.

Rayner, P. (1991). Colors. In *Food Additive User's Handbook*, J. Smith (ed.). Blackie, London.

Sankaranarayanan, R. (1981). Food colors. *Ind. Food Packer 35*:25–28.

Santhanakrishnan, T. S. (1981). Food colors and their future. *Ind. Food Packer 35*:19–22.

Settipane, G. A., Chafee, F. H., and Klein, D. E. (1974). Aspirin intolerance. II. A prospective study in an atopic and normal population. *J. Allergy Clin. Immunol. 53*:200–204.

Sharratt, M. (1971). Unpublished reports. Submitted to WHO, 1975. *Toxicological Eval-*

uation of Some Colors, Enzymes, Flavor Enhancers, Thickening Agents and Certain Food Additives. Food Additive Series No. 6. World Health Organization, 1975, Geneva.

Sharratt, M., Frazer, A. C., and Paranjoti, I. S. (1966). Biological effects of Citrus Red No. 2 in the mouse. *Food Cosmet. Toxicol. 4*:493–502.

Silbergeld, E. K., Lafferman, J. A., and Finkel, T. (1983). *Neurochemical Approaches to Toxicity Testing: Artifical Food Dyes*. NATO Conf. Ser. 1, 5A.

Sobatka, T. J. (1976). *Estimates of Average, 90th Percentile and Maximum Daily Intake of FD&C Artifical Colors in One Day's Diets Among Two Age Groups of Children*. Memorandum of July 30, 1976. U.S. Dept. of Health, Education, and Welfare, Food and Drug Administration, Biochemical and Toxicology Branch, Washington, DC.

Spring, C., and Sandoval, J. (1976). Food additives and hyperkinesis. A critical evaluation of the evidence. *J. Learn. Disability 9*:28–37.

Swanson, J. M., and Kinsbourne, M. (1979a). *Artifical Food Colors Impair the Learning of Hyperactive Children*. Report to the Nutrition Foundation, New York.

Swanson, J. M., and Kinsbourne, M. (1979b). Artifical color and hyperactive behavior. In *Rehabilitation, Treatment and Management of Learning Disorder*, R. M. Knight and D. Bekker (eds.). University Park Press, Baltimore.

Swanson, J. M., and Kinsbourne, M. (1980). Food dyes impair performance of hyperactive children on a laboratory learning test. *Science 207*:1485–1487.

Swanson, J. M., and Logan, W. R. (1980). Effects of food dyes on neurotransmitter accumulation in rat brain homogenate and on the behavior of hyperactive children. *Methods Predict. Toxic. 182*:4.

Tannahill, R. (1973). *Food in History*. Stein and Day, New York.

Taylor, A. J. (1984). Natural colors in food. In *Developments in Food Color—2*, J. Walford (ed.). Elsevier, London.

U.S. FDA. (1974). Termination of provisional listing and certification of FD&C Red No. 2. *Fed. Reg. 41*(28):5823–5825.

U.S. FDA. (1980). FD&C Red No. 2. Denial of petition for permanent listing; final decision. *Fed. Reg.* (Jan. 25):6252.

U.S. FDA. (1982). Toxicological principles for the safety assessment of direct food additives and color additives in foods. In *Red Book*. Food and Drug Administration, Washington, DC.

U.S. FDA. (1983a). *Listing of Color Additives Subject to Certification*. Subpart A. Foods Section 74.302. Citrus Red No. 2. Title 21, Code of Federal Regulation Part 74. Office of the Federal Register, General Services Administration, Washington, DC.

U.S. FDA. (1983b). *Termination of Provisional Listing of FD&C Red No. 1*. Title 21, Code of Federal Regulation, Part 81, Sect. 81.10. Office of the Federal Register, General Services Administration, Washington, DC.

Vorhees, C. V., Butcher, R. E., Brunner, R. L., Wooten, V., and Sobotka, T. J. (1983). A developmental toxicity and psychotoxicity evaluation of FD&C Red dye No. 3 (erythrosine) in rats. *Arch. Toxicol. 53*:253–264.

Weber, R. W., Hoffman, M., Raine, D. A., and Nelson, H. S. (1979). Incidence of bronchoconstriction due to aspirin, azo dyes, nonazo dyes, and preservatives in a population of perennial asthamatics. *J. Allergy Clin. Immunol. 64*:32–37.

Weiss, B., Williams, J. A., Weiss, B., Hicks, W. J, Margen, S., Abrams, B., Caan, B., Citron, L. J., Cox, C., McKibben, J. Ogar, D., and Schultz, S. (1980). Behavioral responses to artifical food colors. *Science 207*:1487–1489.

Wender, E. H. (1977). Food additives and hyperkinesis. *Am. J. Dis. Child. 131*:1204–1208.

WHO. (1975). *Toxicological Evaluation of Some Colors, Enzymes, Flavor Enhancers, Thickening Agents and Certain Other Food Additives*. Food Additive Series No. 6. World Health Organization, Geneva.

WHO/FAO. (1969). *Toxicological Evlauation of Some Food Colors, Emulsifiers, Stabilizers, Anticaking Agents, and Certain Other Substances*. FAO Nutrition Meetings Reports Series No. 46A. WHO/FAO Add 70.36. World Health Organization, Geneva.

Willheim, R., and Ivy, A. C. (1953). A preliminary study concerning the possibility of dietary carcinogenesis. *Gastroenterology 23*:1–19.

Williams, J. I., Cram, D. M., Tausig, F. T., and Webster, E. (1978). Relative effects of drug and diet on hyperactive behaviors. An experimental study. *Pediatrics 61*:811–817.

Zlotlow, M. J., and Settipane, G. A. (1977). Allergic potential of food additives. A report of a case of tartrazine sensitivity without aspirin intolerance. *Am. J. Clin. Nutr. 30*:1023–1025.

5
Curing Agents

John N. Sofos and S. Raharjo*
Colorado State University
Fort Collins, Colorado

I. INTRODUCTION

Curing agents permitted for use in meat, poultry, and fish products include sodium nitrate, potassium nitrate, sodium nitrite, or potassium nitrite and their combinations. Ingredients such as ascorbic acid, isoascorbic or erythorbic acid, sodium ascorbate, sodium erythorbate, fumaric acid, glucono-delta-lactone, sodium acid pyrophosphate, citric acid, or sodium citrate may be used in combination with these curing agents to serve as curing accelerators. In the curing reaction, nitrate can be reduced to nitrite through the action of microorganisms, but microbial conversion is slow and difficult to control. Direct addition of a controlled amount of nitrite to either the pickle (curing solution) or directly to the meat itself facilitates the curing process and reduces the variability in color and flavor of cured meat products (Bard and Townsend, 1971; Binkerd and Kolari, 1975; Sofos et al., 1979e). In general, use of sodium nitrite in cured meat products fixes their color (Okayama et al., 1991), improves their flavor (Noel et al., 1990), inhibits *Clostridium botulinum* growth (Sofos et al., 1979a, b) and toxin formation (Sofos et al., 1979c, d, 1980), and stabilizes lipids against oxidation (Zubillaga et al., 1984). Ascorbate and its isomer, erythorbate, act as curing accelerators and color stabilizers, reduce lipid oxidation, and inhibit formation of carcinogenic *N*-nitroso compounds, which are the product of the nitrite reaction with meat components (Mirvish, 1975a). When nitrite is added to meat, it reacts with the muscle protein myoglobin and with blood hemoglobin (Hb) to form the cured meat color (Dryden and Birdsall, 1980). Initially, the meat pigment is oxidized from the purple-red color of myoglobin to the brown of metmyoglobin. Eventually the pigment is converted to the rather dark red of nitric oxide myoglobin, which, upon heating, is converted to the pink pigment of nitrosylhemochrome (Anonymous, 1987).

---

* *Current affiliation*: Gadjah Mada University, Yogya Karta, Indonesia

Use of curing agents in meat and other muscle foods is regulated at the national or local level of each country and depends on individual products (NAS, 1981; Hotchkiss, 1989a). In the United States, the use of nitrite and nitrate as meat and poultry curing agents is regulated by the U.S. Department of Agriculture (USDA), while in fish products it is regulated by the U.S. Food and Drug Administration (FDA). The regulations permit the use of sodium or potassium nitrite at 2 lb/100 gal of pickling solution at a 10% pump (weight gain after injection of a brine solution) level, 1 oz/100 lb of meat in dry curing, or 0.25 oz/100 lb of meat in chopped-meat products. Sodium or potassium nitrate were permitted at 7 lb/100 gal of pickle solution, 3.5 oz/100 lb of meat in dry curing, or 2.75 oz/100 lb of chopped meat. Levels permitted in fish products are 0.001–0.02%. The use of nitrite and nitrate in combination should not result in more than 0.02% of nitrite in a finished meat product.

Curing accelerators, such as ascorbate and erythorbate, must be used only in combination with curing agents. The regulations allow ascorbic acid or erythorbic acid to be used at 75 oz/100 gal of pickling solution at 10% pump level, 0.75 oz/100 lb of meat or meat byproduct, or 10% solution to surfaces of cured meat cuts prior to packaging. Other ingredients in meat curing may be used as follows: fumaric acid at 0.065% (or 1 oz/100 lb) of the weight of the meat or meat byproduct before processing; glucono-delta-lactone at 8 oz/100 lb of meat or meat byproduct; sodium acid pyrophosphate at a level not to exceed 8 oz/100 lb of meat or meat byproduct, alone or in combination with other curing accelerators or a maximum level of 0.5% in the finished product; sodium ascorbate or sodium erythorbate at 87.5 oz/100 gal of pickling solution at 10% pump level, 0.875 oz/100 lb meat or meat byproduct, or 10% solution to surfaces of cured meat cuts prior to packaging; citric acid or sodium citrate in cured products or in 10% solution used to spray surfaces of cured meat cuts prior to packaging to replace up to 50% of the ascorbic acid, erythorbic acid, sodium ascorbate, or sodium erythorbate that is used (Lewis, 1989).

In the United Kingdom, cured meats are divided into four categories with different levels of nitrite/nitrate permitted for each (Roberts and Dainty, 1991). The first category includes cured meat packed in a sterile pack, whether or not it has been removed from the pack. These products may contain a maximum of 150 mg/kg nitrate and nitrite, of which not more than 50 mg/kg should be nitrite, expressed in both cases as sodium nitrite. The second category includes acidified and/or fermented cured meat products not packed in a sterile pack. A maximum of 400 mg/kg nitrate and nitrite, of which not more than 50 mg/kg may be nitrite, expressed in both cases as sodium nitrite, is permitted in these products. The third category incudes uncooked bacon and ham and cooked bacon and ham that is not (and has not been) packed in any hermetically sealed container. The allowable levels in these products are a maximum of 500 mg/kg nitrate and nitrite, of which not more than 200 mg/kg may be nitrite, expressed in both cases as sodium nitrite. The fourth category includes any cured meat product not specified above. These products may contain a maximum of 250 mg/kg nitrate and nitrite, of which not more than 150 mg/kg may be nitrite, expressed in both cases as sodium nitrite (Roberts and Dainty, 1991).

Two major sources of nitrate in the human diet are water and vegetables. Nitrate may be converted to nitrite in the food or in the human body (Archer,

1982; Hotchkiss, 1989a, b). Naturally present nitrate is generally nontoxic. When reduced to nitrite, however, it can become toxic directly or especially as a precursor of N-nitroso compounds, which are carcinogens (Barnes and Magee, 1954; Archer, 1982). Reduction of nitrate to nitrite occurs in foods and in the saliva. The toxicity of nitrite can be explained by its high degree of reactivity, especially at low pH, where it forms its protonated form of nitrous acid, which acts both as an oxidizing and as a nitrosating agent. Examples of reactions of nitrous acid with organic compounds are: (1) with primary amines to form alcohols and unsaturated derivatives, (2) with secondary and tertiary amines to form nitrosamines, (3) with secondary amides, ureas, and carbamates to form the corresponding N-nitroso derivatives, (4) with compounds containing activated methylene groups to form oximes, (5) with phenols to form nitrosophenols, (6) with alcohols to form alkyl nitrites, (7) with thiols to form thionitrites, and (8) with reductones to form dehydroreductones (Archer, 1982). Major concerns for toxicity, however, involve reaction of nitrite in the body to cause direct toxicity and with secondary and tertiary amines to form N-nitrosamines. Human exposure to N-nitroso compounds in foods and beverages was investigated intensely during the 1970s and 1980s because of their possible association with various human cancers (Bartsch and Montesano, 1984; Preussmann and Eisenbrand, 1984; Anonymous, 1987; Hotchkiss, 1987; Magee, 1989; Tricker and Kubacki, 1992). The discovery of N-nitroso compounds in foods and their carcinogenicity have prompted regulatory agencies and food processors to revise regulations and to develop modified methods in food handling and processing. It is also now known that dietary amines may be nitrosated in vivo, which would provide a constant exposure of humans to carcinogens (Anonymous, 1987; Hotchkiss, 1987).

N-Nitroso compounds can be divided into N-nitrosamines and N-nitrosamides. N-Nitrosamines are either volatile or nonvolatile. Volatile nitrosamines are generally considered to be N-nitrosated derivatives of simple low molecular weight dialkylamines and cyclic compounds that can be isolated from food materials by aqueous distillation under atmospheric or vacuum conditions and subsequently analyzed by gas chromatography without derivatization. The most common volatile N-nitrosamines are N-nitrosodimethylamine, N-nitrosopiperidine, and N-nitrosopyrrolidine. The nonvolatile N-nitrosamines, which, as the name implies, are not isolated by distillation, include N-nitrosohydroxypyrrolodine, N-nitrosated derivatives of amino acids (i.e., hydroxyproline, proline, and sarcosine), amino acid derivatives, and condensation products of amino acids with aldehydes (Hotchkiss, 1987, 1989a, b; Tricker and Kubacki, 1992).

Nitrate, nitrite, and N-nitroso compounds have been implicated as causative agents of various adverse health effects in human and other animals (NAS, 1981). Although nitrate can be legally used as a curing agent for meat in some countries, only the toxicological aspects of nitrite are discussed in detail in this chapter for the following reasons: (1) nitrite is used as an ingredient in all cured meat products, while nitrate is only used in certain dry-cured or fermented meat products; (2) nitrite is a more effective curing agent, while nitrate is converted to nitrite before it can be an active curing agent; and (3) the carcinogenic N-nitroso compounds are produced by the reaction of nitrite with nitrogen compounds. The occurrence of N-nitroso compounds in foods and their toxic effects are also discussed and have been extensively reviewed by Spiegelhalder et al. (1980), Archer (1982), Hotchkiss (1987, 1989a, b), Preussmann (1984), Tricker and Preussmann (1991), Tricker and Kubacki (1992), and the National Academy of Sciences (1981, 1982).

II. TOXICOLOGY OF NITRITE

A. Reactivity and Safety

Nitrite is available as slightly yellowish or white crystals, sticks, or powder with a slightly salty taste (Lewis, 1989). It is soluble in water and very reactive, especially at low pH in its protonated form of nitrous acid (pK_a = 3.4). The safety profile of sodium nitrite was described by Lewis (1989) as human poison by ingestion; experimental poison by ingestion or administration by subcutaneous, intravenous, and intraperitoneal routes; experimental neoplastigen, tumorigen, and teratogen; human systemic effects caused by ingestion including motor activity changes, coma, decreased blood pressure with possible pulse rate increase without fall in blood pressure, arteriolar or venous dilation, nausea or vomiting, and blood methemoglobinemia—carboxyhemoglobinemia; experimental reproductive effects; mutagenic effects; eye irritant; increased cancer risk; and formation of carcinogenic nitrosamines. It should be stated, however, that most of these toxic effects can be induced only at concentrations exceeding those used in curing and often under less than physiological conditions (NAS, 1981, 1982).

Nitrous acid can react both as a nitrosating agent and as an oxidizing agent (Archer, 1982). However, the complete chemistry of interactions between nitrite and meat components including protein and fat has not been adequately explained due to the highly reactive nature of nitrite. When nitrite is used in meat as a curing agent, approximately 50% of the amount added is undetectable after processing, and the amount detected continues to decline during storage. Although the exact reactions of nitrite depletion have not been well defined, the highly reactive nature of nitrite would justify such reduction. It is known that nitrite is reduced to nitric oxide by ascorbate, which reacts further with meat components or escapes as gas (Frouin, 1977). Nitrite also forms nitrous acid, which forms dinitrogen dioxide, which reacts readily with proteins, thiols, cholesterol, hemoproteins, and lipids (Ito et al., 1983; Hotchkiss, 1987; Tricker and Kubacki, 1992). According to Cassens et al. (1977), 5–15% of the nitrite reacts with myoglobin, 1–10% is oxidized to nitrate, 5–10% remains as free nitrite, 1–5% becomes nitric oxide gas, 5–15% is bound to sulfhydryl groups, 1–5% is bound to lipids, and 20–30% is bound to proteins. Other reactions may involve nitrosation of amino compounds and formation of organic nitrites and nitrates (Mottram, 1984).

Formation of N-nitroso compounds in certain cured meat products, such as bacon, was detected in the 1970s and resulted in extensive research efforts to develop alternatives to nitrite in cured meat products (NAS, 1981, 1982; Sofos, 1989). In addition, new regulations were issued controlling use of nitrite in products such as bacon and presence of N-nitroso compounds (e.g., nitrosamines) in these products. No single alternative to nitrite tested was found adequate, however, to fulfill its color, flavor, antimicrobial, and preservative activities in meat products (NAS, 1982; Sofos, 1989; Sofos and Busta, 1980).

B. Acute Toxicity

Nitrate, which is generally unreactive, is not considered toxic, but it can become a hazard through its reduction to nitrite, which is reactive (NAS, 1981; Archer, 1982; Hill, 1991). Nitrite may be toxic either directly or through formation of N-nitroso compounds. The acute toxic effect of the nitrite molecule occurs through its ability to oxidize oxyhemoglobin (ferrous form) to methemoglobin (ferric form), which cannot bind and transfer oxygen in the body. Hemoglobin is an iron-containing complex protein found in erythrocytes, where it functions as a transporter of oxygen. When it combines with oxygen, hemoglobin forms red oxyhemoglobin, which dissociates readily to release oxygen to the tissues (Hill, 1991). Hemoglobin is converted to brown methemoglobin through oxidation by nitrite and becomes unable to bind oxygen. Any oxygen bound to methemoglobin is strongly bound and unavailable. Presence of a certain amount of methemoglobin in the blood also distorts the oxygen dissociation curve of residual hemoglobin so that it transports oxygen less effectively (Archer, 1982). Reducing systems in living cells maintain the level of methemoglobin at 1–2% of total hemoglobin. The most important mechanism that reduces methemoglobin to hemoglobin is through NADH-dependent methemoglobin reductase or diaphorase. Another reductive system that requires NADH as a cofactor is activated by electron carriers such as methylene blue (Archer, 1982). Levels of methemoglobin less than 10% of the total hemoglobin are usually asymptomatic, but above 10%, it causes cyanosis or blue skin (e.g., lips) and brown blood (Hill, 1991). When a high proportion of the hemoglobin is converted to methemoglobin, the affected person goes into anoxia, coma, and may die. Other clinical signs are tachycardia, dyspnea and restlessness, and death from suffocation. Treatment involves intravenous administration of methylene blue, which, as an electron carrier, activates the reductive system of the erythrocytes that requires NADPH as a cofactor. The activated enzyme reduces the dye to its leucoform, which then reduces methemoglobin (Archer, 1982). The generally accepted lethal level of methemoglobin is 60% of total blood hemoglobin (Hill, 1991).

Methemoglobinemia is a more serious problem in infants and young children than in adults and has been examined extensively by Hill (1991). Methemoglobinemia in infants usually occurs as a result of drinking water with high levels of nitrate, an accidental overdose, or consumption of foods with high levels of nitrite. In contrast, vegetables with high levels of nitrate do not appear to be involved in infantile methemoglobinemia, possibly because of their ascorbic acid content and presence of other reducing agents (Archer, 1982). Infant methemoglobinemia is known as "blue-baby syndrome" and is caused not only by nitrite, but also by other compounds, such as sulfonamides, aniline, nitrophenol, acetanilide, phenactin, and potassium chlorate (Bodansky, 1951; Hill, 1991). As indicated above, the cause of the illness is oxygen starvation in the tissues, which is detected as cyanosis and results in cardiovascular/respiratory problems and death.

Conversion of oxyhemoglobin to methemoglobin by nitrite follows the equation described by Kosaka et al. (1979):

$$4HbO_2 + 4NO_2^- + 4H^+ \rightarrow 4Hb^+ + 4NO_3^- + O_2 + 2H_2O$$

This equation is applicable in systems having a large excess (i.e., at least eightfold) of nitrite over hemoglobin, and it is very complex (Doyle et al., 1985; Kosaka and Uozumi, 1986; Hill, 1991).

The lethal dose of nitrite has been estimated to be 2–9 g, with an average of 4 g as sodium nitrite (WHO, 1985). Onset of symptoms after oral nitrite poisoning develop within 15–45 minutes (Aquanno et al., 1981). A study by Kiese and Weger (1969) indicated that humans given 4 mg of sodium nitrite per kg body weight intravenously formed 7% methemoglobin, while at the dose of 12 mg/kg, the methemoglobin level was 25%. Assuming that the dose-response relationship is linear and that lethality occurs at 60% methemoglobin, then the intravenous lethal dose for a 60- to 70-kg human would be 1.5–2.5 g of sodium nitrite (Hill, 1991).

Nichols and Weber (1989) used a nonvascularized fish heart model to assess the oxidation of cardiac myoglobin in vivo by sodium nitrite and other compounds known to cause methemoglobinemia. Buffalo sculpins (*Enophrys bison*) were cannulated from the afferent bronchial artery to permit repeated blood sampling and injected intraperitoneally with sodium nitrite, hydroxylamine, or aniline. Sublethal levels of sodium nitrite (0.1 g/kg) resulted in formation of methemoglobin. Hydroxylamine produced the same effect in less than one hour, but with nitrite the onset was less rapid and the effect was more prolonged. Aniline had no effect on hemoglobin while cardiac myoglobin was also oxidized by nitrite and hydroxylamine, even more than hemoglobin. The implication of the study is that cardiac myoglobin may be oxidized through occupational or other types of exposure to sodium nitrite, hydroxylamine, or similar compounds (Nichols and Weber, 1989).

A single dose of sodium nitrite (0.055 g/kg) via subcutaneous injection on adult male rats resulted in a short-term suppression of locomotor, exploratory, and grooming activities, but the animals successfully recovered their normal activities within 24 hours. Doubling the amount of sodium nitrite administered in adult rats resulted in marked decrease in locomotor and exploratory activities as well as in investigatory time combined with an increase of time spent in relaxation patterns. These results suggested that the delayed behavioral deficits could be due to the secondary structural changes developing in the central nervous system over several days after the exposure to sodium nitrite (Hlinak et al., 1990).

Grudzinski and Szymanski (1991a) studied the effect of acute poisoning with sodium nitrite on the processes of intestinal absorption of D-xylose in rats. Orally administered sodium nitrite at a dose of 80 mg/kg body weight increased the permeability of the gastric mucosa for D-xylose and raised the uptake of oxygen by the mucosa of the small intestine. No changes were observed in the activity of Na^+/K^+ ATPase and alkaline phosphatase. A dose of 10 mg sodium nitrite/kg body weight, however, was not followed by increased absorption of D-xylose. Intakes of nitrate and nitrite have also been associated with spina bifida, vitamin A metabolism, spontaneous abortion, reduced milk production, and thyroid function (Archer, 1982).

C. Long-Term Toxicity

Nitrite may also cause sublethally toxic effects, which sometimes may be associated with nonlethal methemoglobinemia (Cazottes et al., 1981). Extended poisoning of rats with nitrite could produce irreversible changes in the electroencephalographic pattern of brain activity due to damage to certain structures (Shuval and Gruener, 1977). Nitrite has also induced disturbances of thyroid function, which are caused by its effect on iodine metabolism (Bloomfield et al., 1962). Prolonged exposure of rats to sodium nitrite intensified toxic effects by carbaryl and phenitrothion (Podolak-Majczak and Tyburczyk, 1986; Tyburczyk et al., 1989). Simultaneous administration of nitrite and aminopyrine in rats reduced DNA and RNA levels in the liver and increased mortality, potentially due to endogenous formation of N-nitrosodimethylamine (Urbanek-Karlowska and Fonberg-Broczek, 1986).

Grudzinski and Szymanski (1991b) indicated that sodium nitrite had a significant effect on the processes of intestinal absorption of D-xylose and on selected biochemical parameters of the mucosa in the small intestine of rats. It is also worth indicating that reduced activity of Na^+/K^+-ATPase and alkaline phosphatase was observed after 21 days of subchronic poisoning of rats with sodium nitrite (10 mg $NaNO_2$/kg body weight). The intensity of nitrite effects in subchronic poisoning may have been due to possible secretion of nitrite from the blood into the intestinal lumen and greater penetration of sodium nitrite across the changed gastric mucosa. The destabilizing effect of nitrite on the plasma membrane of the erythrocytes provides a potential possibility of reduction of their stability and subsequent changes in the transport function of the membrane (Nalecz and Wojtczak, 1982). Nitrite interaction with proteins and lipids in the membrane is possible and suggests a possible influence of the nitrite on Na^+/K^+-ATPase in the membrane (Kubberod et al., 1974; Mallett et al., 1984; Mellet et al., 1986). However, a direct effect of nitrite on the ATPase complex cannot be ruled out. The potential for reaction of nitrite with sorbic acid and other fatty acids to form mutagens (Sofos, 1981, 1989) is discussed in Chapter 11.

Sodium nitrite administered through the drinking water of rats during pregnancy and lactation severely affected erythropoietic development, growth, and mortality in their offspring (Roth et al., 1987). In this experiment, pregnant rats were provided with 0.5, 1, 2, or 3 g sodium nitrite/L of drinking water throughout their gestation period. There were no significant differences between treated and control litters at birth, but pups of dams treated with 2 and 3 g of nitrite/L gained less weight, progressively became severely anemic, and began to die by the third week postpartum. By the second week postpartum, hemoglobin levels, red blood cell counts, and mean corpuscular volumes of these pups were all drastically reduced compared to controls. Administration of 1 g nitrite/L of drinking water resulted in hematological effects but did not affect growth or mortality, while the level of 0.5 g nitrite/L had no significant effect compared to the control. The treatment also resulted in lactational induction of severe iron deficiency in the neonate (Roth et al., 1987).

Results of epidemiological and animal studies on the correlation of nitrite consumption and cancer development have been contradictory (Grant and Butler, 1989). Thus, the issue of nitrite acting as a direct carcinogen has been controversial. A controversial study indicated that high levels (250–2000 ppm) of nitrite in the drinking water promoted lymphoma incidence in rats, but the lymphoma incidence was also high in the control rats (Newberne, 1979; NAS, 1981, 1982). Other studies, however, found that nitrite was not carcinogenic in laboratory animals (Archer, 1982).

Grant and Butler (1989) carried out a long-term rat feeding study with sodium nitrite, administered as part of a reduced protein diet to groups of 50 male F344 rats (6 weeks old) at dose levels of 0.2 or 0.5% (w/w) for up to 115 weeks, while a control group of 20 male rats received the reduced protein diet alone. Animals on the diet with sodium nitrite exhibited a dose-related decrease in the rates of body weight gain and a corresponding decrease in total body weights throughout the study. Hematological parameters reduced in the first week of the study included red blood cell count, hematocrit, and hemoglobin concentration. The red blood cell count continued to fall for 8 weeks, but it slowly returned to normal by 52 weeks. A dose-related reduction was noted in both the incidence and time of onset of lymphomas, leukemias, and testicular interstitial cell tumors. These results suggested that sodium nitrite was found not to be carcinogenic when fed in the diet to rats for up to 115 weeks, but rather that the incidence of tumors was reduced in a dose-related manner (Grant and Butler, 1989).

The possibility that thiocyanate could catalyze the in vivo formation of carcinogenic nitrosamines from nitrite and amines in foods was tested by feeding a group of 20 male and 20 female rats with a dose of thiocyanate (0.32% w/w) together with sodium nitrite (0.2% w/w) in their drinking water (Lijinsky and Kovatch, 1989). Other groups of rats were given thiocyanate or sodium nitrite alone in their drinking water or were untreated. All treatments lasted most of the lifetime of the rats, at least 2 years. There was no difference in survival between treatments of rats or in the incidence of any tumor that could be related to the treatment. The results indicated that sodium thiocyanate had no carcinogenic effects in rats either alone or when combined with sodium nitrite (Lijinsky and Kovatch, 1989).

When gestating rats were exposed to drinking water containing 2 g sodium nitrite/L throughout the second half of pregnancy, they had inferior auditory and visual discrimination learning paradigm compared to controls. They had also impaired long-term retention of a passive avoidance response, but the acquisition of simple learning tasks was not significantly disturbed. Simultaneous prenatal daily treatment with the calcium antagonist nimodipine at 10 mg/kg body weight interfered with the nitrite neurotoxicity and prevented the development of adult behavioral problems (Nyakas et al., 1990). It is unlikely that such direct toxic effects from nitrite can happen in humans because of the high amounts of nitrite needed for their development.

D. Mutagenicity

According to a National Academy of Sciences committee (NAS, 1981), nitrite, as nitrous acid, may lead to mutations by three mechanisms: (1) deamination of DNA bases by nitrous acid in viruses containing single-stranded DNA, (2) mutagenesis of organisms with double-stranded DNA by creation of intra- or interstrand crosslinks between purine residues leading to helix distortion, and (3) reaction of nitrite with nitrosatable compounds to form N-nitroso compounds, as well as C-nitroso, S-nitroso, and aryl-nitroso carcinogens. It should be noted that deamination can also be spontaneous and that DNA repair systems exist in bacteria and in healthy mammalian cells.

Incubation of human and animal feces in saline with sodium nitrite resulted in formation of mutagens. The detected mutagenicity was reduced by sodium ascorbate and α-tocopherol, and it was probably caused by formation of *N*-nitroso compounds (Rao et al., 1981). Luca et al. (1985) tested the in vivo mutagenic activity of sodium nitrate and found that it induced cytogenic damage in micronuclei of bone marrow cells in mice and chromosomal aberration in rats. Luca et al. (1987) also investigated the mutagenicity of sodium nitrite using in vivo and in vitro experiments. The in vivo experiments were carried out in male rats and mice intragastrically treated twice (at 24-hour intervals) with nitrite at doses of 1.72, 5.18, 15.55, and 46.66 mg/kg body weight and in male rabbits treated with the same doses of nitrite administered daily in their drinking water for 3 months. The authors indicated that nitrite induced increases in aberrant metaphases in all three species of animals. Likewise, in mice it induced increases in the number of micronucleated polychromatic erythrocytes and a light bone marrow depression. The in vitro experiments were carried out on BSC-1 and HeLa cells grown in cultures with nitrite in doses of 0.265 and 0.530 mg/mL for 24 hours. Both doses produced significant increases of the percentage of chromosomal aberrations but without demonstration of positive dose-effect relationships.

When treated with 0.2% (w/w) nitrite, soybean sauce was found to contain mutagenic substances as demonstrated by the Ames test (Lin et al., 1979). However, the mutagenicity test of soy sauce in *Salmonella typhimurium* TA98, TA100 and *Escherichia coli* WP2uvrA was purported to be false-positive due to the presence of L-histidine and L-tryptophan in the condiments. Furthermore, soy sauce with added nitrite was not mutagenic, and its mutagen precursors did become mutagens under physiological conditions (Nagahara et al., 1986). In addition, Ishidate et al. (1984) reported positive results for soy sauce without nitrite treatment using the in vitro chromosomal aberration test with a Chinese hamster fibroblast cell line. In order to reexamine the mutagenicity of soy sauce with or without nitrite treatment, Nagahara et al. (1991) carried out in vitro chromosomal aberration and in vivo micronucleus tests. Soy sauce pretreated with 0.23% (w/w) nitrite caused no more aberrations than the untreated soy sauce in the chromosomal aberration test using a Chinese hamster fibroblast cell line. Soy sauce with or without 2300 ppm nitrite was orally given to male mice at a dose of 14 mL/kg body weight once or 6 mL/kg body weight/d for 5 consecutive days. This oral administration did not induce any significant increase in micronuclei in the in vivo micronucleus test.

II. TOXICOLOGY OF *N*-NITROSO COMPOUNDS

A. Formation

N-Nitroso compounds are formed by nitrosation, which involves replacement of a hydrogen, attached to a nitrogen, by a nitroso group, and are usually divided into *N*-nitrosamines and *N*-nitrosanides (Archer, 1982; Shuker, 1988; Hotchkiss, 1989a; Hill, 1991; Tricker and Kubacki, 1992). Nitrosamines are derived from secondary amines containing dialkyl, alkylaryl, and diaryl substituents. Nitrosamides are formed from nitrosation of *N*-alkylureas, *N*-alkylcarbamates, simple *N*-alkylamides, cyanamides, guanidines, amidines, hydroxylamines, hydrazones, and hydrazines.

N-Nitrosamines are generally stable compounds, while *N*-nitrosamides become unstable as the pH increases above 2, and they decompose rapidly at pH values above 7 and can be destroyed by cooking (Fan and Tannenbaum, 1972; Kakuda and Gray, 1980a, b). Due to limitations in methodology, N-nitrosamides and non-volatile N-nitrosamines have not been extensively studied, especially in foods (Hotchkiss, 1987, 1989a; Sen and Kubacki, 1987). In contrast, volatile nitrosamines have been studied extensively.

Weak, basic secondary amines, such as morpholine, piperazine, and N-meth-ylamine, are the most readily nitrosated compounds, as well as tertiary enamines (i.e., aminopyrine), N-alkylureas, and N-alkylcarbamates. Amines, ureas, and carbamates occur widely as constituents or additives in foods (Mirvish, 1975a, b). The common nitrosating agents of dinitrogen trioxide (N_2O_3), dinitrogen tetraoxide (N_2O_4), and the nitrous acidium ion (H_2O^+NO) are formed from nitrite and nitrous acid (HONO), which is derived from the reaction between nitrite ions (NO_2^-) and protons (H^+ or H_2O^+) (Tricker and Kubacki, 1992). In general, the nitrosating agent (X—N=O) is generated first from HONO and a catalytic nucleophile where X is NO_2, H_2O^+, SCN^-, or Cl^- (Hotchkiss, 1987). Then the nitrosating agent reacts with unprotonated amines or amides to form the N-nitroso compound.

The main nitrosating specie of amides and carbamates is the nitrous acidium ion (Mirvish, 1971; Kubacki and Kupryszewski, 1981; Tricker and Kubacki, 1992). Nitrosation involves an electrostatic interaction between the positively charged nitrosating species (e.g., H_2O^+NO and NO^+) and the carbonyl oxygen, followed by rearrangement of the nitroso group onto nitrogen. O-Nitrosation, which is the first step, is readily reversible, and relatively strong acidic conditions are required for rearrangement to the N-nitroso compound. During nitrosation, proteins, peptides and amino acids form C-, S- and N-nitroso derivatives, and even minor constituents in foods, such as amides or similar compounds (e.g., ureas, guamadines), can serve as precursors of N-nitroso compounds (Mirvish, 1975b; Gray and Dugan, 1975; Bonnett et al., 1975; Berry and Challis, 1984; Yamamoto et al., 1987; Tricker and Kubacki, 1992).

Primary amines are not common precursors of N-nitrosamines because their nitrosation reactions involve diazotization and nucleophilic replacement of the amino group (Shuker, 1988). Nitrosation of methylamine (CH_3NH_2), the simplest aliphatic amine, however, produces a complex mixture of products, including N-nitrosodimethylamine. More complex primary aliphatic amines form elimination, substitution, and rearrangement products (Mende et al., 1989; Tricker and Kubacki, 1992). Nitrosation of weakly basic amines, such as N-alkylaromatic amines, depends on the nitrosating agent. It is slow with N_2O_2 and more rapid with the more reactive H_2O^+NO and NO^+ at low pH (Challis and Challis, 1982). The reactivity of tertiary amines is more complex and difficult to predict. They can form N-nitrosamines after formation of secondary amines by dialkylation. Simple tri-alkylamines react slowly with nitrous acid, while more complex tertiary amines with substitutents other than simple alkyl groups, such as gramine and hordenine in barley malt, are readily nitrosated (Tricker and Kubacki, 1992).

Nitrosation can be catalyzed by anions such as I^-, Br^-, Cl^-, CNS^-, acetate, phthalate, sulfur compounds, and weak acids (Shuker, 1988; Tricker and Kubacki, 1992). The catalytic effect of these ions is related to their relative nucleophilic strengths (Archer, 1982). Nucleophilic anions may also cause a downward shift in the optimum pH for nitrosation. The reason that nitrosation is pH dependent is because only unprotonated amines are reactive (Hotchkiss, 1987, 1989a, b). Although it occurs under mildly acidic conditions, it can also take place under basic conditions in the presence of carboxyl compounds, such as formaldehyde, and because oxides of nitrogen can act as direct nitrosating agents. Formation of nitrous acid is increased at lower pH, but as the pH decreases, amines become protonated and unreactive. The pH for maximum nitrosation depends on the basicity of the amine. Nitrosation of strongly basic amines, such as morpholine, reaches a maximum at pH 3.4, where interaction of unprotonated amines and the nitrosating specie occurs. In contrast, amides and related compounds do not have a maximum pH for nitrosation, and their reaction rate is first order in both amide and nitrous acid but third order overall because of the need for H^+ (Hotchkiss, 1987, 1989a, b).

Formation of nitrosamines is more rapid at high temperatures (e.g., 1980°C) even under conditions of low moisture. Nitrosation of morpholine, however, took place even in frozen conditions and at a rate higher than expected. At temperatures above 0°C, its nitrosation followed the Arrhenius law (Fan and Tannenbaum, 1973). The maximum rate of nitrosation in a model system of freeze-dried carboxyle-methyl-cellulose, however, was at 100–125°C (Ender and Ceh, 1971). In meat products, presence of nitrosamines has been more of a problem in fried bacon because of its fat content and the high temperatures of frying. Nitrosation rates are also accelerated in the presence of surfactants forming micellar aggregates and by nitrosphenols, which are present in smoked products and by polyphenols (Archer, 1982).

Nitrosamine formation may be influenced by microorganisms that (1) reduce nitrate to nitrite, (2) oxidize ammonia to nitrite, (3) convert nitrate to amino acids or ammonia, (4) oxidize nitrite to nitrate, (5) lower the pH, and (6) produce substances that directly catalyze nitrosation (Scanlan, 1975; Archer, 1982; Hotchkiss, 1987). Direct catalysis of nitrosation by microorganisms can be enzymatic or nonenzymatic (Collins-Thompson et al., 1972; Archer, 1982). There are indications that catalysis of nitrosamine formation by bacteria can be a factor in the indirect exposure of humans to N-nitroso compound carcinogens (Hotchkiss, 1987).

The mechanism by which bacteria catalyze nitrosation has not been clearly defined (Fine and Rounbehler, 1975; Mills and Alexander, 1976; Calmels et al., 1985; Leach et al., 1987). Treatments such as freeze-thawing, high temperature, sonication, or treatment with strong acids and strong bases, which disrupt cell integrity, eliminate the ability of the cells to catalyze the nitrosation reaction (Leach, 1988). Although the nitrosating activity of $E.$ $coli$ has been attributed to the enzyme nitrate reductase, $Neisseria$ spp., which lack nitrate reductase activity, can also catalyze nitrosation (Calmels et al., 1985). In addition to nitrate reductase, it appears that there is an association between bacterial nitrosation and denitrification (Garber and Hollocher, 1982). Denitrifying bacteria (e.g., $Pseudomonas$ $aeruginosa$, $Neisseria$, spp., $Alcaligenes$ $faecalis$, $Bacillus$ $licheniformis$) catalyze nitrosation more rapidly than nondenitrifying bacteria (Archer, 1982; Bleakley and Tiedje, 1982; Leach et al., 1987; Hotchkiss, 1987).

In general, endogenous formation of N-nitroso compounds can be catalyzed by acid or by bacteria (Hill, 1988). Acid-catalyzed endogenous nitrosation has an optimum pH of 2–3, which is present in the stomach, and it requires the presence of nitrite. Nitrosatable amines are provided with the diet or are formed endogenously in the colon and in the liver. Nitrite may be introduced with water or food, where it is a natural constituent or added as a preservative, or it can be formed through bacterial reduction of salivary or dietary nitrate. Bacteria that can nitrosate amines are found in the saliva, stomach, infected urinary bladder, infected vagina, and intestines. Simultaneous presence of nitrite, nitrosatable amines, and bacteria should result in nitrosation if the inhibitory effect of other factors can be overcome (Hill, 1988; Leach, 1988; Shuker, 1988).

B. Inhibition of Nitrosation

Formation of N-nitroso compounds in foods and in vivo is difficult to predict because, in addition to factors that catalyze nitrosation, several compounds inhibit the reaction (Shuker, 1988). Phenolic compounds in foods may interact with nitrite under acidic (pH 3) conditions, such as in the stomach, to produce p-nitrosophenol and p- and o-diazoquinones, which may reduce nitrosamine formation (Challis, 1973; Kikugawa and Kato, 1988). Nitrosophenols, however, can also catalyze nitrosamine formation. The catalytic or inhibitory effect of phenols on nitrosation depends on the concentration of nitrosophenol. A large amount of nitrosophenol can overcome the inhibitory effect of phenols and increase nitrosation (Davis and McWeeny, 1977; Archer, 1982). In general, inhibition or catalysis of nitrosation by phenolic compounds depends on pH and the concentrations of the phenolic compound and nitrosating agent, but presence of phenolic compounds in foods makes them important in both in vitro as well as endogenous formation of nitrosamines (Hotchkiss, 1987). A postulated mechanism for the stimulatory effect of p-nitrosophenol on the nitrosation of diethylamine involves interaction of p-nitrosophenol with nitrite to produce an active nitrosating agent for diethylamine (Walker et al., 1979, 1982).

Lipids were thought to inhibit nitrosamine formation by making the nitrosating agent unavailable, but it was also shown that at temperatures above 80°C, the lipid-nitrosating agents reacted with amines to form nitrosamines in products such as fried bacon (Hotchkiss, 1987). Of other foods or food constituents, wheat bran enhanced nitrosamine formation, while soybean products and kiwi fruit juice were inhibitory.

In general, nitrosation of nitrite and nitrosamine formation can be inhibited by any compound that can react with nitrite (Tricker and Kubacki, 1992). Such compounds include primary amines and sulfhydryl and aromatic compounds. The most important inhibitors are reducing compounds, such as ascorbate. These are effective because the reaction rate of nitrous acid as an oxidizing agent is usually greater than its reaction as a nitrosating agent (Archer, 1982). The inhibitory effect of ascorbic acid (or erythorbate, its isomer) is very useful in meat products, because the compound is an acceptable food ingredient as vitamin C (Mirvish et al., 1972; Fiddler et al., 1973). Inhibition of the nitrosation reaction of nitrite with dimethylamine, morpholine, piperazine, methylurea, N-methylaniline, and oxytetracycline by ascorbate can range from 45 to 100%. The mechanism of inhibition involves reaction of ascorbate with nitrite to form nitric oxide and dehydroascorbic acid. Thus, ascorbic acid competes with the nitrogen compound for nitrite. Inhibition depends on the ratio of ascorbate to nitrite and presence of oxygen, because the nitric oxide formed can be oxidized to form more nitrite. Oxygen can also oxidize ascorbates, which makes it ineffective as an inhibitor of nitrosation (Hotchkiss, 1987). Inhibition of nitrosation by ascorbic acid is reduced as the pH decreases, and a higher ascorbate-to-nitrite ratio is needed for inhibition. Ascorbic acid may also inhibit nitrosation in vivo. Esters of ascorbic and erythorbic acid also inhibit nitrosation, as well as bisulfite, tannic acid, thiols, α-tocopherol, phenolic components, azide, hydrazine, NADH, sulfamic acid, aniline, hydroxylamine, and urea (Mirvish, 1975b; Sen et al., 1976; Fiddler et al., 1978; Mergens et al., 1978; Hallet et al., 1980; Archer, 1982; Shuker, 1988).

As indicated above, the ability of ascorbic acid to inhibit formation of N-nitroso compounds and to increase the formation of nitric oxide, which reacts with myoglobin to form the pink color of nitrosomyoglobin, makes it very valuable, not only as an accelerator of the curing reaction (Watts and Lehmann, 1952), but also as an inhibitor of nitrosamine formation in cured meat products (Fiddler et al., 1973, 1978; Mergens et al., 1978; Mirvish, 1986; Izumi et al., 1989). Inhibition of nitrosamine formation is greater when ascorbate and α-tocopherol are used in combination.

C. Metabolism

After administration to animals, N-nitrosamines such as N-nitrosodimethylamine equilibrate rapidly throughout the body and usually induce tumors in specific sites (Magee, 1956). The toxic effects of nitrosamines may depend on metabolism because they induce in vitro mutations only in presence of appropriate sources of metabolic activation. In contrast, N-nitrosamides, as well as nitrosoureas and nitrosoguanidines and their nonenzymatic decomposition products, appear to be direct mutagens (Rowland, 1988). It would therefore appear that the organotropic carcinogenic effects of N-nitrosamines are the result of the combination of at least two factors: (1) activation or detoxification of the compounds by the metabolic activity of different organs, and (2) tissue susceptibility to DNA damage, as well as ability to repair such damage (Rowland, 1988).

The liver appears to be the major site of N-nitroso metabolism, and extensive research has examined their metabolism by hepatic tissue (Rowland, 1988). The dialkylnitrosamines are generally thought to be metabolically activated by the liver forming an alkylating specie, but there is disagreement relative to specific metabolic pathways and enzymes involved (Magee et al., 1981; Gangolli, 1981). Druckrey (1973) postulated that N-nitrosodimethylamine is metabolized by N-nitrosodimethylamine-demethylase (i.e., a cytochrome P-450–dependent mixed-function oxidase), which catalyzes hydroxylation of the α-carbon to form hydroxymethylmethylnitrosamine, followed by dealkylation to methyl diazonium hydroxide, which finally yields methylcarbonium ion. This agent is capable of alkylating cellular macromolecules (Preussmann, 1984; Rowland, 1988). Derivatives of this pathway have been shown to be mutagenic (Bartch, 1981; Mochizuki et al., 1982). Metabolism of certain N-nitroso compounds can also be through denitrosation, which appears to be catalyzed by a cytochrome P-450–dependent monooxygenase and results in deactivation of nitrosamines (Rowland, 1988). Other enzymes, such as demethylases and a microsomal monoamine oxidase, may also be involved in the activation of dialkylnitrosamines (Arcos et al., 1977; Lake et al., 1978; Kroeger-Kopke and Michejda, 1979). Amine oxidase inhibitors and substrates were also determined to protect rats from the hepatotoxic effects of N-nitrosodimethylamine and N-nitrosodieethylamine and to inhibit the mutagenic activity of N-nitrosodimethylamine (Rowland et al., 1980; Gangolli, 1981). This would indicate that an enzymatic *N*-oxidation step was involved in the metabolic activation of dimethyl-nitrosamine to toxic and genotoxic derivatives (Rowland, 1988).

The above apply mostly to simple *N*-nitrosamines (e.g., *N*-nitrosomethylamine and *N*-nitrosodiethylamine), while the longer-chain dialkylnitrosamines may undergo β-hydroxylation to methylalkyl nitrosamines and then α-hydroxylation. Also, β-, γ- and ω-oxidation products of dibutyl-nitrosamine and its derivatives have been detected. Cyclic nitrosamines, such as *N*-nitrosophyrrolidine, appear to be metabolized through ring hydroxylation and α-, β- and γ-hydroxylation (Rowland, 1988).

Metabolism of *N*-nitrosamines appears to differ with animal species. Liver preparations from hamsters were better activators of nitrosamines than those from rats, while the activating capacity of liver preparations from mice was intermediate (Prival et al., 1979; Phillipson and Ioannides, 1984; Rowland, 1988).

The human liver can activate *N*-nitroso compounds to become gerotoxic, but there is large individual variation. Activation of *N*-nitrosomorpholine and *N*-nitroso-*N'*-methylpiperazine to bacterial mutagens was highly variable when hepatic postmitochondrial supernatant fractions from different humans were evaluated (Sabadie et al., 1980). Bartsch and Montesano (1984) reported that metabolism of *N*-nitrosodimethylamine by human liver slices was 45% of that detected in the presence of hamster liver slices. Although there is animal species and individual animal variation in metabolism of *N*-nitroso compounds, Lijinsky (1984) found no evidence that hamsters were more or less susceptible than the rat to carcinogenesis after oral exposure to 50 compounds. Thus, it is difficult to predict the susceptibility of humans to *N*-nitroso compounds, even from results of studies involving activation with tissue preparations derived from humans (Rowland, 1988).

Metabolism of *N*-nitrosamines by the liver is greater than by other tissues, but there is evidence indicating that extrahepatic human tissues are also able to metabolize several *N*-nitrosamines, converting them to forms that bind to or alkylate DNA (Rowland, 1988). These tissues include cell cultures or explants from bladder, colon, bronchus, and esophagus (Harris et al., 1977; Autrup et al., 1978, 1981; Autrup and Stoner, 1982; Castonguay et al., 1983). Thus, humans may be exposed to the genotoxic metabolites of *N*-nitrosamines from food or food additives (Rowland, 1988).

N-Nitrosodimethylamine and *N*-nitrosopyrrolidine are metabolized by the liver and nasal mucosa of rats into products causing injurious effects (Brambilla et al., 1981; Brittebo et al., 1981; Brittebo and Tjalve, 1983; Alldrick et al., 1985; Streeter et al., 1990). Metabolic activation of *N*-nitrosodimethylamine and *N*-nitrosopyrrolidine, resulting in formation of electrophilic intermediates, is mediated by cytochrome P-450 and may form covalent bonds with DNA or other macromolecules (Druckery, 1973; Chen et al., 1978; Miller and Miller, 1981; Harris, 1987). The interaction may result in formation of adducts, leading to mutation (Miller and Miller, 1981; Singer, 1984; Barbacid, 1986). In general, metabolic intermediates may result in formation of toxic and carcinogenic effects (Harris, 1987).

D. Toxicity

Acute Toxicity

Studies on the acute toxicity of *N*-nitroso compounds are limited because they have very little direct commercial use, except for the therapeutic application of some

N-nitrosamides, and because their presence in foods is at low levels. In general, there is more concern due to chronic rather than acute toxic effects. N-Nitroso-dimethylamine at high levels was found to cause acute toxicity in two research chemists, which was expressed as severe symptoms of liver failure, as well as liver necrosis and death in one patient. This toxicity was also confirmed with mice and dogs (NAS, 1981; Hotchkiss, 1987). According to established LD_{50} values, they show a wide range of toxicity with values in the range of 22–7500 mg/kg for N-nitrosomethyl-2-chloroethylamine and N-nitrosodiethanolamine, respectively (Hotchkiss, 1987). Others have reported that the LD_{50} values for a single oral dose of nitrosamines vary in adult male rats from 18 mg/kg for N-nitrosomethylbenzy-lamine to more than 7.5 g/kg for N-nitrosoethyl-2-hydroxyethylamine (Druckrey et al., 1967; Rowland, 1988). N-Nitrosamides also cause necrosis of the liver and damage at the site of application as well as in organs with rapid cell turnover (Leaver et al., 1969). The LD_{50} values of N-nitrosamides range from 180 mg/kg for N-methylnitrosourea to 240 mg/kg for N-methylnitrosourethane (Archer, 1982).

One study (Hard et al., 1984) involved exposure of rats to a single carcinogenic dose (60 mg/kg) of N-nitrosodimethylamine and determination of the sequence of events involved in kidney damage for a period of 2 hours to 3 weeks. The reactive intermediates of N-nitrosodimethylamine, which were formed in the proximal ne-phron, injured mesenchymal cells, resident cortical fibrocytes, and subsequently the peritubular endothelium, suggesting that these cell populations were the origins of the cortical epithelial and mesenchymal tumors induced eventually by N-nitro-sodimethylamine (Rowland, 1988). N-nitrosopyrrolidine was found to be mostly a liver carcinogen in rats and hamsters, but in vitro studies with rat hepatocytes indicated that it was able to induce cytotoxic effects (Alldrick et al., 1985; Berger et al., 1987).

A sequential study of nasal and hepatic lesions in rats induced by N-nitroso-dimethylamine and N-nitrosopyrrolidine was conducted by Rangga-Tabbu and Sleight (1992). Female Sprague-Dawley rats were given an intraperitoneal dose of N-nitrosodimethylamine (10–60 mg/kg) and N-nitrosopyrrolidine (10–100 mg/kg), singly or in combination. Rats were killed at 6 or 12 hours and at 1, 3, 10, or 30 days after treatment. Olfactory epithelium and adjacent Bowman's glands were specifically targeted by each chemical. Lesions were seen as early as 6 hours and were most severe by 3 days. At the high doses (60 mg N-nitrosodimethyl-amine/kg or 100 mg N-nitrosopyrrolidine/kg), regeneration of tissue was not completed by 30 days. Hepatic necrosis was seen at 1 and 3 days with N-nitrosodimethylamine, but was not seen with N-nitrosopyrrolidine. Combination exposure appeared to cause additive effects in both the liver and the nasal cavity. These results indicate that a single intraperitoneal administration of N-nitrosodimethylamine or N-nitro-sopyrrolidine can induce severe and prolonged toxic effects on nasal tissues in rats (Rangga-Tabbu and Sleight, 1992). N-Nitrosamines, however, are better known for their potential to cause carcinogenic effects after long-term exposure to low levels.

Carcinogenicity

It is generally accepted that many nitrosamines are potent carcinogens. Actually, more than 90% of the 300 N-nitroso compounds have been shown to be carcinogenic in several animal species (Preussmann and Stewart, 1984; Lijinsky, 1987; Hotchkiss, 1987, 1989a, b). Actually, more than 40 animal species including mammals, birds, fish, amphibia, and higher primates are susceptible to N-nitroso compound–induced carcinogenesis (Bogovski and Bogovski, 1981; Archer, 1982; Tricker and Preussmann, 1991). Only indirect evidence, however, associates N-nitroso compounds with human cancer (Hotchkiss, 1987), but they have been studied extensively for their involvement in animal carcinogenesis (Rowland, 1988).

Mechanism of Carcinogenesis

Both nitrosamines and nitrosamides may be carcinogenic, but, as indicated above, the former need enzymatic activation, while the latter are inherently active. N-Nitrosamines produce tumors at sites or organs that are usually distant from the point of their application, while N-nitrosamides are direct acting mutagens, producing tumors at the site of application (Hotchkiss, 1987). N-Nitrosamines require metabolic activation by cytochrome P-450–dependent hydroxylation at the carbon adjacent to the N-nitroso group to yield an α-hydroxyalkylnitrosamine (Hotchkiss, 1987; Tricker and Preussmann, 1991). Spontaneous elimination of an aldehyde by cleavage of the carbon-nitrogen bond produces an alkyldiazohydroxide. This loses a hydroxide ion and forms an alkyldiazonium ion, which decomposes to molecular nitrogen, and a carbonium ion that serves as the alkylating agent reacting with proteins, nucleic acids, water, or other nucleophiles (Archer, 1982; Hotchkiss, 1987). N-Nitrosamides are chemically active under physiological pH and decompose to form the same alkyldiazohydroxide species, which is the intermediate step in the production of an electrophilic alkyl diazonium ion. This constitutes the ultimate carcinogen, which can react at nucleophilic sites of various cellular constitutents. Alkylation of DNA by dialkynitrosamines forms modified bases and is generally considered to be the critical cellular target for carcinogens in the initiation of cancer (Archer, 1982; Tricker and Preussmann, 1991).

The most common DNA base modification by nitrosamines is the alkylation of the 7-position of quanine, but it shows no correlation with carcinogenic activity (Tricker and Preussmann, 1991). In contrast, O^6-alkylguanine and O^4-alkylthymine are important base modifications, which result in the incorporation of noncomplementary bases (mis-coding) during polyribonucleotide or polydeoxyribonucleotide synthesis (Pegg, 1983; Dyroff et al., 1986). A large number of alkylated DNA products, however, undergo repair either by hydrolysis or by enzymatic apurination or apyromidation (Tricker and Preussmann, 1991).

Structure-Activity Relationship

There is a relationship between N-nitrosamine structure and organs in which carcinogenesis develops (Hotchkiss, 1987). Symmetrical dialkylnitrosamines are mostly liver carcinogens, while unsymmetrical dialkylnitrosamines are usually esophageal carcinogens. Organ specificity is determined not only by chemical nature, but it may also depend on dose, animal species, and route of administration (Archer, 1982). In the symmetric dialkynitrosamines, except N-nitrosodiethylamine, which is the most potent carcinogen, the carcinogenic potency is inversely related to chain length, with N-nitrosododecylamine apparently being inactive (Lijinsky, 1982; Rowland, 1988). Chain length also determines target organ specificity. Nitrosamines generally cause systemic tumors, while nitrosamides cause local as well as systemic tumors (Tricker and Preussmann, 1991). In general, nitrosamines affect the liver, esophagus, respiratory tract, and kidneys in rats, while nitrosamides affect the nervous system, gastrointestinal tract, and kidneys (Archer, 1982). Specifically, N-nitrosodimethylamine induces liver tumors, N-nitrosodiethylamine liver and esophageal tumors, N-nitroso-di-n-propylamine mostly esophageal tumors, and N-nitroso-di-n-butylamine liver and bladder tumors (Preussmann and Stewart, 1984; Rowland, 1988). Small changes in structure can change the target organ, and target organs for cyclic nitrosamines are less predictable (Hotchkiss, 1987, 1989a, b).

As indicated, the symmetrical compounds induce mostly liver tumors, the unsymmetrical ones are mostly active on the esophagus, while heterocyclic nitrosamines show mixed effects, with some acting on the liver and others on the esophagus (Archer, 1982). The asymmetrical dialkylnitrosamines exhibit distinct organotropic effects. Although N-nitrosomethylethylamine is less potent than N-nitrosodimethylamine or N-nitrosodiethylamine, it causes mostly liver tumors, while N-nitrosomethyl-n-propylamine, -n-butylamine, -n-pentylamine, and -n-hexylamine are very potent esophageal carcinogens in the rat. However, N-nitrosomethyl-n-hexylamine also induces hepatic tumors (Druckrey et al., 1967; Lijinsky, 1983). N-Nitrosomethyl-n-octylamine and its higher even-chain homologs induce bladder tumors (Lijinsky, 1983; Rowland, 1988). Nitrosamides express their carcinogenicity at the site of application, but several structures demonstrate neurotropism, and the C_1 through C_6 N-nitrosoureas are potent neurocarcinogens (Preussmann and Stewart, 1984; Hotchkiss, 1987).

Cyclic nitrosamines with smaller rings, such as N-nitroso-azetidine, -pyrrolidine, and -pyrroline, are weaker carcinogens than those with six-membered rings, such as N-nitroso-piperidine and N-nitroso-morpholine. The most potent cyclic nitrosamines are the N-nitroso derivatives of hexa- and hepta-methyleneimines, which have seven- and eight-membered rings, respectively (Rao et al., 1982). They are the most carcinogenic and cause lung and esophageal tumors in rats (Rowland, 1988).

Variation with Animal Species

As indicated, animals susceptible to tumor formation by N-nitroso compounds include mammals, fish, birds, reptiles, and amphibians, but there are major differences in organs affected between species (Bogovski and Bogovski, 1981; Lijinsky, 1984; Rowland, 1988). Differences may also exist among cell types affected within the same organ (Lijinsky, 1984). Even N-nitroso compounds, not dependent on metabolic activation, such as N-nitrosoalkylureas, may exhibit specificity of action in animal models such as rats and hamsters. N-Nitrosomethylurea induced tumors in many organs and the central nervous system of the rat, but tumors of the nervous system were not detected in hamsters, even though alkylated DNA was present in the brain after treatment with N-nitrosomethylurea. It therefore appears that in addition to alkylation of DNA, other steps necessary for induction of tumors by N-nitroso compounds may include site of alkylation or rate of damage and repair (Rowland, 1988).

Rats are commonly susceptible to induction of tumors by N-nitrosamines in the esophagus, an organ only rarely affected in the hamster (Lijinsky, 1984). Guinea pig is the animal species insensitive to the tumorigenic effects of many N-nitrosamines, probably due to the absence of activating enzymes (Lijinsky, 1984; Rowland, 1988).

Effect of Animal Age

Tumor development and carcinogenic effects may also depend on the age of the animals. Nitrosamines, as well as nitrosamides, can act transplacentally with the effect on the offspring depending on the time of exposure during gestation. Exposure to N-nitroso compounds on days 1–10, 9–16, and 10 to delivery has resulted in embryotoxic, teratogenic, and carcinogenic effects, respectively. Transplacental carcinogenesis has resulted in brain and spinal tumors in rats (Archer, 1982).

Animal neonates exposed to N-nitroso compounds develop significantly more liver tumors within a shorter period of time than their adult counterparts, as was shown with mice treated with N-nitrosodiethylamine alone and rats treated with N-nitrosodimethylamine and N-nitrosodiethylamine (Hard, 1979; Vasselinovitch et al., 1984). When N-nitrosodiethylamine treatment of rats began at 3 weeks of age, the rate of liver tumor incidence was six times higher than when treatment began at 20 weeks (Peto et al., 1984), indicating the potential presence of factors in very young animals which greatly enhance the sensitivity of the liver to N-nitrosodiethylamine (Rowland, 1988). Development of esophageal tumors by N-nitrosodiethylamine, however, after treatment of rats from 3 weeks of age, was only slightly more rapid than for rats treated at 20 weeks of age. It should be noted that in this study, the younger animals were exposed to a higher dose (per kg body weight) because water intake (per kg body weight) is higher in early life (Peto et al., 1984). Age of the animals also affects the type of tumors induced (Rowland, 1988).

Effect of Dose and Route of Administration

In addition to chemical structure, the organotropic effect of N-nitroso compounds is dependent on the dosage level and the route of exposure, especially for N-nitrosamides (Rowland, 1988). The doses needed to produce tumors in laboratory animals are generally low, and sometimes they produce tumors only after a single dose. Doses such as 10 μg/kg in mice and 130 μg/kg in rats have resulted in tumors (Hotchkiss, 1987). When animals were exposed to a low dose of N-nitrosodimethylamine in drinking water, they developed liver tumors, while a single high dose (30–60 mg/kg) administered by gavage resulted in a high incidence of renal tumors (Magee and Barnes, 1962; Hard, 1979). A single intravenous injection of N-nitrosodiethylamine caused kidney tumors in rats, while lifetime exposure through the drinking water resulted in hepatic and esophageal tumors (Mohr and Hilfirch, 1972). Druckrey (1973) showed that oral exposure to N-nitrosomethylurea and N-nitrosomethylurethane induced tumors in the forestomach, while chronic intravenous administration of N-nitrosomethylurea caused brain tumors. Differences in metabolism of N-nitrosamines among species and tissues as well as DNA damage, type of bases affected, and repair could play a role in determining organotropism and susceptibility to tumor induction (Rowland, 1988).

In general, N-nitrosamines are able to induce formation of tumors in laboratory animals, even at very low doses, and no evidence of a threshold for induction of tumors has been determined. The existing evidence indicates, however, that exposure of humans to normal levels of nitrosamines results in an extremely low risk of tumor induction (Rowland, 1988).

Mutagenicity

N-Nitroso compounds are also mutagenic and teratogenic, but in general, N-nitrosamines appear to be less potent as bacterial mutagens than as carcinogens (Montensano and Bartsch, 1976; Rao et al., 1979; Andrews and Lijinsky, 1980; NAS, 1981; Archer, 1982; Rowland, 1988). As for carcinogenicity, nitrosamides are directly mutagenic, while nitrosamines become mutagenic after activation with liver microsomes by oxidation at the carbon atom alpha to the N-nitroso group to form the α-hydroxylnitramine, which also makes them carcinogenic (Archer, 1982).

Bacterial mutagenicity induced by aliphatic N-nitrosamines appears to be directly correlated with alkyl chain length, while the carcinogenic activity may be inversely correlated with the alkyl chain length (Yahagi et al., 1977). Thus, there is no significant correlation between bacterial mutagenicity and carcinogenicity of aliphatic N-nitrosamines (Rao et al., 1982; Andrews and Lijinsky, 1984). The mutagenic activity of cyclic N-nitrosamines, however, appears to be closely related to their carcinogenicity. Since N-nitrosohepta- and N-nitrosohexa-methyleneimines were more active than N-nitrosopiperidine and N-nitrosopyrrolidine, bacterial mutagenicity increased with ring size (Rao et al., 1982). In general, the correlation of bacterial mutagenicity with animal carcinogenicity for many N-nitroso compounds is questionable (Bartsch et al., 1984). N-Nitrosoethylurea was a potent carcinogen in rodents, but it was a weak bacterial mutagen (Rowland, 1988).

Specific genotoxicity effects induced by dialkylnitrosamines in mammalian cell cultures from rats, mice, hamster, and humans include gene mutations, chromosomal aberrations, and chromatid exchanges, but a hepatic fraction was required for activation (Rowland, 1988). In some studies, N-nitrosamine activation was effected by human liver microsomes (Thust, 1982). Potency of induction of gene mutations in cultured mammalian cells by dialkylnitrosamines was inversely correlated with the alkyl chain length, which is indicative of their carcinogenic potency (Jones et al., 1981; Ho et al., 1984; Langenbach, 1986; Rowland, 1988).

N-Nitrosamines have also been found to cause genetic damage in vivo, but in many cases testing yielded negative results for genotoxicity. N-Nitrosodimethylamine and N-nitrosodiethylamine induced a limited number of gene mutations in the mouse spot test after intraperitoneal administration, but the results were negative when assayed with a dominant lethal test in mice after intraperitoneal exposure. N-Nitrosodimethylamine administered subcutaneously, however, resulted in a weak response (Fahrig et al., 1981; Sankaranarayan, 1981). Induction of micronuclei in bone marrow in vivo after intraperitoneal injection of high doses of N-nitrosodimethylamine has been genotoxic, while N-nitroso-diethylamine did not induce micronuclei in bone marrow after intraperitoneal treatment (Jenssen and Ramel, 1978; Matter and Wild, 1981; Watanabe et al., 1982). N-Nitrosodipropylamine and N-nitrosodibutylamine induced sister chromatid exchanges at intraperitoneal doses of 170–300 mg/kg (Inoue et al., 1983; Parodi et al., 1983; Rowland, 1988).

N-Nitrosodimethylamine and N-nitrosodiethylamine have also exhibited mutagenic activity in host-mediated in vivo mutagenicity tests at high doses (Neale and Solt, 1980; Fahrig and Remmer, 1983). These assays involve injection of indicator bacteria or fungi in mice or rats treated with N-nitrosamines (Rowland, 1988).

E. *N*-Nitroso Compounds and Human Cancer

Epidemiological studies have suggested that the biological activity of N-nitroso compounds in humans may not be substantially different from that in experimental animals. Animal experiments, however, usually involve single exposures to high doses, while humans usually undergo a gradual exposure to N-nitroso compounds through various sources, including foods, consumer products, tobacco, and occupational and environmental exposure (Rowland, 1988; Tricker and Preussmann, 1991). Continuous and extended exposure to multiple N-nitroso compounds at probably noncarcinogenic low individual concentrations may be carcinogenic for humans. When evaluating human cancer risk from exposure to N-nitroso compounds, however, the following should be considered: (1) foods may contain preformed N-nitroso compounds or their precursors, as well as catalysts and inhibitors of nitrosation; (2) nitrosation may occur in vivo, leading to exposure to endogenous N-nitroso compounds; and (3) carcinogenesis may be affected by the genetic, nutritional, health, and stress status of the individual. The combination of these confounding factors and variables complicates attempts to establish epidemiological links between exposure to N-nitroso compounds and development of human cancer (Archer, 1982; Hotchkiss, 1989b; Tricker and Preussmann, 1991). As indicated above, however, epidemiological studies have indicated that exposure to N-nitroso compounds may be a risk factor for development of certain human cancers, such as those of the esophagus, nasopharynx, and stomach.

N-Nitroso compounds, particularly N-nitrosamides, have been widely used as a model to study gastric carcinogenesis, probably the most common cancer in the world (Correa et al., 1975; Hill, 1988). Salted, dried, and smoked fish products have been suspected of being etiological agents in human gastric cancer, because amines and amides known to be present in these products can produce carcinogenic N-nitroso compounds upon nitrosation in vivo and several performed N-nitroso compounds have been found in such products (Mirvish, 1983; Tricker and Preussmann, 1991). Studies from countries such as Japan, China, Iceland, Norway, and Finland have associated consumption of salted fish and fish sauce with human carcinogenesis (Bjelke, 1974; Weisburger et al., 1980; Howson et al., 1986; Shuker, 1988; Chen et al., 1992). Some have suggested that certain gastric cancers may be caused at least in part by endogeneously formed, from ingested nitrate and nitrite, if not dietary, N-nitroso compounds (Mirvish, 1983; Hill, 1988). Relative to involvement of nitrate, nitrite, and N-nitroso compounds in development of stomach cancer, a committee of the National Academy of Sciences (NAS, 1981) concluded that this hypothesis is plausible because (1) nitrite, amides, and other precursors can react and form nitrosamides under acidic conditions, (2) nitrosamides are chemically unstable, direct-acting carcinogens, and (3) animal feeding studies with nitrosamides have produced gastric adenocarcinomas.

N-Nitrosamines found to induce esophageal tumors in experimental animals have been detected in several food products such as cured meats, including bacon products (Tricker and Preussmann, 1991). In addition, several epidemiological studies from China, Iran, and Kashmir have reported on the potential involvement of endogenous or dietary N-nitrosamines in development of human esophageal cancer (Yang, 1980; Singer et al., 1986; Ji et al., 1986; Lu et al., 1986; Siddiqi and Preussmann, 1989). Furthermore, nasopharyngeal cancer development has been associated with a virus, but also with consumption of salted fish in China (Tricker and Preussmann, 1991). Other sites of potential carcinogenesis in humans by endogenously formed N-nitroso compounds are the liver, cervix, and colon (Hill, 1988, 1991).

The urine is the route of excretion of a range of nitrosatable amino compounds and of nitrite (Hill, 1988). Therefore, an infected urinary bladder is a potential site for bacterial nitrosation. This potential is increased if one considers that most urinary tract infections are caused by bacteria capable of reducing nitrate, such as *E. coli*, *Proteus* spp., and *Klebsiella* spp. Thus, bacterial infection of the bladder may increase the risk of bladder cancer through *N*-nitroso compounds in the urine (Hill, 1988). In addition, chronic bacterial infection of the stomach or the vagina may lead to endogenous nitrosation and development of cancer. In general, continuous and extended exposure to dietary and/or endogenously formed *N*-nitroso compounds has been suggested as a risk factor for development of carcinogenesis in humans.

F. Human Exposure to *N*-Nitroso Compounds

Exposure of humans to *N*-nitroso compounds may be from exogenous and endogenous sources (Hill, 1988). Sources of exogenous *N*-nitroso compounds are foods and beverages, cigarette smoke, exhaust fumes, industrial processes, and the air. Endogenous formation of *N*-nitroso compounds is catalyzed by acids or by microorganisms. In general, humans may be exposed to *N*-nitroso compounds from a large variety of sources. Specific exogenous sources of nitrosamines include food, tobacco, cosmetics, drugs, pesticides, indoor air, household goods, and occupational exposure such as rubber manufacturing, leather tanning, metal works, and chemical industries. Endogenous exposure in the body involves nitrosation of dietary or endogenously synthesized amines and amides (Preussmann and Eisenbrand, 1984; Hotchkiss, 1987, 1989a; Shuker, 1988).

Extent of endogenous nitrosation is difficult to estimate, but humans are believed to be exposed to higher levels of endogenous than exogenous nitrosamines (Hotchkiss, 1989a). Mechanisms of endogenous nitrosation have been discussed by Leach (1988). There is also evidence that food components, such as vitamins C and E, modulate the carcinogenic effects of nitrosamines or their precursors or that endogenous nitrosation is inhibited (Pearson et al., 1993). According to the United States National Academy of Sciences, estimated daily exposures for residents of the United States in μg/day/person are (1) from fried bacon, <0.17, (2) from beer, 0.34, (3) from Scotch whiskey, <0.03, (4) from automobile interiors, 0.2–0.5, (5) from cigarettes, 17, and (6) from occupational exposure, up to 440 (NAS, 1981; Hotchkiss, 1989a, b). These exposures, depending on the source, are through ingestion or inhalation.

N-Nitroso compounds, especially volatile nitrosamines, have been detected in a large variety of food products, including raw and fried bacon, other cured meat products, dried and smoked fish products, milk and cheese products, beer and other alcoholic beverages, and fermented vegetables. Because they are potent carcinogens, however, people should try to minimize their intake of nitrosamines from any source (NAS, 1981). Thus, *N*-nitrosamines are mostly found in fried products such as bacon, in malted or products dried by flame-heated air, and in foods coming in contact with materials containing *N*-nitrosamines. Commonly isolated compounds include *N*-nitrosodimethylamine, *N*-nitrosodiethylamine, *N*-nitrosopyrrolidine, and *N*-nitrosopiperidine at levels in the range of 1–200 μg/kg (Archer, 1982; Anonymous, 1987; Hotchkiss, 1987, 1989a, b; Tricker and Kubacki, 1992). Studies isolating nitrosamines from foods have been conducted in several countries including the United States, United Kingdom, Japan, Germany, and

Canada. The data of several surveys led Hotchkiss (1987) to conclude that the average contribution of the diet is less than 1 μg of N-nitrosamine per day per person. This exposure is minor compared to other known sources such as tobacco smoke. Awareness of nitrosamine toxicity, progress in science, and technological developments have continuously led to reduction of N-nitrosamine levels in the food supply.

One cured meat product that received extensive notoriety and testing for nitrosamines in the United States is bacon (Robach et al., 1980; Archer, 1982). Raw and fried bacon, especially its fat, was found to consistently contain detectable levels of volatile N-nitrosamines, especially N-nitrosodimethylamine, N-nitroso-pyrrolidine, N-nitrosothiazolidine, and N-nitrosopiperidine (Tricker and Kubacki, 1992). In order to control and minimize nitrosamine levels in bacon, the Food Safety and Inspection Service of the United States Department of Agriculture not only monitors levels present, it also requires additions of sodium ascorbate (550 mg/kg) together with sodium nitrite (100–120 mg/kg) or addition of only 40 mg/kg nitrite together with sugar and lactic acid bacteria, which reduces residual nitrite and nitrosamine formation, but still inhibits C. botulinum. The limit of permissible levels of N-nitrosamines in fried bacon is set at 10 μg/kg, with an action level of 17 μg/kg. Evidence also exists that certain nonvolatile N-nitrosamines, such as N-nitrosamino acids, may be found in raw and fried bacon (Hotchkiss, 1987). Detection of N-nitrosamides in bacon has been limited by the lack of appropriate analytical methodology. The chemistry of nitrosation to form these N-nitroso compounds in bacon has been reviewed by Hotchkiss (1987). In addition to bacon, N-nitrosamines have been found sporadically in many other smoked or cured meat products (Tricker and Kubacki, 1992).

In addition to fried bacon, N-nitrosamines have been found consistently in malt and malted beverages. Although lower than those found in bacon, N-nitrosamine levels in beer could constitute a greater threat to human health because the higher beer consumption may result in greater overall exposure than from consumption of bacon (Hotchkiss, 1987, 1989b). The N-nitrosamine most commonly found in beer is N-nitrosodimethylamine, which is derived from the malt, where it can be formed during the kilning process, especially when the malts are dried in kilns with air heated by a direct open flame. Methods developed to reduce the N-nitrosamine content of malts include (1) modification of the kiln to avoid direct heating of drying gases by an open flame, (2) use of low temperature gas burners, and (3) treatment of malt with sulfur dioxide during the kilning process, which may be reducing nitrosamine formation by reducing the pH of the malt and by reducing nitrogen dioxide to nitric oxide, which is a poorer nitrosating agent (Hotchkiss, 1987). In addition to beer, low levels (<1 μg/kg) of N-nitrosamines have been found in other products of malt or dried products such as Scotch whiskies, nonfat dried milk, instant coffee, infant formulas, soy protein isolates, and salted, dried, or cooked fish products.

In addition to direct formation in foods, N-nitrosamines have entered into foods by indirect contact with nonfood materials. Such materials include rubber products used in baby bottle nipples and pacifiers, rubber nettings and spice mixtures used in meat products such as hams, and paper-based packaging materials (Tricker and Kubacki, 1992). Other indirect sources of N-nitrosamines include pesticides and environmental formation (Hotchkiss, 1987).

IV. SUMMARY

Addition of nitrite converts perishable meats, poultry, and fish products into unique cured products such as bacon, ham, and sausages, which have desirable flavor and appearance characteristics and longer shelf life. In addition, nitrite and its precursor, nitrate, are found as natural constituents of vegetables and water. Nitrite in cured meats inhibits formation of neurotoxins by the most dangerous foodborne bacterium, *C. botulinum*. Nitrite itself, however, at excessive levels is an acute or chronic toxic agent for humans and animals. In addition, nitrite may react with nitrogenous compounds in foods or in vivo to form carcinogenic *N*-nitroso compounds, such as nitrosamines. The *N*-nitroso compounds represent an important class of carcinogens, which have been implicated to cause tumor development in animal and human studies. The potency of the *N*-nitroso compounds is determined by several factors including types of animal species, types of tissues, age of the animal, doses, and route of administration. Therefore, it is difficult to draw generalized conclusions about the toxicology of such a diverse group of *N*-nitroso compounds. There is epidemiological evidence indicating that exposure to *N*-nitroso compounds may lead to development of cancer in humans. Therefore, continuous and extended exposure to low concentrations of several different *N*-nitroso compounds in the diet may be an etiological risk factor for certain human cancers. There is considerable evidence that the mechanism of action of *N*-nitroso compounds in carcinogenesis is by DNA damage, probably via alkylation of nucleic acids. Such damage alone, however, may not be sufficient for tumor induction, because other factors such as site of damage at the molecular level and the extent of repair in the DNA are also influential. *N*-Nitrosamines have to be metabolically activated in order to exert any damage in the DNA. The pathways involved, however, are still the subject of controversy even for the simple dialkylnitrosamines. In general, *N*-nitroso compounds can be considered as potential contributors to human carcinogenesis only in cases of continuous and extended exposure. A normal diet, including a variety of foods, should not be a risk factor for development of carcinogenesis from nitrate, nitrite, and *N*-nitroso compounds.

REFERENCES

Alldrick, A. J., Cottrell, R. C., Rowland, I. R., and Gangolli, S. D. (1985). The role of DNA repair processes in *N*-nitrosopyrrolidine-induced mutagenesis. *Carcinogenesis* 6:105–108.

Andrews, A. W., and Lijinsky, W. (1980). The mutagenicity of 45 nitrosamines in *Salmonella typhimurium*. *Terato. Carcino. Mutagen.* *1*:295–330.

Andrews, A. W., and Lijinsky, W. (1984). *N*-Nitrosamine mutagenicity using the *Salmonella*/mammalian microsome mutagenicity assay. In *Genotoxicology of N-Nitroso Compounds*, T. K. Rao, W. Lijinsky, and J. L. Epler (eds.). Plenum Press, New York, pp. 13–43.

Anonymous. (1987). Nitrate, nitrite, and nitroso compounds in foods. *Food Technol.* *41*(4):127–135.

Aquanno, J., Chan, K. M., and Dietzler, D. (1981). Accidental poisoning of two laboratory technicians with sodium nitrite. *Clin. Chem.* 27:1145–1146.

Archer, M. C. (1982). Hazards of nitrates, nitrite, and *N*-nitroso compounds in human nutrition. In *Nutritional Toxicology*, Vol. 1, J. N. Hathcock (ed.). Academic Press, New York, pp. 327–381.

Arcos, J. C., Davies, D. L., Brown, C. E. L., and Argus, M. F. (1977). Repressible and inducible enzymic forms of dimethylnitrosamine-demethylase. *Z. Krebsforsch. 89*:181–199.

Autrup, H., and Stoner, G. D. (1982). Metabolism of *N*-nitrosamines by cultured rat and human oesophagus. *Cancer Res. 42*:1307–1311.

Autrup, H., Harris, C. C., and Trump, B. F. (1978). Metabolism of acyclic and cyclic *N*-nitrosamines by cultured human colon. *Proc. Soc. Exp. Biol. Med. 159*:111–115.

Autrup, H., Grafstrom, R. C., Christensen, B., and Kieler, J. (1981). Metabolism of chemical carcinogens by cultured human and rat bladder epithelial cells. *Carcinogenesis 2*:763–768.

Barbacid, M. (1986). Oncogenes and human cancer. *Carcinogenesis 7*:1037–1042.

Bard, J., and Townsend, W. E. (1971). Meat curing. In *The science of meat and meat products*, J. F. Price and B. S. Schweigert (eds.). W. H. Freeman Co., San Francisco, pp. 452–483.

Barnes, J. M., and Magee, P. N. (1954). Some toxic properties of dimethylnitrosamine. *Br. J. Ind. Med. 11*:167–174.

Bartsch, H. (1981). Detection of *N*-nitroso compounds as bacterial mutagens: past experience. In *Safety Evaluation of Nitrosable Drugs and Chemicals*, G. G. Gibson and C. Ioannides (eds.). Taylor and Francis, London, pp. 185–205.

Bartsch, H., and Montesano, R. (1984). Relevance of nitrosamines to human cancer. *Carcinogenesis 5*:1381–1393.

Bartsch, H., Malaveille, C., Tomatis, L., Brun, G., and Dodet, B. (1984). Quantitative comparison between carcinogenicity, mutagenicity and electrophilicity of direct-acting *N*-nitroso compounds, and other alkylating agents. *IARC Sci. Publ. 41*:525–532.

Berger, M. R., Schmahl, D., and Zerban, H. (1987). Combination experiments with very low doses of three genotoxic *N*-nitrosamines with similar organotropic carcinogenicity in rats. *Carcinogenesis 8*:1635–1643.

Berry, C. N., and Challis, B. C. (1984). Denitrosation and deamination of *N-n*-butyl-*N*-nitrosoacetamide in aqueous acids. *J. Chem. Soc.* (London), *Perkin Trans. II*:1638–1644.

Binkerd, E. F., and Kolari, D. F. (1975). The history and use of nitrate and nitrite in curing of meat. *Food Cosmet. Toxicol. 13*:655–661.

Bjelke, E. (1974). Epidemiological studies of cancer of the stomach, colon and rectum: with special emphasis on the role of diet. *Scand. J. Gastroenterol. 9*:1–235.

Bleakley, B. H., and Tiedje, J. M. (1982). Nitrous oxide production by organism other than nitrifiers or denitrifiers. *Appl. Environ. Microbiol. 44*:1342–1348.

Bloomfield, R. A., Welsch, C. W., Garner, G. B., and Muhrer, M. E. (1962). Thyroid compensation under the influence of dietary nitrate. *Proc. Soc. Exp. Biol. Med. 111*:288–290.

Bodansky, O. (1951). Methemoglobinemia and methemoglobin-producing compounds. *Pharm. Rev. 3*:144–196.

Bogovsky, P., and Bogovsky, S. (1981). Animal species in which *N*-nitroso compounds induce cancer. *Int. J. Cancer 27*:471–474.

Bonnett, R., Holleyhead, R., Johnson, B. L., and Randall, E. W. (1975). Reaction of acidified nitrite solutions with peptides derivatives: Evidence for nitrosamine and thiocyanate formation from ^{15}N n.m.r. studies. *J. Chem. Soc.* (London), *Perkin Trans I*:2261–2264.

Brambilla, G., Cavanna, M., Pino, A., and Robbiano, L. (1981). Quantitative correlation among DNA damaging potency of six *N*-nitroso compounds and their potency in inducing tumor growth and bacterial mutations. *Carcinogenesis 2*:425–429.

Brittebo, E. B., and Tjalve, H. (1983). Metabolism of *N*-nitrosamines by the nasal mucosa. In *Nasal Tumors in Animals and Man: Experimental Nasal Carcinogenesis*, Vol. III, G. Reznik, and S. F. Stinson (eds.). CRC Press, Boca Raton, FL, pp. 234–250.

Brittebo, E. B., Lofberg, B., and Tjalve, H. (1981). Extrahepatic sites of metabolism of *N*-nitrosopyrrolidine in mice and rats. *Xenobiotica 11*:619–625.

Calmels, S., Ohshima, H., Vincent, P., Gounot, A.-M., and Bartsch, H. (1985). Screening of microorganisms for nitrosation catalysis at pH 7 and kinetic studies on nitrosamine formation from secondary amines by *E. coli* strains. *Carcinogenesis 6*:911–915.

Cassens, R. G., Woolford, G., Lee, S. H., and Gouteforgea, R. (1977). Fate of nitrite in meat. In *Proceedings of the Second International Symposium on Nitrite in Meat Products*, B. J. Tinbergen and B. Krol (eds.). Wageningen Center for Agriculture, Wageningen, The Netherlands, pp. 95–109.

Castonguay, A., Stoner, G. D., Schut, A.-J., and Hecht, S. S. (1983). Metabolism of tobacco-specific *N*-nitrosamines by cultured human tissues. *Proc. Natl. Acad. Sci. 80*:6694–6697.

Cazottes, C., Fritsch, P., Gas, N., and de Saint Blanquat, G. (1981). Nitrates and nitrites: nutritional impacts in the rat. *Ann. Nutr. Metab. 25*:182–193.

Challis, B. C. (1973). Rapid nitrosation of phenols and its implications for health hazard from dietary nitrites. *Nature* (London) *244*:466.Challis, B. C., and Challis, J. A. (1982). *N*-Nitrosamines and *N*-nitrosoimines. In *The Chemistry of Amino, Nitroso, and Nitro-Compounds and Their Derivatives*, S. Patai (ed.). John Wiley & Sons, Inc., New York, pp. 1151–1223.

Chen, C. B., McCoy, G. D., Hecht, S. S., Hoffmann, D., and Wynder, E. L. (1978). High pressure liquid chromatographic assay for α-hydroxylation of *N*-nitrosopyrrolidine by isolated rat liver microsomes. *Cancer Res. 38*:3812–3816.

Chen, C. S., Pignatelli, B., Malaveille, C., Bouvier, G., Shuker, D., Hautefeuille, A., Zhang, R. F., and Bartsch, H. (1992). Levels of direct-acting mutagens, total *N*-nitroso compounds in nitrosated fermented fish products, consumed in high-risk area for gastric cancer in southern China. *Mutation Res. 265*:211–221.

Collins-Thompson, D. L., Sen, S. P., Aris, B., and Schwinghamer, L. (1972). Nonenzymatic in vitro formation of nitrosamines by bacteria isolated from meat products. *Can. J. Microbiol. 18*:1968–1971.

Correa, P., Haenszel, W., Cuello, C., Archer, M. C., and Tannenbaum, S. R. (1975). A model for gastric cancer epidemiology. *Lancet ii*:58–60.

Davis, R., and McWeeny, D. J. (1977). Catalytic effect of nitrosophenols on *N*-nitrosamine formation. *Nature* (London) *266*:657–658.

Doyle, M. P., Herman, J. G., and Dykstra, R. L. (1985). Autocatalytic oxidation of hemoglobin induced by nitrite: activation and chemical inhibition. *J. Free Radicals Biol. Med. 1*:145–154.

Druckrey, H. (1973). Specific carcinogenic and teratogenic effects of 'indirect' alkylating methyl and ethyl compounds, and their dependency on stages of ontogenic development. *Xenobiotica 3*:271–303.

Druckrey, H., Preussmann, R., Ivankovic, S., and Schmahl, D. (1967). Organotrope carcinogene Wirkungen bei 65 verschiedenen *N*-nitroso-Verbindungen an BD-ratten. *Z. Krebsforsch 69*:103–201.

Dryden, F. D., and Birdsall, J. J. (1980). Why nitrite does not impart color? *Food Technol. 34*(7):29–42.

Dyroff, M. C., Richardson, F. C., Popp, J. A., Dedell, M. A., and Swenberg, J. A. (1986). Correlation of O⁴-ethyldeoxythymidine accumulation, hepatic initiation and hepatocellular carcinoma induction in rats continuously administered diethylnitrosamine. *Carcinogenesis 7*:241–246.

Ender, F., and Ceh, L. (1971). Conditions and chemical reaction mechanisms by which nitrosamines may be formed in biological products with reference to their possible occurrence in food products. *Z. Lebensm. Uters. Forsch. 145*:133–142.

Fahrig, R., and Remmer, H. (1983). The organo-specific activity of six *N*-nitroso compounds in the host mediated assay with yeast and rats. *Teratogenesis Carcinog. Mutagen. 3*:41–49.

Fahrig, R., Dawson, G. W. R., and Russell, L. B. (1981). Mutagenicity of selected chemicals in the mammalian spot test. *Environ. Sci. Res. 24*:709–727.

Fan, T. Y., and Tannenbaum, S. R. (1972). Stability of *N*-nitroso compounds. *J. Food Sci. 37*:274–276.

Fan, T. Y., and Tannenbaum, S. R. (1973). Factors influencing the rate of formation of nitrosomorpholine from morpholine and nitrite: acceleration by thiocyanate and other anions. *J. Agric. Food Chem. 21*:237–240.

Fiddler, W., Pensabene, J. W., Piotrowski, E. G., Doerr, R. C., and Wasserman, A. E. (1973). Use of sodium ascorbate or erythorbate to inhibit formation of *N*-nitrosodimethylamine in frankfurters. *J. Food Sci. 38*:1084.

Fiddler, W., Pensabene, J. W., Piotrowski, E. G., Phillips, J. G., Keating, J., Mergens, W. J., and Newmark, H. L. (1978). Inhibition of formation of volatile nitrosamines in fried bacon by the use of cure-solubilized α-tocopherol. *J. Agric. Food Chem. 26*:653–656.

Fine, D. H., and Rounbehler, D. P. (1975). Trace analysis of volatile *N*-nitroso compounds by combined gas chromatography and thermal energy analysis. *J. Chromatogr. 109*:271–279.

Frouin, A. (1977). Nitrates and nitrites: reinterpretation of analytical data by means of bound nitric oxide. In *Proceedings of the Second International Symposium on Nitrite in Meat Products*, B. J. Tinbergen and B. Krol (eds.). Wageningen Center for Agriculture, Wageningen, The Netherlands, pp. 115–120.

Gangolli, S. D. (1981). Metabolic activation and detoxication of nitroso compounds. In *Safety Evaluation of Nitrosable Drugs and Chemicals*, G. G. Gibson and C. Ioannides (eds.). Taylor and Francis, London, pp. 157–171.

Garber, E. A. E., and Hollocher, T. C. (1982). ^{15}N, ^{18}O Tracer studies on the activation of nitrite by denitrifying bacteria. *J. Biol. Chem. 257*:8091–8097.

Grant, D., and Butler, W. H. (1989). Chronic toxicity of sodium nitrite in the male F344 rat. *Food Chem. Toxicol. 27*: 565–571.

Gray, J. I., and Dugan, L. R. (1975). Formation of *N*-nitrosopyrrolidine from proline and collagen. *J. Food Sci. 39*:484–487.

Grudzinski, I., and Szymanski, A. (1991a). The effect of acute poisoning with potassium nitrate and sodium nitrite on the process of intestinal absorption of D-xylose in rats. *Arch. Environ. Contam. Toxicol. 21*:453–461.

Grudzinski, I., and Szymanski, A. (1991b). The effect of subchronic poisoning with potassium nitrate and sodium nitrite on the process of intestinal absorption of D-xylose in rats. *Arch. Environ. Contam. Toxicol. 21*:447–452.

Hallett, G., Johal, S. S., Meyer, T. A., and Williams, D. L. H. (1980). Reactions of nitrosamines with nucleophiles in acid solution. In *N-Nitroso Compounds: Analysis, Formation, and Occurrence*, E. A. Walker, L. Griciut, M. Castegnaro, and K. Borzsonyi (eds.). IARC Scientific Publication No. 31, International Agency for Research on Cancer, Lyon, France, pp. 31–41.

Hard, G. C. (1979). Effect of age at treatment on incidence and type of renal neoplasm induced in the rat by a single dose of dimethylnitrosamine. *Cancer Res. 39*:4965–4970.

Hard, G. C., Mackay, R. L., and Kochhar, O. (1984). Electron microscopic determination of the sequence of acute tubular and vascular injury induced in the rat kidney by a carcinogenic dose of dimethylnitrosamine. *Lab. Invest. 50*:659–672.

Harris, C. C. (1987). Biochemical and molecular effects of *N*-nitroso compounds in human cultured cells: an overview. In *Relevance of N-Nitroso Compounds to Human Cancer: Exposures and Mechanisms*, H. Bartsch, I. K. O'Neill, and R. Schulte-Hermann (eds.). IARC Scientific Publication No. 84, International Agency for Research on Cancer, Lyon, France, pp. 20–25.

Harris, C. C., Autrup, H., Stoner, G., McDowell, E., Trump, B., and Schafer, P. (1977). Metabolism of acyclic and cyclic *N*-nitrosamines in cultured human bronchi. *J. Natl. Cancer Inst. 59*:1401.

Hill, M. J. (1988). *N*-Nitroso compounds and human cancer. In *Nitrosamines: Toxicology and Microbiology*, M. J. Hill (ed.). Ellis Horwood Ltd., Chichester, pp. 142–162.

Hill, M. J. (1991). Nitrates and nitrites from food and water in relation to human disease. In *Nitrates and Nitrites in Food and Water*, Ellis Horwood Ltd., New York, pp. 163–193.

Hlinak, Z., Krejci, I., Hondlik, J., and Yamamoto, A. (1990). Behavioral consequences of sodium nitrite hypoxia in male rats: amelioration with alaptide treatment. *Methods Find. Exp. Clin. Pharmacol. 12*:385–393.

Ho, T., San Sebastian, J. R., and Hsie, A. W. (1984). Mutagenic activity of nitrosamines in mammalian cells. Study with the CHO/HGPRT and human leukocyte SCE assay. In *Genotoxicity of N-Nitroso Compounds*, T. K. Rao, W. Lijinsky, and J. L. Epler (eds.). Plenum Press, New York, pp. 129–147.

Hotchkiss, J. A. (1987). A review of current literature on *N*-nitroso compounds in foods. *Adv. Food Res. 31*:53–115.

Hotchkiss, J. A. (1989a). Preformed *N*-nitroso compounds in foods and beverages. *Cancer Surv. 8*:295–322.

Hotchkiss, J. A. (1989b). Relative exposure to nitrite, nitrate, and *N*-nitroso compounds from endogenous and exogenous sources. In *Food Toxicology: A Perspective on the Relative Risks*, S. L. Taylor and R. A. Scanlan (eds.). Marcel Dekker, New York, pp. 57–100.

Howson, C. P., Hiyama, T., and Wynder, E. L. (1986). The decline in gastric cancer: epidemiology of an unplanned triumph. *Epidemiol. Rev. 8*:1–27.

Inoue, I. K., Shibanta, T., and Abe, T. (1983). Induction of sister-chromatid exchanges in human lymphocytes by indirect carcinogens with and without metabolic activation. *Mutation Res. 117*:301–309.

Ishidate, M. Jr., Sofuni, T., Yoshikawa, K., Hayashi, M., Nohmi, T., Sawada, M., and Matsuoka, A. (1984). Primary mutagenicity screening of food additives currently used in Japan. *Food Chem. Toxicol. 22*:623–636.

Ito, T., Cassens, R. G., Greaser, M. L., Lee, M., and Izumi, K. (1983). Lability and reactivity of nonhaem protein bound nitrite. *J. Food Sci. 48*:1204–1207.

Izumi, K., Cassens, R. G., and Greaser, M. L. (1989). Reaction of nitrite with ascorbic acid and its significant role in nitrite-cured food. *Meat Sci. 26*:141–153.

Jenssen, D., and Ramel, C. (1978). Factors affecting the induction of micronuclei at low doses of X-rays, MMS and dimethylnitrosamine in mouse erythroblasts. *Mutation Res. 58*:51–65.

Ji, C., Xu, Z. H., Li, M. X., Li, G. Y., and Li, J. L. (1986). A new *N*-nitroso compound, *N*-(2-methylpropyl)-*N*-(1-methylacetonyl) nitrosamine, in moldy millet and wheat flour. *J. Agric. Food Chem. 34*:628–632.

Jones, C. A., Marlino, P. S., Lijinsky, W., and Huberman, E. (1981). The relationship between the carcinogenicity and mutagenicity assay. *Carcinogenesis 2*:1075–1077.

Kakuda, Y., and Gray, J. S. (1980a). *N*-Nitrosamides and their precursors in food systems. 1. Formation of *N*-substituted amides. *J. Agric. Food Chem. 28*:580–583.

Kakuda, Y., and Gray, J. S. (1980b). *N*-Nitrosamides and their precursors in food systems. 2. Kinetics of the nitrosation reaction. *J. Agric. Food Chem. 28*:584–587.

Kiese, M., and Weger, N. (1969). Formation of ferrihaemoglobin with aminophenols in the human for treatment of cyanide poisoning. *Eur. J. Pharmacol.* 7:97–105.

Kikugawa, K., and Kato, T. (1988). Formation of a mutagenic diazoquinone by interaction of phenol with nitrite. *Food Chem. Toxicol.* 26:209–214.

Kosaka, H., and Yozumi, M. (1986). Inhibition by amines indicates involvement of nitrogen dioxide in autocatalytic oxidation of oxyhemoglobin by nitrite. *Biochim. Biophys. Acta* 871:14–18.

Kosaka, H., Imaizumi, K., Inai, K., and Tyuma, I. (1979). Stoichiometry of the reaction of oxyhemoglobin with nitrite. *Biochim. Biophys. Acta* 581:184–188.

Kroeger-Kopke, M. B., and Michejda, C. J. (1979). Evidence for several dimethylase enzymes in the oxidation of dimethylnitrosamine and phenylmethylnitrosamine by rat liver fractions. *Cancer Res.* 39:1587–1591.

Kubacki, S. J., and Kupryszewski, G. (1981). The formation, chemistry and stability of *N*-nitrosocarbaryl under simulated gastric conditions. In *N-Nitroso Compounds, Analysis, Formation and Occurrence*, A. E. Walker, L. Griciute, M. Castegnaro, and M. Borzsonyi (eds.). IARC Scientific Publication No. 31, International Agency for Research on Cancer, Lyon, France, pp. 245–257.

Kubberod, G., Cassens, R. G., and Greaser, M. L. (1974). Reaction of nitrite with sulfhydryl groups of myosin. *J. Food Sci.* 39:1228–1230.

Lake, B. G., Phillips, J. C., Cottrell, R. C., and Gangolli, S. D. (1978). The possible involvement of amicrosomal amine oxidase enzyme in hepatic dimethylnitrosamine degradation in vitro. In *Biological Oxidation of Nitrogen*, J. W. Gorrod (ed.). Elsevier, Amsterdam, pp. 131–135.

Langenbach, R. (1986). Mutagenic activity and structure-activity relationships of short-chain dialkyl *N*-nitrosamines in hamster hepatocyte V79 cell-mediated system. *Mutation Res.* 163:303–311.

Leach, S. A., Thompson, M., and Hill, M. (1987). Bacterially catalyzed *N*-nitrosation reactions and their relative importance in the human stomach. *Carcinogenesis* 8:1907–1912.

Leach, S. A. (1988). Mechanism of endogenous *N*-nitrosation. In *Nitrosamines: Toxicology and Microbiology*, M. J. Hill (ed.). Ellis Horwood Ltd., Chichester, pp. 69–87.

Leaver, P. D., Swann, P. F., and Magee, P. N. (1969). The induction of tumors in the rat by a single oral dose of *N*-nitrosomethylurea. *Br. J. Cancer* 23:177–187.

Lewis, R. J., Jr. (1989). *Food Additives Handbook*. Van Nostrand Reinhold, New York.

Lijinsky, W. (1982). Chemical structural effects in carcinogenesis by nitrosamines. *IARC Sci. Publ.* 41:533–542.

Lijinsky, W. (1983). Species specificity in nitrosamine carcinogenesis. *Basic Life Sci.* 24:63–75.

Lijinsky, W. (1984). Species differences in nitrosamine carcinogenesis. *J. Cancer Res. Clin. Oncol.* 108:46–55.

Lijinsky, W. (1987). Structure-activity relations in carcinogenesis by *N*-nitroso compounds. *Cancer Met. Rev.* 6:301–356.

Lijinsky, W., and Kovatch, R. M. (1989). Chronic toxicity tests of sodium thiocyanate with sodium nitrite in F344 rats. *Toxicol. Ind. Health* 5(1):25–29.

Lin, J. Y., Wang, H.-I., and Yeh, Y.-C. (1979). The mutagenicity of soy bean sauce. *Food Cosmet. Toxicol.* 17:329–331.

Lu, S. H., Montesano, R., Zhang, M. S., Feng, L., Luo, F. J., Chui, S. X., Umbenhauer, D., Saffhill, R., and Rajewsky, M. F. (1986). Relevance of *N*-nitrosamines to oesophageal cancer in China. *J. Cell Physiol.* 4(Suppl.):51–58.

Luca, D., Raileanu, L., Luca, V., and Duda, R. (1985). Chromosomal aberrations and micronuclei induced in rat and mouse bone marrow cells by sodium nitrate. *Mutation Res.* 155:121–125.

Luca, D., Luca, V., Cotor, F., and Raileanu, L. (1987). In vivo and in vitro cytogenicity damage induced by sodium nitrite. *Mutation Res. 189*:333–339.

Magee, P. N. (1956). Toxic liver injury: the metabolism of dimethylnitrosamine. *Biochem. J. 64*:676–682.

Magee, P. N. (1989). The experimental basis for the role of nitroso compounds in human cancer. *Cancer Surv. 8*:207–240.

Magee, P. N., and Barnes, J. M. (1962). Induction of kidney tumors in the rat with dimethylnitrosamine (*N*-nitrosodimethylamine). *J. Pathol. Bacteriol. 84*:19–31.

Magee, P. N., Jensen, D. E., and Henderson, E. E. (1981). Mechanism of nitrosamine carcinogenesis: an overview and some recent studies on nitrosocimetidine. In *Safety Evaluation of Nitrosable Drugs and Chemicals*, G. G. Gibson and C. Ioannides (eds.). Taylor and Francis, London, pp. 118–140.

Mallett, A. K., Rowland, I. R., Cottrell, R. C., and Gangolli, S. D. (1984). Nitrosoproline formation in control and antibiotic-treated rats given nitrate and proline. *Cancer Lett. 25*:231–235.

Matter, B. E., and Wild, D. (1981). Mutagenicity of selected chemicals in the mammalian micronucleus tests. *Environ. Sci. Res. 24*:657–680.

Mellet, P. O., Noel, P. R., and Goutefongea, R. (1986). Nitrite-tryptophan reaction: evidence for an equilibrium between tryptophan and its nitrosated form. *J. Agric. Food Chem. 34*:892–895.

Mende, P., Spiegelhalder, B., Wacker, C. D., and Preussmann, R. (1989). Trapping of reactive intermediates from the nitrosation of primary amines by a new type of scavanger reagent. *Food Chem. Toxicol. 27*:469–473.

Mergens, W. J., Kamm, J. J., Newmark, H. L., Fiddler, W., and Pensabene, J. (1978). Alpha-tocopherol: uses in preventing nitrosamine formation. In *Environmental Aspects of N-Nitroso Compounds*, E. A. Walker, M. Castegnaro, L. Griciut, and R. E. Lyle (eds.). IARC Publication No. 19, International Agency for Research on Cancer, Lyon, France, pp. 199–212.

Miller, E. C., and Miller, J. A. (1981). MEchanisms of chemical carcinogenesis. *Cancer 47*:1055–1064.

Mills, A. L., and Alexander, M. (1976). *N*-Nitrosamine formation by cultures of several microorganisms. *Appl. Environ. Microbiol. 31*:892–895.

Mirvish, S. S. (1971). Kinetics of nitrosamide formation from alkyureas, *N*-alkylurethanes and alkylguanidines: possible implications for the etiology of human gastric cancer. *J. Natl. Cancer Inst. 46*:1183–1193.

Mirvish, S. S. (1975a). Blocking the formation of *N*-nitroso compounds with ascorbic acid in vitro and in vivo. *Proc. NY Acad. Sci. 258*:175–180.

Mirvish, S. S. (1975b). Formation of *N*-nitroso compounds: chemistry, kinetics and in vivo occurrence. *Toxicol. Appl. Pharmacol. 31*:325–351.

Mirvish, S. S. (1983). The etiology of gastric cancer: intragastric nitrosamide formation and other theories. *J. Natl. Cancer Inst. 71*:631–647.

Mirvish, S. S. (1986). Effects of vitamins C and E on *N*-nitroso compound formulation, carcinogenesis, and cancer. *Cancer 58*:1842–1850.

Mirvish, S. S., Wallcave, L., Eagen, M., and Shubik, P. (1972). Ascorbate-nitrite reaction: possible means of blocking the formation of carcinogenic *N*-nitroso compounds. *Science 177*:65–68.

Mochizuki, M., Ango, T., Takd, K., Suzuki, E., Skiguchi, N., Hugang, G. F., and Okada, M. (1982). Chemistry of mutagenicity of alpha-hydroxy nitrosamines. *IARC Sci. Publ. 41*:552–559.

Mohr, U., and Hilfirch, J. (1972). Effects of a single dose of *N*-diethylnitrosamine on the rat kidney. *J. Natl. Cancer Inst. 49*:1729–1731.

Montesano, R., and Bartsch, H. (1976). Mutagenic and carcinogenic N-nitroso compounds: possible environmental hazards. *Mutation Res. 32*:179–228.

Mottram, D. A. (1984). Organic nitrates and nitrites in the volatile of cooked cured meats. *J. Agric. Food Chem. 32*:343–345.

NAS (National Academy of Science). (1981). *The Health Effects of Nitrate, Nitrite, and N-Nitroso Compounds*. National Academy Press, Washington, DC.

NAS (National Academy of Science). (1982). *Alternatives to the Current Use of Nitrite in Foods*. National Academy Press, Washington, DC.

Nagahara, A., Ohshita, K., and Nasuno, S. (1986). Relation of nitrite concentration to mutagen formation in soy sauce. *Food Chem. Toxicol. 24*:13–15.

Nagahara, A., Ohshita, K., and Nasuno, S. (1991). Investigation of soy sauce treated with nitrite in the chromosomal aberration test in vitro and the micronucelus test in vivo. *Mutation Res. 262*:171–176.

Nalecz, M. J., and Wojtczak, L. (1982). Surface charge of biological membranes and its regulatory functions. *Post. Biochem. 28*:191–225.

Neale, S., and Solt, A. K. (1980). Factors affecting the induction of bacterial mutations by dimethylnitrosamine in mice. *Chem. Biol. Interact. 31*:221–225.

Newberne, P. M. (1979). Nitrite promotes lymphoma incidence in rats. *Science 204*:1079–1081.

Nichols, J. W., and Weber, L. J. (1989). Oxidation of cardiac myoglobin in vivo by sodium nitrite or hydroxylamine. *Arch. Toxicol. 63*:484–488.

Noel, P., Briand, E., and Dumont, J. P. (1990). Role of nitrite in flavour development in uncooked cured meat products: sensory assessment. *Meat Sci. 28*:1–8.

Nyakas, C., Markel, E., Bohus, B., Schuurman, T., and Luiten, P. G. (1990). Protective effect of the calcium antagonist nimodipine on discrimination learning and impaired retention behavior caused by prenatal nitrite exposure to rats. *Behav. Brain Res. 38*:69–76.

Okayama, T., Fujii, M, and Yamanone, M. (1991). Effect of cooking temperature on the percentage colour formation, nitrite decomposition, and sarcoplasmic protein denaturation in processed meat products. *Meat Sci. 30*:49–57.

Parodi, S., Zunino, A., Ottaggio, L., Ferrari, M. D., and Santi, L. (1983). Quantitative correlation between carcinogenicity and sister chromatid exchange induction in vivo for a group of 11 N-nitroso derivatives. *J. Toxicol. Environ. Health 11*:337–346.

Pearson, A. M., Sleight, S. D., Brooks, R. I., and Gray, J. I. (1993). Further studies on N-nitrosopyrrolidine and its precursors: effects of ascorbic acid and vitamin E on tumor development in mice as related to consumption of cured meat. *Meat Sci. 33*:111–120.

Pegg, A. E. (1983). Alkylation and subsequent repair of DNA after exposure to diethylnitrosamine and related compounds. In *Reviews in Biochemical Toxicology*, E. Hogdson, J. R. Bend, and R. M. Philpot (eds.). Elsevier, New York, pp. 83–133.

Peto, R., Gray, R., Brantom, P., and Grasso, P. (1984). Nitrosamine carcinogenesis in 5120 rodents: chronic administration of sixteen different concentrations of NDEA, NDMA, NPYR and NPIP in the water of 440 inbred rats, with parallel studies on NDEA alone of the effect of age of starting (3, 6 or 20 weeks) and of species (rats, mice or hamsters). *IARC Sci. Publ. 57*:627–665.

Phillipson, C. E., and Ioannides, C. (1984). A comparative study of the bioactivation of nitrosamines to mutagens by various animal species including man. *Carcinogenesis 5*:1091–1095.

Podolak-Majczak, M., and Tyburczyk, W. (1986). Effect of joint action of sodium nitrite and carbaryl on rats organisms. Part 4. Hepatotoxic action. *Bromat. Chem. Toksykol. 19*:161–166.

Preussmann, R. (1984). Carcinogenic N-nitroso compounds and their environmental significance. *Naturwissenschaften 71*:25–30.

Preussmann, R., and Eisenbrand, G. (1984). *N-Nitroso Carcinogens in the Environment*. ACS Monograph 182, American Chemical Society, Washington, DC, pp. 829–867.

Preussmann, R., and Stewart, B. W. (1984). *N-Nitroso Carcinogens*. ACS Monograph 182, American Chemical Society, Washington, DC, pp. 643–828.

Prival, M. J., King, V. D., and Sheldon, A. T. (1979). The mutagenicity of dialkylnitrosamines in the salmonella plate assay. *Environ. Mutagen* 1:95–105.

Rangga-Tabbu, C., and Sleight, S. D. (1992). Sequential study in rats of nasal and hepatic lesions induced by *N*-nitrosodimethylamine and *N*-nitrosopyrrolidine. *Fund. Appl. Toxicol. 19*:147–156.Rao, T. K., Young, J. A., Lijinsky, W., and Epler, J. L. (1979). Mutagenicity of aliphatic nitrosamines in *Salmonella typhimurium*. *Mutation Res. 66*:1–7.

Rao, B. G., MacDonald, I. A., and Hutchison, D. M (1981). Nitrite-induced volatile mutagens from normal human feces. *Cancer 47*:889–894.

Rao, T. K., Epler, J. L., and Lijinsky, W. (1982). Structure activity studies with *N*-nitrosamines using *Salmonella typhimurium* and *Escherichia coli*. *IARC Sci. Publ. 41*:543–551.

Robach, M. C., Owens, J. L., Paquette, M. W., Sofos, J. N., and Busta, F. F. (1980). Effects of various concentrations of sodium nitrite and potassium sorbate on nitrosamine formation in commercially prepared bacon. *J. Food Sci. 45*:1280–1284.

Roberts, T. A., and Dainty, R. H. (1991). Nitrite and nitrate as food additives: rationale and mode of action. In *Nitrates and Nitrites in Food and Water*, M. J. Hill (ed.). Ellis Horwood, London, pp. 113–130.

Roth, A. C., Herkert, G. E., Bercz, J. P., and Smith, M. K. (1987). Evaluation of the developmental toxicity of sodium nitrite in Long-Evans rats. *Fundam. Appl. Toxicol. 9*:668–677.

Rowland, I. R. (1988). The toxicology of *N*-nitroso compounds. In *Nitrosamines: Toxicology and Microbiology*, M. J. Hill (ed.). Ellis Horwood Ltd., Chichester, pp. 117–141.

Rowland, I. R., Lake, B. G., Phillips, J. C., and Gangolli, S. D. (1980). Substrates and inhibitors of hepatic amine oxidase inhibit dimethylnitrosamine-induced mutagenesis in *Salmonella typhimurium*. *Mutation Res. 72*:63–72.

Sabadie, N., Malaviielle, C., Camus, A.-M., and Bartsch, H. (1980). Comparison of hydroxylation of benzo(a)pyrene with the metabolism of vinyl chloride, *N*-nitrosomorpholine and *N*-nitroso-*N'*-methylpiperazine to mutagens by human and rat liver microsomal fractions. *Cancer Res. 40*:119–126.

Sankaranrayan, K. (1981). Comparative mutagenicity of dimethylnitrosamine and diethylnitrosamine. *Environ. Sci. Res. 24*:787–855.

Scanlan, R. A. (1975). *N*-Nitrosamines in foods. *CRC Crit. Rev. Food Technol. 5*:357–402.

Sen, N. P., and Kubacki, S. J. (1987). Review of methodologies for the determination of nonvolatile *N*-nitroso compounds in foods. *Food Addit. Contamin. 4*:357–383.

Sen, N. P., Donaldson, B., Seaman, S., Iyengar, J., and Miles, W. F. (1976). Inhibition of nitrosamine formation in fried bacon by propyl gallate and L-ascorbyl palmitate. *J. Agric. Food Chem. 24*:397–401.

Shuker, D. E. G. (1988). The chemistry of nitrosation. In *Nitrosamines*, M. J. Hill (ed.). Ellis Horwood, Ltd., Chichester, pp. 48–67.

Shuval, H. I., and Gruener, N. (1977). Infant methemoglobinemia and other health effects of nitrates in drinking water. *Prog. Wat. Technol. 8*:183–193.

Siddiqi, M., and Preussmann, R. (1989). Esophageal cancer in Kashmir—an assessment. *J. Cancer Res. Clin. Oncol. 115*:111–117.

Singer, B. (1984). Alkylation of the O^6 of guanidine is only one of many chemical events that may initiate carcinogenesis. *Cancer Invest 2*:233–238.

Singer, G. M., Ji, C., Roman, J., Li, M. H., and Lijinsky, W. (1986). Nitrosamines and nitrosamine precursors in foods from Linxian, China, a high incidence area for oesophageal cancer. *Carcinogenesis* 7:733–736.

Sofos, J. N. (1981). Nitrite, sorbate and pH interaction in cured meat products. In *Proceedings of the 34th Reciprocal Meat Conference*, June 19–22, Oregon State University, Corvallis, OR, Vol. 34, pp. 104–120.

Sofos, J. N. (1989). *Sorbatic Food Preservatives*. CRC Press, Boca Raton, FL.

Sofos, J. N., and Busta, F. F. (1980). Alternatives to the use of nitrite as an antibotulinal agent. *Food Technol.* 34(5):244–251.

Sofos, J. N., Busta, F. F., and Allen, C. E. (1979a). Sodium nitrite and sorbic acid effects on *Clostridium botulinum* spore germination and total microbial growth in chicken frankfurter emulsions during temperature abuse. *Appl. Environ. Microbiol.* 37:1103–1109.

Sofos, J. N., Busta, F. F., and Allen, C. E. (1979b). *Clostridium botulinum* control by sodium nitrite and sorbic acid in various meat and soy protein formulations. *J. Food Sci.* 44:1662–1667.

Sofos, J. N., Busta, F. F., Bhothipaksa, K., and Allen, C. E. (1979c). Sodium nitrite and sorbic acid effects on *Clostridium botulinum* toxin formation in chicken frankfurter-type emulsions. *J. Food Sci.* 44:668–672.

Sofos, J. N., Busta, F. F., and Allen, C. E. (1979d). Effect of sodium nitrite on *Clostridium botulinum* toxin production in frankfurter emulsions formulated with meat and soy proteins. *J. Food Sci.* 44:1267–1271.

Sofos, J. N., Busta, F. F., and Allen, C. E. (1979e). Botulism control by nitrite and sorbate in cured meats: A review. *J. Food Protect.* 42:739–770.

Sofos, J. N., Busta, F. F., Bhothipaksa, K., Allen, C. E., Robach, M. C., and Paquette, M. W. (1980). Effects of various concentrations of sodium nitrite and potassium sorbate on *Clostridium botulinum* toxin production in commercially prepared bacon. *J. Food Sci.* 45:1285–1292.

Spiegelhalder, B., Eisenbrand, G., and Preussmann, R. (1980). Volatile nitrosamines in food. *Oncology* 37:211–216.

Streeter, A. J., Nims, R. W., Sheffels, P. R., Heur, Y.-H., Yang, C. S., Mico, B. A., Gombar, C. T., and Keefer, L. K. (1990). Metabolic denitrosation of N-nitrosodimethylamine in vivo in the rat. *Cancer Res.* 50:1144–1150.

Thust, R. (1982). Interindividual variation in carcinogen activation by human liver homogenates. A study using dimethylnitrosamine (DMN) and cyclophosphamide (CP) as precursor genotoxic agents and clastogenicity and induction of sister chromatid exchanges in Chinese hamster V79-E cells as endpoints. *Arch. Geschwulstforsch.* 52:97–104.

Tricker, A. R., and Kubacki, S. J. (1992). Review of the occurrence and formation of nonvolatile N-nitroso compounds in foods. *Food Add. Contam.* 9:39–69.

Tricker, A. R., and Preussmann, R. (1991). Carcinogenic N-nitrosamines in the diet: Occurrence, formation, mechanisms and carcinogenic potential. *Mutation Res.* 259:277–289.

Tyburczyk, W., Borkowska, J., Klimek, K., and Galicki, D. (1989). Effect of combined action of sodium nitrite and phenitrotione on certain biochemical parameters in rat blood. *Rocan. PZH.* 40:58–64.

Urbanek-Karlowska, B., and Fonberg-Broczek, B. (1986). Effect of sodium nitrite and amidopyrine administration on hepatic level of nucleic acids in the rat. *Roczn. PZH.* 37:228–234.

Vasselinovitch, S. D., Koka, M., Mihailovich, N., and Rao, K. V. N. (1984). Carcinogenicity of diethylnitrosamine in newborn, infant and adult mice. *J. Cancer Res. Clin. Oncol.* 108:60–65.

Walker, E. A., Pignatelli, B., and Castegnaro, M. (1979). Catalytic effect of *p*-nitrosophenol on the nitrosation of diethylamine. *J. Agric. Food Chem. 27*:393–396.

Walker, E. A., Pignatelli, B., and Friesen, M. (1982). The role of phenols in catalysis of nitrosamine formation. *J. Sci. Food Agric. 33*:81–88.

Watanabe, M., Honda, S., Hayashi, M., and Matsuda, T. (1982). Mutagenic effects of combination of chemical carcinogens and environmental pollutants in mice as shown by the micronucleus test. *Mutation Res. 97*:43–48.

Watts, B. M., and Lehmann, B. T. (1952). The effect of ascorbic acid on the oxidation of hemoglobin and the formation of nitric oxide hemoglobin. *Food Res. 17*:100–108.

Weisburger, J., Marquardt, H., and Hirota, N. (1980). Induction of cancer of the glandular stomach in rats by extract and nitrite treated fish. *J. Natl. Cancer Inst. 64*:163–167.

WHO (World Health Organization). (1985). *Health Hazards from Nitrates in Drinking Water*. Report of WHO Working Party.

Yahagi, T., Nagao, M., Seino, Y., Matsushima, T., Sugimura, T., and Okada, M. (1977). Mutagenicities of *N*-nitrosamines on *Salmonella. Mutation Res. 48*:121–130.

Yamamoto, M., Ishiwata, H., Yamada, T., Yoshinira, K., and Tanimura, A. (1987). Studies in the guinea-pig stomach on the formation *N*-nitrosomethylurea, from methylurea and sodium nitrite and its disappearance. *Food Cosmet. Toxicol. 25*:663–668.

Yang, C. S. (1980). Research on oesophageal cancer in China: a review. *Cancer Res. 40*:2633–2644.

Zubillaga, M. P., Maerker, G., and Foglia, T. A. (1984). Antioxidant activity of sodium nitrite in meat. *J. Am. Oil Chem. Soc. 61*:772–775.

6
Flavoring Agents

Robert Leslie Swaine, Jr.
The Procter & Gamble Company
Cincinnati, Ohio

I. INTRODUCTION

The objective of this chapter is to provide the toxicologist with insight and perspective as to the origin, manufacture, use, and safety considerations of flavoring agents. It is not a toxicology reference manual, rather it is written for the toxicologist who wants to obtain an introduction to flavoring agents. The chemical nature and derivation of flavoring substances will be stressed, and while several examples of known toxins will be discussed, the safety and toxicological data for all flavoring agents is beyond the scope of this chapter. For comprehensive individual toxicological studies, the reader is referred to resources such as *The National Toxicology Program Technical Report Series* and *The Registry of Toxic Effects of Chemical Substances*, available through the U.S. Department of Health and Human Services.

It is appropriate, if not ironic, to include flavoring agents (flavorings) in this endeavor since many flavoring agents are pharmacologically active and, of course, according to the dose, may be toxic to some organisms, even humans. For example, vanilla extract is toxic to humans, but the LD_{50} is estimated to be 4.0 pounds (Hodge and Downs, 1961). Actually, much of modern flavor chemistry has its roots in the early pharmaceutical industry. A search of official compendia, some as late as NF XII, reveals the codification of many of today's flavorings and flavoring agents not only for their organoleptic value but also for their pharmaceutical actions (Table 1). Some flavorings still exist in current compendia. Their use, however, is almost exclusively as a flavoring, more specifically as a masking agent for unpalatable medicinal principles. Exceptions include clove bud oil, used as a local anesthetic for toothaches, and enteric-coated peppermint oil, used for irritable bowel syndrome (Evans and Rhodes, 1979).

The reasons for using flavorings and flavoring agents may appear obvious, but a closer examination of such agents reveals perhaps as many subtleties and nuances

Table 1   Early Flavoring Agents Codified as Pharmaceuticals

Agent	Action
Anethole	Calmative
Anise oil	Calmative
Caraway oil	Calmative
Cardamom oil	Calmative, aromatic, stomachic
Cinnamon oil	Calmative
Clove oil	Aromatic
Coriander oil	Stomachic
Ethyl vanillin	Preservative
Eucalyptol	Antiseptic, inhalant
Eucalyptus oil	Bacteriostat, expectorant
Fennel oil	Calmative
Lavendar oil	Calmative, aromatic
Methyl salicylate	Counterirritant
Nutmeg oil	Calmative, G.I. stimulant
Peppermint oil	Calmative, antiseptic, local anesthetic
Phenyl ethyl alcohol	Antibacterial
Pine needle oil	Inhalent
Rosemary oil	Rubifacient
Spearmint oil	Calmative
Tolu balsam	Expectorant

as a good flavoring itself. Flavor is that property of a food or beverage that causes the simultaneous reaction of taste on the tongue and odor in the olfactory center of the nose. Flavoring agents are those substances that, when added to a food or beverage, impart flavor, i.e., evoke those simultaneous responses. The classical flavorist, then, uses flavorings with one of three main objectives (Swaine, 1972):

1. To impart the characteristic flavor of the flavoring: e.g., vanillin to give the flavor of vanilla to ice cream
2. To augment, complement, or modify a flavor: e.g., vanillin to modify the flavor of chocolate or cocoa
3. To mask the original flavor: e.g., anise to cover bitter medicinals

Recently the use of flavorings has been expanded to include interesting new roles.

1. Antioxidant
    Various spices and herbs and their extracts have been shown to exhibit antioxidant properties in a variety of food systems (Simon, 1990). These include:

Allspice	Clove
Mace	Cinnamon
Ginger	Oregano
Black pepper	White pepper
Bay	Coriander
Sage	Rosemary

The compounds responsible for the antioxidant activity in extract of rosemary are phenolic in nature. One such compound, rosmaridiphenol and the mechanisms of antioxidants are shown in Figure 1.

2. Antimicrobial (Bactericidal)

Both clove bud oil and cinnamon oil have long been used in oral care and skin care preparations. Today they are common components in dentrifices and oral rinses. Garlic oil, because of its selective bactericidal action, is part of the current revival of folk-type medicines. Garlic oil acts selectively in food systems such as salami to prevent the growth of unwanted bacteria while permitting desirable microbes to flourish and produce the desired flavor and color.

Kubo et al. (1991) have demonstrated antimicrobial activity in the 10 most abundant chemicals in cardamom. These constituents—1,8-cineole, α-terpinyl acetate, linalool, linalyl acetate, geraniol, limonene, α-terpinene, safrole, methyl eugenol, and eugenol—are all common flavoring agents or constituents of flavoring (essential) oils.

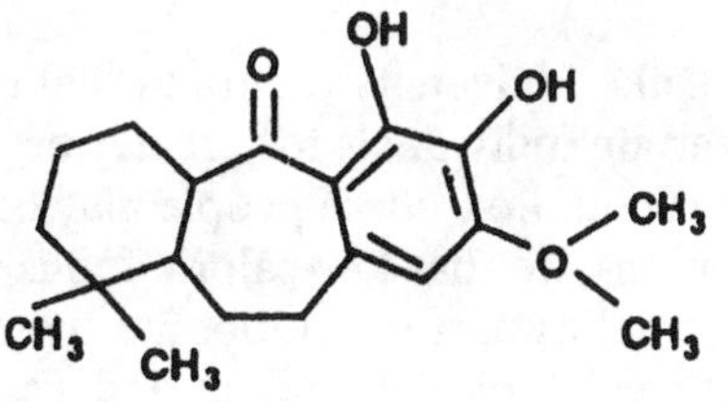

These phenolic compounds interrupt free radical formation by donating a hydrogen ion to a free radical to reform the original molecule.

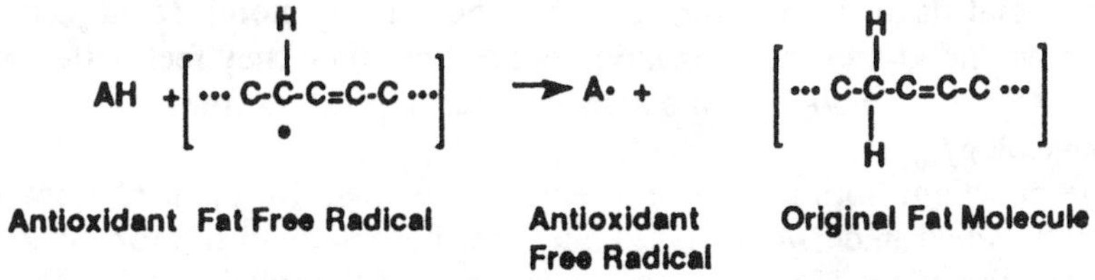

| Antioxidant | Fat Free Radical | Antioxidant Free Radical | Original Fat Molecule |

They also may donate hydrogen ions to peroxides, forming hydroperoxides and preventing free radical formation in other molecules.

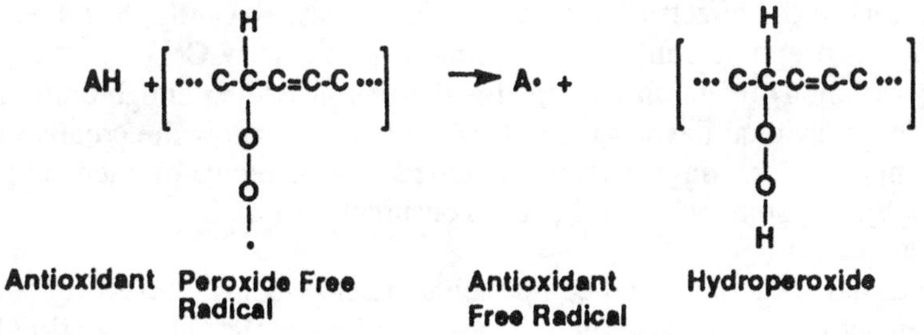

| Antioxidant | Peroxide Free Radical | Antioxidant Free Radical | Hydroperoxide |

Fig. 1   Natural phenolic antioxidant.

Pellecuer et al. (1983) have established the antibacterial spectrum for certain gram-positive and gram-negative bacterial flora using thyme oil, rosemary oil, and lavender oil. Antimicrobial activity may allow the food scientist to reduce or eliminate added preservatives. This may have significant economic and consumer implications.

3. Color

Paprika and turmeric, both as ground spices and as extracts, are used to add color to culinary items.

4. Enzymatic Activity

Certain herbs and spices contain proteolytic and lipolytic enzymes. These are involved in flavor generation in many traditional dishes and ripened foods, such as certain Scandinavian fish preparations.

5. Physiological Effects

Several herbs and spices are used for their side effects as well as for their characteristic flavor. Digestive beverages and breath fresheners, especially common in Europe, make use of cardamom, caraway, sweet marjoram, and thyme. Mustard also has been reported to stimulate the digestive process. Procter & Gamble (Tsai et al., 1990) has demonstrated that extracts of green tea ameliorate the state of anxiety and agitation induced by caffeine.

6. Health Benefits

Schiffman (1986) at Duke University theorizes that obesity may be caused by the requirement of certain individuals for greater organoleptic signals, such as taste and odor in their food, i.e., obese people may have an exaggerated flavor setpoint. The implications are that low-calorie foods with high intensity flavor profiles may be beneficial as part of antiobesity therapy.

Providing a more palatable, appealing and varied diet is important in insuring the consumption of sufficient nutrients. Lyman (1989) has shown in preliminary experiments that eating in general makes one happier. The effect, however, was dependent on the subject's initial mood. Generally his results suggest that flavor associations enhance the existing mood. If subjects are in a positive mood and the association is positive, then they feel better; if they are in a negative mood and the association is unpleasant, they will feel worse!

7. Aromacology

While olfaction, both from a biochemical and cognitive point of view, is still not completely understood, researchers in the new field of aromacology are studying the effect of aromas on the function of the mind and the body (van Toller, 1991). Common biological measurements such as skin potential level, eye movement, pupil dilation, pulse wave, and blood pressure are unreliable indicators of the effects of aromas and flavorings. Recently, however, the use of electroencephalographic measurement, particularly CNV (contingent negative variation), of brain electrical activity is providing enlightening insights. Data on individual flavoring agents will eventually allow the creative flavorist to compound flavorings that, when added to a beverage or chewing gum, for example, will stimulate or relax the consumer.

8. Therapeutic Agent

Several flavoring oils or oil components are now being studied for their anticancer activity. Organosulfur compounds from garlic oil may stimulate the activity of anticancer enzymes in the liver. d-Limonene, the major component in citrus oils, has been implicated in breast cancer prevention in animals. Other flavoring agents with antioxidant properties may also find application in anticancer therapy. Antioxidants have been shown to exhibit anticancer effects, most probably by complexing with free radicals prior to any deleterious effects on the body cells nucleic acids (Cheetham and Lecchini, 1988).

The impact of flavorings on the food and beverage industry is dynamic and involves more applications than one could have envisioned even a few decades ago.

II. HISTORY AND INDUSTRY PERSPECTIVE

The discovery and evolution of flavoring agents and subsequently the flavor industry was most probably serendipitous. While the exact origins are still unknown, archeologists and flavor chemists alike can speculate as to the historical role of flavoring agents.

Archeologists do, however, believe that the knowledge and use of seasonings can be traced as far back as 50,000 years. Primitive experiences with flavoring agents could have been when humans cooking meat over different types of wood observed the variation in flavor (Swaine, 1972). Early humans may also have used leaves to protect food from dirt only to discover that upon heating (cooking) a most enjoyable flavor resulted from certain leaves. They probably also learned, probably too late, that certain flora were to be avoided. This most likely led people to gather other leaves, roots, and berries, perhaps blending them in unique proportions or mixing them with wild honey, thus preparing some of the first flavorings. These crude flavoring agents added variety to the rather monotonous diet. They may even have discovered that certain concoctions or processes made palatable food that may have otherwise been unfit for human consumption, a custom that was to be practiced for centuries to come.

Spices played an important part in several religions. Spices are referred to in the scriptures of the Assyrians (ca. 3000 B.C.). There are numerous references in the Bible to spices and the spice trade. When the Queen of Sheba visited King Solomon (I Kings 10) (ca. 1000 B.C.) she brought offerings of spice (Hodson, 1981).

In the Orient spices were used to introduce variety into a diet consisting mainly of rice. Cassia, for example, was known as early as 2700 B.C.

In the main, spices that have come to be significant items of commerce were indigenous to the East, India, Ceylon, Sumatra, Java, Bali, and the Molucca Islands. The spice trade that developed between the Mediterranean region (the ancient Greek and Roman civilizations) and the East was most likely the beginning of the flavor industry as we know it today. Among the more popular spices (flavoring agents) of the ancient Greeks and Romans were pepper, cassia, cinnamon, ginger, anise, caraway, fennel, coriander, and mint.

The Greek and Roman cultures spread throughout Europe and with them the appreciation for and knowledge of spices. Mustard, for example, was introduced into England in 50 B.C. by Roman soldiers. These new spices were not only flavorings but also valuable barter. The trade between Europe and the Orient ceased with the decline of the great civilizations of the ancient world. During this period the Islamic empire was rapidly expanding. Its newly found control over the spice trade ensured and strengthened its commercial position and religious posture. The

Muslims held captive the spice market for several hundred years. It was in the tenth century A.D. that the European spice trade enjoyed a revival. Spices were quite dear to the Europeans. One must be mindful that the diet at this point in history was at best monotonous and more often than not putrid or at least partially spoiled. Spices provided a welcome change and even a sense of adventure and romance since the spices came from faraway lands whose origins were shrouded in mystery. Further, the spices made spoiled food palatable.

During the late thirteenth century the monopoly on spice trade ended. Following his expeditions through the New East, Central and South Asia, and the exotic Pacific islands, Marco Polo recounted his exploits including his rediscovery of spices: ginger in China, cinnamon in Ceylon, pepper in Borneo, and nutmeg in the Pacific islands. The next several centuries saw exploration by sea and new trade routes develop in the East, Central America, and the Caribbean. New spices such as paprika, cayenne, and allspice were introduced into the kitchens of Europe.

The Middle Ages saw the early use of chemistry to develop flavoring agents. The alchemist in his search for "the elixir of life" used distillation to prepare or to concentrate essences from herbs. History actually credits Avicenna, an Arab physician in the tenth century, as being the first to isolate volatile oils from plant material using distillation. These extracts or volatile oils became increasingly more important to the alchemist, the druggist, the doctor, and finally to the creative flavorist. By the beginning of the sixteenth century only 13 volatile oils were widely used (Short, 1973): benzoin, rosemary, calamus, sage, cedarwood, spike (Lavender), costus, turpentine, mastic, juniperwood, rose, frankincense, and cinnamon. During the next century 66 volatile oils were used, and by the mid-1700s the number of oils had reached 100.

The crystallization of vanillin from an extract of vanilla beans in 1858 and the subsequent synthesis of vanillin in 1876 by Tiemann and Haarmann signaled the beginning of modern flavor chemistry. The organic chemist now began to assemble for the creative flavorist a much larger palette, containing both natural isolates and synthetic flavor chemicals. The advent of affordable sophisticated analytical instruments led to the identification of literally thousands of volatile aroma and flavor chemicals for foods and beverages. At last count some 6200 compounds had been identified in 320 foods (Maarse and Visscher, 1990). Figure 2 demonstrates the proliferation of flavor chemicals and patents during the past 2½ decades. The compounds identified still vastly outnumber the chemicals listed in the United States as generally recognized as safe (GRAS) for flavorings when used under conditions of intended use in accordance with Good Manufacturing Practices as defined by the Food, Drug and Cosmetic Act, section 182.1. The permutations of natural products and synthetic compounds seem, however, limited only by the imagination of the creative flavorist.

The flavor industry today records sales in excess of $3 billion per year. Since many flavor houses are still privately held, exact turnover is impossible to establish. Best estimates place third-party sales of compounded flavorings at $1.7 billion for 1986, $2.3 billion for 1987, and most recently $3.2 billion for 1990, $4.5 billion if one includes the sale of essential oils as well as of compounded flavorings (Broekhof, 1987; Matheis, 1989a; Unger, 1989; Abderhalden, 1991). Figure 3 demonstrates the use of flavoring according to industry. The 10 largest flavor houses account for approximately one third of this business. Aroma chemicals required

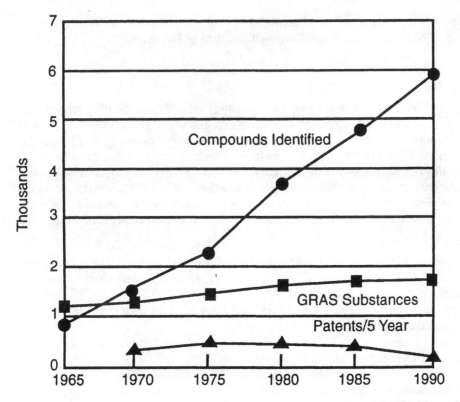

Fig. 2 Proliferation of flavor chemicals and patents. (From Maarse and Visscher, 1990.)

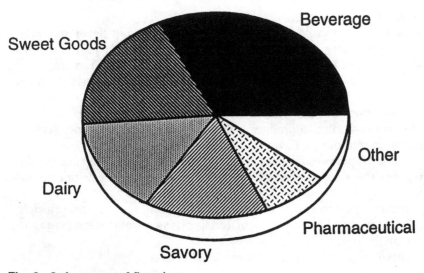

Fig. 3 Industry use of flavorings.

to support this volume may total another $750 million per annum. A healthy growth of 5–6% per year is anticipated through the turn of the century.

III. LEXICON

The flavor industry has developed a terminology reflective of the idiosyncrasies of the flavor chemist. Since certain terms are expressions of subjective observations and measurements, it may be difficult to define them. For example, is the essential oil of lemon citrusy, fruity, or is it refreshing? This may become clearer as individual terms are defined. Often research chemists and creative flavorists must discuss specific project requirements and review or develop new vocabulary at the inception of a project. The following are arbitrary definitions based on common industry practice and specific work in the Flavor Technology Laboratory of Procter & Gamble.

Absolute A highly concentrated form of plant material whose flavor is extremely similar to the starting material. An absolute is prepared by removing the alcohol-soluble portion of a concrete.

Accord A group of flavor notes that blend together to form one unique and harmonious composition.

Agrumen Flavor notes characteristic of citrus: orange, lemon, lime, tangerine, grapefruit, bergamot, and bitter orange.

Aldehydic Note from aliphatic fatty aldehydes containing 8–12 carbons. They possess fatty, waxy, and floral notes.

Aldehyde (So-Called) A potent flavor chemical, for example, γ-decalactone (aldehyde C14), or γ-nonalactone (aldehyde C 18). Many early synthetic flavoring agents were true aldehydes. They possessed great strength and diffusiveness. Flavorists came, therefore, to also call several new, potent flavor chemicals aldehydes.

Animalic Odor and flavor character of civet and castoreum. It is sometimes known as fecal.

Anosmia Loss of the sense of smell.

Aromatic Chemical A volatile chemical that has an odor and flavor property. This is a flavorist's term and should not be confused with a pure chemist's definition. It does not have to contain the typical benzene ring structure.

Balsamic A sweet, warm note typified by cinnamic alcohol or resinous plant exudates.

Blender A compound that has the ability to smooth or round a flavor, tying together the various notes to produce a harmonious effect. A blender such as vanilla may even introduce a flavor of its own.

Bottom Note The evaporative residue; the aroma present when the top and middle notes are gone. These tend to be higher molecular weight chemicals or resinous compounds.

Bulking A method used to ensure uniformity of flavoring agents. This principle is extremely important with natural raw materials that vary from season to season. Usually materials from various lots are mixed.

Burnt A charred or scorched note, or a smoky character.

Camphoraceous Fresh, clean medicinal flavor notes characterized by a resemblance to camphor.

Caramel Flavor of browned or burned sugar. Furaneol® is an example.

Compound 1. A true chemical compound. 2. A flavoring or part of a flavoring composed of two or more individual flavorings.

Concrete A waxy solid or semisolid extract produced by extraction, usually with a hydrocarbon solvent. It contains the essential oil, waxes, pigments, and fixed oil. The term concrete usually applies to flower material.

Deepener As with β-ionone in raspberry, a compound that enhances or reinforces the main theme.

Diffusive Flavor or odor that most rapidly permeates the air. Ylang Ylang is quite diffusive.

Earthy The odor of moist soil or a damp basement.

Essence A concentrated flavoring agent containing alcohol.

Essential Oil A volatile oil, usually possessing the characteristic odor and flavor of the plant from which it was isolated. These oils were once thought to be essential to the plant's life processes or communication.

Ethereal A spiritous, sharp, penetrating aroma.

Extract A water-soluble solution obtained by passing alcohol or a hydroalcoholic mixture through a substance. These should not be confused with official extracts, where the solvent is removed and the active constituent or flavoring subsequently standardized.

Fatigue Loss of the sensation of smell with respect to a specific odorant or flavoring. This is usually caused by continued exposure in sufficient concentration to an odorant.

Fixative A compound that reduces the overall volatility of a flavoring and results in a reduction in the loss of more volatile compounds.

Floral Odor reminiscent of flowers.

Fold Denotes the strength of a flavoring agent, particularly an essential oil or an extract.

Green A class of flavor notes characterized by intense fresh leafy odor. Six-carbon alcohols and aldehydes are green.

Isolate A chemical or fraction composed of several chemicals obtained from a natural source. Citronellal may be chemically isolated from citronella oil.

Main Note This is also known as the heart or the middle note. It is characteristic for a particular flavor system.

Masking Agent A compound that covers unwanted odors and flavors, e.g., as lemon oil covers fishiness.

Modifier A compound that changes (slightly) the overall character of a flavoring, e.g., citral in an orange composition.

Note A singular characteristic of a flavoring agent. Any flavoring, however, may be a blend of several notes and accords.

Oleoresin A resinous plant extractive prepared by extraction with a nonaqueous, usually hydrocarbon solvent. An oleoresin contains both the volatile fraction and the nonvolatile fraction, which may include pigments, waxes, fixed oils, gums, and resins. The nonvolatile portion contains, in the case of ginger and pepper, the pungent principles.

Safety   Reasonable certainty that a substance is not harmful under the conditions of use. This is a most difficult thing to determine on an absolute scale.

Tinctures   Cold alcoholic or hydroalcoholic solutions prepared from vegetable materials, essential oils, or chemical substances.

Topnote   The volatile note first observed upon exposure to a flavoring. It may be smelled or tasted and is usually suggestive of the flavor identity.

Woody   Flavor note provided by certain natural woods and their isolates. These have excellent fixative properties.

Many terms, especially those used to describe flavor sensations, are subjective. Commonly available chemicals and natural products that exemplify key flavor notes are shown in Table 2.

IV. FLAVOR PROCESSES

A. General Considerations

This section will discuss methods to commercially isolate or generate flavoring agents from natural raw materials. Natural raw materials in this context are botanical or animal products containing flavorful compounds or the precursors to flavoring agents. It is not the intention here to define natural products of flavorings for any legal or regulatory purpose. Flavor-labeling regulations still vary among

Table 2 Flavor Notes

Flavor note	Examples
Aldehydic	Decanal, undecanal, dodecanal
Alliacious	Allyl disulfide, onion oil, garlic oil
Almond	Benzaldehyde
Animalic	Civet, indole
Anise	Anethole
Balsamic	Balsam Peru, benzyl cinnamate
Bite	Capsicum, oleoresin black pepper
Brown	Maltol
Buttery	Diacetyl
Camphoracous	Isobornyl acetate, marjoram
Citrus	Orange oil, lemon oil
Peachy	Aldehyde C14 (so called)
Phenolic	Guaiacol, clove bud oil
Roast	2,3-Dimethyl pyrazine
Skunky	Dimethyl sulfide
Smoky	Guaiacol
Soapy	Decanal
Spicy	Eugenol, cinnamic aldehyde
Sweet	Vanillin
Vegetable	Galbanum, maté
Violet	β-Ionone, methyl octyne carbonate
Waxy	2,4-Decadienal
Woody	Sandalwood, Vetiver, γ-methyl ionone

many countries, and even within a specific country they may be subject to interpretation. Interpretation and renderings are better left to the legal or regulatory divisions of individual companies or trade organizations.

The objective of the preparation of a flavoring agent is to reproduce or develop with the highest degree of fidelity that odor and flavor quality possessing the desirable characteristic of a certain raw material (e.g., orange oil from orange juice and rind) or finished food (e.g., roast beef from amino acid and reducing sugar precursors). The following sections will describe some of the factors that govern the means by which flavoring agents are processed and the implications of these choices on quality.

Tradition

The means used to grow, harvest, and process a particular botanical all influence the flavor quality. In certain locales it may be traditional to harvest crops manually or to process by means of an established but outdated technology. The flavor quality generated by this means may, however, be the industry standard and unattainable by other means.

Resources Available

It is not always convenient or practical to transport freshly harvested botanicals from an agricultural center to a processing or industrial center. In these instances processing must be done on site, and under these circumstances state-of-the-art equipment is not always available. Processing must be done within a very well-prescribed period of time, or postharvest deterioration of the harvested materials and a corresponding deterioration in flavor quality can result. In some instances a partial processing is done, and this partially processed material is then shipped to a site equipped with more sophisticated apparatus where the processing is completed. One must also consider the technical expertise and cost of labor at processing sites and in agricultural regions.

Economics

When one considers that the yield of an essential oil can be maximized by harvesting only at a particular time of day, it is readily apparent that every decision that is made in the isolation of flavoring agents from natural sources has serious economic repercussions. Partial production at a remote site may positively influence economics. The production of a concrete at one location near or in the growing region and its shipment to a second area for further processing reduces the amount of raw material that has to be transported, an obvious cost savings.

The final application for a flavoring should greatly influence the processing. Elaborate isolation techniques such as industrial-scale gas chromatography or supercritical fluid extraction are among emerging technologies that can produce exquisite flavoring agents. These techniques, however, carry with them in most instances extreme burdens of cost. The question must always be asked: Is the perceived value of a flavoring the same as the market value? Not all food and beverage formulations can afford the most elaborately processed flavoring. Similarly, the purity of a processed botanical can influence cost, and again the final use governs the cost. A chemically pure isolate may be required in perfumery work, while a more complex, less pure fraction may do quite well for most flavor applications.

Alternate processing methods can deliver different yields, as well as a variety of byproducts. The ability to identify byproduct streams and find industrial application aids the financial considerations of the basic flavoring. The fractionation of citrus peel oils is a good example. The preparation of a more concentrated version of an orange oil, a 5× (5-fold), yields 20 pounds of the more valuable, more flavorful 5× orange oil and 80 lb of orange terpenes. Rather than treating these terpenes as waste to discard, essential oil manufacturers found a market for the terpene byproduct. Terpenes are used in flavor-cloud emulsions for beverages. They are also sold to the perfume industry. Assume that orange peel oil costs an essential oil manufacturer $1.65/kg, and that the value of this 1× oil to a third party is $2.75/kg, and that the value of 5× and terpenes are $7.75 and $2.45/kg, respectively. From the sale of 100 kg of 1× oil the essential oil manufacturer would receive $275, whereas $155 from 20 kg of 5× oil plus $196 from the sale of 80 kg of terpenes would increase the total to $351.

Application

The final application impacts the method of manufacture not only economically but also functionally. A cloudy citrus beverage would require a citrus oil containing a high concentration of terpenes, while a clear (Up-type) citrus beverage would require a citrus oil with a high degree of water solubility, hence an oil with diminished terpene content.

Ease of Recovery of Flavoring Agents

The anatomical location of the volatiles within the plant (or animal) and the ease of removal is also a factor in determining the processing method. Essential oils may be located in soft tissues (cold pressed orange oil) that are easily ruptured or abraded to yield the flavorful oil. The converse may also be true. Volatiles may be "locked away" in hard tissues that must be comminuted, macerated, or heated to affect the release of volatile flavorings, for example, cinnamon.

Origin

The country and even the region within a given country can greatly influence the chemical and hence the flavor properties of a natural product. Crop-to-crop and seasonal variations may be at least partially overcome by bulking raw materials. The time of year and even the time of day a botanical is harvested influences the final flavor. The climate, growing conditions, and soil all influence volatile formation. For this reason it is always wise to specify with as much accuracy as possible the source of a naturally processed flavoring. This not only ensures consistency but also assures that the purchaser receives the quality contracted. Boelens and Jimenez (1990) identified qualitative differences in lemon oils from Spain and Italy (Table 3). Flavorists measure quality of lemon oils by the citral content. Applying this measurement of quality to the Spanish and Italian lemon oils, it is apparent that the Italian oil, with a citral content of 2.905% vs. 1.520% for the Spanish oil, should be more highly valued. (Citral is the sum of the isomers neral and geranial.)

Roberts et al. (1983) demonstrated gross difference in the gas chromatographic profile of geranium essential oil produced in China and the United States (Table 4).

Table 3 Comparative Chemical Composition (%) of Spanish and Italian Lemon Oil

Compound	Spanish oil	Italian oil
α-Thujene	0.351	0.239
α-Pinene	1.580	2.082
Camphene	0.065	0.210
Sabinene	1.287	1.700
β-Pinene	8.908	12.172
Myrcene	1.929	1.183
α-Phellandrene	0.099	0.102
δ-3-Carene	0.002	0.066
α-Terpinene	0.172	0.176
p-Cymene	0.070	0.101
Limonene	70.362	67.577
(E)-β-Ocimene	0.588	t[a]
γ-Terpinolene	8.716	6.979
Terpinolene	0.458	0.393
Octanal	0.090	0.171
Nonanal	0.118	0.092
Decanal	0.033	0.055
(E,Z)-2,4-Decadienal	0.008	0.005
(E,E)-2,4-Decadienal	0.005	0.003
Undecanal	0.015	0.026
Dodecanal	0.027	0.010
Myrtenal	t	0.031
Citronellal	0.090	0.069
Neral	0.572	1.227
Geranial	0.948	1.678
Perillaldehyde	0.038	0.047
Linalool	0.114	0.852
Terpinen-4-ol	0.021	0.033
α-Terpineol	0.167	0.176
Nerol	0.017	0.066
Geraniol	0.045	0.269
Citronellol	0.011	0.016
α-Terpinyl acetate	0.026	0.019
Neryl acetate	0.264	0.346
Geranyl acetate	0.261	0.233
Citronellyl acetate	t	0.016
p-Mentha-1,8-dien-10yl acetate	t	t
Sesquiterpene HC	1.405	0.695

Source: Boelens and Jimenez, 1990.
[a]t = trace.

Chemical Nature of Flavoring Agents

Knowledge of the chemical properties including volatility, solubility, thermal liability, and reactivity are essential in determining the processing of a flavoring. For example, if an essential oil contains components that are thermally labile, it may be wise to use a solvent extraction rather than a thermally intensive process such

Table 4 Distribution (%) of Components of Geranium Oil

	China	United States
α-Pinene	0.35	0.30
Z-rose oxide	2.25	1.09
E-rose oxide	1.04	0.71
Menthone	1.94	0.69
Isomenthone	4.51	6.30
Linalool	3.79	1.89
Citronellyl formate	17.45	24.40
Geranyl formate	2.20	4.97
Citronellyl propionate	2.20	5.48
Citronellol	44.39	29.23
Geranyl propionate	0.60	1.29
Geraniol	6.40	7.41
Geranyl butyrate	0.73	1.96
10 Epi-γ eudesmol	2.03	2.77
Geranyl tiglate	1.64	1.40

Source: Roberts et al., 1983.

as distillation to recover the oil. The choice of solvents is now important, as a solvent can result in selective extraction of components and the tailoring of an odor profile. It should also be noted that extraction is useful in removing less volatile compounds that don't easily distill (e.g., vanilla). If the products to be isolated are sufficiently volatile and thermally stable, then distillation may be used. Again, however, there are choices to be made. Flavoring agents containing significant proportions of compounds (e.g., esters) that decompose readily under heat and aqueous conditions should not be isolated using simple water distillation. Here steam distillation may be the process of choice. Flavorings containing extremely volatile but labile compounds may require molecular distillation.

Storage and Handling

Since great care has of necessity gone into the processing of flavorings from natural products, an equal amount of thought should be applied to the manner in which these flavorings are stored. The containers must be inert so as not to enter into reactions with the flavoring. Containers should occlude light and oxygen, which can accelerate deterioration. The headspace should be minimized or filled with an inert gas. It is wise, where practical, to store flavoring components at reduced temperatures. Special precautions are required to maintain the integrity of certain flavoring agents. Antioxidants may be added to terpene-containing or aldehydic oils. Compounds such as z-3-hexenal, which tend to isomerize, or acetaldehyde (ethanal), which polymerize, are best stored as dilutions in the appropriate solvents at refrigerated conditions. Acetaldehyde (7) is known to polymerize to paraldehyde (8) (see Fig. 4).

Paraldehyde is one of the oldest hypnotics known. It also irritates the throat and gastric mucosa. The amount of acetaldehyde used in a flavoring will, however, generally be consumed at less than 10 ppm.

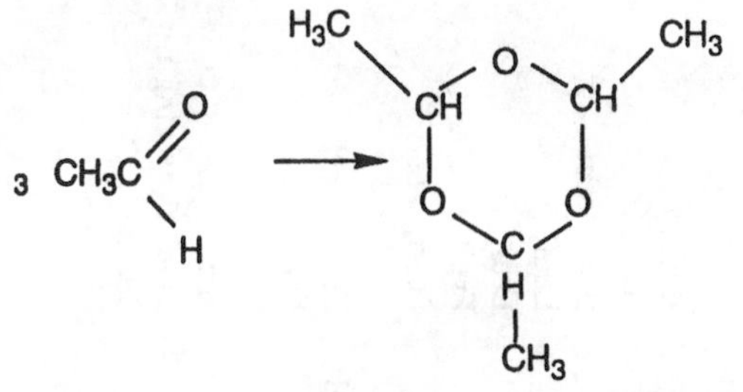

Fig. 4 Polymerization of acetaldehyde.

If preblends are stored for any length of time prior to dilution, interactions may occur. For example, patchouly essential oil and clove bud essential oil can cause a dark color change. Anthranilates and aldehydes, if not properly diluted, will form viscous, brightly colored aldimines.

B. Whole and Ground Spices and Herbs

This first group of flavoring agents represents the oldest and most fundamental class. As a class they are multifunctional. They are highly aromatic and colorful; several possess antioxidant activity, and several possess hot or pungent principles. Spices are defined rather broadly as the products of dried (aromatic) plant materials essentially used for their flavoring properties in foods. This would also include herbal material, perhaps viewed as a subset of this class and defined as soft-stemmed plants whose main stem dies down to ground level. The plants may be annuals, biennials, or perennials. Spices may be used as whole or ground seasonings. Herbs likewise may be used whole (fresh or dehydrated) or may be screened (broken, rubbed). Spices generally contain higher quantities of volatile oil and coloring matter. While spices do not represent the economic significance they did to international commerce in the Middle Ages, they are still a popular form of flavoring and, perhaps due to the increasing popularity of ethnic foods beginning in the 1970s, are enjoying a rebirth.

Herbs are processed and sold in several different forms (Fig. 5). Herbs are first cleaned. The cleanliness of the incoming herbs is a major concern to the processor. The clean, whole herb is the first herb form marketed. After cleaning the herb is sliced. The leaves are cut into 3- to 6-mm-diameter pieces. The herbs are then ready for transport for further processing. The next step involves removing the hard stems by coarsely screening the leaves and other soft herbaceous parts, a process known as rubbing. The resultant product is a very commonly marketed form of herb. The broken or rubbed herbs may be further processed by grinding to a specific particle size. Various forms of herbs may be combined to form unique, proprietary seasoning blends or sold individually. During each step of processing, loss of volatiles is a major concern.

Spices too may be sold as whole spices, in the ground form, or as seasoning blends. Like herbs, they may be used for their flavoring properties or, as with

Table 5 Principal Culinary Herbs and Spices

Biotanical	Herb/Spice	Scientific name	Geographical source	Part used
Allspice	Spice	*Pimenta dioica*	Jamaica, Guatemala Honduras, Mexico	Fruit (berry)
Anise	Spice	*Pimpinella anisum*	Europe, CIS	Seed
Basil	Herb	*Ocimum basilicum*	Mediterranean, United States, Madagascar, Comores	Leaf
Bay laurel	Herb	*Laurus nobilis*	Mediterranean	Leaf
Capsicum	Spice	*Capsicum frutescens*	Europe, South America	Fruit
Caraway	Spice	*Carum carvi*	Netherlands, Poland, Egypt, Hungary	Fruit
Cardamom	Spice	*Elettaria cardamomum*	India, Guatemala, Costa Rica, Sri Lanka, El Salvador	Seed
Cassia	Spice	*Cinnamomum cassia*	China, Vietnam, Burma	Bark
Cinnamon	Spice	*Cinnamomum zeylanicum*	Sri Lanka, Seychelles, Vietnam, Brazil	Bark
Clove	Spice	*Syzygium aromaticum*	Tanzania, Sri Lanka	Bud, stem
		Euginia caryophyllus	Malaysia, Malagassy Republic	Leaf
Coriander	Spice	*Coriandrum sativa*	CIS, India, North Africa	Fruit
Cumin	Spice	*Cuminum cyminum*	Mediterranean, India, CIS	Fruit
Dill	Spice	*Anethum graveolens*	United States, CIS, Hungary, Poland, Egypt, Bulgaria	Seed, weed
Fennel	Spice	*Foeniculum vulgare*	Egypt, Spain, China, CIS, Bulgaria, Italy	Fruit, seed
Ginger	Spice	*Zingiber officinale*	Jamaica, China, India, West Africa, Australia	Rhizome
Mace	Spice	*Myristica fragrans*	Graneda, Sri Lanka	Aril
Marjoram	Herb	*Majorana hortensis*	Morocco, Egypt	Leaf, flowering tip
Mustard	Spice	*Brassica nigra* (black) *B. juncea* (brown) *B. hirta* or *alba* (white)	Southwest Asia, Europe, California	Seed

Common Name	Type	Scientific Name	Origin	Part
Nutmeg	Spice	Myristica fragens	West Indies, Indonesia, Sri Lanka	Seed
Origanum	Herb	Origanum spp.	Spain, Albania	Leaf, floral parts
Paprika	Spice	Capsicum annuum	Central America, Hungary, Spain	Fruit
Parsley	Spice	Petrosilinum sativa	UK, United States, Germany, Hungary	Seed
		P. crispum		Top
Pepper	Spice	Piper nigrum	India, Malaysia, Singapore, Indonesia, West Africa, Sri Lanka, Brazil, Vietnam	Fruit
Peppermint	Herb	Mentha piperita	United States, Eastern Europe, Italy	Leaf
Rosemary	Herb	Rosmarinus officinalis	Spain, Tunisia, Morocco	Leaf
Saffron	Spice	Crocus sativas	Spain, China, France	Stigma
Sage	Herb	Salvia triloba (Greek)	CIS, United States	Leaf
		S. officinalis (Dalmation)	Albania, Yugoslavia	
		S. lavandularfolia (Spanish)	Spain	
Savory	Herb	Satureia hortensis	Spain, Morocco, Yugoslavia	Leaf, flowering top
Spearmint	Herb	Mentha spicata	United States, China	Leaf
Tarragon	Herb	Artemisia dracunculus	Central, East Europe	Leaf
Thyme	Herb	Thymus vulgaris	Spain	Leaf, floral parts
Turmeric	Spice	Curcuma longa	India, Sri Lanka, Malaysia	Rhizome

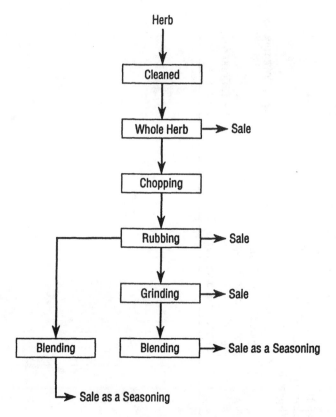

Fig. 5 Processing of whole and ground herbs.

sesame seeds or allspice, to provide visual and textural aesthetics. Few spices, however, can be directly incorporated into foods. They must therefore be milled or ground. Precautions such as subambient processing must be employed to avoid volatile loss during milling and comminution. Cleanliness is also a major concern to the processor. Spices are a rich source of viable bacteria, thermophilic aerobic bacteria and spores, yeasts, and molds, some of which may be pathogenic (Krishnaswamy et al., 1979). A bacterial count for an untreated ground spice is as high as $1 \times 10^7/g$. It is necessary, therefore to eliminate this contamination by use of sterilizing gases (ethylene oxide, propylene oxide, dichlorofluoromethane), heat processing, or exposure to gamma irradiation. Alternatively, the flavor, pungent, or color principles may be isolated from the spice.

A compilation of the major culinary herbs and spices may be found in Table 5. This class of flavoring agent, while finding diverse application as both a flavoring agent and a garnish, has both advantages and limitations. These can be summarized (Swaine, 1972; Heath and Reineccius, 1986) as follows:

Advantages	Disadvantages
May contain natural antioxidants	Weak flavor
May contain some antibacterial activity	Introduces color (sometimes undesirable)

Maintains flavor integrity	Batch-to-batch variation (both strength and profile)
Flavor fidelity	Longer time to reach equilibrium with surroundings
Ease of handling	High microbiological load
Gradual flavor release during thermal processing	Readily adulterated
	Presence of enzymes
	Limited shelf life (loss or change of flavor)
	Poor flavor distribution
	Dusty

Whole and ground herbs and spices are used today in a diverse range of products, which includes picked products, baked goods, confections, soups, sauces, gravies, catsup, processed meat, pizza, salad dressing, chili, condiments, entrees, and croutons.

C. Expression and Recovery of Citrus Flavorings

Citrus fruits have most desirable aromas and flavors. Their aroma is refreshing and connotes health, wholesomeness, and vitality. Citrus fruits have been eaten for centuries. While they are an integral part of a healthy diet (Kramer in 1732 first reported antisorbitic activity in citrus fruits), they were probably first enjoyed for their sweet appealing flavor. The flavoring agents obtained from citrus are mainly byproducts. The development of the TASTE (thermally accelerated short time evaporator) evaporator shortly after World War II and the essence recovery unit pioneered by Dr. James B. Redd have greatly enhanced the citrus processor's ability to process fruit and recover valuable flavorings as byproducts.

Since citrus peel oil is located in oil glands near the surface of the peel or rind (the flavedo), oil is easily recovered by rupturing, scarification, or grating. This is a much gentler process than was first practiced in the Middle Ages, when oils were prepared by distillation. The subepidermal layer of the flavedo consists of several layers of small cells and then several layers of larger cells that fill in the areas between the oil glands. Oil glands enlarge as fruit ripens. Commercially the peel oil is recovered during the processing of the citrus fruit. A schematic diagram depicting typical orange juice processing is shown as Figure 6. Since the expression and recovery of citrus oils is an integral part of citrus juice concentration, an overview of orange juice manufacture will add perspective.

The fruit is first washed and graded. Some manufacturers choose to remove the majority of the peel oil following the grading and prior to the fruit sizing. This is shown in Figure 6 as option 1 and is classified as extraction from the whole fruit. The Brown Oil Extractor (BOE) is widely used for this type of extraction. The BOE has a bed of rollers equipped with sharp needles partially submerged in a tank of water. The fruit is passed through this tank and has its flavedo abraded or pierced by the metal discs containing pointed teeth or needles. Peel oil is released and forms an emulsion with the water. The oil is then separated by centrifugation, sometimes with the aid of enzymes used to crack the emulsion. The fruit is then ready for extraction. It is sliced in half and reamed to liberate or extract the juice. Juice is next sent to a series of finishers to remove pulp. An alternate method (Fig. 6, option 2) uses simultaneous peel oil and juice extraction. In this process (FMC)

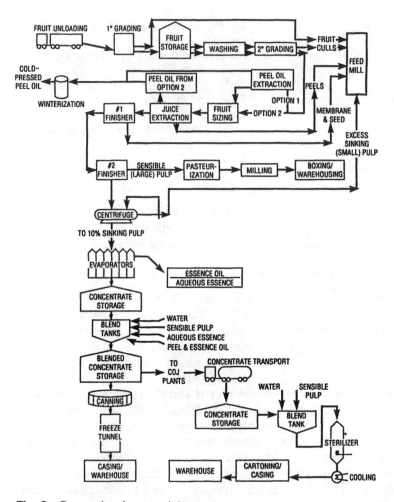

Fig. 6 Conventional orange juice process.

the fruit proceeds from sizing to extraction. The FMC machine uses a single piece of equipment to both "squeeze" the fruit, liberating juice, and rupture oil cells in the peel. Juice is collected and distributed to finishers while the oil-water emulsion is sent to centrifuges.

The process is now similar for both oil-extraction options. The oil is stored for several months at reduced temperatures (0–40°F). This process is called winterization. It removes waxes and other higher molecular weight nonvolatiles. Peel oil is then sold or further processed to make folded oils or specialties. Following a final centrifugation to standardize the pulp, the juice is concentrated. The most common means is the TASTE evaporator. Other evaporators such as the Schmidt have also been used. During the evaporation additional flavorings are recovered. A substantial quantity of aromatics are present in the first 25% of the juice that is evaporated. Recovery units (essentially a fractionating distillation unit equipped with multiple condensers) condense, collect, and concentrate vapors from the TASTE. The condensate is separated into an oil phase, known as essence or phase oil, and an aqueous phase, known as the aqueous essence or water phase essence. These recovered oils and essences are becoming increasingly more important and popular as they provide the fresh, juice topnotes that are lacking in processed juices and juice-based beverages. Essence oils are differentiated from peel oils by the inclusion of low molecular weight esters such as ethyl acetate and ethyl butyrate and the greater quantity of sesquiterpenes such as valencene. A comparison of peel and essence oils from orange is shown in Table 6 (Swaine and Swaine, 1988). The orange aqueous essence is characterized by Lund and Bryan (1977) in Table 7. It contains primarily acetaldehyde, which imparts a pungent, sharp, fresh flavor, and ethyl butyrate, which imparts a fresh fruitiness to juice.

Typically the yield of peel oil (also known as cold-pressed peel oil) is 0.10–0.35% for orange oils, 0.05–0.10% for grapefruit and tangerine oils, and 0.005–0.015% for lime oil. A mass balance of flavorings from orange and grapefruit is shown in Figure 7 (Johnson and Vora, 1983).

The majority of citrus peel oil is manufactured by expression. Lime oil, however, may be processed by expression as described above or by distillation. Al-

Table 6 Comparison of Orange Essence and Peel Oils (%)

	Florida, Valencia CP	California, Navel CP	Florida, Essence	California, Essence
Ethyl butyrate	0.006	0.004	0.052	
α-Pinene	0.454	0.513	0.494	0.394
β-Pinene	0.010	0.031	0.022	0.042
Hexanal		0.004	0.028	0.028
Myrcene	1.773	1.890	1.690	1.590
e-2-Hexenal		0.002	0.007	0.022
d-Limonene	90.600	77.600	88.600	88.500
γ-Terpinene	0.002	0.031	0.015	0.036
para-Cymene	0.002	0.016	0.033	0.351
Octanal	0.590	0.196	0.375	0.003
Hexanol	0.096	0.002		0.055
Nonanal	0.077	0.032	0.066	0.044
Citronellal	0.087	0.052	0.036	0.510
Decanal	0.523	0.202	0.285	0.430
Linalool	0.372	0.228	0.379	0.075
Octanol	0.039	0.012	0.042	
β-Caryophyellene	0.045	0.027	0.018	0.040
Neral	0.077	0.052	0.044	
α-Terpineol	0.064	0.046	0.047	
d-Carvone	0.012	0.009	0.047	
Geranial	0.122	0.048	0.061	0.067
Dodecanal	0.068	0.026	0.033	0.053
Valencene	0.058	0.079	0.241	0.620
Geraniol	0.006	0.007	0.003	0.005
Nootkatone	0.014	0.012	0.090	

Source: Swaine and Swaine, 1988.

Table 7 Orange Aqueous Essence

Compound	mg/100 ml
Methanol	800
Acetaldehyde	120
Ethanol	11,000
Ethyl butyrate	4
Hexanal	0.14
1-Penten-3-ol	0.3
3-Methybutan-1-ol + limonene	1.3
n-Amyl alcohol	0.09
trans-2-Hexenal	0.07
Octanal	0.5
1-Hexanol	0.08
cis-3-Hexen-1-ol	0.3
trans-Linalool oxide	0.2
cis-Linalool oxide	0.2
Linalool	2.6
1-Octanol	0.2
Terpinen-4-ol	0.2
trans-2,8-p Menthadien-1-ol	0.03
Ethyl-3-hydroxy-hexanoate	6
α-Terpineol	0.28
trans-Carveol	0.08
Unidentified compounds	1.5

Source: Lund and Bryan, 1977.

though this is obviously not an expressed-type oil, it is described here because it, along with orange, lemon, and grapefruit, is a commonly used citrus flavoring. Distilled lime oil is commonly prepared by distillation of the acidic juice from the lime fruit presses. The chemical consequences of this method as compared to expression are great. Aldehydes (especially citral) and β-pinene are more plentiful in the expressed oil. The distilled-type contains much more α-terpineol (10), the ACHD compound formed from the degradation of d-limonene (9) (Fig. 8). This difference is quite apparent in Table 8 (Haro and Faas, 1985).

Expressed citrus oils commonly used as flavoring agents are orange, tangerine, mandarin, grapefruit, bitter orange, and lemon. Representative chemical composition of these oils is provided in Table 9 (Hussein and Pidel, 1976; Staroscik and Wilson, 1982; Vora et al., 1983; Swaine and Swaine, 1988; Boelens and Jimenez, 1989; Dugo et al., 1990).

The predominant class of chemicals in citrus oils is terpene hydrocarbon, and the major terpene is d-limonene. Common terpenes include d-limonene (9), γ-terpinene (11), myrcene (12), α-pinene (13), and β-pinene (14) (Fig. 9).

d-Limonene may account for as much as 95% of the aroma volatiles in expressed citrus oils. Terpenes, and particularly d-limonene, are part of the overall flavor profile. d-Limonene is weak for a flavoring agent and certainly is not the characterizing component in citrus oils. Flavorists consider that small amounts of citrus terpenes are required to complete the profile and impart a fresh citrusy character.

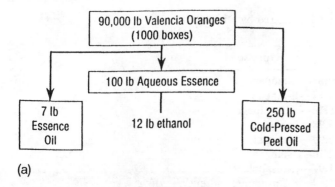

(a)

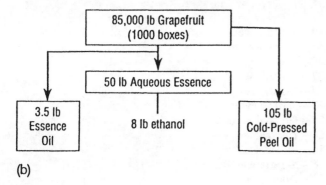

(b)

Fig. 7 (a) Mass balance of orange flavorings. (b) Mass balance of grapefruit flavorings. (From Johnson and Vora, 1983.)

Fig. 8 Acid-catalyzed hydration dehydration of limonene.

Certainly they are not required in the amounts present in $1 \times$ oil. In fact, d-limonene may in many instances be potentially detrimental to the flavor of a food or beverage. Terpenes are not very soluble in aqueous or hydroalcoholic mixtures. The high degree of unsaturation renders them very susceptible to oxidative transformation and the formation of deleterious compounds. They exhibit poor stability with respect to light and temperature. Further, in the presence of hydrogen ions, an acid-catalyzed hydration-dehydration reaction occurs with limonene, forming potent terpenols. This reaction was documented earlier in the discussion of distilled lime oil. Additional key reactions that lead to the formation of untoward aromas

Table 8 Comparison of Lime Oil Prepared by Distillation
or Expression (%)

Distilled	Expressed
48.00	47.87—Limonene
2.23	19.54—β-Pinene
10.91	8.10—γ-Terpinene
	3.28—Sabinene
0.04	2.99—Geranial
1.19	2.16—α-Pinene
1.42	1.97—β-Bisabolene
1.11	1.89—β-Sesquiphellandrene
0.02	1.82—Neral
0.83	1.20—α-Bergamotene
0.62	1.16—β-Caryophyllene
1.28	1.15—Myrcene
1.00	0.80—1,8-Cineole
0.12	0.51—Neryl acetate
7.75	0.40—Terpinolene
0.02	0.37—α-Thujene
6.26	0.30—α-Terpineol
1.79	0.27—*para*-Cymene
0.08	0.25—Geranyl acetate
	0.24—Decanal
0.05	0.16—Linalool
2.53	0.16—α-Terpinene
	0.12—Dodecanal
	0.12—1-Octanol
0.48	0.09—Camphene
	0.07—Geraniol
	0.07—Hexadecanal
	0.07—Octanal
0.01	0.05—Nonanal
0.37	0.05—α-Phellandrene
	0.04—Citronellal
	0.04—Nerol
0.84	0.04—Terpinen-4-ol
	0.04—Tetradecanal
	0.03—6-Methyl-5-hepten-2-one
	0.03—Undecanal
	0.01—δ-3-Carene
1.00	0.01—1,4-Cineole
	0.01—Pentadecanal
0.69	β-Terpineol
0.94	γ-Terpineol
1.00	δ-3-Carene
0.66	α-Fenchol
0.42	Borneol

Source: Haro and Faas, 1985.

Table 9 Composition of Citrus Oils (%)

Compound	Orange, Florida, Valencia	Tangerine, Florida	Mandarin, Italy	Grapefruit, Florida	Lemon, United States	Bitter orange, Italy
Limonene	95.17	91.23	69.51	83.41	68.72	92.21
Myrcene	1.51	2.03	1.71	1.37	1.51	2.01
α-Pinene	0.42	1.01	2.36	0.38	1.72	0.55
Octanal	0.36	0.21	0.11	0.62	0.07	0.12
Decanal	0.28	0.11	0.09	0.41	0.04	0.14
Linalool	0.25	0.62	0.11		0.14	0.34
Sabinene	0.24		0.26	0.42	1.65	0.15
Geranial	0.11	0.01	0.05	0.06	1.22	0.02
Dodecanal	0.07	0.02	0.02	0.02	0.02	0.03
Neral	0.07	0.03	0.01	0.04	0.76	0.01
Citronellal	0.05	0.04	0.03	0.09	0.07	0.02
Phellandrene	0.05	0.03	0.11		0.04	
Valencene	0.05			0.01		
1-Octanol	0.03		0.01	0.09	0.01	
β-Sinensal	0.03					
α-Terpineol	0.03	0.02	0.14	0.04	0.22	0.26
β-Caryophyllene	0.02	0.01	0.11	0.24	0.24	0.13
β-Copaene	0.02					
β-Farnesene	0.02		0.17			
Nonanal	0.02	0.02	0.03	0.07	0.12	0.02
α-Sinensal	0.02	0.07				
Undecanal	0.02		0.01			0.01
Nootketone	0.01			0.11		0.13
Octyl Acetate	0.01					
Perillaldehyde	0.01	0.03			0.01	
1,8-Cineol		0.63				0.01
β-Pinene		0.44	1.68	0.02	10.13	0.21
Terpinolene		0.13	0.87		0.39	0.06
Geranyl Acetate		0.05	0.01		0.43	0.15

Table 9 Continued

Compound	Orange, Florida, Valencia	Tangerine, Florida	Mandarin, Italy	Grapefruit, Florida	Lemon, United States	Bitter orange, Italy
α-Terpinene		0.05	0.44		0.32	0.01
Thymol		0.03	0.05			
d-Carvone		0.02	0.01		0.01	
Neryl Acetate		0.02	0.01	0.06	0.51	0.05
Benzyl Alcohol		0.01				
Camphene		0.01	0.02		0.05	0.01
Z-Carveol		0.01				
E-Carveol		0.01				
Citronellol		0.01				0.02
1-Decanol		0.01				
1-Dodecenol		0.01				
Geraniol		0.01	0.01	0.01	0.04	0.02
1-Heptanol		0.01				
Z-3-Hexen-1-ol		0.01				
6-Methyl-5-heptene-2-one		0.01			0.01	
Nerol		0.01	0.02		0.04	0.01
1-Nonanol		0.01				
Sabibene hydrate		0.01	0.07			
1-Undecanol		0.01				
α-Thujene			0.89		0.38	0.01
Methyl-N-methyl-anthranilate			0.45			
para-Cymene			0.33	0.02		
Terpinene-4-ol			0.04		0.04	
E-Ocimene			0.02		0.14	
α-Copaene			0.01			0.75
α-Cubebene			0.01			
β-Cubebene			0.01			

α-Humulene	0.01		0.02	0.04
Perillyl Alcohol	0.01			
γ-Terpinene	19.85		8.55	0.01
E-2-Hexanal		0.01		
Ethyl Butyrate		0.01		
E-β-Bergamotene		0.01	0.37	
β-Bisabolene			0.56	
Citronellyl Acetate			0.02	
δ-3-Carene			0.01	
Nonyl Acetate			0.01	
Meranzin				0.41
Nerolidol				0.23
Ethanal				0.11
Ethanol				0.11
Germacrene D				0.11
Methanol				0.11
Acetone				0.05
Ethyl Acetate				0.05
Z-Ocimene				0.05
1-Propanol				0.05
E-2-Decenal				0.02
Farnesols				0.02
Limonene Oxide				0.02
α-7-epi-Selinenone				0.02
E,E-2,4-Decadienal				0.01
E,Z-2,4-Decadienal				0.01
δ-Elemene				0.01
Tetradecanal				0.01
Tridecanal				0.01

Source: Hussein and Pidel, 1976; Staroscik and Wilson, 1982; Vora et al., 1983; Swaine and Swaine, 1988; Boelens and Jimenez, 1989; Dugo et al., 1990.

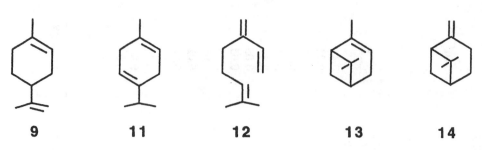

Fig. 9 Common terpene hydrocarbons.

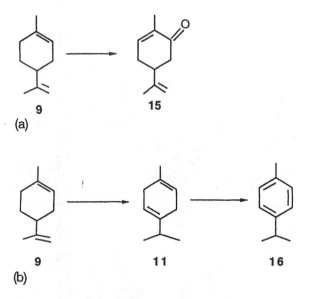

Fig. 10 Off-flavor formation in citrus oils: (a) oxidation of d-limonene; (b) isomerization of d-limonene.

are (1) oxidation of d-limonene (9) to form d-carvone (15) and (2) the isomerization of d-limonene (9) to form gamma-terpinene (11), and the subsequent dehydrogenation to form *para*-cymeme (16) (Fig. 10).

Character-significant compounds in citrus are the oxygenated compounds such as aliphatic aldehydes, terpene alcohols, and terpene aldehydes. In applications such as beverages or gelatin desserts where stability or solubility is important, it may be necessary to use citrus oils that have had the terpenes partially or totally removed. These are called folded and terpeneless oils, respectively. Deterpenization may be performed using several different processes: fractional distillation, solvent extraction, or chromatography. Table 10 summarizes key points about citrus oils.

D. Extraction

Many of the negative attributes associated with natural products such as variability, reduced strength, and microbiological liability may to a great extent be eliminated

Table 10 Citrus Oils

Essential oil	Botanical source	Geographical source	Flavor (odor) characteristics	Chemical constituents	Utility	Chemical characteristics	Sensitivities			
							Heat	Light	Oxygen	Acid
Bergamot	C. aurantium; bergamia: rind	S. Calabria, Italy	Sweet, fresh, lemon—bitter orange topnote, rich, herbaceous, floral	Limonene, linalool linallyl acetate nerol α-terpineol 4-terpineol	Topnote Blender Modifier	Less reactive than other citrus	High	High	High	Low
Lemon	Citrus limomum: rind	California, Florida, Sicily, S. Africa, Spain, Israel	Fresh, sharp, sweet, lemon-citrus clean, refreshing	Limonene, citral (neral: geranial), octanal, decanal, neryl acetate, geranyl acetate	Modifier Blender Body Character	Rapid deterioration on exposure to heat, air, and light; increase in viscosity upon aging	High	Moderate	High	Moderate
Orange (bitter)	C. aurantium, amara, rind, semiripe fruit	West Indies, Guinea, Spain, Italy	Fresh, citrus: floral, aldehydic	Limonene, citral, decanal, linalool, α-terpineol	Body Modifier Topnote	Rapid deterioration on exposure to heat, air, and light; increase in viscosity upon aging	High	High	High	Moderate
Orange (sweet)	C. aurantium, dulcis: rind	Florida, California, Brazil, Italy, S. Africa, Israel	Fresh, citrus, orange, sweet, fruity, adehydic	Limonene, citral, octanal, decanal, linalool, methyl anthranilate	Body Modifier Topnote Character	Rapid deterioration on exposure to heat, air, and light; increase in viscosity upon aging	High	High	High	Moderate

Table 10 (*Continued*)

Essential oil	Botanical source	Geographical source	Flavor (odor) characteristics	Chemical constituents	Utility	Chemical characteristics	Sensitivities			
							Heat	Light	Oxygen	Acid
Lime (distilled)	*Citrus aurantifolia,* Swingle: steam distillation	West Indies, Mexico, Guatemala	Fresh, sharp, citrus-terpeny, floral-lilac, "lime"	Limonene, dipentene, citral, octanal, nonanal, decanal, linalool, geraniol, α-terpineol	Blender Modifier Topnote Body	Rapid deterioration on exposure to heat, air, and light; increase in viscosity upon aging	High	Moderate	High	Low
Lime (expressed)	*C. aurantifolia,* Swingle, rind		Fresh, citrus-lemon				*High	Moderate	High	Moderate
Grapefruit	*Citrus papadisi:* rind	Florida, Texas, West Indies, California, Brazil	Fresh citrus, bittersweet grapefruit	Waxes, octanal, decanal, geraniol, citral, demethyl anthranilate, nootkatone, 1-*p*-menthene-8-thiol	Body Blender Modifier Character	Rapid deterioration on exposure to heat, air, light; increase in viscosity upon aging	High	High	High	Moderate
Mandarin tangerine	*Citrus reticulata:* rind	Mediterranean, Florida, Brazil	Sweet-citrus fresh, orangelike	Decanal, *p*-cymene, linalool, α-terpineol, nerol terpenyl acetate, octanal, nonanal, dodecanal, citronellal, dimethyl anthranilate	Modifier Topnote Character	Rapid deterioration on exposure to heat, air, and light; increase in viscosity upon aging	High	High	High	High

Source: Adapted from Swaine and Swaine, 1988.

by removing the flavoring agent from the inert matter in which it resides. Most flavoring principles are present in extremely small proportions in natural products. One is reminded of the patience it must take to gather and process 9,000,000 jasmine flowers, the amount required to yield only one kilogram of jasmine absolute. The intention of solvent extraction is to isolate, concentrate, or render soluble active flavoring materials from either a botanical or an animal source. Extracts are convenient methods to incorporate poorly soluble flavoring agents. This may be accomplished by preparation of the parent substance and treatment with the appropriated solvent. The solvent is sometime removed from the final flavoring. Perhaps the purist would include distillation in a broad definition of extraction, since separation can be affected by steam. The subject of distillation, however, will be addressed in the next section.

The physical and chemical properties of both the raw material and the solvent as well as the final use for the extractive must be considered when deciding on a process. Some variables to be considered are moisture and fat content of the raw material, size and hardness of raw material, intercellular location and concentration of volatiles, thermal and chemical liability of volatiles, polarity of solvent, boiling point of solvent (Table 11), viscosity of solvent, and latent heat of evaporation of solvent.

Tinctures and Pharmaceutical Extractions

While many of the once-codified flavoring agents are no longer official, the methods used to prepare them form the basis for extraction processes still in use today. Historians recorded the use of extractives as early as the second century A.D. The Greek physician Galen extracted active principles from inert plant material. In the centuries that followed, extracts were known as galencals. They were placed into five principal categories: maceration, percolation, digestion, infusion, and decoction. A generalized scheme for the production of the extractives is shown in Figure 11 and is described below.

Table 11 Solvents Used in the Preparation of Flavoring Agents

	Boiling point (°C) at 760 mm
Acetone	0.35
Cyclohexane	2.25
Dichloromethane	1.04
Ethanol	1.94
Ethyl Acetate	4.51
Ethylene chloride	3.79
Glycerol	17.45
Hexane	2.20
Isopropanol	2.20
Methanol	44.39
Pentane	0.60
Propylene glycol	6.40
Trichloroethane	0.73

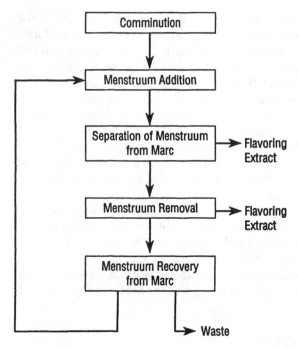

Fig. 11 Generalized scheme for the processing of tincture and extracts.

All of these processes begin with the preparation of the raw material to be extracted. Vegetable matter must be comminuted or ground to a coarse powder. The degree to which the material is powdered depends on the nature of the tissues, size of the cells, ducts, and intercellular spaces where the flavoring principles reside, as well as the chemical nature of the menstruum (solvent) and the solubility of the flavoring actives. Too coarse a grind, hence a small surface area, does not permit adequate exposure of the raw material to the menstruum, while too fine a grind may form a mass that plugs percolation equipment and releases fixed oils.

Maceration is the crudest extraction process. It simply involves the steeping of the raw material in an aqueous or hydroalcoholic solution at ambient temperatures for a prolonged period of time. With maceration the cellular structure of the raw material is thoroughly penetrated by the menstruum and the soluble portions are softened and dissolved. The raw material and all of the menstruum are placed in a closed vessel for a period of 2–14 days. The vessel must be closed so as to prevent loss of volatile menstruum and concentration variability. During maceration the product is "shaken" or mixed periodically to disperse the saturated layer of menstruum and allow fresh menstruum to come in contact with raw material particles. In some instances the pH may be adjusted to facilitate the solution of certain chemical species. After the prescribed period of time the liquid is strained from the marc (extraction residue). The marc may also be pressed to remove any absorbed menstruum. Some processes call for a second steeping of the marc for a shorter period of time and with a different menstruum. The liquids from the various streams are then combined and, if desired, clarified by filtration.

Percolation is a more preferred technique. Also known as lixiviation, percolation extracts flavoring principles by the descent of a suitable solvent through a comminuted raw material that has been packed into a column. This process was first used to decolorize syrups with charcoal in 1813. Fundamentally, a powder is placed in a conical or cylindrical vessel with a porous diaphragm and is treated from above with a solvent capable of dissolving a portion of the substance. The portion of the liquid first in contact with the substance and passing downward exercises a solvent power on the successive layers of powder. Eventually, the liquid is saturated and is impelled down by the combined forces of its own gravity and that of the column liquid above it, less the capillary force of the powder attempting to retain it.

A more expedient form of maceration, *digestion* employs the use of heat to facilitate the extraction. Gentle heat, about 68°C, is applied to increase the solvent powers of the menstruum. Pressure is sometimes used. Some extractions, especially in the case where the menstruum is very volatile at the operating temperatures, employ the use of a reflux condenser to recover and return the menstruum. Quality is always a concern when heat is used in the isolation of botanical flavoring agents.

Most *infusions* are prepared by moistening a comminuted botanical with cold water for a very short period of time (15 min), followed by the addition of boiling water. This mixture is allowed to macerate for 30 minutes and then strained. In isolated instances, with quassia, for instance, where the actives are sufficiently water soluble, cold water may be used. The difficulty in standardization and the microbial susceptibility of infusions means they are rarely used.

Decoction is generally only used for flavorings that are very water soluble and very heat stable. The process involves boiling the raw material, cooling, and straining. Decoctions have almost entirely disappeared from use.

The extracts prepared by the above processes are classified according to strength and residual solvent as either tinctures, fluid extracts, or solid extracts. Tinctures are alcoholic or hydroalcoholic solutions prepared by extraction of vegetable, animal, or chemical substances. Official tinctures represent the activity of 10–20 g of active per 100 ml. Some tinctures, e.g., sweet orange peel, may be more potent. This makes standardization following extraction and assay critical. Fluid extracts again have their roots in the pharmaceutical industry and represent 1 g of active per one ml. Solid extracts are concentrated preparations of fluid extracts (vegetable or animal) having had all or most of the solvent removed by evaporation.

These types of extracts find use in the flavor industry today and are especially valuable as blenders, modifiers, and fixatives in both alcoholic and nonalcoholic beverages. The pharmaceutical and tobacco industries also use these products as masking agents and flavorings. Common botanical sources for flavoring extracts are angelica, bitter orange peel, lemon peel, red clover, elderflower, ginseng, white horehound, limeflowers, sarsaparilla, savory, yerba santa, fenugreek, juniper, gentian, hops, locust bean (carob), chicory, licorice, quassia, taraxacum, wild cherry bark, kola, tea, coffee, cocoa, tamarind, chrysanthemum, rhubarb, elderberry, castoreum,* civet,* and, of course, vanilla. Because of its economic significance, a closer examination of vanilla extract is in order before leaving this section.

---

* From animal sources.

Vanilla comes from the extraction of properly cured and harvested dried fruit pods (the vanilla beans) of *Vanilla planifolia* Andrews and *Vanilla tahitensis* Moore. The former is grown in Madagascar, Indonesia, and the Comores and the Reunion Islands, and the latter, which is economically much less significant, is grown in Tahiti. After harvesting, the beans are cured, a process that may take several months. It is during this curing process that flavor development occurs. Beans are then sorted for processing. The beans are cut and loaded into perforated baskets and placed in a percolator. The extraction process is essentially a percolation. The menstruum, ethanol and water, is pumped through a system (containing a heating coil to maintain temperature at about 90–120°C) from the bottom of the percolator to the top, where it then is sprayed over the cut beans. The soluble solids and volatile flavorings are extracted as the menstruum flows down through the beans. The circulation is continuous. The heat is turned off at the prescribed time, and the menstruum cools to ambient temperature. The menstruum is eventually drained from the beans, removed from the percolator, strained, and pasteurized.

Alcohol Extraction of Citrus Oils

The next three sections will address nonthermal intensive processes that are used to concentrate flavorings recovered from natural products. Recall that singlefold citrus oils are composed of about 95% terpene hydrocarbons, which in higher doses are undesirable due to their instability toward oxidation and acid-catalyzed degradation and their water immiscibility. It is desirable therefore to greatly diminish the terpene hydrocarbons subsequently enriching the flavorful oxygenated compounds. Alcohol has been used since about 800 A.D. as a solvent for extraction. Dilute ethanol is commonly used to (partially) deterpenate citrus oils, especially for use in beverages. This method involves the dissolution of the citrus oil (other terpene-containing essential oils may also be used) in 95% ethanol. Water is added to this solution to produce an attenuated ethanol concentration of about 60%. This mixture is then agitated for a minimal period of time and allowed to stand for 1–3 days. The mixture separates into a predominantly terpene (top) layer and hydroalcoholic (lower) layer of oxygenated compounds and some terpenes. Following segregation of these layers, the hydroalcoholic extract is filtered. The terpene layer, also known as washed oil, has application in the fragrance, cosmetic, and flavor industry. Variation in either the ethanol:water ratio or the solvent:citrus oil ratio results in a spectrum of volatile profiles. This traditional method can be expensive, time consuming, and inefficient. As much as 50% of the flavor volatiles may remain with the washed oil.

Chromatography

Commercial-scale gas-liquid chromatography and high pressure liquid chromatography have been reported to be successful in the deterpenation of essential oils (Bonmati and Guiochon, 1978; Jones, 1988). This is rarely practiced today. A chromatographic method more popular today is preparative adsorptive chromatography (PAC). Several processes have been reported.

    Tzamtzis et al. (1990) described the deterpenation of lemon and orange oils using PAC. Glass columns were packed with silica gel. Slurry packing used in this method is hypothesized to reduce the initial reactivity of the column. This reduces the risk of isomerization of polymerization of labile compounds. A mixture of hexane and ethyl alcohol was used to elute the terpene hydrocarbons. Ethyl acetate was the used to elute the oxygenates.

German patent DE 3834988 teaches a similar procedure for the deterpenation of citrus oils. In this variation the terpene-containing essential oil is adsorbed onto a polar adsorbent. Solids that can be used include silica gel, aluminum oxide, diatomaceous earth, cellulose, or bentonite. Ten to sixty percent polar adsorbent is used. The majority of the oxygenates are adsorbed from the solid matter, and the terpenes remain in the liquid phase. Sixty to ninety percent of the oxygenates are adsorbed. The next step involves the separation of the oxygenated loaded adsorbent from the terpenes in the liquid phase. This is done with centrifugation or filtration. In the final stage the oxygenate (aroma phase)-loaded adsorbent is subjected to high-pressure extraction with carbon dioxide. The oxygenates are effectively desorbed or extracted.

The poroplast technique of PAC has been described by Fleisher (1990) and by Kozhin et al. (1972). This technique may be applied to hydrocarbon containing essential oils (Fig. 12) as well as dilute aqueous fruit and vegetable essences (Fig. 13). In the case of terpene-containing oils, a poroplast (polytetrafluoroethylene) column is charged with an oil and aqueous ethanol. During the 15-minute cycle time oxygenated aroma compounds are transferred to the alcohol phase. An efficiency of >90% is claimed. The liquid phases are separated after elution from the column. The terpene hydrocarbon phase is continually discharged. The enriched

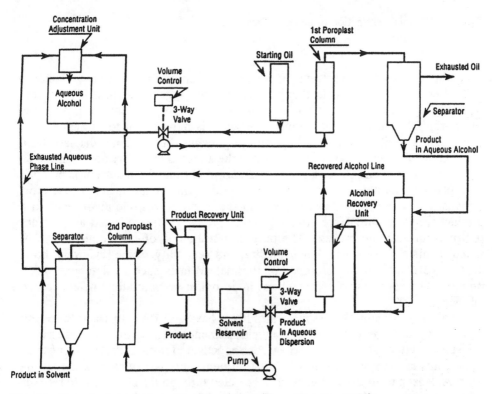

Fig. 12 Poroplast extraction of hydrocarbons. (From Fleisher, 1990).

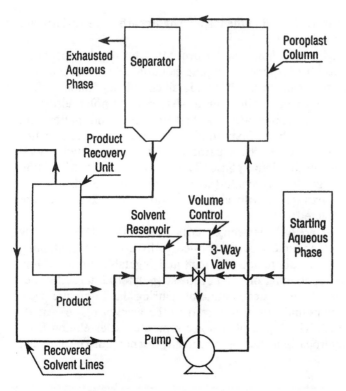

Fig. 13 Poroplast extraction of aqueous flavorings.

alcohol phase is sent to a solvent recovery unit. Evaporators reduce the alcohol to 30%. Recovered alcohol is further processed. The oxygenated phase is recovered from the aqueous dispersion. For aqueous systems an organic solvent is added to the poroplast column and the aqueous essence is pumped on to the column. It makes contact with the solvent held on the polymer, but does not displace from the column. The active flavor compounds in the aqueous phase are now transferred to the organic solvent. After a prescribed period of time, fresh solvent is pumped in, replacing saturated solvent. The eluted liquids form two layers in the deaerator. Exhaust aqueous phase is discharged and the enriched organic phase goes to a product recovery unit. Here aromatic flavor principles are collected and solvent returned through the process. The poroplast technique offers the advantage of speed, minimal solvent use, flavor fidelity, and versatility. Some reviewers, however, have identified the presence of thermal artifacts such as limonene oxide isomers, d-carvone, and dihydrocarbone in poroplast-prepared terpeneless orange oil (Moyler, 1991).

Procter & Gamble (Persson et al., 1990) has used PAC to fractionate and improve the flavor properties of aqueous citrus essences. The citrus aqueous essence is first passed through a solid adsorbent such as activated carbon. Part of the essence compounds exit the adsorbent in the first effluent, and part remain on the adsorbent. At least part of the first effluent is recycled through the adsorbent to recover a fraction of the remaining compounds and produce a second effluent.

Styrene-divinylbenzene (SDVB) resins have been reported by Ericson et al. (1992) to be valuable in the recovery of citrus oils from wastewater streams. Grapefruit oil wastewater was passed through an upward flow column extraction system. Ethanol 95% was used to desorb flavoring volatiles.

Countercurrent Extraction

The technique of countercurrent extraction (CCE) was introduced to the flavor industry in 1939 with the teachings of a patent awarded to van Wijk and van Dijk. The patent was a result of a joint effort between the Dutch flavor house Naarden (now Quest) and the Batavian Petroleum Company (now Royal Dutch Shell). Their patent described the manufacture of deterpenated essential oils by a double solvent extraction process. The equipment consisted of a horizontal extractor equipped with six mixing chambers separated by perforated vertical chamber walls. At the lower half of one end of the extractor, methanol or another low molecular weight polar solvent was introduced. On the other end of the extractor at the upper half, petroleum ether or another nonpolar solvent was introduced. A bottom inlet supplied the essential oil to one of the two mixing chambers. The countercurrent flow of the solvents and the intense agitation in the chambers resulted in a continuous extraction. Terpene hydrocarbons were absorbed by the polar solvent, and the oxygenated flavorings were dissolved by the polar solvent. Polar solvent removal by distillation under high vacuum yielded the pure terpeneless oil. Variations to the original process may include a tubular apparatus containing mixing and separating chambers in place of a horizontal extractor, the use of proprietary solvents or solvent mixtures, the introduction of polar solvents at the column top, nonpolar solvent at the bottom, and introduction of essential oil in the middle of the column.

Other recent innovations practiced by Universal Flavors, Ltd. (Bletchley, UK) have been described by Moyler (1991) (Fig. 14). In this CCE process the citrus oil is partitioned by pumping against a flow of hydroalcoholic solvent being pumped in the opposing direction. A motor-driven rotor disperses the oil into microscopic droplets through centrifugal force. The result is a high degree of contacting efficiency. After phase separation, the solvent is removed under vacuum. Any residual solvent is removed by molecular distillation. Figure 15 compares the profile of a deterpenated orange oil prepared by CCE to one prepared by fractional distillation. Note the more balanced profile in the CCE sample. This process offers many advantages to traditional concentration process such as alcohol washing, and distillation. These include efficiency, speed, minimal thermal abuse, and high yield, and, depending on the solvents used, deterpenated oils may retain naturally occurring antioxidants.

Oleoresins

Oleoresins are thick, viscous extracts usually prepared from spices. The general process for the preparation of spice oleoresins calls first for cleaning and grinding (or macerating) the raw material. Oleoresins are prepared by percolation with a volatile solvent. Solvents should be as pure as possible, free from off-odors, and sufficiently volatile enough so as to facilitate desolventization after the extraction (see Sec. IV.A). Common solvents used in the preparation of oleoresins are alcohols, hexane, acetone, and chlorinated hydrocarbons. Contact time between the comminuted spice and the solvent must be long enough to ensure sufficient diffusion

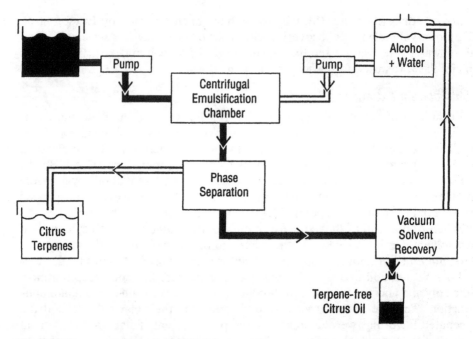

Fig. 14 Countercurrent schematic diagram. (Courtesy of Universal Flavors, Ltd.)

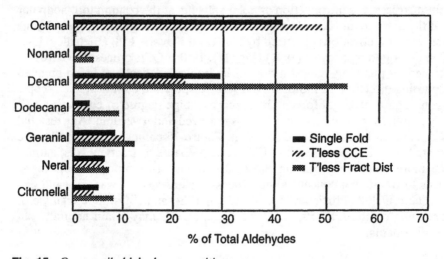

Fig. 15 Orange oil aldehyde composition.

of solvent through the spice and extraction. The amount of solvent varies and of course is proprietary. Generally one may assume that three to four volumes of solvent are required to exhaust the vegetable matter. The solvent is removed by vacuum distillation. Some manufacturers ensure that desolventization is as complete as needed by the sparging with nitrogen under high vacuum. Adequate solvent removal is a critical safety concern regulated by individual countries. The United

States (*Federal Register*, 1980), for example, limits residual solvent amounts in oleoresins to:

Compound	ppm
Acetone	20
Chlorinated solvents	30
Hexane	25
Isopropanol	50
Methanol	50

Procedures for determining residual solvent are disclosed in the Food Chemicals Codex (1981).

Oleoresins may be sold as is, bulked with previous batches to ensure uniformity, mixed with a solvent or emulsifying agent to aid in handling, or blended with other oleoresins to form seasonings or flavorings. Another practice is to remove the volatile oil prior to percolation. This prevents volatile loss during extraction and aids in standardization.

The solvent removes not only the essential (volatile oil) but also anything else miscible in that particular solvent. This may include resins, gums, sugars, color bodies, or pungent nonvolatile flavorings. Spices such as turmeric and paprika are valued for their color. Spice oleoresins from ginger and pepper contain in addition to the volatile oil the characteristic hot or pungent principles associated with those spices. The resulting oleoresin is used at one-fifth to one-tenth the level of the corresponding spice.

Oleoresins offer distinct advantages over whole spices. These include more product uniformity, cleanliness and hygiene, economy, improved shelf life, potency, versatility, and nonenzyme activity. In addition, oleoresins may offer advantages such as fullness of flavor profile and stability during thermal food processing. Be mindful, however, that the flavor is not an exact reproduction of the original spice.

Concretes and Absolutes

A concrete is an extractive perhaps more widely used by the perfumer but still of value to the creative flavorist. A concrete is the extract prepared from nonresinous or low-resinous plant matter using a volatile solvent (Fig. 16). It consists of the essential oil, wax, fat, fixed oil, and other nonvolatile matter soluble in the usually hydrocarbon solvent. Concretes are almost exclusively prepared from once-living tissue, bark, flower, herb, leaf, or root and should not be confused with resinoids, products made by similar process but using exudates (nontissue material) as a feedstock. Flowers such as jasmine, ylang ylang, lavender, oakmoss, rose, orange flower, and orris root are examples of common concretes. Concretes are usually solid or semisolid waxy materials with very sparing solubility in alcohol and insoluble in water. Their high wax content, however, aids in stability towards oxidation. Because of this stability a major use is in the production of absolutes, especially when the absolute is to be at a location a significant distance from the manufacture of the concrete.

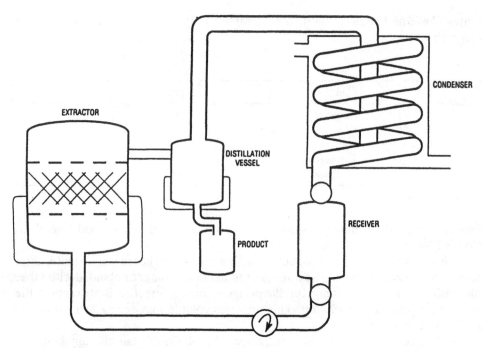

Fig. 16 Solvent extraction.

An absolute is the highly concentrated form of nonresinous extract. It exhibits complete solubility in alcohol and improved solubility in water. An absolute is prepared by successive extractions of warm alcohol in an apparatus known as a batteuse. Alcoholic extracts are bulked and filtered. The alcohol is removed by vacuum distillation. As one might expect, because the preparation of absolutes is time and labor intensive and the yield of aroma concentrate so small, the price of absolutes is dear indeed.

Concretes and absolutes are used in flavorings mainly as blenders. They are extremely useful in "round-off" rough chemical notes, especially in synthetic flavorings. They add warmth, body, and naturalness.

Supercritical Fluid Extraction

Solubilities of organic compounds in supercritical fluids were first studied during the early 1900s. It was not, however, until the 1970s with the increased concern about solvent residues, environmental impact, energy consumption, "naturalness," and heightened awareness of the safety of food ingredients that supercritical fluid extract of flavoring substances became more widely recognized as a viable means with which to produce flavoring agents.

The supercritical fluid state of gas is that set of conditions of temperature and pressure under which gaseous matter is compressed to a density that approximates that of a liquid. Figure 17 shows a phase diagram. By regulating temperature and pressure, highly selective solvating behavior of supercritical fluids may be secured. The density and hence solvating power increase to the point where the dense gas can dissolve a diverse range of materials. Large quantities of a substance perhaps

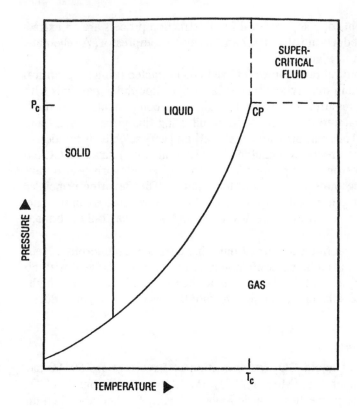

Fig. 17 Pure phase component diagram.

Table 12 Physicochemical Data of Various Gases

Gas	bp (1 bar) (°C)	T_c (°C)	p_c (bar)	ρ_c (g/cm³)
Ethylene	−103.7	9.5	50	0.200
Trifluoromethane	−81.4	28.8	39	0.580
Carbon dioxide	−78 (subl.)	31.3	73	0.448
Ethane	−88	32.4	48	0.201
Nitrous oxide	−89	36.5	71	0.457
Propylene	−47.4	91.8	45	0.220
Propane	−44.5	96.8	42	0.220
Difluorodichloromethane	−29.8	111.8	39	0.558

only sparingly soluble in the liquid or normal gaseous phase may be dissolved in a supercritical fluid at a high density. CO_2, for example, compressed under extreme pressure above its triple point becomes a supercritical fluid and now essentially possesses the characteristics of both a liquid and a gas, i.e., the density of a liquid and the high diffusivity of a gas, thus permitting rapid mass transfer and faster extraction rates. Table 12 lists the physicochemical data of gases used for extraction.

The main components of a supercritical fluid extraction process are an extraction vessel, a pressure reduction valve, a separator, and a compressor. A schematic representation is shown in Figure 18.

Several classes of natural raw materials have been extracted using supercritical CO_2. Essential oils contain mainly low molecular weight lipophilic materials with relatively high vapor pressure. The toxin β-thujone, a component of the herb wormwood, can be separated from the essential oil using this process (Stahl and Gerard, 1983). Essential oils may also be very sharply and very selectively fractioned using supercritical fluids. Procter & Gamble (Japikse et al, 1987) has used CO_2 to isolate selected positive aroma compounds from citrus juices. Flavorings also have been extracted from vegetables, fruits, and their juices. The flavoring principles show good solubility in supercritical CO_2, while inert fruit or vegetable components such as sugars, cellulose, or protein are insoluble and water has only a limited solubility.

The use of supercritical fluids to extract flavoring agents has numerous advantages. CO_2, for example, is an inert, nonflammable, nonexplosive solvent with no solvent residues. It has no "still" off-notes, is a cheap, readily available, high-purity, nontoxic solvent displaying selectivity, versatility, low viscosity, and reduced thermal artifacts.

Subcritical Carbon Dioxide

Parameters for the use of liquid CO_2 for extraction of flavorings are 50–80 bar pressure and 0–10°C temperature (Moyler, 1991). It is at these conditions that CO_2 liquefies and exhibits the properties of a nonpolar solvent. A schematic diagram is shown in Figure 19. In addition to the advantages over conventional extraction with supercritical CO_2, liquid CO_2 offers an extract with much fewer thermal artifacts, such as terpene hydrocarbons, and the retention of more volatile top

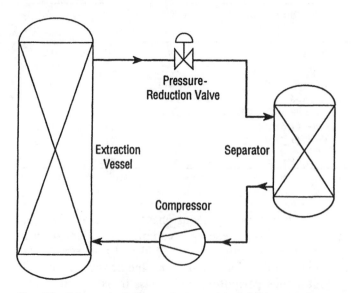

Fig. 18 Schematic diagram of supercritical fluid extraction.

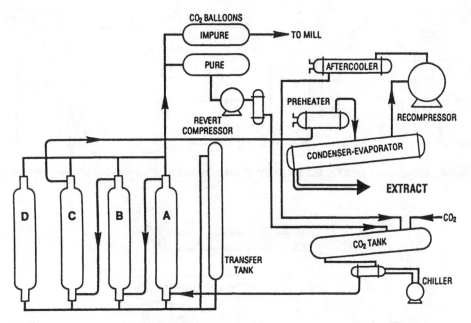

Fig. 19 Schematic diagram of liquid CO_2 extraction. (Courtesy of Universal Flavors, Ltd.)

notes. Since liquid CO_2 can extract the less volatile compounds, more bottom notes are present and a more complete profile is realized.

E. Distillation

Although distillation is an ancient method used to separate essential oils from plant material, it still represents the most widely used method of essential oil production. The equipment is more sophisticated than covered pots heated by open flames and condensers consisting of copper tubes immersed in the nearby stream, but the principles remain the same. The volatile material is converted into a vapor, condensed, and collected. Prerequisites for the use of distillation for the recovery or isolation of a flavoring are volatility and immiscibility in water. Materials to be distilled are usually pretreated by drying or grinding. These operations increase the yield and increase the surface area, permitting better contact with the turbulent water or steam and rupturing cells. The flavor industry prepares distilled essential oils by three methods:

1. Water Distillation—The materials to be distilled is entirely immersed in boiling water and mildly agitated. A mixture of steam and volatile (essential) oil is passed over into the condenser and collected in Florentine receivers where, depending on the density of the essential oil, it is separated from the water (Fig. 20). In some instances the condensed water is returned to the still. This process is quite time consuming so is only recommended for those oils whose components would be sufficiently stable when subjected to prolonged heating in water. Lavender oil, for instance, with its high ester content, would not be

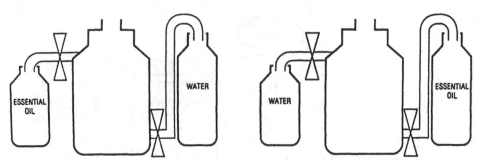

Fig. 20 Florentine flasks for the recovery of essential oils: (a) for oils lighter than water; (b) for oils heavier than water.

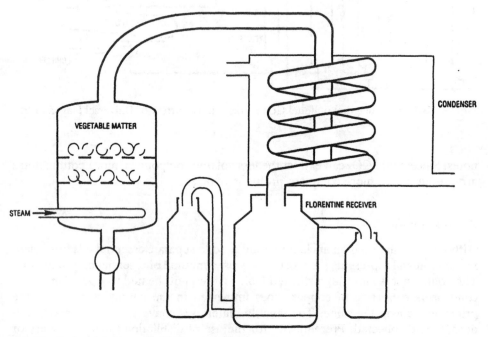

Fig. 21 Industrial steam distillation process.

a good candidate for water distillation. Clove oil, on the other hand, would be.

2. Water and Steam Distillation—With this process the material, usually herbaceous, is supported on a frame or grid above boiling water. The product to be distilled now comes into contact only with the steam. Herbaceous materials such as thyme or mints are distilled by this method.

3. Steam Distillation—The previous two methods used a liquid phase. This process does not. Here the vegetable raw material is added to the still, and live steam is injected into the pot. A typical commercial still is shown in Figure 21. The charge is placed within the still on perforated supports. These ensure

maximum steam circulation and prevent direct contact between the charge and steam pipes. Steam circulates throughout and initially will condense on a portion of the charge and, due to the latent heat release, produce a large heating effect. This heating accompanied by charge moistening results in rapid heat tissue penetration and efficient release of the essential oil. Distillation occurs at a rapid rate, so is ideal for sensitive materials such as lavender.

The yield of essential varies considerably. Table 13 shows the essential oil content of several common flavorings.

Distilled essential oils are concentrated, clean, and convenient forms of flavorings that are characteristic of the starting material. They are, however, not exact replications. Loss of compounds due to volatilization, loss of delicate top notes, formation of thermal artifacts, or loss of very water-soluble compounds will all result in some change in the flavor profile. This can be minimized with techniques such as cryogenic traps or recovery of cohabation water. Still odors may also be present in freshly distilled oils. These are extremely unpleasant vegetable odors caused by the breakdown of proteinaceous material. They dissipate upon standing over a period of time. This process may be sped up by passing oxygen through the oil. The consequences of this may not be totally desirable, however.

Distillation is also used to prepare smoke flavorings. For example, hardwoods may be subjected to dry distillation at temperatures between 300 and 800°C. The condensed vapors are used to impart a smoky flavor to foods. The formation of polycylic aromatic hydrocarbons in these products must be monitored very closely.

Fractional distillation is a very common method used to prepare deterpenated citrus oils. It is relatively inexpensive and fast and therefore finds considerable application in the processing of citrus oils for the beverage, candy, and dessert industries. This method does have the drawback of producing a skewed profile (see Fig. 15). Other drawbacks to distillation include possible loss of very volatile

Table 13 Yield of Essential Oil (%)

Allspice	3.0–5.0
Angelica seed	0.5–1.5
Anise	1.5–4.0
Bois de Rose	0.5–1.5
Cinnamon bark	0.5–0.8
Clove Bud	15–21
Coriander	0.2–1.0
Davana	0.1–0.5
Fennel	4.0–6.0
Ginger	0.25–3.0
Lavender	0.5–1.0
Nutmeg	6.0–15.0
Peppermint	0.3–0.7
Rose	0.03–0.05
Thyme	0.5–1.5
Tumeric	1.5–5.0

and very nonvolatile compounds, thermal degradation, hard-to-separate compounds with close boiling points, hard- or expensive-to-recover trace compounds,
and inefficiency with trace compounds in aqueous media.

Key data relevant to common botanical sources of flavorings not already covered in discussions of herbs, spices, or citrus oils are contained in Table 14.

F. Flavor Chemicals

The creative flavorist's ability to develop more sophisticated and characterizing
flavorings was greatly enhanced with the advent of modern organic chemistry and
the development of aroma chemicals. Initially the flavorist's "palate," which consisted only of natural products, was supplemented with isolates from natural raw
materials. Cinnamic aldehyde was isolated from cinnamon oil in 1834, and 3 years
later benzaldehyde was isolated from bitter almond oil. These two compounds were
synthesized in 1856 and 1863, respectively. Aliphatic aldehydes were first synthesized about 1853, vanillin in 1874, and ionones in 1893. By the turn of the century
100 or so synthetics were available to the flavorist—a great advance but a far cry
from the roughly 2000 chemicals in use today!

Flavor chemicals may be classified by two systems. The first groups them
according to the contribution they make to a finished flavoring.

Orange flavoring is composed of a complex amalgam of chemicals, none of which
alone imparts the flavor of orange but whose combination is characteristic of
orange.

Butter flavoring is composed of only a few compounds, diacetyl and lactones, which
dominate the flavor.

Vanilla is instantly recognized by the use of a single compound, vanillin. Such
compounds are known as character impact compounds and include (Fig. 22)
almond (17), benzaldehyde; anise (18), anethole; apple (19), ethyl-2-methyl-
butyrate; banana (20), isoamyl acetate; bergamot (21), linalyl acetate; bleu
cheese (22), methyl amyl ketone; blueberry (23), isobutyl butenaote; caramel
(24), 2,3-dimethyl-4-hydroxy-3-(2H)furanone; caraway (15), d-carvone; cassia
(25), cinnamic aldehyde; cassie (26), *p*-mentha-8-thio-3-one; celery (27), pro-
pylidene phthalide; cherry (17), benzaldehyde; clove (28), eugenol; cocoa (29),
5-methyl-2-phenyl-2-hexenal; coconut (30), γ-nonalactone; coffee (31), α-fur-
furyl mercaptan; concord grape (32), methyl anthranilate; coriander (33), linalool; cucumber (34), E-2-Z-6-nonadienal; eucalyptus (35), eucalyptol; garlic
(36), diallyl disulfide; grapefruit (37), nootkatone; green bell pepper (38),
methoxy isobutylpyrazine; hazelnut (39), methyl thiomethylpyrazine; horseradish (40), 1-pentene-3-one; jasmine (41), benzyl acetate; lemon (42), citral;
maple (43), 5-ethyl-3-hydroxy-4-methyl-2(5H)-furanone; melon (44); 2,6-di-
methyl-5-heptenal; mushroom (45), 1-oceten-3-ol; mustard (46), allyl isothiocyanate; peanut (47), methyl methoxypyrazine; pear (48), ethyl-2-Z-4-deca-
dienoate; peppermint (49), menthol; pineapple (50), allyl caproate; potato (51),
methional; prune (52), dimethyl benzyl carbinyl isobutyrate; raspberry (53),
p-hydroxyphenylbutanone; spearmint (54), 1-carvone; smoke (55), guaiacol;
thyme (56), thymol; and wintergreen (57), methyl salicylate.

Flavor chemicals may also be classified, by means of their origin, as isolates, semisynthetic, synthetic, or biochemical.

Table 14 Botanical Sources of Flavoring Agents

Common name	Significant chemical components	Producing region	Parts used
Almond-bitter:FFPA	Benzaldehyde	Southern Europe, Middle East, United States	Kernels
Aloe	Aloin, barbaloin	South Africa	Juice
Ambrette	Farnesol, ambrettolide	Java, Martinique	Seed
Amyris	β-Caryophyllene, amyrol, cadinene	Haiti, Jamaica, South America	Wood
Angelica	Phellandrene	France, Germany	Seed, root, leaf
Angostura	Galipol	South America	Bark
Apricot (Persic Oil)	Benzaldehyde	Southern Europe, Middle East, United States	Kernel
Artemisia	Thujone	Central Europe	Herbal tops
Balsam Peru	Benzyl cinnamate, benzyl benzoate	Central America	Oleoresin-gum
Balsam Tolu	Cinnamic acid, benzyl cinnamate, benzoic acid, benzyl benzoate	South America	Exudate-gum
Benzoin Siam	Coniferyl benzoate	Indochina	Oleoresin-gum
Birch (sweet)	Methyl salicylate	North America, Eastern Europe, CIS	Bark
Bois de Rose	Linalool	South America	Wood
Boronia	β-Ionone	Australia, New Zealand	Leaf
Buchu	Diosphenol, diosmin	South Africa	Leaf
Cacao (Cocoa)	Methyl phenyl hexenal	Africa, Central and South America	Seed
Camomile	Chamazulene	Australia, Asia, United States, Europe	Flower
Cananga	Cadinene	Java, East Indies	Flower
Carrot	Carotol	France	Seed
Cassie	Farnesol	West Indies, Mediterranean	Flowers
Celery seed	Limonene, sedenene, sedanolide	Europe, India	Fruit
Cherry	Benzaldehyde	North America, Europe	Bark
Citronella	Citronellal, geraniol, citronellol	Sri Lanka, Java	Leaf, herb
Coffee	Caffeine, furfuryl mercaptan, pyrazines	South America, India	Seeds
Cognac	"Ethyl oenanthate"	France	Wine lees

Table 14 Continued

Common name	Significant chemical components	Producing region	Parts used
Cola	Caffeine	Jamaica	Seed
Copaiba	Caryophyllene	South America	Resin
Costus	Splotnyene, myrcene, linalool, β-Ionone	Nepal	Root
Cubeb	Sabinene	Africa, Indonesia	Berry
Davana	Davanones, bicyclogermacrene, spathulenol, lavender lactone	India	Flowers (herb)
Dill	1-Carvone	India, United States, Eastern Europe	Fruit
Elder	Sambunigrin	Europe, Asia	Leaf, flower
Elemi	Phellandrene, dipenene, elemicin	Philippines	Resin
Eucalyptus	Eucalyptol, terpineol	Australia	Leaf
Fenugreek	Anethole	Asia, Europe	Seed
Galbanum	Pinenes	Middle East	Gum-resin
Garlic	Diallyl disulfide	United States	Bulbs
Geranium	Geraniol, citronellol	Reunion, North Africa, Europe	Leaf
Guaiacwood	Guaiol	Jamaica, South America	Wood
Hops	Humulone, myrcene	Europe, North America	Flower
Hyssop	1-Pinocamphene, α-pinene	Southern Europe	Herb
Immortelle	Neryl acetate, nerol	Mediterranean	Flower
Jasmine	Benzyl acetate, nerol, terpineol, jasmone	Mediterranean	Flower
Juniper	α-Pinene, camphene	North America, Europe	Berry
Labdanum	Terpene hydrocarbons	Spain	Gum-resin
Lavindin	Linallyl acetate	France	Flower
Lavender	Linallyl acetate, linalool	U.K., Mediterranean	Flower
Lavender spike	Linalool, linallyl acetate	France, Spain	Flower
Lemongrass	Citral	West India, Guatemala, Malagasy	Herb
Licorice	Glycyrrhizin	South and Eastern Europe	Root
Litsea cubeba	Citral	Asia	Fruit
Mate	Caffeine, tannic acid	South America	Leaf
Myrrh	Δ-Elemone, β-elemene, α-copaene	Ethiopia	Oleoresin-gum

Table 14 Continued

Common name	Significant chemical components	Producing region	Parts used
Nerol	Linalool, linalyl acetate, methyl anthranilate	Sicily, Spain	Flower
Oak	Tannins	Middle East, Central and Eastern Europe	Wood
Olibdanum	Pinenes, borneol, verbenol	Somaliland	Gum-Exudate
Onion	Propyl disulfide	U.K., United States, Europe	Bulb
Orris	Methyl ionone	Italy	Rhizome
Palmarosa	Geraniol	India, Indonesia, Seyehelles	Herbaceous top
Parsley	Apiole, 1,3,8-*p*-menthatriene, myrcene, β-Phellandrene	Europe, United States	Seed and herbaceous top
Patchouly	Patchouli alcohol α-bulnesene, α-guaiene, seychellene	Brazil, Indonesia, Malaysia	Leaf
Petitgrain	Linalyl acetate	United States, South America	Leaf, twig
Rose	Geraniol, nerol	Bulgaria, France, Turkey	Flower
Sandalwood (East Indian)	α- and β-Santalol	India	Wood
Tagetes	Ocimene	Australia, India, Mexico, South America	Flowering top
Tuberose	Geraniol, nerol	France, Morocco	Flower
Ylang Ylang	Linalool, beraniol, methyl benzoate, eugenol	Reunion, Malagasy, Philippines	Flower

Source: Gildemeister and Hoffman, 1913; Guenther, 1948; Arctander, 1960; Lawrence, 1979, 1981, 1982, 1985; Wilson and Mookherjee, 1983; Klimes and Lamparsky, 1986; Shaath et al., 1986; Nguyen et al., 1989.

Isolates are obtained from natural materials, usually essential oils. Isolation may be either by chemical or physical process. Purity now is usually >95%. Table 15 contains a list of several chemical isolates frequently used by the flavorist. Common methods of preparation are:

Fractional Distillation—Cedrol (cedarwood), citral (lemon grass, or litsea cubeba), octanal from orange and pinenes (turpentine) may be isolated by fractional distillation.

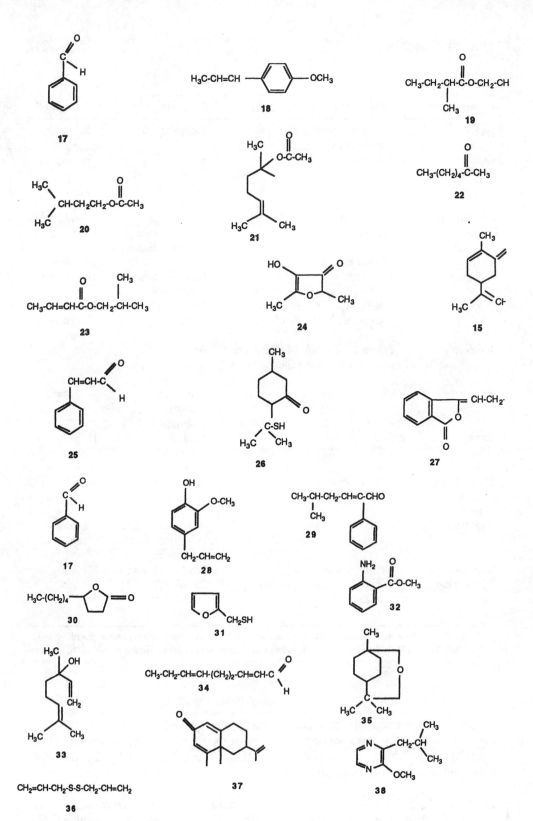

Fig. 22   Character impact compounds.

318

Fig. 22 Continued

Table 15 Flavor Chemical Isolates

Chemical	Origin
Octanal	Orange, grapefruit
Nonanal	Orange, grapefruit
Decanal	Orange, grapefruit
Dodecanal	Orange
Perillaldehyde	Orange
E-2-Hexenal	Mint
Nootkatone	Grapefruit
Valencene	Orange
Linalool	Bois de Rose, orange, grapefruit, ho
α-Terpineol	Orange, lime
3-Octanol	Mint
Sabinene hydrate	Mint
Eugenol	Clove leaf
Geraniol	Palmasosa
Methyl-methylanthranilate	Petitgrain mandarin
Methyl cinnamate	Eucalyptus
Cinnamic aldehyde	Cassia
Citral	Lemongrass, *Litsea cubeba*
1,8-Cineole	Eucalyptus
Citronellal	Citronella, eucalyptus
Cedrol	Cedarwood
Menthol	Peppermint
Pinenes	Turpentine

Chemical Reaction—Figures 23, 24, and 25 represent three chemical processes to isolate flavor chemicals.

Alkali Treatment (Fig. 23)—Phenolic oils such as clove leaf oil (containing eugenol 28) form water-soluble salts when reacted with alkalis. The aqueous eugenyl salt is separated and washed with an immiscible solvent. Treatment with acid liberates eugenol. Commercial eugenol is then rectified.

Bisulfite Addition (Fig. 24)—Aldehydes such as citral (42) form soluble addition complexes with aqueous sodium bisulfite. Following extraction of the complexed carbonyl, it is liberated with acid. The regenerated citral is washed and rectified.

Hydrolysis (Fig. 25)—Essential oils containing large proportions of esters can be used as a source for alcohols. Cinnamyl esters can be alkali hydrolyzed to yield cinnamyl alcohol (58).

Crystallization—Chilling and subsequent centrifugation is used to isolate menthol (49) from cornmint or peppermint oil.

Semisynthetic flavor chemicals are produced by chemical modification of compounds isolated from natural raw materials. Figure 26 shows the transformation of d-limonene (9) isolated from orange oil by fractional distillation to 1-carvone (54). This is the basis for a great many terpene-based flavor compounds. Figure 27 shows the derivation of several very high-volume flavor compounds derived from turpentine oil (Griffin, 1969; Muller, 1984; Bauer and Garbe, 1985). These include

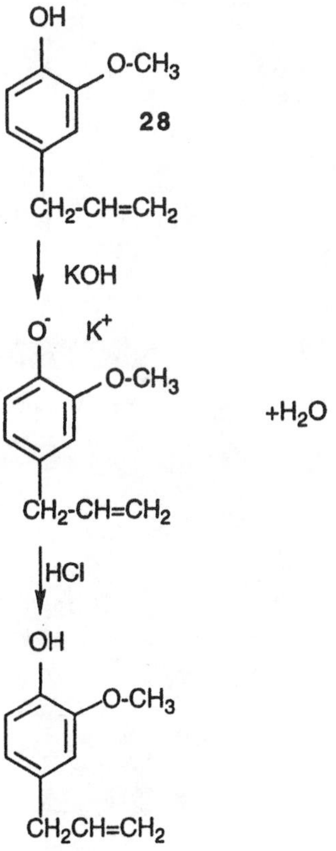

Fig. 23 Isolation of eugenol by alkali treatment.

α-pinene (13), β-pinene (14), α-terpineol (10), camphene (59), isobornyl acetate (60), citronellol (64), citronellal (65), menthol (49), menthone (66), hydroxycitronellal (67), citral (42a, geranial, 42b, neral), β-ionone (68), myrcene (12), α-terpinene (69), γ-terpinene (11), *para*-cymene (16), methyl chavicol (70), and anethole (18).

Synthetic flavor compounds are compounds produced solely from organic chemical feedstocks. Linalool (and esters), geraniol (and esters), citronallol (and esters), citral, and ionones may also be synthesized from petrochemicals, i.e., acetylene or isobutylene. Benzene (Fig. 28) and toluene (Fig. 29) are important feedstocks. From them cumin aldehyde (71), phenyl ethyl alcohol (72), acetophenone (73), phenylacetaldehyde (74), methyl phenyl glycidic acid ethyl ether (75), styryl alcohol (76), and styryl acetate (77) from the former and benzyl alcohol (78), benzaldehyde (17), cinnamic aldehyde (25), cinnamic alcohol (58), benzoic acid (79), methyl acetophenone (80), and phenyl acetic acid (81) from the latter are produced.

Phenol (Fig. 30) is the feedstock for anisole (82), anethole (18), parahydroxyphenylbuanone (53), anisic aldehyde (83), anisyl alcohol (84), phenoxyethyl isobutyrate (85), methyl salicylate (57), ethyl vanillin (86), vanillin (87), heliotropine (88), isoeugenol (89), eugenol methyl ether (90), eugenol (28) and isoeugenol methyl ether (91). Other phenolic starting materials include *meta*-cresol, from which

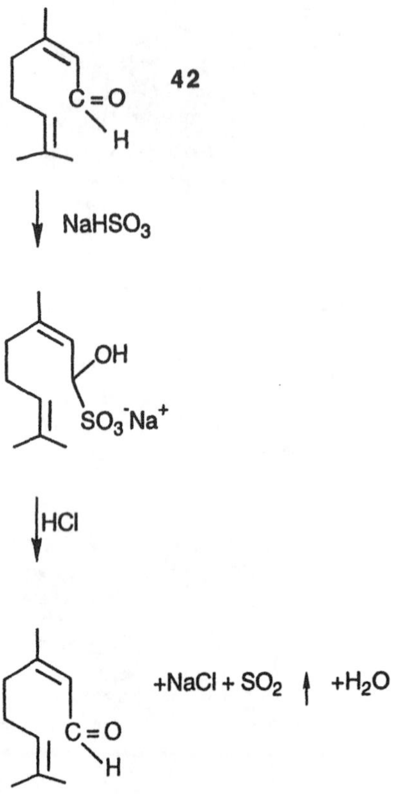

Fig. 24 Isolation of citral by bisulfite addition.

thymol (59), menthol (52), and menthone (69) are produced, and *para*-cresol, from which anisic compounds are produced.

Methyl anthranilate (32) and methyl-*n*-methyl anthranilate (92) are produced from naphthalene through phthalic and anthranilic acids (Fig. 31).

Biochemically derived flavor chemicals are now being produced on industrial scale using biosynthetic processes, e.g., enzymolysis or microbiological fermentation. These processes (Fig. 32) mimic or accelerate many of the reactions that occur during the biogenesis of food and beverage aromas. After all, humans made use of enzymes and microbial processes to improve texture, flavor, stability, and nutritional quality of foods and beverages long before they understood the biological mechanisms. Wine, for example, was made as early as 3200 B.C. in Egypt. Beer was made in Babylon in 2800 B.C. Cheese may have been discovered by a shepherd purely by accident when milk was stored in the stomachs of slaughtered animals. I'm sure that our ancestors who unknowingly discovered that the fermentation of sugar in a fruit juice resulted in a more stable product and pleasing flavor were also surprised to notice a physiological reaction! Today fermented foods and beverages alone are a $50 billion per year industry. The sale of pharmaceuticals, enzymes, and chemicals is estimated at another $5.9 billion (Faust and Prave, 1985).

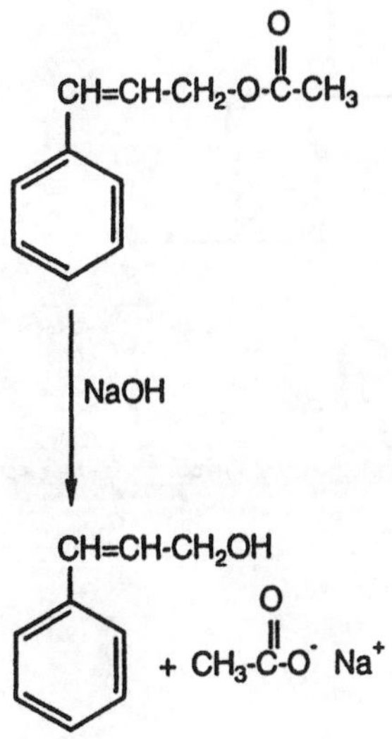

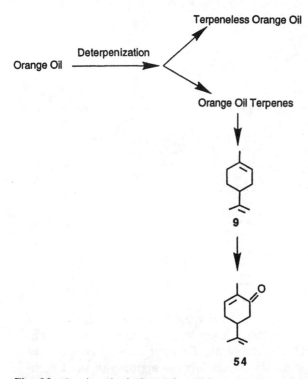

Fig. 25 Isolation of cinnamic alcohol by hydrolysis.

Fig. 26 Semisynthetic formation of I-carvone from d-limonene.

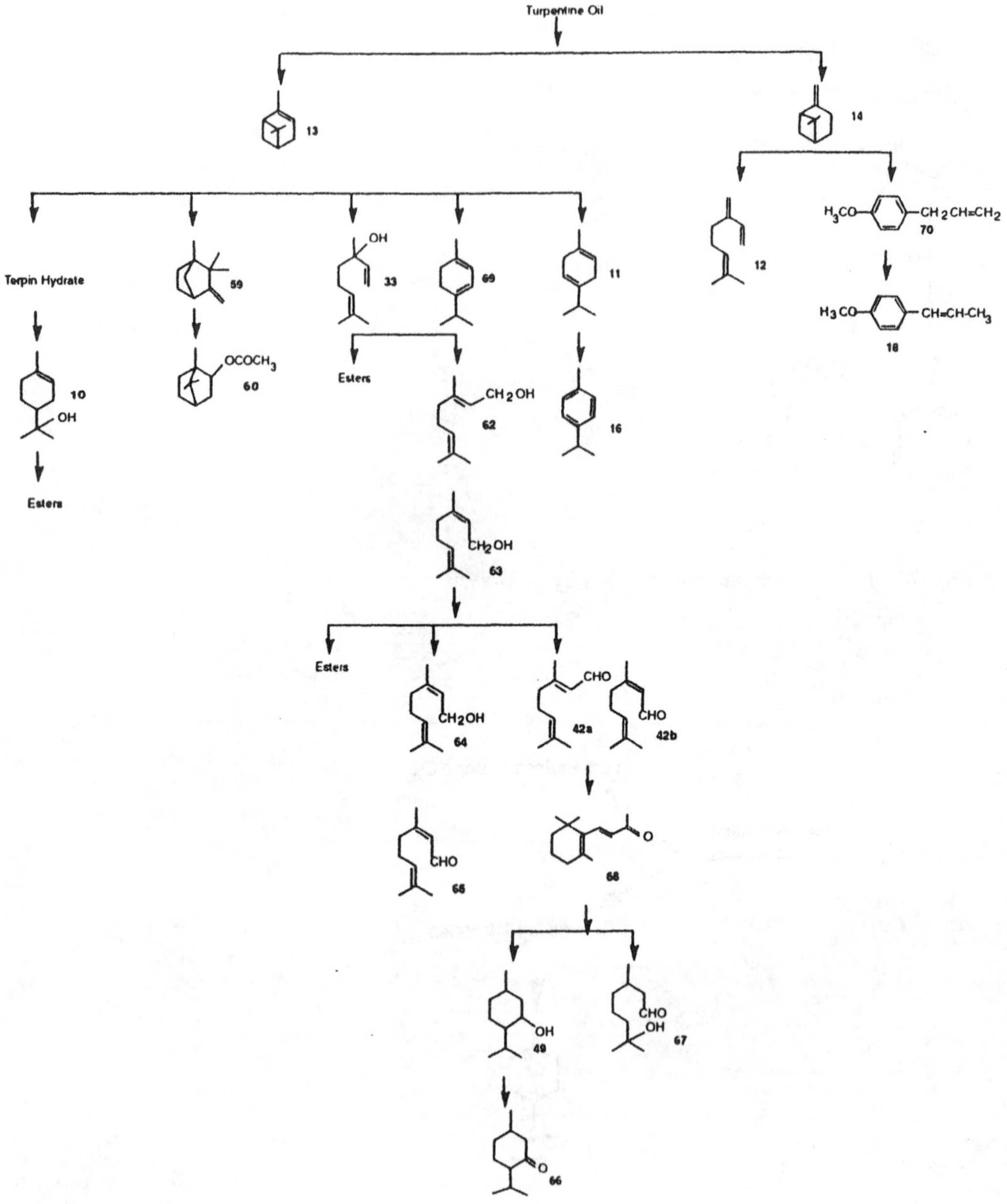

Fig. 27 Turpentine oil derivatives.

Since fermentation customarily requires lengthy, expensive separation and purification, biochemicals cannot compete with many high-volume synthetic chemicals, nor are all applications suited for biochemicals. They appear useful in a limited but ever-increasing number of applications. Certainly the majority of these compounds find use in value-added products or in the production of hard-to-synthesize

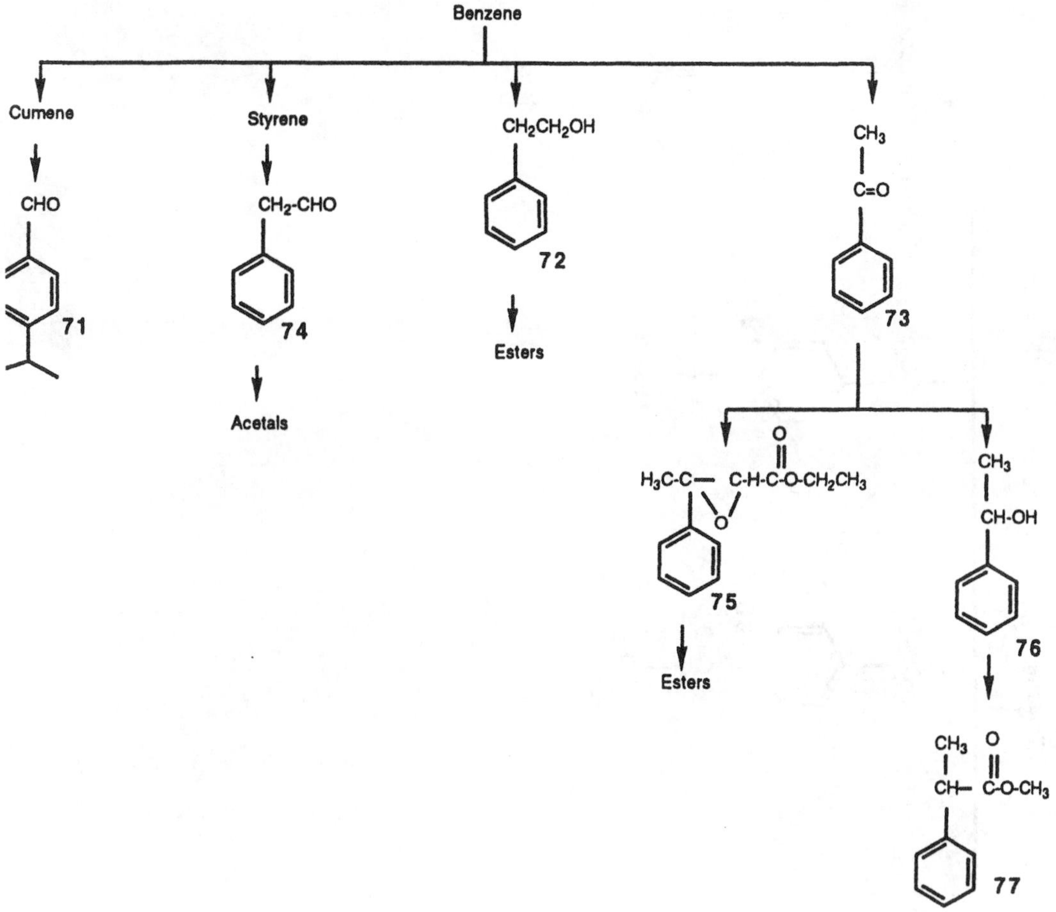

Fig. 28 Benzene derivatives.

chemicals. Other considerations are the limited aqueous solubility of precursor material and toxicity of flavor compounds to the producing cells. Several reasons or sets of circumstances have made the development of flavor chemicals via biochemical process viable commercially. Probably the greatest impetus came from consumer chemophobia and the desire of the food and beverage industries to market products containing natural flavorings. Although the term natural, as applied to food labeling, may be defined differently in individual countries, a common interpretation considers flavorings resulting from fermentation and enzymolysis as natural. Therefore, even though these products may be present in low yield or bear added costs, they have become new ingredients for the flavor industry. Bioflavorings do offer some advantages both to classical natural flavorings or chemical synthesis (Armstrong and Yamazaki, 1986). They are not influenced by any political, social, environmental, or climatic concerns in a specific growing region; consequently they are not subject to price fluctuations. In some cases yield, uniformity, and purity of biochemicals is favorable. One does not have to worry about exhausting finite natural raw materials since some bioprocesses use renewable

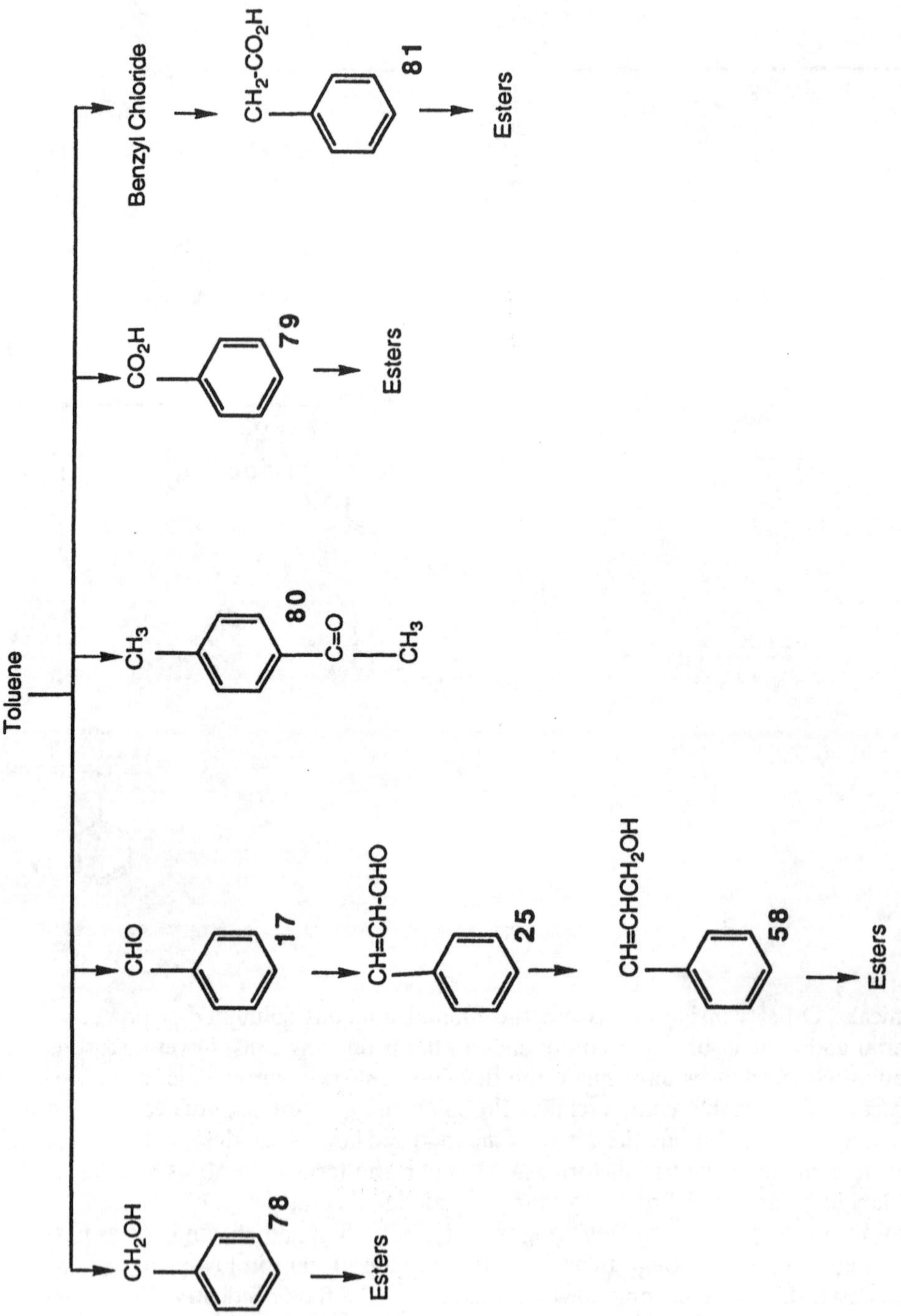

Fig. 29 Toluene derivatives.

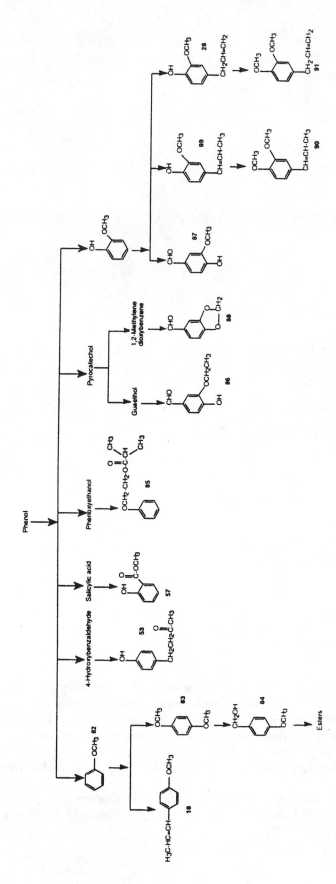

Fig. 30 Phenolic derivatives.

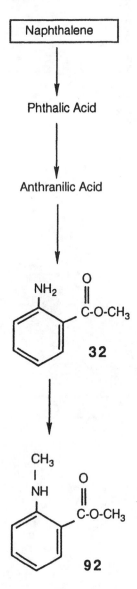

Fig. 31 Synthesis of methyl anthranilate.

resources. Novel aroma quality may be superior. The high substrate and reaction specificity guarantees a definite stereochemistry. Microbial enzymes are chemoselective, regioselective, diastereoselective, and enantioselective. Microbial catalysts have the ability to synthesize flavorants de novo from inexpensive nutrients. Microorganisms can perform multistep conversions reducing the steps in a synthesis, many times under mild conditions (such as atmospheric pressure and temperatures of 20–50°C).

It appears that the flavor industry has now entered into a third phase of biological production—the use of microbially produced secondary metabolites. The

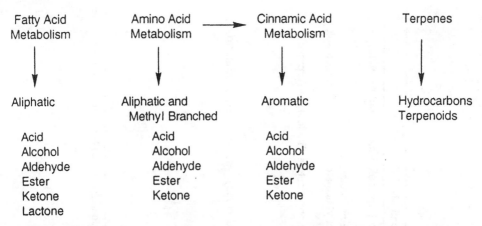

Fig. 32 Flavor chemicals from metabolic processes. (Adapted from Matheis, 1990.)

first two phases were fermented food production (cheese) and microbial primary metabolite production (ethanol). The range of chemicals currently capable of being produced by microbial fermentation is impressive. Indeed, the creative flavorist one generation removed must be envious. The range of chemicals includes esters, aldehydes, ketones, alcohols (interestingly, this first group of four accounts for about 85% of the chemicals used in the flavor and fragrance industries), fatty acids, lactones, terpenes, and heterocyclic compounds. Several examples of chemicals isolated from microbial fermentations are included in Table 16.

Fermentation isolates may be used as flavorings, blended to form proprietary mixtures, or used as precursors for additional flavor chemicals.

Castor oil is converted to γ-hydroxydecanoic acid using *Yarrow lipolytica*. Lactonization of the acid results in γ-decalatone. Cheetham and Lecchini (1988) described the formation of 5-ketogluconic acid from glucose by bacterial oxidation (Fig. 33). The acid is subsequently heated to form 4-hydroxy-5-methyl-3-(2H)-furanone (Fig. 33). This is a potent flavor chemical used in fruit flavorings, brown (caramel) flavorings, and as a precursor in meat flavorings.

The use of isolated enzymes is also being practiced by the flavor industry. Enzymes catalyze a wide variety of organic reactions, typically most effectively. Table 17 lists several common classes of flavorings processed with enzymes. A disadvantage to the use of enzymes is their relative instability. This may be overcome by bonding to a solid carrier (immobilization). Gillies et al. (1987) absorbed *Candida culindracea* lipase to silica gel and, when hydrated and shaken with *n*-heptane, containing substrates (butyric acid and ethanol), produced a series of flavor esters. These included ethyl propionate, ethyl butyrate, ethyl hexanoate, ethyl heptoate, ethyl octanoate, ethyl laurate, ethyl isobutyrate, ethyl isovalerate, isobutyl acetate, isoamyl acetate, and isoamyl butyrate.

Langrand et al. (1990) were able to prepare 35 flavor esters in an organic solvent using lipases from *Mucor miehi, Aspergillus* sp., *Candida rugosa*, and *Rhizopus arrhizus*, C2, C3, C4, C5, C6 acids and ethanol, butanol, iso-pentanol, hexanol, citronellol, and geraniol. Each lipase preparation tested presented a reaction selectivity according to the acid or alcohol moiety of the ester. *Aspergillus*

Table 16 Aroma Chemicals Isolated from Microorganisms

Microorganism	Chemicals
Ceratocystis moniliformis	Geraniol, citronellol, nerol, linalool, α-terpineol, 3-methyl butylacetate, γ-decalactone
Trametes odorata	Geraniol, citronellol, nerol, methyl phenylacetate
Ceratocystis coerulescens	Geranyl acetate, neryl acetate, citronellyl acetate, linalool, nerol, geraniol, nerolidol, farnesol
Trichothecium roseum	Linallyl acetate, citronellyl acetate, geranyl acetate, linalool, α-Terpineol, nerol, citronellol, nerolidol
Trichoderma virde	γ-Octalactone
Sporobolomyces odorus	γ-Decalactone
Sporobolomyces salmonicolor	γ-Decalactone, δ-Decalactone
Pityrosporum sp.	γ-Hexalactone, γ-heptalactone, γ-octalactone, γ-nonalactone, γ-decalactone, γ-undecalactone
Pseudomonas perolens	Methoxyisopropylpyrazine
Bacillus subtilis	Tetramethylpryrazine
Streptococcus lactus	Methylbutanol
Penicillium sp.	1-Octen-3-ol
Candida utilis	Ethanal, ethyl acetate
Pseudomonas fragi	Ethyl butyrate
Lasiodiplodia theogbromae	β-Ionone

Source: Pereira and Morgan, 1958; Tahara et al., 1972, 1973; Tahara and Mizutani, 1975; Jourdain et al., 1985; Armstrong, 1986; McIver and Reineccius, 1986; Scharpf et al., 1986; Manley, 1987; Montville et al., 1987.

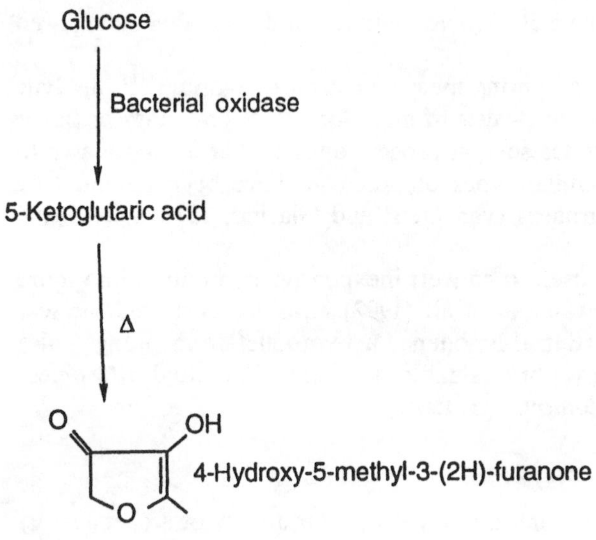

Glucose

| Bacterial oxidase

5-Ketoglutaric acid

Δ

4-Hydroxy-5-methyl-3-(2H)-furanone

Fig. 33 Biochemical production of furanones.

Table 17 Flavorings Produced by Enzymes

Precursor	Enzyme	Flavoring
Fat, protein	Lipase, proteinase	Cheese flavoring
Alcohol, carboxylic acid	Lipase	Ester
Hydroxycarboxylic acid	Lipase	Lactone
Alcohol	Alcohol dehydrogenase	Aldehyde
Alcohol	Alcohol dehydrogenase	Ketone

Source: Adapted from Matheis, 1989b.

lipase was very selective for very short chain acids and alcohols. *C. rugosa* lipase was more selective of propionic acid, butyric acid, butanol, hexanol, and isopenanol. The lipases from *M. miehi* and *R. arrhizus* were more selective of long-chain acids and not greatly influenced by the alcohols.

The development, enhancement, or intensification of cheese flavorings using enzymes is practiced on an industrial scale. Moskowitz et al. (1977) used an esterase from *M. miehi* to produce Italian-type cheese flavorings on a variety of substrates such as triglycerides, sorbitol esters of fatty acids, and animal and vegetable fats. They demonstrated activity over a wide pH and temperature range. Other dairy flavorings have been prepared with lipases from *Aspergillus niger, Penicillium camemberti, Penicillium cyclopium, Penicillium roqueforti, Pseudomonas fluorescens, Candida regusa, Candida cylindracea, Candida lipolytica, Humicola lanuginosa, Mucor javanicus, M. miehi, Rhizopus delemar, Rhizopus japonicus*, and *Geotrichum candidum*. Selection of enzyme is critical because of the specificities. Certain of the above enzymes, *A. niger*, for example, liberate considerable mono- and diglycerides. According to Trepanier et al. (1992) maturation was greatly enhanced in Cheddar cheese with one of *Lactobacillus casei* subsp. casei L2A.

Sensory evaluation demonstrated a 50% increase in flavor development compared to a control.

Enzymes are also useful in preparing meat and savory flavorings. Proteolytic enzymes are used to prepare flavor digests of meat for use as flavorings or flavor precursors. Figure 34 demonstrates several process options that use proteases to generate chicken flavorings. Similar types of processes have been patented by International Flavors and Fragrances (van Delft and Giacino, 1978) and Nestlé (Gasser, 1972).

Enzymic processes may be used to convert inexpensive byproducts into more valuable flavor chemicals. Cadwallader et al. (1992) have demonstrated the feasibility of enzymatically converting d-limonene, a byproduct from orange juice manufacture, into α-terpineol, a more valuable flavorant. They used α-terpineol dehydrates isolated from *Pseudomonas gladioli*.

Chemical Structure and Flavor Properties

It would be ideal to be able to predict the flavor or odor quality of a chemical by structural inspection. To this end numerous theories have been formulated; none, however, can fully explain this phenomenon. The following are general assumptions and observations about classes of chemicals commonly used in the preparation of flavoring agents.*

To have odor properties, a compound should have a molecular weight less than 300.
The odor intensifies until the molecular weight approaches 300.

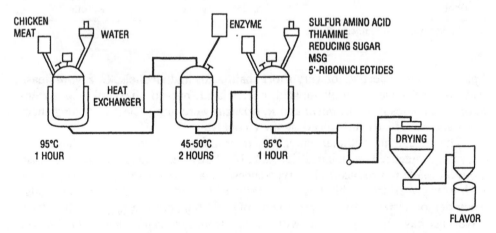

Fig. 34 Enzymatic preparation of meat flavorings. Enzymes: papain, bromelin, pepsin, trypsin.

---

* For a complete list of chemicals used in flavorings, the reader is referred to *Flavor and Fragrance Materials* (Allured Publishing, 1991, and for detailed characterization of flavor chemicals to *The Handbook of Food Additives*, 2nd ed. (CRC Press, 1972, Chapter 11) and *The Handbook of Food Additives*, 2nd ed., Vol. II (1980, pp. 256–306).

Odor is associated with osmophoric groups. In foods, nitrogen, oxygen, and sulfur are important, especially in the form of carbonyls, esters, lactones, amines, imines, lactames, and hydroxyls.

Introduction of a second hydroxyl variety reduces or eliminates the odor.

Substitution of a hydroxyl moiety by a ketone usually enhances the aroma.

Substitution of two hydroxyl groups by two ketone groups enhances the aroma in small molecules and removes it in large molecules.

Going from a plastic, aliphatic compound to a rigid, cyclic compound increases the odor.

Cis isomers usually are more potent than *trans* isomers.

Higher concentrations are required for odor than for taste.

There is no correlation between chain length and odor threshold.

Introduction of one double bond increases the threshold, while introduction of a second double bond decreases the threshold.

There is an alternating effect regarding the threshold of compounds within a homologous series. For example, with the series of 2-E-enals, C6 has a higher threshold than C5 and C7 has a lower threshold than C6.

Terpene Hydrocarbons

The chemical properties of the major compounds in this class have been discussed in the citrus extraction section. Their flavor characters are d-limonene (9, mild citrus), myrcene (12, disinfectant, herbal balsamic), α-pinene (13, turpentine, piney), β-pinene (14, woody, piney), and γ-terpinene (11, herbaceous, turpentine). Other frequently used terpene hydrocarbons are camphene (59, camphoraceous) and *para*-cymene (16, kerosene). This class is the most widely distributed in nature, and d-limonene is the most common hydrocarbon. This group also represents an important group of feedstocks for the synthesis of other flavor chemicals. α-Pinene and the enantiomeric limonenes are important starting materials for compounds in the *p*-menthane series. Ocimene (93) has seen more use as the popularity of reconstructed tropical flavorings has become more popular (Fig. 35).

Sesquiterpenes

These compounds have higher molecular weights and as such introduce characteristic sustainable aromas. Valencene (94) is isolated from orange essence oil and

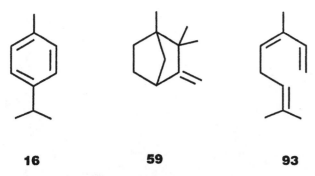

16   **59**   **93**

Fig. 35 Additional terpene hydrocarbons used in flavorings.

helps to distinguish essence oil from peel oil. It has a sweet, woody character. Valencene is also used to produce nootkatone (37).

Nootkatone has a warm, woody, grapefruit odor and is claimed by many flavorists to be the character impact compound for grapefruit. Other researchers, however, claim that 1-p-menthene-8-thiol (95) is responsible for the fresh grapefruit note (Demole et al., 1982). The compounds responsible for grapefruit flavor are shown in Figure 36.

Commercial preparations of both valencene and nootkatone range from 65 to 95% purity, so impurities can affect the odor quality of these compounds as they are currently used by the creative flavorist. Bisabolene (96) has been identified in grapefruit and bergamot oils. It has a sweet balsamic character. Cadinene (97), found in spice oils and tropical fruits, has a dry, woody, spice flavor. Caryophyllene (98) has a mild, woody, spice-clove odor (Fig. 37).

Fatty Acids

The flavor of short- to medium-chain saturated fatty acids ranges from sharp and pungent, for lower molecular weight compounds, to fatty and finally soapy and waxy, for the higher molecular weights (Table 18). The addition of a side chain, 2-methyl hexanoic acid, for example, introduces a fruity note. Unsaturated fatty acids, such as linoleic (99), common in vegetable oils, and arachidonic acid (100), common in chicken fat, are useful as precursors to flavoring compounds (van den Ouweland and Swaine, 1980; Manley, 1987). The formation of potent fresh green notes [E-2-hexenal (101), hexanol (102)] from linolenic acid and chicken flavor

Oxidation of Valencene to Nootkatone

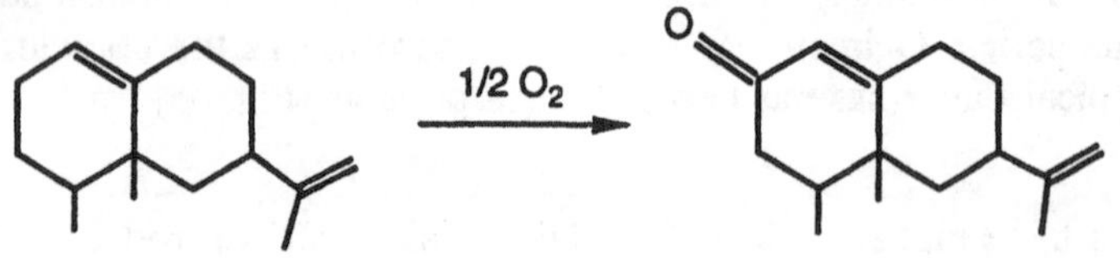

$$\text{94} \quad \xrightarrow{1/2\,O_2} \quad \text{37}$$

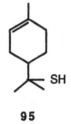

95

Fig. 36 Compounds important to grapefruit flavor.

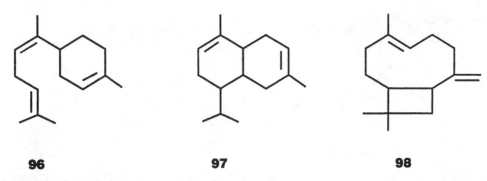

Fig. 37 Sesquiterpenes used in flavoring.

Table 18 Saturated Fatty Acids

Name	Structure	Characteristics
Acetic	CH_3CO_2H	Sharp pungent, winey, vinegar, grape, rum, topnote
Propionic	$CH_3CH_2CO_2H$	Sour, fatty, dairy, emmenthal
Butyric	$CH_3(CH_2)_2CO_2H$	Fatty, dairy, sour, rancid
Valeric	$CH_3(CH_2)_3CO_2H$	Sour, rancid, sweaty, chocolate
Caproic	$CH_3(CH_2)_4CO_2H$	Fatty, rancid, oily, soapy, goaty
Heptanoic	$CH_3(CH_2)_5CO_2H$	Fatty, sour
Caprylic	$CH_3(CH_2)_6CO_2H$	Fatty, sour, fruity
Capric	$CH_3(CH_2)_8CO_2H$	Fatty
Lauric	$CH_3(CH_2)_{10}CO_2H$	Soapy
Myristic	$CH_3(CH_2)_{12}CO_2H$	Soapy
Palmitic	$CH_3(CH_2)_{14}CO_2H$	Soapy, waxy
Stearic	$CH_3(CH_2)_{16}CO_2H$	Soapy, waxy

aldehydes using controlled oxidation of arachidonic acid are shown in Figures 38 and 39.

Alcohols

The function of some members of this class may be that of flavoring, flavor enhancer, or solvent. Ethanol, propylene glycol, and glycerin are common solvents for flavorings. Generally water solubility decreases as the molecular weight increases. Water solubility increases as hydroxyl or branched chains are introduced. As the number of hydroxyl moieties increase, the boiling point and sweetness increase. Ethanol may also enhance or alter the flavor profile of beverage flavors. Williams and Rooser (1981) demonstrated that there was a physiochemical effect of ethanol on the vapor pressure of volatiles in apple cider and that the fruity flavor of cider could be enhanced with specific concentrations of ethanol.

Low molecular weight alcohols have a light, spirituous, even solventlike aroma, while higher homologs become progressively fatty and citrusy. Figure 40 catalogs this effect with saturated straight-chain alcohols. Branched alcohols like isoamyl alcohol (103) have fermented character. Unsaturated alcohols such as Z-3-hexenol

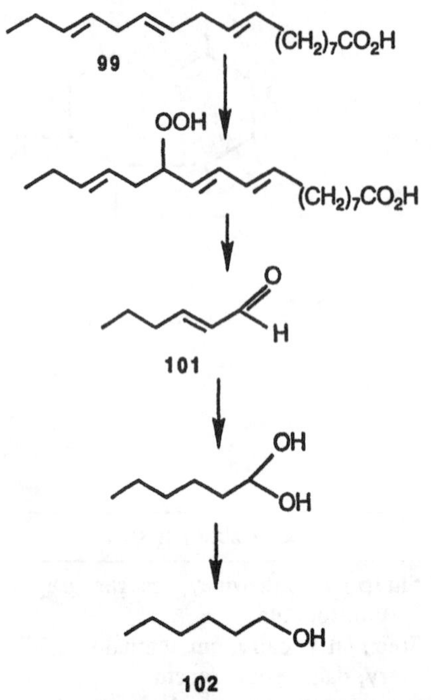

Fig. 38 Unsaturated fatty acid precursor to green notes.

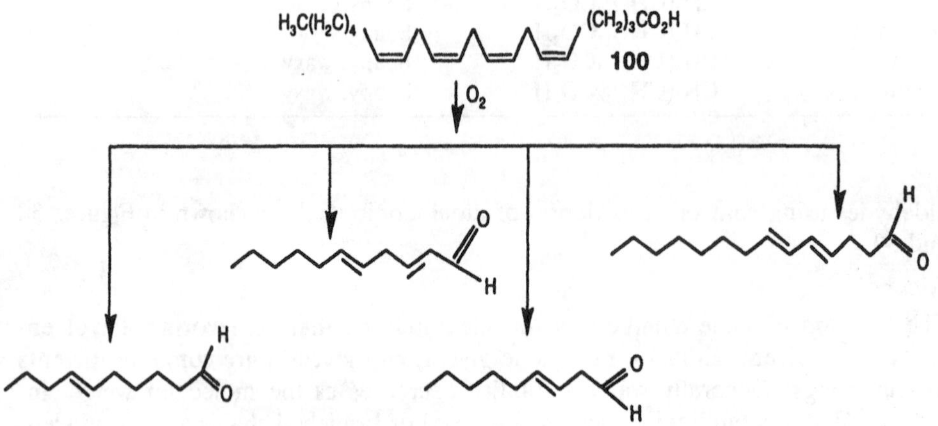

Fig. 39 Formation of chicken-flavor aldehydes by oxidation of arachidonic acid.

(104), commonly referred to as leaf alcohol, and E-2-Z-6-nonadienol (105) have green aromas.

Menthol (49) is an interesting compound. It is the major constituent in peppermint and cornmint oils and possesses not only the characteristic minty aroma but also the cooling mouthfeel. Aromatic alcohols are also commonly used. Phenyl

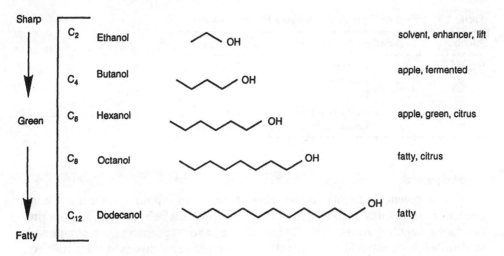

Fig. 40 Saturated straight-chain alcohols.

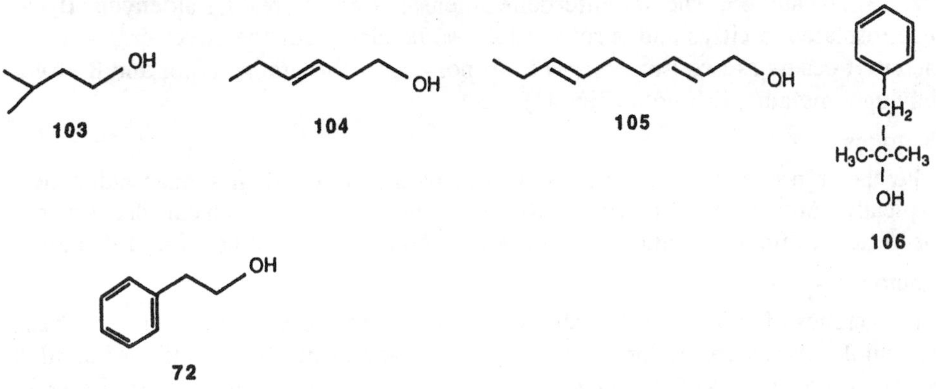

Fig. 41 Alcohols used in flavorings.

ethyl alcohol (72) has a floral-rosy, honey flavor. Dimethyl benzyl carbinol (106) also has a floral aroma. Structures 103 through 106 are shown in Figure 41.

Esters

These are the most diverse and most widely used class of chemicals in the flavor industry. About 40% of the chemicals used are esters. Esters are more volatile than the corresponding acids or alcohols. Generally, lower molecular weight esters are floral and higher molecular weight ones are fruity. Table 19 demonstrates this with the esters of benzyl alcohol. Several of the more common esters and their flavor characteristics are listed in Table 20.

Ethers

The odor of an ether is usually more intense and lighter than the corresponding alcohol. Common flavoring ethers are catalogued in Table 21.

Table 19 Effect of Fatty Acid on Ester Flavor Quality

Alcohol	Fatty acid (carbons)	Flavor
Benzyl	Formate	Floral
	Acetate	Jasmine
	Propionate	Floral-Fruity
	Isobutyrate	Fruity
	Laurate	Odorless

Aldehydes

These are potent and reactive flavoring agents. The instability of certain compounds, most notably acetaldehyde (7) and phenylacetaldehyde (74), require precautions in handling and storage. Frequently the flavorist prepares these compounds as solutions, uses antioxidants, and refrigerates reactive aldehydes to aid in stability. Acetals, perhaps a bit more floral, are sometimes prepared in an attempt to produce a more stable aldehyde flavoring.

Several classes of aldehydes are popular for flavor creation. The more common fatty, unsaturated, terpenic, and aromatic aldehydes are characterized in Tables 22, 23, 24, and 25. The sesquiterpene sinensal is an interesting aldehyde. It has been isolated in citrus and is responsible, some claim, for the sweet orange character. It occurs as two isomers: α (107), possessing the orange note, and β (108), having a metallic, fish note (Fig. 42).

Ketones

The flavor property of ketones is, in the main, milder than similar aldehydes, typically fruity, herbal, and woody. Ketones range, however, from dairylike (cheese or butter) to floral to minty. The more common ketones are listed in Table 26.

Lactones

The lactones of concern to the creative flavorist are the γ- and δ-lactones. These intramolecular esters are formed naturally from acyclic precursors such as bounded γ-hydroxy acids (Fig. 43). They generally possess sweet, creamy notes. Table 27 contains characterizations of the most commonly used lactones.

Phenols

Several phenolics are used in flavoring, but there are very few true phenolics. Most compounds in this class also contain other functional groups, for example, vanillin (87) or 4-vinyl guaiacol (109) (Fig. 44). Generally phenolics have characteristic medicinal notes. Thymol (56), the character impact compound for thyme oil, is a true phenolic.

Heterocyclic Compounds

This class of compounds originates predominantly from the thermal processing of foods and is covered in the sections on Maillard reaction products, hydrolyzed vegetable protein, and autolyzed yeast extracts.

Thermally Processed Flavoring Agents

No discussion of the thermal generation of aroma or flavor could begin without an understanding of the Maillard reaction, perhaps more correctly termed Maillard

Table 20 Flavor Esters

Ester	Structure	Flavor characteristics
Ethyl acetate		Ethereal, topnote, fruit, wine, rum
Ethyl acetoacetate		Green-fruity, apple, strawberry
Ethyl benzoate		Topnote, floral-ylang, fruity-pineapple
Ethyl butyrate		Tutti-fruiti, ethereal, topnote, orange juice
Ethyl cinnamate		Sweet-jammy, peach, strawberry
Ethyl-*trans*-2, *cis*-4-decadienoate	$CH_3\text{-}(CH_2)_4\text{-}CH{=}CH\text{-}CH{=}CH\text{-}C\text{-}O\text{-}CH_2\text{-}CH_3$	Pear, apple
Ethyl caproate		Fruity-banana, pineapple, grape
Ethyl caprylate		Fatty-fruity, winey, grape, rum
Ethyl caprate		Wine, grape, cognac
Ethyl isovalerate		Apple, pineapple, rum
Ethyl-2-methyl butyrate		Apple, strawberry
Ethyl-3-methylthiopropionate		Pineapple

Table 20 Continued

Ester	Structure	Flavor characteristics
Ethyl-*cis*-4-octenoate		Green-fruity, apple, tropical
Ethyl sorbate		Prune
Allyl cyclohexanepropionate	$-(CH_2)_2-C-O-CH_2-CH=CH_2$	Pineapple
cis-3-Hexenylacetate		Green, banana
Methyl anthranilate		Foxy, concord grape
Linallyl acetate		Bergamot, lavender
Isoamylacetate		Banana

reactions, since it is actually a series of complex reactions in foods or model food systems that are responsible for potent flavor compounds characterized by nitrogen, sulfur, and oxygen heterocyclics and aldehydes that give rise to baked, roasted, fried, and boiled flavors. The Maillard reaction is also referred to as nonenzymatic browning. The first scientific study of what up to that time was a flavor problem, i.e., the browning of foods, was undertaken in 1912 by Dr. Louis-Camille Maillard at the University of Nancy. In attempting to study the biological synthesis of proteins, Maillard observed a gradual browning and odor reminiscent of baked bread or roasted meat when he heated solutions of glucose with amino acids. It is now generally agreed that reducing compounds readily combine with amino acids, proteins, and peptides to generate aroma compounds and color bodies in foods and beverages—the Maillard reaction.

The Maillard reaction proceeds through several stages. The initial step, shown in Figure 45 (Hodge, 1953), involves the formation of *N*-glycosides by the con-

Table 21 Flavor Ethers

Ether	Structure	Flavor characteristics
Anethole	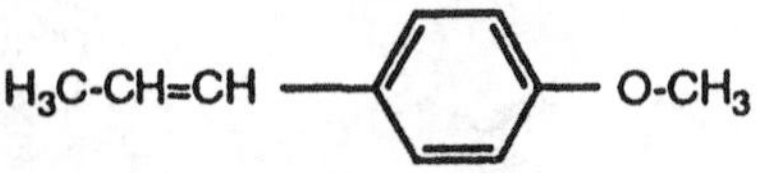 $H_3C\text{-}CH=CH$ —⟨benzene ring⟩— $O\text{-}CH_3$	Anise, fennel
Anisole	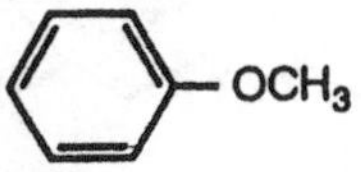 ⟨benzene ring⟩— OCH_3	Sharp, anise
Benzyl ethylether	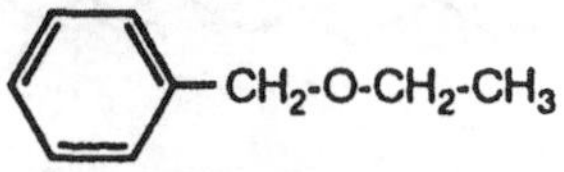 ⟨benzene ring⟩— $CH_2\text{-}O\text{-}CH_2\text{-}CH_3$	Pineapple
Dimethyl hydroquinone	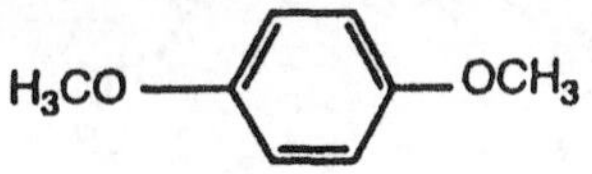 H_3CO —⟨benzene ring⟩— OCH_3	Nutty, hyacinth
Estragole	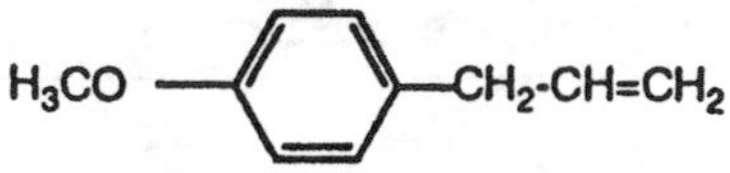 H_3CO —⟨benzene ring⟩— $CH_2\text{-}CH=CH_2$	Basil, anise
Yara yara	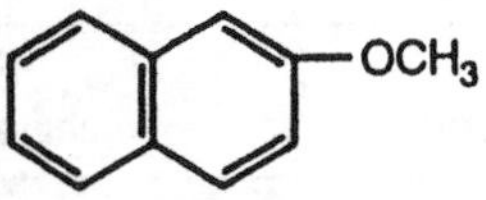 ⟨naphthalene ring⟩— OCH_3	Orange blossom acacia
Nerolin II	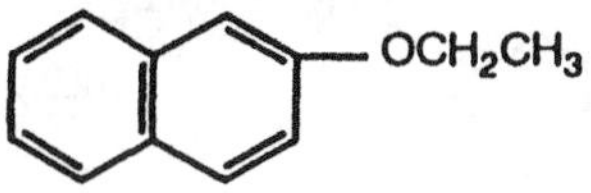 ⟨naphthalene ring⟩— OCH_2CH_3	Orange blossom

Table 22 Fatty Aldehydes

Flavor characteristic	Carbons	Name	Formula
Sharp	C2	Ethanal (acetaldehyde)	CH_3CHO
Penetrating	C3	Propionaldehyde	CH_3CH_2CHO
	C4	Butyraldehyde	$CH_3(CH_2)_2CHO$
	C5	Valeraldehyde	$CH_3(CH_2)_3CHO$
Green	C6	Hexanal	$CH_3(CH_2)_4CHO$
	C7	Heptanal	$CH_3(CH_2)_5CHO$
Fatty (citrus)	C8	Octanal	$CH_3(CH_2)_6CHO$
	C9	Nonanal	$CH_3(CH_2)_7CHO$
Waxy	C10	Decanal	$CH_3(CH_2)_8CHO$
	C11	Undecanal	$CH_3(CH_2)_9CHO$
	C12	Dodecanal	$CH_3(CH_2)_{10}CHO$

densation of the free carbonyl group of the reducing sugar and the free amino moiety of the protein or amino acid, dehydration, the formation of an aldimine, and cycilization. This may occur under mild conditions. Spontaneous conversion of the N-glycosides into isomeric forms (the Amadori rearrangement, the reaction of a ketose, and an amine proceeds through the Heyn's rearrangement) yields

Table 23 Unsaturated Aldehydes

Aldehyde	Structure	Flavor characteristics
trans-2-Hexenal		Green, penetrating, sharp, intense, apple
cis-3-Hexenal		Green
trans-2-*cis*-6-Nonadienal		Green, cucumber
cis-4-Heptenal		Green, fatty, tomato
2-4-Octadienal		Fatty, citrus, poultry

Table 24 Terpene Aldehydes

Aldehyde	Structure	Flavor characteristics
Citral	neral ① geranial ②	① Lemon ② Green, grassy
Citronellal		Lemon, rose, citronella

Amadori compounds. These compounds, 1-amino-1-deoxy-2-ketoses, are nonvolatile precursors of flavor and have been the subject of flavor patents (Doornhos and van den Ouweland, 1977).

Thermal degradation of Amadori compounds results in the formation of active intermediates. At low pH, the reaction proceeds through a 3-deoxyhexosone and results in compounds such as 5-hydroxyfurfural (110) (Fig. 46). At higher pH the reaction proceeds through a 1-deoxyhexosone and results in compounds such as maltol (111) and isomaltol. Breakdown of Amadori compounds produces reductones, which in turn mediate the oxidative degradation of amino acids. This pathway (Fig. 47) results in flavor aldehydes, some of which have been patented for use in

Table 25 Aromatic Aldehydes

Aldehyde	Structure	Flavor characteristics
Phenylacetaldehyde	CH_2CHO benzene ring	Floral: hyacinth, fruity, green
Cinnamic aldehyde	$CH=CH-CHO$ benzene ring	Cinnamon, cassia
Benzaldehyde	CHO benzene ring	Cherry, almond, marzipan
α-Amyl cinnamic aldehyde	$CH=C-CHO$ $CH_2(CH_2)_3-CH_3$ benzene ring	Floral: jasmine, waxy

foods, e.g., methyl phenylhexenal in cocoa flavor (van Praag and Stein, 1971). Aminoketones (Fig. 48) undergo dehydration and dehydrogenation reactions to form pyrazines, many of which are responsible for roast flavor in meat, nuts, bread, and coffee.

The goal for the creative flavorist, therefore, is to use the Maillard reaction either alone or in combination with other precursors to mimic, in concentrated form, those reactions responsible for characteristic flavors from heated foods. Flavorings may take the form of concentrated model systems that, when thermally processed either pre- or postaddition to the food, react to impart desirable flavor, or the identification, isolation, and subsequent synthesis of single chemicals responsible for a particular flavor or individual flavor note. To date the most successful systems employ precursor-model systems. This field of flavor chemistry was

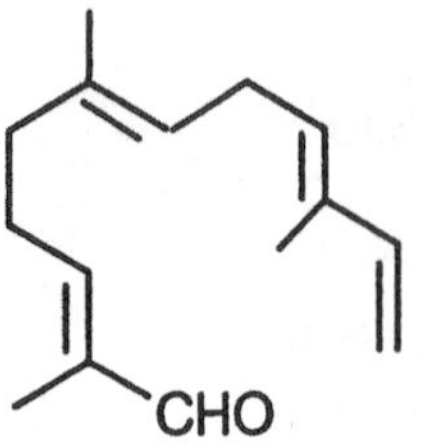

Fig. 42 Sesquiterpene aldehydes.

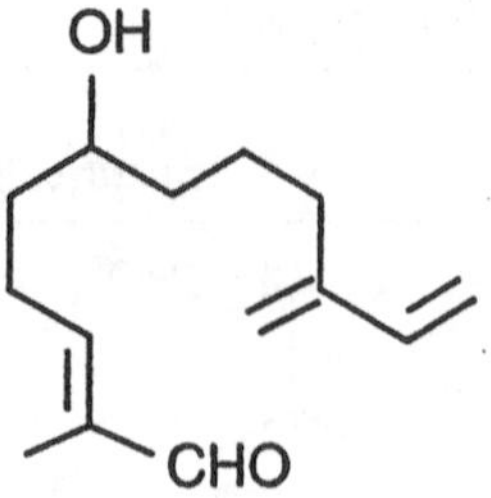

pioneered during the early 1960s by Unilever Research. Early patents (May, 1960; Morton et al., 1960) taught the use of reducing sugars and sulfur-containing amino acids to generate meat flavorings. Herz and Schallenberger (1960) observed the following aromas when amino acids were heated with glucose: aspartic (candy, caramel), threonine (chocolate), serine (maple), glutamic acid (caramel, burnt sugar), proline (baked goods), glycine (caramel), alanine (caramel), valine (rye bread), isoleucine (fruity, aromatic), leucine (chocolate). This technology is currently used to prepare meat, chocolate, maple, caramel, coffee, and nut flavoring agents.

While the Maillard reaction deals with amino acids and sugars, there are several other classes of precursor compounds that the creative flavorist uses to generate flavorings. These include lipids, vitamins, and ribonucleotides.

Lipids, especially fatty acids, contribute to flavor through oxidation, hydrolysis, dehydration, or decarboxylation reactions and are especially important in recreating the species specific flavor of meats. The precursors used in the nonenzymatic browning meat flavorings are predominantly low molecular weight, water-soluble, dializable compounds that when heated generate general meaty aromas common to several cooked meats. Table 28 contains the aldehydes that are formed from heating meat. The fatty acid precursors are shown in Figure 49 (van den Ouweland and Swaine, 1980). The importance of arachidonic acid in the phospholipid fraction of chicken as a precursor of unsaturated aldehydes characteristic of chicken flavor was discussed earlier (see Fig. 35). Thermal oxidative compounds such as aldehydes, ketones, and lactones are used by the flavorist to compound meat flavor. Gamma and deca C5–C15 lactones have been identified in beef fat and gamma C5 and C9 lactones in pork (Wasserman, 1972).

Thermal degradation of vitamins also results in meat and other processed flavors. The most studied and often used vitamin is thiamine. It gives rise to thiazoles, thiazolines, hydrogen sulfide, acetyl mercaptopropanal, and 3-mercaptopropanol. The incorporation of pantothenic acid accentuates the formation of potent flavor compounds from thaimine. Ascorbic acid has also been used as a precursor for the formation of cooked meat and chocolate flavorings. Ascorbic acid decomposition leads initially to highly reactive dicarbonyl intermediates, which give rise to potent aromas. Such compounds include glyoxal, glyceraldehyde, furfural, 3-hydroxyfurfural, 5-methyl-4-hydroxy-3-furanone, 3-hydroxy-2-pyrone, and

Table 26 Flavoring Ketones

Ketone	Structure	Flavor characteristics
Methyl amyl ketone	$CH_3(CH_2)_4\text{-}\overset{\displaystyle O}{\overset{\|}{C}}\text{-}CH_3$	Bleu cheese
Methyl nonyl ketone	$CH_3(CH_2)_8\text{-}\overset{\displaystyle O}{\overset{\|}{C}}\text{-}CH_3$	Cheese
Benzophenone		Grape
Acetophenone		Sweet
Methyl-β-naphthyl ketone		Neroli
Menthone		Peppermint
Allyl ionone		Pineapple
α-Ionone		Violet, orris, raspberry

Table 26 Continued

Ketone	Structure	Flavor characteristics
β-Ionone		Raspberry, fruity-woody
β-Damascone		Berry, floral
β-Damascenone		Berry, floral
Oxanone		Raspberry, blackberry
Isojasmone		Jasmine
Jasmone		Jasmine
Diacelyl		Butter
α-Irone		Orris waxy

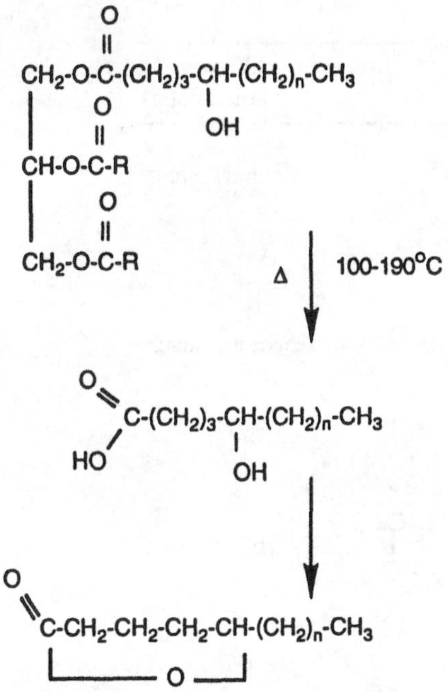

Fig. 43 Lactone formation from bounded γ-hydroxy acid.

2-acetylfuran. These may further react with amino acids. Figure 50 contains information about flavor formation from vitamins (Mikova and Davidek, 1974; Schutte, 1976).

Ribonucleotides present in both meat and yeast extract and derivatives of ribonucleotides are useful in generating both caramel and meat flavors. Figure 51 describes the formation of furanones by a nucleophilic-catalyzed beta elimination of phosphate from ribose-6-phosphate. Furanones possess a variety of caramel and brothy aromas and, when further reacted with labile sulfur compounds, give rise to potent meat flavors (van den Ouweland and Peer, 1975).

Hydrolyzed Proteins

The two main categories of hydrolyzed proteins are acid-hydrolyzed vegetable protein (HVP or HPP) and autolyzed yeast extracts (AYE). These products are versatile flavoring agents capable of inferring or enhancing characteristic savory flavors. HVP has its origins in Europe during the Napoleonic wars as a replacement for meat extract and in Japan, about 1912, where it was found to be an economical source of monosodium glutamate. AYE has been used only more recently, originating as a brewery byproduct.

HVP is produced commercially by acid hydrolysis. This process results in a more complete hydrolysis and preferred flavor profile than either enzymatic or alkaline hydrolysis. It is prepared from feedstocks containing from 50 to 80% protein. Common raw materials are defatted oilseeds (peanut and soy) and gluten (wheat, corn, and rice). Less common substrates include potato, casein, and yeast. The choice of protein source, processing aids, and process influences the final

Table 27 Flavoring Lactones

Lactone	Structure	Flavor characteristics
γ-Octalactone		Coconut, sweet
γ-Nonalactone		Coconut, peach fatty
γ-Decalactone	$CH_3\text{-}(CH_2)_5\text{-}CH\text{-}CH_2\text{-}CH_2\text{-}C{=}O$ with O ring	Peach
γ-undecalactone ("aldehyde C14")		Peach
6-Methyl coumarin		Coconut tonka
δ-Decalactone	$CH_3\text{-}(CH_2)_4\text{-}CH\text{-}(CH_2)_3\text{-}C{=}O$ with O ring	

flavor and the end use of the HVP. A typical process for the manufacture of HVP is shown in Figure 52.

The protein source is hydrolyzed with hydrochloric acid, generally for a period of up to 8 hours at temperatures of 110–130°C. HCl has been found to give the cleanest, most desirable flavor. The hydrolysate is cooled and then neutralized to pH 5–6 with sodium carbonate or sodium hydroxide. Again the choice of base is based on concerns for flavor quality. Potassium hydroxide is sometimes used to produce so-called "low-salt" HVP. The bitter metallic flavor is regarded by the flavorist as inferior. Humin, insoluble carbohydrate degradation products, are removed by filtration and the resulting hydrolysate is bleached or refined. One to three percent activated charcoal is used to standardize the color and flavor. Less refined HVP is dark brown in color and has strong roasted and bitter flavor, while the more refined HVP is a lighter, golden brown and milder in flavor. Following

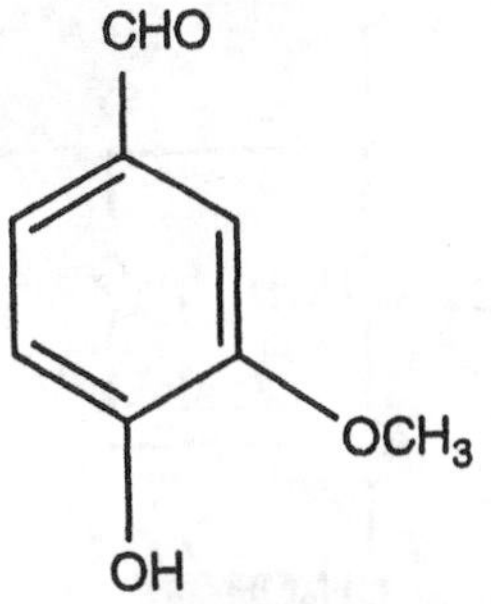

Fig. 44 Phenols used in flavorings.

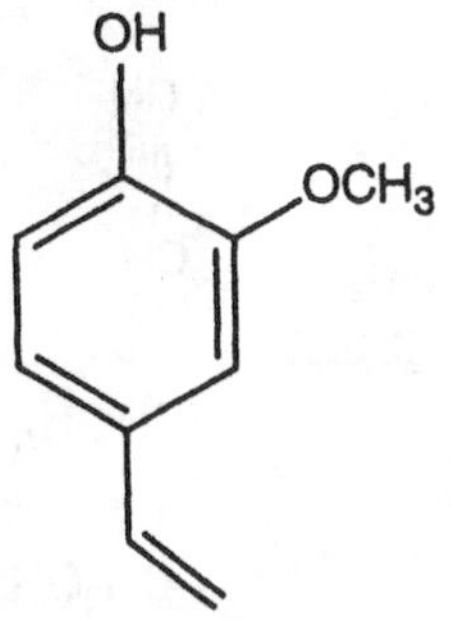

the removal of carbon by filtration the commercial HVP of about 40% solids may be sold: mixed with spices, flavorings, color, flavor enhancers (MSG, 5′-ribonucleotides); mixed with amino acids and reducing compound precursors and further thermally processed; or dried to a powder. The composition and amino acid profile of commercial HVPs are shown in Table 29 and Figure 53.

HVPs are used in a wide variety of foods such as meat analogs, bouillons, gravies, soups, snacks, reformed meats, and sauces in levels that range from 0.1 to 3.0%. Manley and Swaine (1979) have classified HVP according to chemical and sensory properties.

Figure 54 contains a flowchart for the manufacture of AYE. Primary AYE is produced from yeast cream grown on a substrate such as molasses or whey. Secondary AYE is produced from brewery byproduct yeast cream. In the case of secondary AYE, bitter isohumulones must first be at least partially removed. This is done by mild base extraction. The resulting product must have the pH adjusted, for example, with phosphoric acid, to about 5.5. The yeast cream is autolyzed (hydrolyzed) by endogenous enzymes that are liberated by rupturing the cell walls of the yeast. Thermal conditions are generally milder than those used for HVP— 40–50°C. Cell wall material is removed by centrifugation. At this point, as with HVP, the AYE liquid may be standardized with salt, flavor enhancers, or seasonings, may have precursors added and further processed, or be concentrated to a powder. The chemical composition and amino acid profiles may be found in Table 30 and Figure 55 (Manley et al., 1981). The uses of AYE are similar to those for HVP. An additional application for AYE is as a cheese flavor enhancer or extender. The presence of sulfur-containing amino acids and vitamins, especially thiamine and pantothenic acid, make AYE particularly useful in meat and cheese flavorings.

The volatile flavor of hydrolyzed proteins is generated from thermally induced chemical transformations of carbohydrates, proteins, and amino acids, primarily through amino-mediated degradation of reducing sugars. Lignin has also been indicated as a precursor for flavorings. This chemistry is summarized in Figure 56 et al., (Manley and Fagerson, 1970a, 1971; Manley et al., 1981). Nonvolatile flavorants include salt and the flavor enhancers monosodium glutamate and nucleotides.

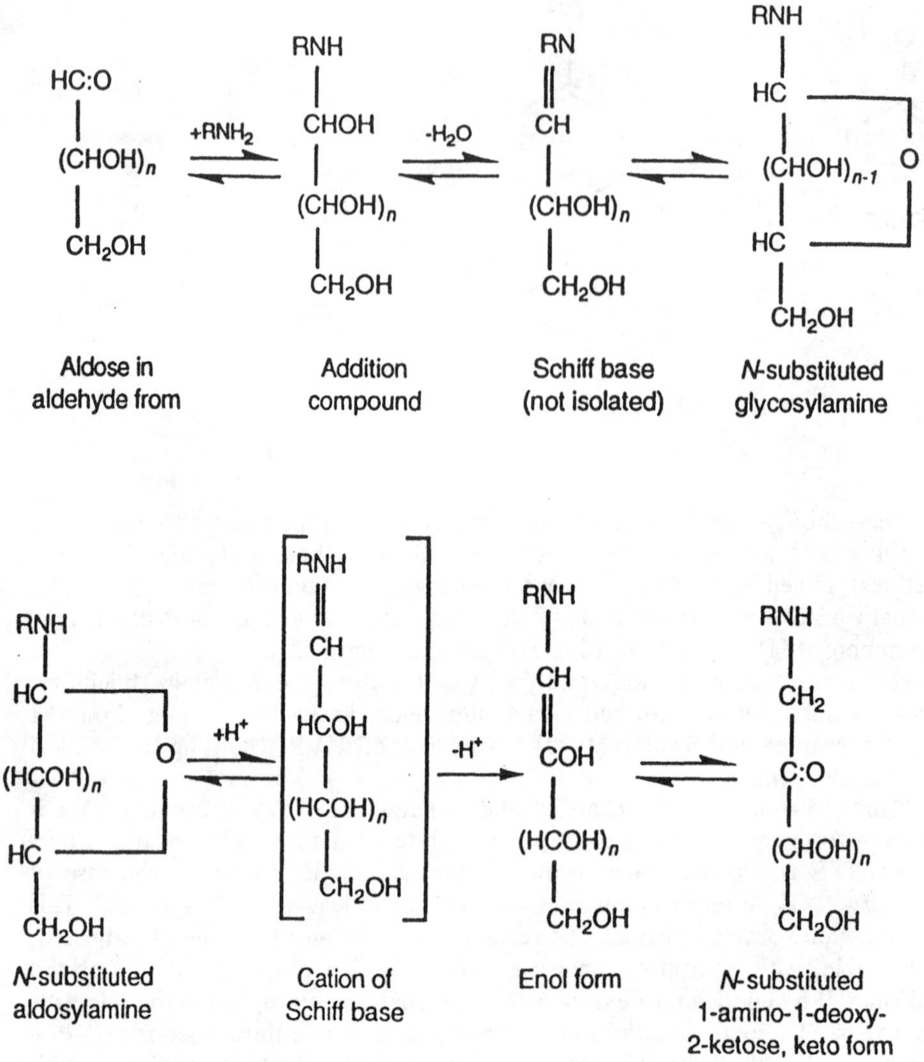

Fig. 45 Maillard reactions (early stages). (From Hodge, 1953.)

V. SAFETY AND TOXICOLOGY

A. Safety Considerations

It is ironic that flavoring agents, the very food additives responsible for the characteristics that most often influence our choice of food or drink, are also so often the center of great concern and even controversy. The safe efficacious use of flavoring agents must therefore be the principal concern of the flavor industry. But it is not solely flavoring agents that are singled out for scrutiny; food additives, food systems, and in fact diet in general are all of concern to the consumer, food scientist, and the regulator. Certainly, however, food additives and especially flavorings, perhaps because of their mystique and chemical origin, are more often

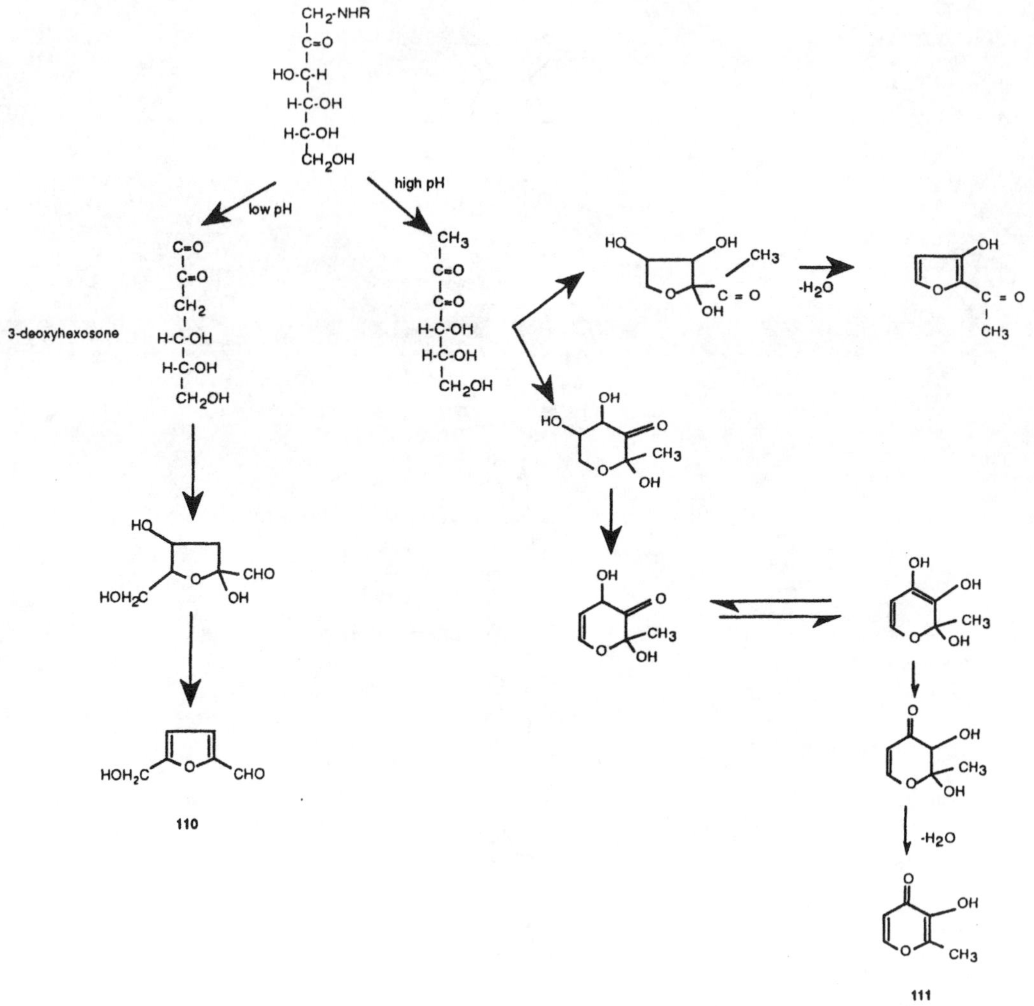

Fig. 46 Thermal generation of flavorings from amadori compounds.

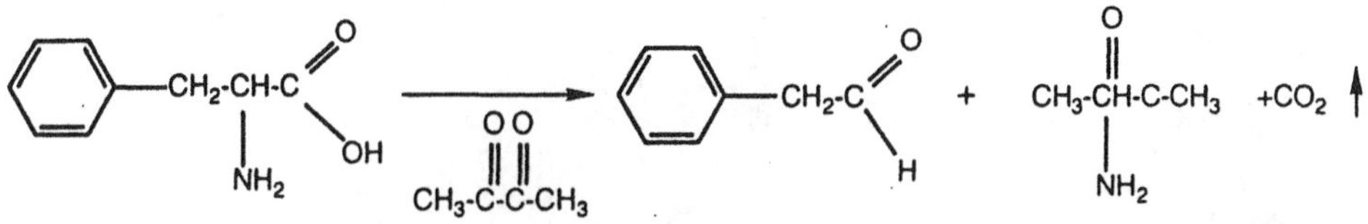

Fig. 47 Strecker degradation of phenylalanine by diacetyl.

the first to be questioned. According to Hall (1973, 1979, 1988, 1992), there are several classifications of perceived and actual risks associated with the food supply:

Microbiological—Estimates for the bacteriological contamination of food are as high as 10% of the U.S. population per year. This contamination is due pre-

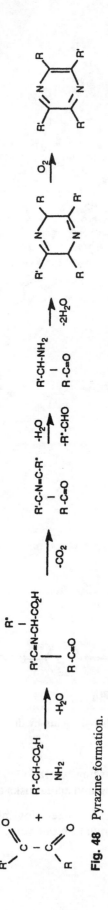

Fig. 48 Pyrazine formation.

Table 28   Aldehydes Identified in Heated Beef Fat, Chicken Fat, and Pork Fat

Aldehyde	Beef	Chicken	Pork
C5	+	−	−
C6	+	+	+
C7	+	+	−
C7 2t	+	+	+
C7 2t 4C	−	+	+
C8	+	−	+
C8 2t	+	+	+
C9	+	+	+
C9 2t	+	+	+
C9 2t 4C	−	+	+
C10	−	+	+
C10 2t	+	+	+
C10 4C	−	+	−
C10 2t 4C	+	+	+
C10 2t 4C 7C	−	+	−
C11	−	−	+
C11 2t	+	+	+
C11 2t 5C	−	+	−
C12 2t	−	+	−
C12 2t 6C	−	+	−
C12 2t 6t	−	+	−
C13	−	+	−
C13 2t	−	+	−
C13 2t 4C	−	+	−
C13 2t 4C 7C	−	+	−

Source: van den Ouweland and Swaine, 1980.

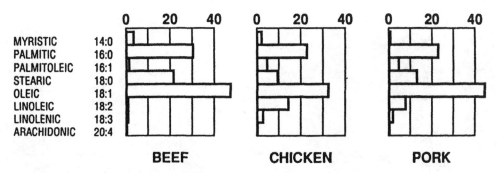

Fig. 49   Percentage of main fatty acids in lipid fraction of meat species.

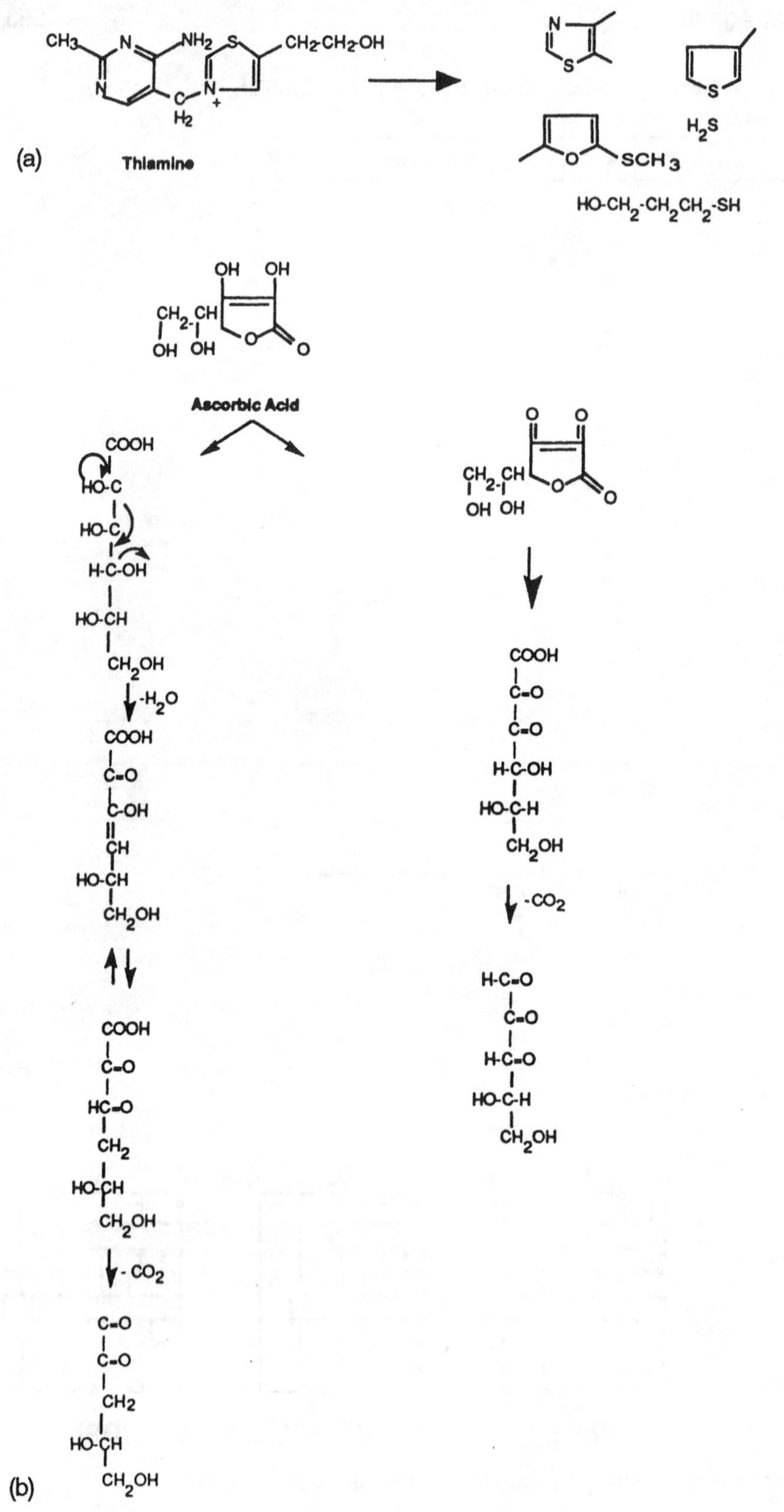

Fig. 50 (a) Contribution of thiamine to meat flavor. (b) Contribution of ascorbic acid to meat flavor. (From Mikova and Davidek, 1974; Schutte, 1976.)

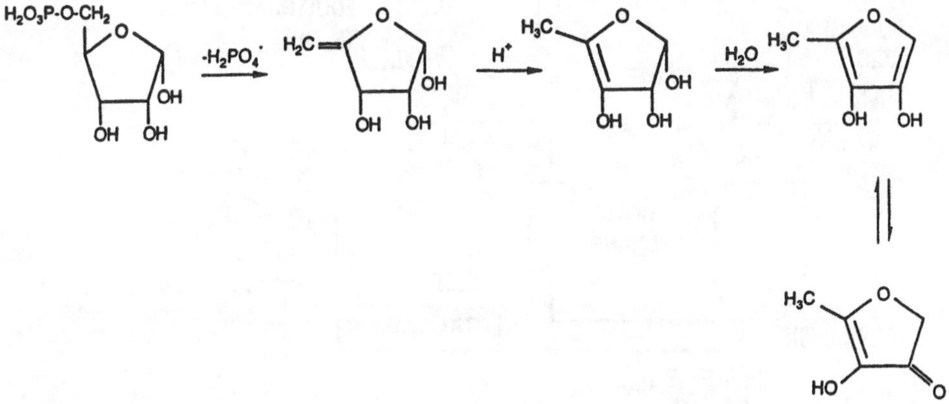

Fig. 51 Formation of 4-hydroxy-5-methyl-3(2H)-furanone from ribose-5-phosphate.

dominantly to unsanitary food-handling practice and occurs not only in restaurants or food service situations but also with regularity in the home. Too many U.S. kitchens practice unsafe food handling and preparation.

Environmental Contaminants—This category is particularly worrisome since the contaminant may be directly ingested by inhalation or transported across the skin or indirectly through the food chain. For a pollutant to "survive" to enter the food system, it must be quite resistant to change. Polychlorinated biphenyls (PCBs) are an example.

Nutrition—There is increasing evidence and concern for the role of diet in both acute and chronic disease states. Consumer and regulatory regard for this area has prompted the food industry to respond with a more varied selection that addresses current issues as well as increased access to information regarding food choices. Nutritional concerns include such issues as excess dietary fat, calories, and sodium and micronutrients deficiencies.

Natural Toxins—This is particularly interesting category, since virtually every food contains one or more species with toxic capabilities. It is of course, the relationship of dose and effect, *Dosis sola factit veneum* (what makes a poison is the dose), that is important. Heavy metal micronutrients, such as zinc, while essential to the life process in trace quantities, can exhibit mortally toxic effects in sufficient concentrations. Common table salt, a constituent of most savory flavorings, has an LD_{50} of 0.7 lb for the average adult male. As with most flavoring agents, however, its use is self-limiting. The list of common food constituents that are toxic includes such entities as enzyme inhibitors, lectins, phytates, and hemmagglutinins in legumes, coumarin, saponins, and oxylates in spinach, vicene and concine in fava bean, goitrogens in soybean and groundnut, cyanogenic glycosides in almond, chlorogenic acid in apple, mineral corticoid stimulant in licorice, vasopressor amines in cheese and red wine, and thiamine antagonist in berries. While this list is very interesting, taken out of context it could be very misleading. Because of the awareness of natural toxins, the variety of diet in developed countries, and the ability of the food industry

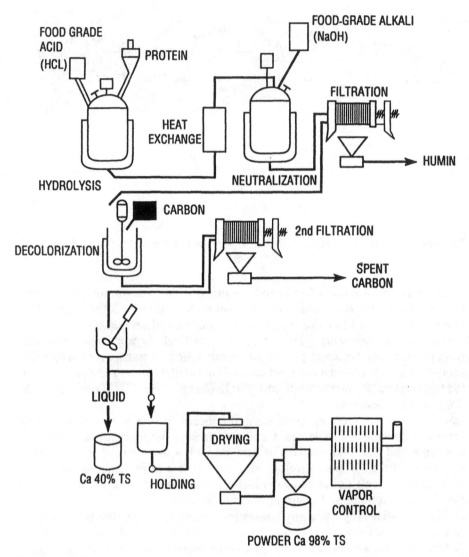

Fig. 52 HVP process.

to render many of these toxins innocuous by processing, natural toxins should present a decreased risk.

Pesticides—Proper use of pesticides assures a varied and economical diet in developed countries and the vital necessities for developing nations. A heightened concern lately of pesticide use has occurred in response not to known toxic occurrences so much as to a lack of data and general skepticism.

Food Additives—The days of *The Jungle* and the flagrant misuse of food additives for economic adulteration are, due to increasing analytical sophistication and enhanced regulatory scrutiny, behind us. Food additives, and most particularly flavoring agents, should, therefore, be considered a minor risk.

Table 29 Composition of HVP % by Weight

	Wheat	Soy
Water	2.0–4.0	2.0–4.0
Sodium chloride	39.0–44.0	42.0–45.0
Fat	0.2–0.5	0.2–0.5
α-Amino acids	42.0–52.0	26.0–52.0
Carbohydrates	0.1–0.2	0.5–0.7
Organic acids[a]	6.0–7.0	8.0–9.0
Ammonium chloride	4.0–6.0	1.0–3.0
Aroma volatiles	<0.01	<0.01
pH	4.5–5.0	5.0–5.5

[a]The major organic acid is levulenic acid. Other acids present are lactic, succinic, acetic, formic, and pyrroglutamic.

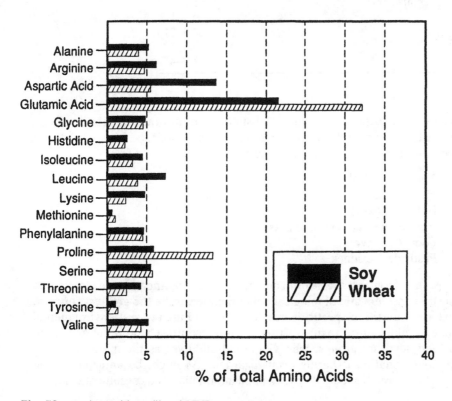

Fig. 53 Amino acid profile of HVP.

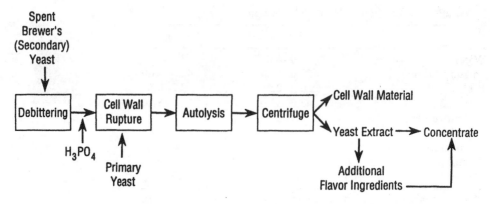

Fig. 54 Manufacture of autolyzed yeast extract.

Table 30 Chemical Composition of Autolyzed Yeast Extract

Material	AYE (%)
Total nitrogen (N)	8–10.5
Salt (NaCl)	2.1–3.6
α-Amino acids	28
Organic acids	2.0–4.0
Nucleic acid components	1.1
Fat	0.1–0.3
Carbohydrate	12.0–21.0
NH_4Cl	0.6–1.0
Water	2.0–4.0

Additional risks associated with the food supply are misbranding, fertilizer use, and product tampering. Hall's most recent prioritization of food hazards (1992) is as follows: (in order of decreasing priority):

Class I   Microbiological
             Nutritional
Class II   Natural Toxins
             Environmental Contaminants
Class III   Food Additives
             Pesticide Residues

It is interesting to contrast this list of concerns or risks to others. For example, the food industry considers microbiological contamination to be the greatest concern. They next rank nutrition, pesticide residue, food additives, and environmental contamination and natural toxins. This is in stark contrast to the lay and more fanatical food advocate groups, who view food additives as the major concern. Microbial contamination is hardly even regarded. As might be anticipated, the U.S. political concerns are fed both by scientific information and constituent emotion.

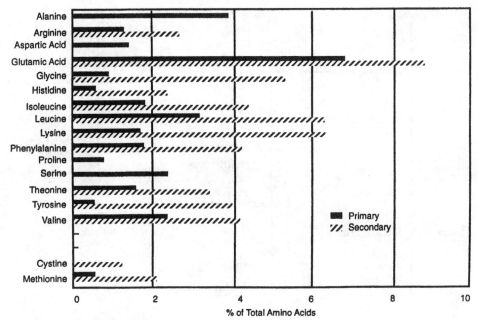

Fig. 55 Amino acid profile of AYE.

Congressional concerns range from microbiological contamination to nutrition, food additives, pesticide residues, environmental contamination, and natural toxins.

Several idiosyncrasies of flavoring agents warrant special consideration relative to other food additives:

1. Flavoring agents represent a large number and diverse range of additives. More flavoring agents (>2000) are used than any other category of food additive. Routine regulatory efforts would require a considerable increase in effort and staffing. The additional testing required would elevate the cost of flavorings well beyond what is reasonable to expect and would tie up valuable but limited laboratory resources. It has been estimated that the cost for toxicological testing of a new food additive is $500M–1MM for acute and chronic studies and $250–500M for teratogenic and mutagenicity studies (Jones, 1992). Time to complete this level of testing is estimated to be in excess of 5 years.

2. Most flavorings are based on natural food components and traditional methods used to prepare foods and beverages. The novel or fantasy flavorings such as Coca-Cola® are in the minority. Ford (1989) has estimated that 85% of all flavoring agents have been found in nature, and while this cannot be meant to imply their safety, it does illustrate that the majority of flavor chemicals are consumed by eating traditional foods. New flavor chemicals not (yet) found in nature in the main possess chemical structures analogous to previously identified compounds. Ethyl vanillin, not reported in vanilla extract, is a more potent homolog of vanillin, the character impact compound of vanilla.

3. The exposure level to flavoring agents is very low due to remarkably low use levels. The thresholds for flavoring agents range from a relatively weak compound d-limonene at 0.21 ppm (Ahmed et al., 1987) to a potent compound

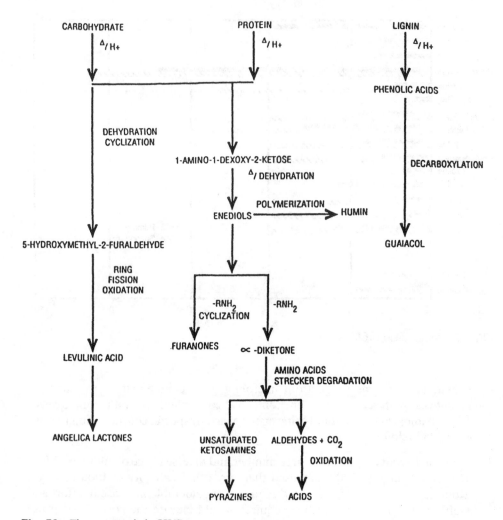

Fig. 56 Flavor genesis in HVP.

1-*p*-mentene-8-thiol at 1×10^{-7} ppm (Demole et al., 1982). The volume of flavoring agents sold annually in the United States and the estimated dose of flavorings are graphically depicted in Figures 57 and 58 (Oser and Ford, 1991). Only about 22% of the flavorings are used in concentrations that exceed 100 ppm. The majority of these are such ingredients as MSG, AYE, or HVP. The majority of flavor chemicals are produced in volumes less than 100 kg annually. These data are in sharp contrast to the use of most food additives. According to Hall and Merwin (1981) the estimated annual per capita consumption for the majority of flavoring agents was less than 10 mg. Consumption of essential oils and higher-volume flavorings, such as vanillin, is 10–100 mg. Salt consumption is estimated to be 7–10 kg, and sugar in excess of 50 kg.

4. The distinct aroma or taste provided by a flavoring makes its use self-limiting. Excessive use or overdosing of a flavoring results in a most unpalatable but memorable product.

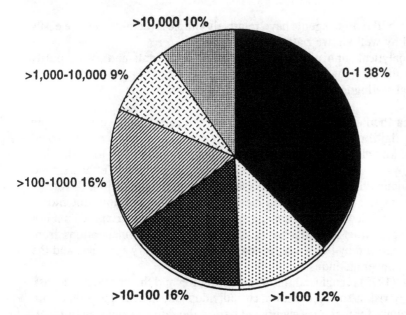

Fig. 57 Annual usage volumes of GRAS flavoring agents (kg/y). (From Oser and Ford, 1991.)

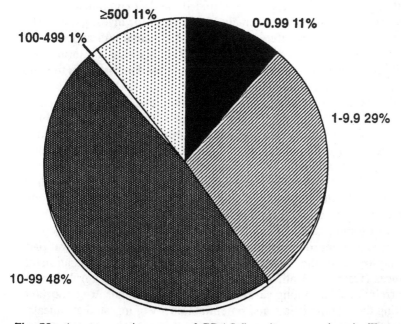

Fig. 58 Average maximum use of GRAS flavoring agents (ppm). (From Oser and Ford, 1991.)

5. The majority of flavoring agents have relatively simple structures that are easily metabolized by well-known pathways.
6. Increased analytical sophistication can detect contaminants and assure purity of flavor chemicals.
7. Toxicological testing is now more reliable and sensitive.

What criteria then should be used to evaluate the safety of flavorings? Some would argue for rigid, mandatory testing of every compound, while others would contend that the knowledge that a substance is normally present in food that has been consumed by human beings for ages without apparent untoward effects should be sufficient evidence to allow the incorporation of that substance in a flavoring. Rather than reviewing all rationales and methods of safety evaluation, one model will be discussed: the decision tree approach as practiced by the Expert Panel of FEMA (Flavoring Extract Manufacturers Association). Recommendations from this panel are recognized by the scientific community, regulatory agencies, and the food, flavor, and beverage industries.

Cramer et al. (1978) recognized this unique situation and the unachievable task of accessing every risk associated with each individual substance. They therefore proposed a procedure for making a significant part of the safety evaluation rational, public, and explicit. Priorities were established, as were sensible limits for investigation. Available toxicological and metabolic data for a substance, elucidation of chemical structure, and knowledge of the chemical properties of a substance and exposure data were used to validate this procedure, which consists of a "decision tree" of 33 questions, each answered solely yes or no. Each question leads to another and ultimately results in the substance being classified into one of three classes. Each class reflects a presumption of toxicity. Class I substances have structures and data that suggest a low order of oral toxicity and, if combined with low human exposure, should require an extremely low priority for investigation. The criteria for adequate evidence of safety would also be minimal. As exposure increased, so would the priority for additional study. Class II includes intermediate substances. While they are less clearly innocuous than Class I substances, they do not offer the basis either of the positive indication of toxicity or the lack of knowledge characteristic of Class III substances. The decision tree allows knowledgeable investigators to provide a "protection index" related to exposure, to establish priorities, and to define the appropriate protocol. Priority classification is assigned based on these three classifications and exposure data. The highest-priority substance to be tested therefore would be one whose structure is suggestive of high presumed toxicity combined with high-volume use. This procedure has been applied to a large number of pesticides, drugs, food additives, and industrial chemicals and has not resulted in any underestimation of toxicity. It is useful with pure chemicals or mixtures such as essential oils and oleoresins.

The decision tree procedure for evaluating ingredient safety is an integral part of the criteria employed by the Expert Panel of FEMA for the evaluation of flavoring substances (Oser and Hall, 1976). As practiced here, structural characteristics and interrelationships among various classes of compounds are important factors in predicting the metabolic fate and potential toxicity of ingested chemicals. The Expert Panel was formed more than 30 years ago in response to consumer, governmental, and industry needs. Though at the time new U.S. legislation, food additives were defined and regulated, the Food and Drug Administration (FDA) alone could not deal adequately with efficiently accessing the safety of numerous flavoring agents, i.e., flavorings Generally Recognized as Safe (GRAS). The flavor industry could not afford to satisfy the stringent requirements of a food additive petition for each flavoring agent. To this end an independent (expert) panel was established to determine the safety of flavoring agents and to make recommendations to the FDA. The criteria used by the Expert Panel for the establishment of the GRAS status of flavoring substances can be used as a model for flavor safety evaluation. The major considerations upon which the panel judged the safety of substances were:

1. Toxicity data
2. Biochemical and metabolic data
3. Occurrence of the substance in natural foods
4. Analogies with chemically related substances (toxicologically and metabolically)
5. The nature, level, and volume of use
6. Toxicological significance of the levels of use

All these criteria must be mutually supportive of and agreed upon for a safety recommendation to be received. No single factor is used to the exclusion of others. Principal precepts are potential toxicity and metabolic fate based on chemical structure and properties and exposure to the population. The three categories used by the expert panel are:

Class I—Compounds of simple organic structure that are readily handled by known metabolic pathways and are without adverse biochemical, physiological, or pharmacological effect. This class includes many naturally occurring flavorings, macronutrient metabolites, or compounds present in the body biochemical processes.

Class II—Compounds structurally analogous to those in Class I and whose metabolic fate can also reasonably be assured not to be associated with adverse biochemical, physiological, or pharmacological effect. Substances in this class may be less common in food or are in smaller units of food components. Examples are alicyclic compounds and terpenoids.

Class III—Compounds with structures so different from Class I or II that reasonable assumptions regarding metabolic fate and freedom from the possibility of adverse effects are precluded. Clearly the chemical structures of this class, heterocyclic compounds or polycyclic compounds, for example, are either uncommon or extremely complex, and scientific evidence is required for assessment of safety or definition of toxicological protocol.

Stofberg and Kirschman (1985) also recognized the impracticality of testing thoroughly all components commonly used as flavorings. They have reviewed the consumption ratio (CR) as a mechanism for establishing priority for safety evaluation. The CR relies on the facts that most flavoring agents are components of natural foods widely used in the traditional preparation of meals and that exposure or dose of such a substance is paramount to its toxicity. The CR is the ratio between the quantity of flavoring agent that is consumed as an ingredient of basic and traditional foods and the quantity of that same substance consumed as a component of added flavorings by the same population over the same period of time (Stofberg, 1983). A flavoring agent would be said to be food predominant if the CR is greater than 1, i.e., the consumption of this substance is predominantly as a component of traditionally prepared food. Conversely, a CR of less than 1 would indicate that a flavoring agent was consumed predominantly as an ingredient in added flavorings. Stofberg (1983) has proposed the use of the CR as a means of classification for safety evaluation. Several examples of common flavoring agents and their consumption ratios are included in Table 31.

B. Toxicological Considerations

The following will present several cases of flavoring agents or constituents of flavoring extracts that are regarded as toxic, have chemical structures analogous to toxic compounds, and are used in high volumes. It is not the purpose of this section to present detailed toxicological profiles or protocols, rather several cases will be presented to gain insight into the structure activity relationship of toxic compounds that have been identified in flavoring agents. Unless otherwise noted, all structures will be found in Figure 59. Toxicity of flavorings must be considered in concern with dose, occurrence, and exposure. For example, onion and garlic, two common seasoning ingredients, contain numerous sulfur compounds responsible for the characteristic flavor and aroma of *Allium* species. Several sulfides have been shown to affect iodine uptake in rats (Cowen et al., 1967). When onions are consumed as a major part of the diet, such as in the valleys of Lebanon, they are implicated in the high incidence of goiter (Saghir et al., 1966). There is little evidence that these sulfur compounds present in *Allium* species are harmful when consumed in traditional, varied diets.

Allyl Isothiocyanate

Allyl isothiocyanate (46) (Fig. 22) is a component of spice seasonings and condiments. It is most commonly known for the hot-pungent character it imparts to mustard and horseradish. It is formed from the glycoside precursor sinigrin upon the moistening and crushing of mustard seeds. It is a most potent irritant both by skin contact and inhalation. Experiments involving high dietary concentrations resulted in adverse reactions—epithelial hyperplasia and ulcers of the stomach, minor inflammatory foci in the liver (dogs), increase mitotic activity (mice), and toxicity (rabbits) (Cordier and Cordier, 1951; Rusch et al., 1955; Hagen et al., 1967). Ingestion of large amounts of isothiocyanate has been implicated in persons suffering from goiter—a minor and seemingly isolated population. The minor exposure in the normal human diet and the self-limiting factor account for an adequate margin of safety for continued use in the human diet.

Bay Laurel

The California bay laurel should not be mistaken for or used in place of bay leaves or laurel (*Laurus nobilis*), the more traditional hazard-free species. Bay Laurel was used as a condiment. The essential oil is 0.5–4.0% of the spice. Umbellone (112) is the major constituent of the oil, present at 50 ± 10%. It was reported by Drake and Stuhr (1935) that contact with the oil or inhalation of the vapor may cause severe headaches, skin irritation, and even unconsciousness. Interperitoneal

Table 31 Consumption Ratio of Flavoring Agents

Flavoring agent	Annual consumption (kg) via food	Annual consumption (kg) as a flavoring	Consumption ratio	Food predominant
Acetaldehyde	39,543.7	597.0	66.24	+ +
Benzaldehyde	57,945.9	156,738.0	0.37	—
Ethyl butyrate	37,478.0	137,259.0	0.24	—
3-Ethyl-2,6-dimethylpyrazine	9,655.2	5.4	1,788.00	+ +
Limonene	1,300,995.1	68,403.0	19.02	+ +
Methyl anthranilate	61,731.4	27,768.0	2.22	+
Vanillin	20,674.7	475,650.0	0.042	—

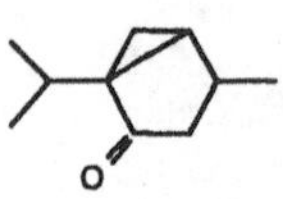

112

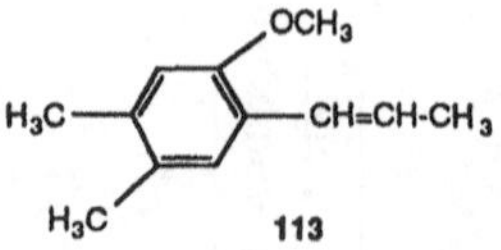

113

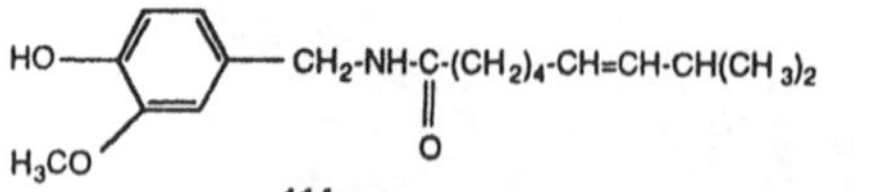

114

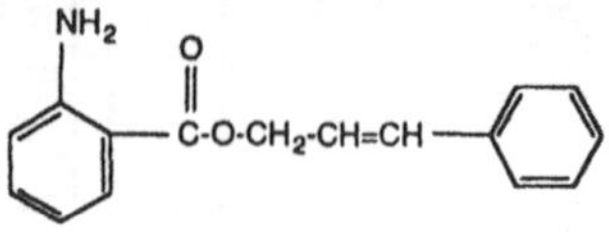

115

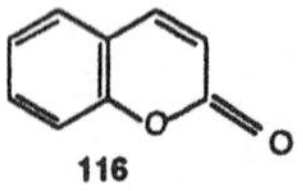

116

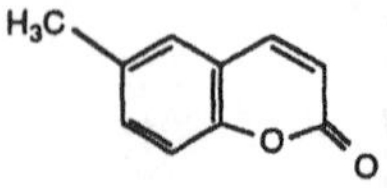

117

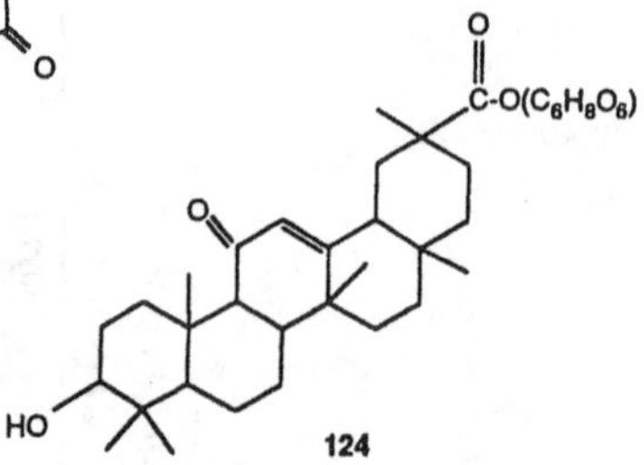

124

HCN

119

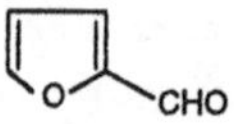

118

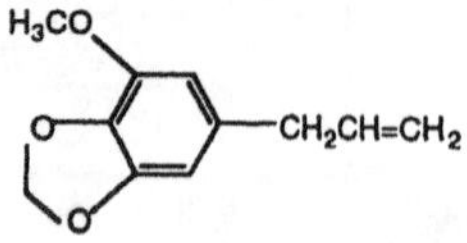

125

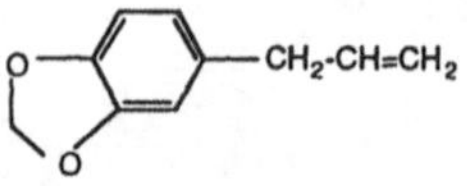

126

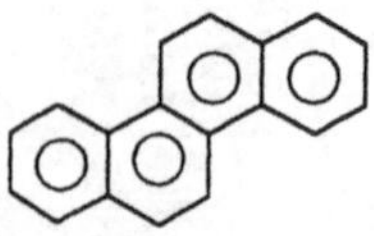

127

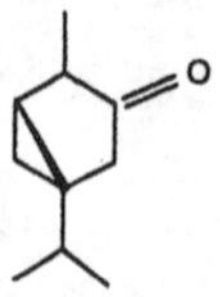

128

Fig. 59 Toxic agents.

injection of 2 ml of a 0.1% olive oil solution three times a week for 6 weeks in guinea pigs showed it to be markedly hemolytic. Umbellone has atropinelike effects on the nerves and muscle fibers of frogs. They concluded that umbellone blocks pulmonary circulation.

Calamus

The essential oil of calamus root (*Acorus calamus* L.) contains 5–90% asarone (113). This serves as another example of the variation of flavor components due to geographical origin. Italian oil has higher asarone content. Until Hagen et al. (1967) reported that ingestion of calamus oil could produce growth depression and increased mortality caused by accumulation of fluid in the abdomen, heart and hepatic abnormalities, and malignant intestinal tumors in rats, calamus was a common ingredient in bitters flavorings used in liqueurs and wines. Calamus is no longer permitted for use in U.S. flavorings, and its use is restricted in other locations.

Capsaicin

Capsaicin (114) is the nonvolatile pungent or hot principle found in the oleoresin of capsicum. Recall that oleoresins contain not only the aroma volatiles but also the nonvolatiles responsible for taste and trigeminal stimulation. Capsaicin has been suggested to activate perfusion of the gastric mucous membranes, movements of the intestinal fimbria, and the reabsorption of glucose. Ingestion may also induce sweating and salivation. It is a vesicant when applied in concentrated form to the skin.

Cinnamyl Anthranilate

Cinnamyl anthranilate (115), cinnamyl-2-aminobenzoate, is a synthetic flavoring agent used since the 1940s. It possesses fruity balsamic notes somewhat reminiscent of grape and cherry. It was withdrawn as a GRAS flavoring agent in the United States after the National Cancer Institute reported that it caused cancer in rats and mice. Prior to its withdrawal approximately 1000 kg were used annually in the United States in artificial flavorings. The NCI reported malignant tumors of the liver in mice and of the pancreas in rats.

Coumarin

Coumarin (116), 2H-1-benzopyran-2-one, is a common constituent of many natural flavoring materials. It is found in concentrations as low as 0.02% in osmanthus absolute to greater than 15% in the oil of cassia leaf. It has also been reported in spike lavender oil, cassia bark, tea extract, tonka beans, cassie absolute, lovage oil, and woodruff oil. Coumarin has not been used in foods or beverages in the United States since 1954. Prior to that time it was a common constituent of many flavorings, particularly vanilla. Coumarin was shown by Hazelton et al. (1956) and Sporn (1960) to be hepatotoxic in rats. Hagen et al. (1967), demonstrated chronic toxicity manifested by growth retardation, testicular atrophy, and liver damage in dogs fed high doses of coumarin. They observed enlargement of the liver, fatty changes, bile duct proliferation, and fibrosis. In humans coumarin is converted predominantly to 7-hydroxycoumarin. Only traces of o-hydroxyphenylacetic acid were found as human metabolites whereas this is the major metabolite in rats (Shilling et al., 1969). o-Hydroxyphenylacetic acid is a potent inhibitor of glucose-6-phosphate in hepatic microsomes, while 7-hydroxycourmarin is inactive.

An analog of coumarin, 6-methylcoumarin (117), has been shown to exhibit potential for producing photoallergic reactions and may cause dermatitis after skin contact in the sunlight. Coumarin does not exhibit this effect.

Furfural

Furfural (118) is naturally occurring in many natural flavorings, especially those such as coffee, maple, beer, bread, and meat that are thermally processed. Furfural is also a component of several essential oils—labdanum, myrrh, octea, camphor, and myrtle—in ranges of 0.03–1.45%. Although furfural is food predominant and currently has GRAS status in the United States, the Joint Expert Committee on

Food Additives (JECFA) has failed only recently to grant an acceptable daily intake (ADI) for furfural.

Hydrogen Cyanide

Hydrocyanic acid (119) is a well-known toxin, a potent respiratory inhibitor. The inhibition occurs in the enzyme cytochrome oxidase, the terminal respiratory catalyst of aerobic organisms. In the flavor industry HCN is encountered as a byproduct of the production of natural bitter almond oil. Bitter almond oil has almost become a generic term for natural benzaldehyde (18) evolved from pit oils such as almond, peach, and apricot. Figure 60 shows the biochemical conversion of benzaldehyde and HCN from the cyanogenetic glycoside amygdalin. Glycosides such as amygdalin are usually present at a level equivalent to 3% HCN. Treatment with the appropriate hydrolytic enzyme or acid liberates benzaldehyde and, as a contaminant, HCN. Commonly produced pit oils are treated to remove HCN and are then termed free from prussic acid (FFPA). The use of alternate methods to produce benzaldehyde, such as toluene oxidation, and the hydrolysis of activated olefinic aldehydes and ketones by heat, pressure, and steam will soon make the manufacture of benzaldehyde from pit oils obsolete. .

Hydrolyzed Vegetable Protein (HVP)

The high-volume use and chemical nature of acid-hydrolyzed proteins have caused HVP (Fig. 61) to come under considerable scrutiny lately. Unfortunately, much of the adverse publicity is the result of miscommunication or an attempt by certain flavor manufacturers to capitalize on preliminary or insufficient data. Much of the objection to the use of HVP is due to its normally high content of monosodium glutamate (MSG). MSG will be discussed later.

An unusual dipeptide, lysinoalanine (120), has been found in HVP in amounts ranging from 40 to 500 ppm. It is formed by the interaction of individual amino acids during hydrolysis and has been implicated in renal lesions in rats. Another class of suspicious compounds is diketopiperazines (DKP). Eriksen (1978) reported the presence of cyclo: valyl-valyl, isoleucyl-valyl, isoleucyl-isoleucyl, phenylalanyl-valyl, phenylalyl-leucyl, tyrosyl-leucyl, and prolyl-seryl in HVP. While certain DKPs have been shown to produce uterine polyps in female rats, the DKPs from HVP have not been implicated. Toxic chlorohydrins, 3-chloro-1-propanol (121), 2,3-dichloro-1-propanol (122), and 1,3-dichloro-2-propanol (123) have been isolated from HVP by Velisek et al. (1978, 1979). They were identified in ranges from 0.17 to 0.94 mg/kg. Esters of glycerol chlorohydrins were postulated as the precursors.

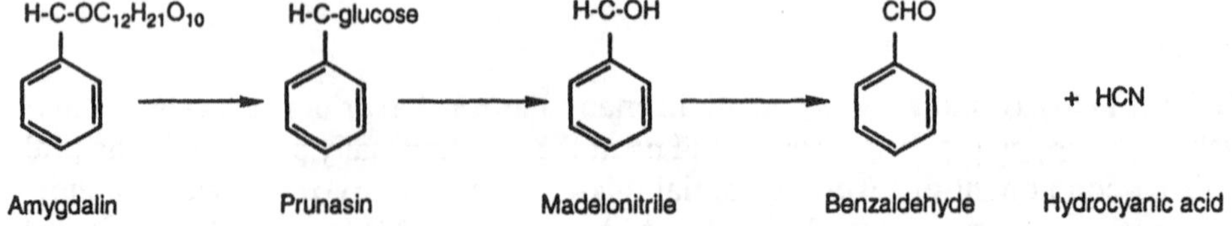

Fig. 60 Benzaldehyde and hydrocyanic acid production from amygdalin.

1. Lysinoalanine

$$\underset{\underset{HOOC-CH-(CH_2)_4-NH-C-C-CH_3}{|}}{\overset{NH_2}{|}} \qquad \overset{O\ NH_2}{\underset{}{|\ |}} \qquad \mathbf{120}$$

2. Diketopiperazines Formed From Dipetides

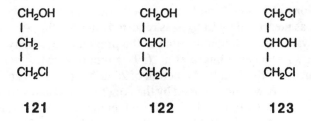

3. Chlorhydrins

$$\begin{array}{c} CH_2OH \\ | \\ CH_2 \\ | \\ CH_2Cl \end{array} \qquad \begin{array}{c} CH_2OH \\ | \\ CHCl \\ | \\ CH_2Cl \end{array} \qquad \begin{array}{c} CH_2Cl \\ | \\ CHOH \\ | \\ CH_2Cl \end{array}$$

121   **122**   **123**

Fig. 61 Toxins isolated from hydrolyzed proteins.

Chlorohydrins cause sharp and chronic intoxications in rats and mice. The presence of these compounds in such small concentrations in HVP, which in turn is diluted as a flavoring prior to consumption, makes experts feel that these compounds do not represent much of a hazard.

Licorice

The extract of the licorice root (*Glycyrrhiza glabra*) has been used both as a medicine for its demulcent and expectorant properties and as a flavoring agent to mask unpleasant medicines. It has also seen use in general, nonpharmaceutical flavored products. About 5–10% of the root is a glycoside consisting of two glucuronic acid units and a polycyclic moiety, the steroidal aglycone glycyrrhetinic acid. The salt of the glycoside, known as glycyrrhin (124), has a pleasant licorice flavor and a sweet, lingering taste about 50 times sweeter than sucrose. When it is taken in large enough quantities, physiological effects such as hypertension, sodium retention, and heart enlargement may occur (Koster and David, 1968; Conn et al., 1968). Because of the steroidal nature of glycyrrhizin, neither this nor the deoxycorticosterone activity should be a surprise. Occasional consumption in a balanced diet should have no untoward effects. Consumption of large amounts by those with kidney or heart disease may be hazardous.

d-Limonene

d-Limonene (9) is ubiquitous in natural flavorings. It is the major component of all citrus oils and is predominant in spice and herb oils. The National Toxicology Program of the United States concluded that d-limonene was carcinogenic in the male rat. No carcinogenic activity was noted in the female rat or mice of either species. Ford (1987) postulated that d-limonene and other hydrocarbons interact with α-2-U-globulin. This protein is found in significant quantities in the male rat but not in the female rat or in mice. Further, it is not found in humans. Evidence has been cited linking this interaction with kidney tumors in male rats. JECFA recently (February 1992) assigned an ADI of 1.5 mg/kg to d-limonene. JECFA acknowledged that male rat kidney tumors were male rat specific and should not be considered in human risk assessment.

Maillard Reaction Products (MRPs)

The objective in using MRPs as flavorings is to produce high-fidelity, concentrated flavorings via mechanisms that closely resemble those used in traditional food preparation and using traditional foods or components of basic foods as precursors. Therefore, one would expect to introduce compounds inherent to the normal diet. The toxicological implications of MRPs have been studied. According to Krug et al. (1959), greater toxicity, as measured by LD_{50}, was reported after heating amino-carbonyl model systems. Lysine premelanoidins, due to the pronounced activity of lysine, were the most toxic substances. Omura et al. (1983) reported that several weak mutagens were produced by the Maillard reaction of 20 different amino acids with sugars at 100°C. Mutagenicity was determined by the Ames method and varied with pH and thermal exposure. Compounds implicated in mutagenicity were 5-hydroxymethyl furfural, E-(2-formyl-5-(hydroxymethyl)pyrrol-1-yl) norleucine and methylthiazolidine. Products of triose reductones with amino acids or nucleic acid substances also displayed mutagenicity. Evidence of the formation of mutagens from model systems made with creatinine, glucose, and alanine or glycine has also been reported (Jagerstad et al., 1983). Barnes et al. (1983) reported that much of the powerful mutagenic activity in fried and broiled meat can be partitioned into a basic fraction. Several structures are known; specifically, they are heterocyclic amines and use carboline or imidazolquinoline derivatives. Model browning systems exhibit mutagenic activity similar to the activity in cooked meat.

Menthol

Menthol (52) (Fig. 22), both as a chemical entity and as a naturally occurring constituent of peppermint oil (about 50%), is widely used as a flavoring, especially in chewing gum, candy, and dentifrices. Menthol can cause sensitization reactions in the form of uticaria. Several other, more serious reactions have been reported (Thomas, 1962; Luke, 1962), including heart fibrillation after prolonged high consumption of candies and toxic psychosis from mentholated cigarettes. In both instances, symptoms disappeared when the menthol source was withdrawn.

Monosodium Glutamate (MSG)

MSG is the sodium salt of glutamic acid. Glutamate is present in the bound form linked to proteins and in the free form in a large number of foods, most especially proteinaceous foods and vegetables. MSG is a common flavor enhancer that intensifies the original flavor impact and creates the umami sensation of rich mouth-fillingness. The use of glutamate goes back more than 2000 years when Asian cooks used a certain seaweed containing MSG to prepare soups. It was not until 1908 that Professor Ikeda of the University of Tokyo isolated MSG and identified it as the flavor-enhancing component of seaweed. Today MSG is used as a chemical additive, produced by fermentation of molasses from beet or cane sugar, or as a constituent of a natural flavoring such as HVP. Oser et al. (1975) studied the effect of MSG on four species of neonatal and infant animals. A uniform dose of one g/kg body weight was given to mice, rats, dogs, and monkeys by intragastric or subcutaneous administration. In no species were any adverse effects on growth, appearance, or behavior noted. They concluded that the risk associated with MSG was extremely small and that except for persons sensitive to MSG, food containing MSG would present no hazard to older children or adults. Safety in use was reinforced by Anantharaman (1978). In a three-generation study involving doses 300–360 times human consumption, no incidence of pathological change was demonstrated. In spite of this evidence MSG seems to be constantly attacked in the lay press and is the subject of controversy even in the food industry. Several flavor houses now advertise MSG-free meat flavorings. The reason no doubt is glutamate hypersensitivity, more commonly referred to as Chinese Restaurant syndrome (CRS), a condition estimated to affect 0.2% of the U.S. population. The symptoms of CRS in hypersensitive individuals are tightness, warmth, tingling, and a feeling of pressure in the upper body. These symptoms, however, are transient. Kenney (1978) theorizes that the mechanism underlying glutamate sensitivity is esophagitis, similar to common heartburn, and that hypersensitive individuals would be predisposed to this response if they ingest a large concentration of MSG, if they lack sufficient saliva flow to dilute MSG, or if they have a tendency toward gastric esophageal reflux.

Myristicin

Oil of nutmeg and oil of mace contain less than 4% myristicin (125). Minor amounts are present in black pepper, carrot, parsley, dill, and celery. Truitt and Ebersberger (1962) have reported that myristicin is a weak monoamine oxidase inhibitor. Myristicin also has narcotic and psychomimetic properties (Truitt et al., 1961; Truitt, 1967). Large doses of nutmeg or mace have resulted in states comparable to alcoholic intoxication. Headaches, nausea, abdominal pain, delirium, hypotension, and stupor have been observed. Interestingly enough, the action of the spices is greater than the equivalent amount of pure myristicin. Very high doses result in liver damage and death.

Safrole

Safrole (126) is a component of many natural essential oils. It is found in trace concentrations in massoia bark to an excess of 90% in ocotea (Brazilian sassafras). It is also found in oils of camphor, wintergreen, nutmeg, cinnamon leaf, litsea cubeba, mace, black pepper, and ylang ylang. Safrole was a common flavoring in beverages, especially root beer, but this practice was discontinued after safrole was determined to induce liver damage in rats. Miller et al. (1983) have confirmed the carcinogenicity of an oxidized metabolite of safrole, 1'-hydroxysafrole. This compound is considerably more toxic than safrole.

Smoke

Smoke flavorings are used to impart a smoky flavor characteristic of specific woods or reminiscent of barbecuing. They are prepared by controlled burning of selected hardwoods, dry distillation, or treatment with superheated steam and subsequent condensation and concentration of vapors. Pyroorganic compounds produced by carbonization contain compounds that infer charred flavor and toxic polycyclic aromatic hydrocarbons (127). These compounds, of which benzo(a)pyrene is an example, are potent carcinogens. It has been recommended by the International Organization of the Flavor Industry (IOFI) that foods contain less than 0.03 ppm polycyclic aromatic hydrocarbons. Pyrolysis at lower temperatures greatly reduces the amounts formed.

Thujone

Thujone (128) is the major volatile in wormwood oil. It is also found in sage and rosemary, but only as a minor component. Wormwood was a major ingredient in the liqueur absinthe, but its use was discontinued when thujone was shown to be a convulsant (Balavoine, 1952). Convulsions associated with lesions of the cerebral cortex were reported. Wormwood has also demonstrated choleretic activity.

Yeast

Nucleic acid material is present in yeast and yeast extracts (AYE). Ingestion of high levels of nucleic acid components is associated with high blood levels of uric acid (Reed, 1981). Humans lack the enzyme urate oxidase, and elevated uric acid can lead to gout. Pharmacologically active amines, tyramine, for example, known to elevate blood pressure are formed during the fermentation of yeast. Tyramine is formed from tyrosine by tyrosine decarboxylase. This should be of concern only to individuals on a regime of monoamine oxidase (MAO) inhibitors.

ACKNOWLEDGMENTS

The author wishes to express his gratitude to the following people: K. A. Leavell and T. J. Roa, creative flavorists, Procter & Gamble; J. C. Grimm, Manager Sensory Laboratory, Procter & Gamble; M. A. Siklosi for her assistance in research; P. S. Adams and L. M. Chapman for the preparation of the manuscript; L. Tucker-O'Brien for the illustrations; K. A. Swaine for editorial assistance; and especially to R. L. Swaine, Sr.

REFERENCES

Abderhalden, H. (1991). The future of the Flavor Business. *Perfumer and Flavorist 16*:31.
Ahmed, E. M., Dennison, R. A., Dougherty, R. H. and Shaw, P. E. (1987). Flavor and odor threshold in water of selected orange juice compounds. *J. Agric. Food Chem.* *26*:187.
Anantharaman, K. (1978). International symposium on biochemistry and physiology of glutamic acid.
Arctander, S. (1960). *Perfume and Flavor Materials of Natural Origin*. Det Hoffensbergske Establissement, Denmark.

Armstrong, D. W. (1986). Selective production of ethyl acetate by *Candida utilis*. In *Biogeneration of Aromas*, T. H. Parliment and R. Croteau (Eds.). American Chemical Society, Washington, DC, p. 254.

Armstrong, D. W., and Yamazaki, H. (1986). Natural flavor production: a biotechnological approach. *Trends Biotechnol 4*:264.

Balavoine, P. (1952). Thujonein absinthe and its imitations. *Mitt. Geb. Lebensm. Hyg. 43*:195.

Barnes, W., Springarn, N. E., Garvie-Gould, C., Vuolo, L. L., Wany, Y. Y., and Weisburger, J. H. (1983). Mutagens in cooked foods: possible consequences of the Maillard reaction. In *The Maillard Reaction in Foods and Nutrition*, G. R. Waller, M. S. Feather (Eds.). American Chemical Society, Washington, DC.

Bauer, K., and Garbe, D. (1985). *Common Fragrance and Flavor Materials*. VCH Verlagsgesellschaft, Weinheim, Germany.

Boelens, M. H. and Jiminez, R. (1990). The chemical composition of some Mediterranean citrus oils. *J. Ess. Oil Rec. 1*:151.

Boelens, M. H. and Jiminez, R. (1989). The chemical composition of peel oils from unripe and ripe fruit of bitter orange. *Flav. Frag. J. 4*:139.

Bonmati, R. G. and Guiochon, G. (1978). Gas chromatography as an industrial process operation—application to essential oils. *Perfumer Flavorist 3*:17.

Broekhof, M. (1987). Natural flavorings—a marketing perspective. *Perfumer Flavorist 12*:23.

Cadwallader, K. R., Braddock, R. J., and Parish, M. E. (1992). Isolation of alpha-terpineol dehydratase from *Pseudomonas gladioli*. *J. Food Sci. 57*:241.

Cheetham, P. S. J., and Lecchini, S. M. A. (1988). A foretaste of flavors of the future. *Food Technology International Europe*, p. 257.

Conn, J. W., Rovner, D. R., and Cohen, E. L. (1968). Licorice induced pseudoaldosteronism, hypertension, hypokalemia, aldosteronism, and suppressed plasma rennin activity. *J. Am. Med. Assoc. 205*(7):492.

Cordier, D., and Cordier, G. (1951). Mode of action of bis (z-chloroethyl) sulfide of the cardiovascular system: effects of chemically similar compounds. *C. R. Soc. Biol. 145*:1310.

Cowen, J. W., Saghir, A. R. and Salji, J. P. (1967). Antithyroid activity of onion volatiles. *Aust. J. Biol. Sci. 20*:683.

Cramer, G. M., Ford, R. A., and Hall, R. L. (1978). Estimation of toxicological hazards—a decision tree approach. *Food Cosmet. Toxicol. 16*:255.

Demole, E., Enggist, P., and Ohloff, G. (1982). 1-p-Menthene-8-thiol: a powerful flavor impact constituent of grapefruit juice. *Helv. Chim. Acta 65*:1785.

Doornhos, T., and van den Ouweland, G. A. M. (1977). Flavoring with amadori compounds. U.S. Patent 4,022,920.

Drake, M. E., and Stuhr, E. T. (1935). Some pharmacological and bactericidal properties of umbellone. *J. Am. Pharm. Assoc. Sci. Ed. 24*:196.

Dugo, G., Cotroneo, A., Verzera, A., and Dugo, G. (1990). Tangelo essential oil. *Flavor Frag. J. 5*:205.

Ericson, A. P., Matthews, R. F., Teixeira, A. A., and Moye, H. A. (1992). Recovery of grapefruit oil constituents from processing waste water using styrene divinylbenzene resins. *J. Food Sci. 57*:186.

Eriksen, S. (1978). Protein hydrolysates: types and flavor aspects. *Dansk Kemi 59*:3.

Evans, B. K., and Rhodes, J. (1979). Treating irritable bowel syndrome with peppermint oil. *Br. Med. J. 2*:835.

Faust, U., and Prave, P. (1985). Biotechnology as a principle method for the production of natural substances. In *Topics in Flavor Research*, R. G. Berger, S. Nitz, and P. Schreier (Eds.), H. Eichhorn, p. 374.

Fleisher, A. (1990). The poroplast extraction technique in the flavor industry. *Perfumer Flavorist 15*:27.

Food Chemicals Codex, 3rd ed. (1981). National Academy Press, Washington, DC, p. 528.

Ford, R. A. (1987). Research Institute for Fragrance Materials.

Ford, R. A. (1989). General principles in the regulation of flavorings. In *International Food Regulatory Handbook, Policy, Science, and Law*, R. D. Middlekauf and R. Shubik, (Eds.). Marcel Dekker, New York, p. 241.

Gasser, R. J. (1972). Meat flavoring composition. U.S. Patent 3,645,753.

Gildemeister, E., and Hoffman, F. R. (1913). *The Volatile Oils*, Vols. 1–4. E. John Wiley and Sons, Inc., New York.

Gillies, B., Yamazaki, H., and Armstrong, D. W. (1987). Production of flavor esters by immobilized lipase. *Biotechnol. Lett. 9*:709.

Griffin, R. W. (1969). *Modern Organic Chemistry*. McGraffin, New York.

Guenther, E. (1948). *The Essential Oils*, Vols. 1–6. van Nostrand Co., Inc., New York.

Hagen, E. C., Hanson, W. H., Fitzhugh, D. G., Jenner, P. M., Jones, W. I., Taylor, J. M., Long, E. L., Nelson, A. A., and Brouwer, J. B. (1967). Food flavorings and compounds of related structure. II. Subacute and chronic toxicity. *Food Cosmet. Toxicol. 5*:141.

Hall, R. L. (1973). Food additives. *Nutrition Today*:20.

Hall, R. L. (1979). Food ingredients and additives. In *Food Science and Nutrition—Current Issues and Answers*, F. M. Clydesdale (Ed.). Prentice Hall, Inc., Englewood Cliffs, NJ, p. 146.

Hall, R. L. (1988). Food science in the year 2000. Speech at IFT/AMA Conference. Washington, D.C.

Hall, R. L. (1992). Toxicological burdens and the shifting of burden of toxicology. *Food Technol. 46*:109.

Hall, R. L., and Merwin, E. J. (1981). The role of flavors in food. *Food Technol. 35*:50.

Haro, L., and Faas, W. E. (1985). Comparative study of the essential oils of key and Persian lime oils. *Perfumer Flavorist 10*:67.

Hazelton, L. W., Tussing, T. W., Zeitling, B. R., Thiessen, R., and Murer, H. K. (1956). Toxicity of coumarin. *J. Pharmacol. Exp. Ther. 118*:348.

Heath, H. B., and Reineccius, G. (1986). *Flavor Chemistry and Technology*. AVI, Westport, CT, p. 185.

Herz, W. J., and Schallenberger, R. G. (1960). Some aromas produced by simple amino acid sugar reactions. *Food Res. 2*:491.

Hodge, H. C., and Downs, W. L. (1961). The approximate oral toxicity in rats of selected household products. *Toxicol. Appl. Pharmacol. 3*:689.

Hodge, J. E. (1953). Chemistry of browning reactions in model systems. *J. Agr. Food Chem. 1*:928.

Hodson, J. A. (1981). The herb and spice trade. *Perfumer Flavorist 6*:53.

Hussein, M. M., and Pidel, A. R. (1976). Gas chromatographic analysis of tangerine peel oils and characterization of their geographic origins. Institute of Food Technologists Meeting.

Japikse, C. H., van Brocklin, L. P., Hembree, J. A., Kitts, R. R., and Meece, D. R. (1987). Orange flavor and aroma compositions made by dense gas extraction of organic orange flavor and aroma compounds. U.S. Patent 4,693,405.

Jagerstad, M., Laser, A., Oste, R., Dahlguist, A., Grivias, S., Olssom, K., and Nyhammer, T. (1983). Creatinine and Maillard reaction products as precursors to mutagenic compounds formed in fried beef. In *The Maillard Reaction in Foods and Nutrition*, G. R. Waller, M. S. Feather (Eds.). American Chemical Society, Washington, DC.

Johnson, J., and Vora, J. D. (1983). Natural citrus essences. *Food Technol. 37*:92.

Jones, J. M. (1992). *Food Safety*. Eagan Press, St. Paul, MN, p. 38.

Jones, K. (1988). A review of very large scale chromatography. *Chromatographia 25*:547.

Jourdain, N., Goli, T., Jallageas, J. C., Crouzet, C., Ghrommidh, C. H., Navarro, J. M., and Crouzet, J. (1985). Aroma components production by immobilized microbial cells. In *Topics in Flavor Research*, H. Eichhorn, Wurzburg, Germany.

Kenney, R. (1978). International Symposium of Biochemistry and Physiology of Glutamic Acid.

Klimes, I., and Lamparsky, D. (1986). Analytical results concerning the essential oil of *Artimisia pallens*. In *Progress In Essential Oils*, E. J. Brunke (Ed.). Walter de Gruyer and Co., Berlin, p. 197.

Koster, M., and David, G. K. (1968). Reversable severe hypertension due to licorice ingestion. *N. Engl. J. Med. 278*(25):1368.

Kozhin, S., Fleisher, A., and Smirnov, A. (1972). USSR Patent 321,860.

Krishnaswamy, M. A., Patel, J. D., Parthasarathy, N. J. and Nair, K. K. S. (1979). Microbiological quality of certain species. *J. Plantation Crops I* (Suppl.):200.

Krug, E., Prellwitz, W., Schaeffner, E., Kiekebusch, W., and Lang R. (1959). Thermische Eiweissveränderungen und biologische Wertigkeit. *Naturwissenschaften 46*:534.

Kubo, I., Himejima, M., and Muroi, H. (1991). Antimicrobial activity of flavor components of Cardamom Elattaria cardamum (Zingiberaceae) seed. *J. Agric. Food Chem. 39*:1984.

Langrand, G., Rondot, N., Triantaphylides, C., and Baratti, J. (1990). Short chain flavor esters synthesis by microbial lipases. *Biotechnol. Lett. 12*:581.

Lawrence, B. M. (1979). *Essential Oils 1976–1978*. Allured Publishing Corp., Wheaton, IL.

Lawrence, B. M. (1981). *Essential Oils 1979–1980*. Allured Publishing Corp., Wheaton, IL.

Lawrence, B. M. (1982). The chemical composition of parsley seed oil. *Perfumer Flavorist 6*:43.

Lawrence, B. M. (1985). Essential oils of the *Tagetes* genus. *Perfumer Flavorist 10*:73.

Luke, E. (1962). Addiction to mentholated cigarettes. *Lancet 1*:110.

Lund, E. D., and Bryan, W. L. (1977). Commercial orange essence: comparison of composition and methods of analysis. *J. Food Science 42*:385.

Lyman, B. (1989). *A Psychology of Foods*. Van Nostrand Reinhold, New York.

Maarse, H., and Visscher, C. A. (1990). *Volatile Compounds in Foods*. TNO Biotechnology and Chemistry Institute, AJ Zeist, The Netherlands.

Manley, C. H. (1986). Flavor Benefits. Speech at Procter & Gamble, Cincinnati, OH.

Manley, C. H. (1987). Processing and biotechnology as a source of flavors. *Perfumer Flavorist 12*:11.

Manley, C. H., and Fagerson, I. S. (1970a). Major volatile neutral and acid compounds of hydrolyzed soy protein. *J. Food. Sci. 35*:286.

Manley, C. H., and Fagerson, I. S. (1970b). Major volatile compounds of the basic fraction of hydrolyzed soy protein. *J. Agr. Food Chem. 18*:340.

Manley, C. H., and Fagerson, I. S. (1971). Aspects of the aroma and taste characteristics of hydrolyzed vegetable protein. *Flavor Industry 2*:635.

Manley, C. H., and Swaine, Jr., R. L. (1979). Higher meat prices, product trends give HVP new roles in product development. *Food Prod. Devel.*

Manley, C. H., McCann, J. S., and Swaine, Jr., R. L. (1981). The chemical bases of the taste and flavor enhancing properties of hydrolyzed protein. In *The Quality of Foods and Beverages*, Vol. I, G. Charalambuus and G. Inglett (Eds.). Academic Press, New York, p. 61.

Matheis, G. (1989a). Natural flavors and their raw materials. *Dragaco Rep. 2*:43, 52.

Matheis, G. (1989b). The use of enzymes in the flavor industry. *Dragaco Rep. 4*:115.

Matheis, G. (1990). Biogenesis of fruit flavors. *Dragaco Rep. 4*:131.

May, C. G. (1960). Process for preparing a flavoring substance. U.S. Patent 2,934,435.

McIver, R. C., and Reineccius, G. (1986). Synthesis of 2-methoxy-alkylpyrazines by Pseudomonas perolens. In *Biogeneration of Aromas*, T. H. Parliment and Croteau (Eds.). American Chemical Society, Washington, DC, p. 266.

Mikova, K., and Davidek, J. (1974). Degradacni produkty kyseliny-askorbove. *Chem. Listy* *68*:715.

Miller, E. C. (1983). Structure activity studies of the carcinogenetics in the mouse and rat of some naturally occurring and synthetic alkenylbenzene derivatives related to safrole and estragole. *Cancer Res. 43*:1124.

Montville, T. J., Hsu, A. H., and Meyer, M. E. (1987). High efficiency conversion of pyruvatate to acetoin by *Lactobacillus plantarum* during pH controlled and batch fed fermentations. *Appl. Environ. Microbiol* 53:1798.

Morton, I. D., Akroyd, P., and May, C. G. (1960). Flavoring substances and their preparation. U.S. Patent 2,934,437.

Moskowitz, G. J., Shen, T., West, I. R., Cassaigne, R., and Feldman, L. I. (1977). Properties of the esterase produced by Mucor miehei to develop flavoring dairy products. *J. Dairy Sci. 60*:1260.

Moyler, D. A. (1991). Oleoresins, tinctures and extracts. In *Food Flavorings*, P. R. Ashurst (Ed.). Van Nostrand Reinhold, New York, p. 80.

Muller, J. (1984). *The H & R Book of Perfume*. Johnson Publications, Ltd., London, p. 77.

Nguyen, X. D., Leclercq, P. A., Thai, T. H., and La, D. M. (1989). Chemical composition of patchouli oil of Vietnam. *Fragrances Flavors 4*:99.

Omura, H., Jahan, N., Shinohara, K., and Murkami, H. (1983). Formation of mutagens by the Maillard reaction. In *The Maillard Reaction in Foods and Nutrition*, G. R. Waller and M. S. Feather (Eds.). American Chemical Society, Washington, DC, pp. 537–563.

Oser, B. L., and Ford, R. A. (1991). FEMA Expert Panel: 30 years of safety evaluation for the flavor industry. *Food Technol. 45*:84.

Oser, B. L., and Hall, R. L. (1976). Criteria employed by the Expert Panel of FEMA for the GRAS evaluation of flavoring substances. *Food Cosmet. Toxicol. 25*: 457.

Oser, B. L., Morgareide, K., and Carson, S. (1975). MSG studies of four species of neonatal and infant animals. *Food Cosmet. Toxicol. 12*:7.

Pellecuer, J., Dehauzun, U., Attiso, M., Simeon de Buochberg, M., Jacob, M., and Iderne, M. (1983). A study of producing and the quality of essential oils obtained by a new process of extraction: hydrodiffusion. *Proceedings of the Ninth International Congress of Essential Oils*, Book V, p. 115.

Pereira, J. N., and Morgan, M. E. (1958). *J. Dairy Sci. 41*:1201.

Persson, L. T., van Broklin, L. P., Morrison, L. R., Smith, C. A., and Meece, D. R. (1990). Process for making improved citrus aqueous essence and product produced therefrom. U.S. Patent 4,970,085.

Reed, G. (1981). Use of microbial cultures: yeast products. *Food Technol. 35*:89.

Roberts, D., Lemberg, S., and Wiese, E. (1983). Development of new essential oils in the U.S. *Proceedings of the Ninth International Congress of Essential Oils*, Singapore, Book I, p. 30.

Rusch, H. P., Bosch, D., and Boutweil, R. K. (1955). The influence of irritants on the mitotic activity and tumor formation in mouse epidermis. *Acta. Unio. Int. Contra. Cancrum 11*:699.

Saghir, A. R., Cowan, J. W., and Salji, J. P. (1966). Goitrogenic activity of onion volatiles. *Nature 211*:87.

Scharpf, L. G., Seitz, E. W., Morris, J. A., and Farboud, M. I. (1986). Generation of flavor and odor compounds through fermentation processes. In *Biogeneration of Aromas*, T. H. Parliment and R. Croteau (Eds.). American Chemical Society, Washington, DC, p. 333.

Schutte, L. (1976). American Chemical Society Symposium, Washington, D.C.

Shaath, N. A., Griffin, P., Dedeian, and Paloympis, L. (1986). The composition of Egyptian parsley seed absolute and herb oil. In *Flavors and Fragrances: A World Perspective*, Lawrence, B. M., Mookherjee, B. D.,and Willis, B. J. (Eds.). Elsevier, Amsterdam, p. 715.

Shilling, W. H., Crampton, R. F., and Longland, R. C. (1969). Metabolism of coumarin in man. *Nature 221*:664.

Short, G. R. A. (1973). Littlejohn Memorial Lecture 1972. *Flavor Industry 4*:80.

Simon, T. (1990). Herbs and spices are not just flavorings. *Liysmedelsteknik 32*:28.

Sporn, A. (1960). Toxicity of coumarin as a flavoring agent. *Igiena 9*:121.

Stahl, E., and Gerard, D. (1983). Hochdruckextraktion von Naturstoffen mit Überkvitischen verflussigten Gaseu. *Z. Lebensm. Unters. Forsch. 176*:1.

Staroscik, J. A., and Wilson, A. A. (1982). Quantitative analysis of cold-pressed lemon oil by glass capillary chromatography. *J. Agric. Food Chem. 30*:507.

Stofberg, J. (1983). Consumption ratio and food predominance of flavoring materials—first series. *Perfumer Flavorist 8*:61.

Stofberg, J., and Kirschman, J. C. (1985). The consumption ratio of flavoring materials; a mechanism for setting priorities for safety evaluation. *Food Chem. Toxicol. 23*:857.

Swaine, R. L. (1972). Natural and synthetic flavorings. In *Handbook of Food Additives*, T. Furia (Ed.). CRC Press, Cleveland, OH, p. 457.

Swaine, R. L., and Swaine, Jr., R. L. (1988). Citrus oils: processing, technology, and application. *Perfumer Flavorist 13*:1.

Tahara, S., and Mizutani, J. (1975). Lactones produced by *Sporobolomyces odorus. J. Agric. Biol. Chem. 39*:281.

Tahara, S., Fujiwara, K., and Mizutani, J. (1973). Neutral constituents of volatiles in cultured broth of *Sporobolomyces odorus. J. Agric. Biol. Chem. 37*:2585.

Tahara, S., Fujiwara, K., Ishizaka, M., Mizutani, J. and Obata, Y. (1972). Decalactone one of the constituents of the volatiles in cultured broth of *Sporobolomyces odorus. J. Agric. Biol. Chem. 36*:2855.

Thomas, J. G. (1962). Peppermint fibrillation. *Lancet 1*:222.

Trepanier, G., Il Abboudi, M., Lee, B. H., and Simard, R. E. (1992). Accelerated maturation of cheddar cheese. *J. Food Sci. 57*:345.

Truitt, E. B. (1967). The pharmacology of myristicin and nutmeg. In *Ethnopharmacologic Search for Psychoactive Drugs*. D. H. Efron (Ed.) USPHS Publ. No. 1645. U.S. Health Service, Washington, D.C., pp. 215–222.

Truitt, E. B., Callaway, E., Brande, M. C., and Krantz, J. C. (1961). The pharmacology of myristicin. *J. Neuropsychiatr. 2*:205.

Truitt, E. B. and Ebersberger, E. M. (1962). Evidence of monoamine oxidase inhibition by myristicin in nutmet in vivo. *Fed. Proc. 21*:418.

Tsai, C. H., Heckert, D. C., Kuznicki, J. T. (1990). Beverages. U.S. Patent No. 4,946,701.

Tzamtzis, N. E., Liodakis, S. E., and Parissakis (1990). The deterpenation of orange and lemon oils using preparative absorption chromatography. *Flav. Frag. J. 5*:57.

Unger, L. (1989). Base business trends in the worldwide flavor and fragrance industry. *Perfumer and Flavorist 14*:42.

U.S. Federal Register. (1980). Food Additive Regulations 173.210–173.290.

van Delft, V., and Giacino, C. (1978). Edible compositions having a meat flavor and process for making same. U.S. Patent 4,076,852.

van den Ouweland, G. A. M., and Peer, H. G. (1975). Components contributing to beef flavor. Volatile compounds produced by the reaction of 4-hydroxy-5-methyl-3(214)-furanone and its thio analog with hydrogen sulfide. *J. Agric. Food Chem. 23*:501.

van den Ouweland, G. A. M., and Swaine, Jr., R. L. (1980). Investigation of the species specific flavor of meat. *Perfumer Flavorist 5*:15.

van Praag, M., and Stein, H. S. (1971). Cocoa flavoring composition containing 2-phenyl-2-alkenals and method of using same. U.S. Patent 3,582,360.

van Toller, S. (1991). The application of EEG measurements to the study of sensory responses to odors. *Trends Food Sci. Technol. 2*:173.

Velisek, J., Davidek, J., Hajslova, J., Kubelka, V., Janicek, G., and Mankova, B. (1978). Chlorohydrins in protein hydrolysates. *Z. Lebensm.Unters. Forsch. 167*:241.

Velisek, J., Davidek, J., Kubelka, V., Barasova, F., Tuckova, A., Hajslova, J., and Janicek, G. (1979). Formation of volatile chlorohydrins from glycerol, triacetin, tributyrin, and hydrochloric acid. *Lebensm. Wiss. Technol. 12*:234.

Vora, J. D., Matthews, R. F., Crandall, P. G., and Cook, R. (1983). Preparation and chemical compositions of orange oil concentrates. *J. Food Sci. 48*:1197.

Wasserman, A. E. (1972). Thermally produced flavor components in the aroma of meat and poultry. *J. Agric. Food Chem. 20*:737.

Williams, A. A., and Rosser, P. R. (1981). Aroma enhancing effects of ethanol. *Chem. Senses 6*:149.

Wilson, R. A., and Mookherjee, B. D. (1983). Characterization of aroma donating components of myrrh. Ninth International Congress of Essential Oils, Singapore.

7
Flavor Potentiators

Joseph A. Maga
Colorado State University
Fort Collins, Colorado

I. INTRODUCTION

Modifying or enhancing the flavor associated with food has been a centuries-old goal that formed the basis for early world explorations in search of unique spices and herbs that would have potential commercial applications. It is a well-accepted fact that even simple compounds, such as salt, when used at low concentrations, can dramatically improve or intensify certain food flavors.

However, through the years only a handful of compounds have been identified that truly enhance certain food flavors. From a commercial standpoint, three such compounds are currently in use. They include monosodium glutamate (MSG) and two nucleotides, namely, inosine 5'-monophosphate (IMP) and guanosine 5'-monophosphate (GMP). IMP in turn is also known as inosinic acid, 5'-inosinic acid, hypoxanthine ribose phosphoric acid, inosine 5'-phosphate, and disodium 5' inosinate, while GMP has been referred to as 5'-guanylic acid, guanosine 5'-phosphate, and disodium 5' guanylate.

As a group, these three compounds have been collectively known as "flavor potentiators," "flavor enhancers," or "umami." They apparently possess the unique ability, upon the addition of relatively small amounts to various food systems, to modify through intensification the original taste or flavor properties of the food in question.

The mechanism by which this reaction occurs is far from understood, which is compounded by the fact that the utilization of one or a combination of all three compounds is not effective in all foods. On the other hand, compound synergism is usually evident in foods in which they are effective. Their stability during subsequent food-processing steps can also be of potential concern since, as is true for any compound, degradation products can be quite reactive or potentially harmful.

Research has demonstrated that these compounds are naturally occurring in various food systems. In addition, convenient methods of synthesis have been developed, and thus these compounds have found widespread application as direct food additives in a vast array of foods. This in turn has raised questions regarding their safety, especially among infants and individuals where significant amounts of these compounds are routinely ingested on a daily basis. Compound sensitivity is also a potential concern among certain individuals.

Therefore, the major objectives of this chapter are to review the natural occurrence of these compounds as well as their manufacture and chemical, sensory and physiological properties relative to their safety as food additives.

II. HISTORICAL BACKGROUND

Through the years various Asian cultures have chosen food ingredients that resulted in the preparation of foods with enhanced flavor properties. For example, the use of the dried seaweed kombu (*Laminaria japonica*) in the preparation of soup stock has been on record since the eighth century. It was held in such high regard that it was offered in religious ceremonies and as a special gift during formal engagements. Likewise, dried bonito fish (katsuobushi) was found to have special flavor potentiation properties and thus was used in special ceremonies. The simmering of vegetables along with meat and bones was also discovered to provide a soup stock that had pleasant and intensifying flavor properties.

Research during the early part of this century, in an effort to chemically define the agent responsible for flavor potentiation in kombu soup bouillon, resulted in the identification of MSG as the responsible agent (Ikeda, 1909). The unique taste effect produced by MSG was called "umami," which is the Japanese word for "deliciousness." At that time it was suggested that umami should be considered to be another of the basic tastes, along with sweet, salt, sour, and bitter. In Chinese, the word "xianwei," which represents the background taste of fish and meat, corresponds to the Japanese umami.

Once identified, the commercialization of MSG was begun (Ikeda, 1908) via the isolation of glutamic acid from wheat gluten, from which glutamic acid was first isolated in 1866. Currently, approximately 400,000 tons of MSG are produced annually in 15 countries, with the major producers in decreasing order of production being Japan, Taiwan, Korea, United States, Italy, Thailand, France, China, Indonesia, and the Philippines.

In 1913 the compound inosinic acid (IMP) was isolated and identified as a umami compound in dried bonito tuna (Kodama, 1913), however, it was not commercially produced until the early 1960s, when the structural relationship of IMP to GMP, the latter of which was isolated from several types of mushrooms (Kuninaka, 1960), was resolved. Currently, Japan is the major producer of flavor potentiators composed of IMP and GMP, with an annual production of approximately 5000 tons.

It is interesting to note that the three flavor potentiators that are currently commercially successful were first isolated from naturally occurring products traditionally utilized as special food sources. In addition, these sources were marine associated. This has led some researchers to postulate that all marine-based products probably contain naturally occurring flavor precursors due to the presence of both glutamic acid and nucleotides (Hashimoto, 1965).

Due to their potency and synergistic effects, the intentional addition of flavor potentiators to most foods occurs at levels well below several tenths of a percent, but even at this level, the use of flavor potentiators in foods in the United States currently represents a business worth over $300 million.

Since the first identification of flavor potentiator compounds occurred over 80 years ago, a vast array of scientific literature has accumulated, and although other naturally occurring and synthesized compounds have been identified that possess flavor potentiation properties, only the three mentioned above are in commercial use. Interestingly, a good deal of this literature centers around the physiological responses associated with the intentional consumption of such compounds added to our food supply. However, it must be kept in mind that the three compounds in question are also naturally occurring in our food supply, and thus one must consider natural intake in addition to intake by intentional addition if one is to completely understand the potential health effects of flavor potentiators.

On the other hand this category of food additives is relatively easy to study since only three flavor potentiator compounds are intentionally added to our food supply, whereas in the case of flavor additives, for example, literally thousands of individual compounds can be intentionally incorporated into food. This in turn has made the design and analysis of most studies in the flavor potentiation area relatively easy to conduct.

III. MONOSODIUM GLUTAMATE

A. Food Occurrences

Since monosodium glutamate (MSG) represents the sodium salt of glutamic acid (Fig. 1), it is not surprising that MSG can be found naturally occurring, in all probability, in any protein-containing food, since glutamic acid is usually one of the major amino acids present in most types of protein. Protein can be degraded or hydrolyzed via numerous common means during various forms of food processing and storage conditions. This in turn can result in the formation of free glutamic acid, which can readily react in the presence of sodium ions to produce MSG. Therefore, MSG can be found especially in protein-rich foods such as various dairy products, meat, fish, and poultry, where it can form upon heating. However, it can also be found in the free glutamic acid form in foods that are not especially high in protein, such as tomatoes. This concept can perhaps best be appreciated by viewing the data presented in Table 1. Here it can be seen that foods high in protein (cheeses) have comparatively high levels of both bound and free glutamate,

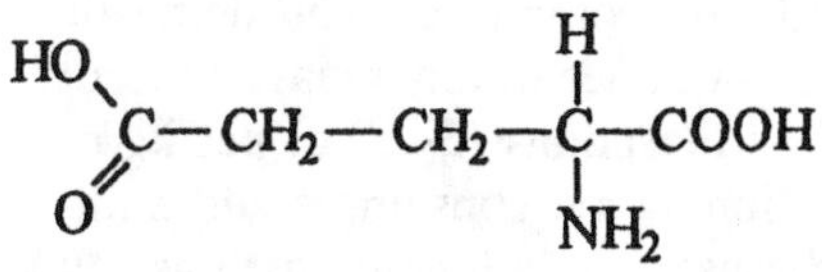

$$HO\diagdown \underset{O}{\overset{}{C}} - CH_2 - CH_2 - \underset{NH_2}{\overset{H}{C}} - COOH$$

Fig. 1 MSG structure.

Table 1 Bound and Free Glutamate Levels in Various Foods

Food	Bound glutamate (g/100 g)	Free glutamate (g/100 g)
Parmesan cheese	9.847	1200
Camembert cheese	4.787	390
Cow milk	0.560	1.9
Human milk	0.170	22
Eggs	1.600	23
Chicken meat	3.700	44
Beef	2.500	33
Pork	3.200	23
Green peas	1.100	75
Sweet corn	0.500	100
Tomatoes	0.260	246
Spinach	0.300	47

Source: Sugita, 1990.

whereas foods low in protein (tomatoes) can have high levels of free glutamate. Since free glutamate can readily form MSG, foods with high free glutamate levels can act as natural sources for the formation of MSG. The free glutamate levels in a wide range of animal-based foods are summarized in Table 2, while similar data are presented in Table 3 for plant-based foods.

B. Food Applications

Aside from relying upon the utilization of foods that naturally contain significant amounts of MSG, food processors and chefs traditionally have intentionally added pure MSG to various foods for the specific purpose of increasing characteristic flavor.

Interestingly, the flavor potentiation effect of MSG apparently does not function in all food systems, and thus the intentional addition of MSG has found its greatest application in various meat- and vegetable-based soups and broths as well as in sauces, gravies, flavorings, and spice blends. It has also found widespread use in various canned and frozen meats, poultry, and vegetables both when processed alone or in combination. As can be seen from Table 4, addition levels are usually relatively low, except in certain food systems such as dehydrated soup mixes where addition levels can approach 20% on a dry weight basis. In most cases these dehydrated products are diluted 10–60 times with water before consumption, however, exceptions can occur. For example, dehydrated soup mixes can be diluted only several times when they serve as the base for snack dips. In this situation, MSG may be directly consumed in the 5–10% range.

Another significant use of MSG is associated with commercial and domestic food preparation. Many times the amount added is not accurately measured, but it has been reported (Sugita, 1990) to average 1–2 teaspoons (5–10 g) per kg of meat or per 8–12 servings of vegetables. In addition, some consumers add additional MSG just prior to consumption through the use of condiments such as soy sauce.

Table 2 Free Glutamate Levels in Various Animal-Based Foods

Food group/Food	Free glumamate (%)
Meat Products	
Beef	0.013–0.088
Bologna	0.004
Chicken	0.051–0.056
Duck	0.064
Eggs	0.029
Frankfurters (boiled)	0.001
Lamb	0.003
Mutton	0.008
Pork	0.012–0.029
Milk products	
Cow milk	0.0008–0.003
Human milk	0.005–0.024
Cheeses	0.495–2.755
Fish products	
Abalone	0.138
Albacore	0.007
Carp	0.009–0.022
Clams	0.121–0.316
Cod	0.011
Corbicula	0.029
Crab	0.032–0.072
Croaker	0.016
Halibut	0.065
Lobster	0.028
Mackerel	0.024–0.075
Octopus	0.046
Oyster	0.037
Prawn	0.065
Sea bream	0.191
Sea urchin	0.012–0.024
Squid	0.004–0.056
Tuna	0.005–0.025
Protein products	
Actin	18.8
Albumin	20.9
Casein	28.5
Myosin	26.6

Source: Maga, 1983.

C. Total Consumption

Various attempts have been made to estimate daily MSG intake considering all dietary sources. As shown in Table 5, cultural differences can account for consumption amounts that vary by approximately a factor of 10.

Recently (Rhodes et al., 1991) the dietary intake of MSG has been evaluated in the Western diet (England). Preliminary evaluation identified 502 commercially

Table 3   Free Glutamate Levels in Various Plant-Based Foods

Food group/Food	Free glutamate (%)
Fruits	
Apple	0.005
Grapes	0.044–0.330
Grapefruit	0.146–0.236
Kumquat	0.019
Lemon	0.009
Nectarine	1.219
Oranges	0.015–0.026
Peach	0.041
Pear	0.020
Persimmon	Trace
Plum	0.100
Prunes	0.017–0.022
Strawberry	0.055
Vegetables	
Asparagus	0.051–0.076
Beans	0.005–0.076
Beets	0.038
Broccoli	0.213
Carrot	0.001
Corn	0.004–0.165
Cucumber	0.001
Eggplant	0.001
Garlic	0.002
Ginger	0.001
Mushrooms	0.025–0.635
Okra	0.038
Onion	0.001
Peas	0.152–0.254
Potato	0.051–0.254
Pumpkin	0.004
Radish	0.002
Spinach	0.002–0.031
Tomatoes	0.005–0.724
Miscellaneous products	
Sea tangle	2.26–5.36
Tea	0.264–0.724
Plant products	
Barley	48.7
Coconut	26.6
Cottonseed	29.9
Flax	26.2
Lupine	34.5
Maize	34.1
Peanut	26.4
Soybean	26.0
Wheat	58.0

Source: Maga, 1983.

Table 4 Added MSG Levels in Various Foods

Food	MSG added (%)
Instant noodle flavoring mix	10–17
Dehydrated soups	5–8
Sauces	1–1.2
Mayonnaise	0.4–0.06
Processed cheese	0.5–0.5
Soy Sauce	0.3–0.6
Dressings	0.3–0.4
Sausage	0.0–0.5
Canned fish	0.1–0.3
Canned ham	0.0–0.2
Snacks	0.1–0.5
Ketchup	0.15–0.3
Vegetable juices	0.0–0.15
Canned soups	0.12–0.18
Canned crab	0.07–0.10
Canned asparagus	0.08–0.16

Source: Maga, 1983.

Table 5 MSG Per Capita Consumption

Country	MSG consumed (g/d)
Taiwan	3.0
Korea	2.3
Japan	1.6
Italy	0.4
United States	0.35

Source: Maga, 1983.

available food items that contained MSG. These foods were divided into five broad categories (meat and meat products, fish, fruit, cereals, miscellaneous) and a total of 228 foods representative of all categories were analyzed for their MSG content. The actual number of samples for each food evaluated ranged from 1 to 26, depending upon the number of brands available. The average of MSG found ranged from 0.06 to 8.70%. Based on the average amount of each food consumed, the authors (Rhodes et al., 1991) calculated that the daily MSG intake per capita intake of MSG was 0.58 g. They also calculated daily MSG intake of extreme consumers, whom they defined as a consumer in the 97.5 percentile region of a normal distribution of consumption for a particular food. In practical terms this represented an individual who consumed three times the average consumption of a particular food. In addition, they calculated MSG intake between school children of two different age groups. Their data are summarized in Table 6. It is interesting to note that they also attempted to evaluate MSG consumption among young adults (15–25 years old), but they lacked sufficient consistent consumption data within this age group to draw reliable conclusions. As seen in Table 6, daily MSG consumption

Table 6 MSG Intake in England

Population group	MSG consumed (g/d)
Whole population	0.58
Extreme consumers	2.34
Schoolchildren (10–11 years)	1.31
Schoolchildren (14–15 years)	1.31

Source: Rhodes et al., 1991.

among children was significantly higher than that of the general population, in all probability due to their greater consumption of snack items.

D. Manufacturing Process

As mentioned previously, MSG can be isolated from naturally occurring sources, but various synthetic pathways have been developed that result in sufficient yields to make biosynthesis more practical from an economic standpoint.

Various strains of glutamic acid producing bacteria belonging to the genera *Corynebacterium* and *Brevibacterium* have been isolated and are in commercial use. These bacteria only produce L-glutamic acid at rates of 30–50 g/L of medium, a vast majority of which is freely released into the medium, which makes subsequent isolation rather simple. It has been determined that L-glutamic acid–producing bacteria are usually gram-positive, non–spore forming, nonmotile, and require biotin for optimum growth. However, the absence of optimum amounts of biotin at the end of their active growth phase results in the loss of cell wall structural integrity, thereby permitting the leakage of glutamic acid into the medium. These bacteria apparently have a different TCA cycle in that they possess low levels of α-ketoglutarate dehydrogenase activity. This in turn results in the buildup of α-ketoglutarate, which via reductive amination results in the formation of glutamate.

The organisms can use various carbohydrate sources including glucose, fructose, sucrose, maltose, ribose, or xylose, which are usually derived from various substrates including starch, cane molasses, beet molasses, or sugar. A nitrogen source is also required, which in practice can be various ammonium salts or urea.

Traditional bacterial strains include *Corynebacterium glutamicum*, which is also known as *Micrococcus glutamicus*, and *Brevibacterium thiogenitalis*. Mutant *Brevibacterium* strains not dependent upon biotin have also been considered, but these require oleic acid for optimum growth (Kanegae et al., 1991). Other strains have also been reported to be effective (Nakadai and Nasuno, 1989; Matsunaga et al., 1991).

The continuous production of MSG utilizing a fluidized bed and immobilized bacteria has also been reported (Henkel et al., 1990). Without question, other advances in bioreactor technology as well as DNA recombination and cell fusion will result in the more efficient production of MSG via fermentation technology.

E. Sensory Properties

Numerous studies have attempted to investigate whether MSG indeed is a separate and independent taste or if it interacts with basic tastes resulting in taste potentiation. From earlier studies (Crocker and Henderson, 1932; Cairncross and Sjostrom, 1948) it was concluded that MSG had the ability to modify the taste intensities of the four commonly accepted basic tastes, namely, sweet, salt, sour, and bitter. However, in more recent years, a vast array of studies, directly or indirectly supported by the manufacturers of MSG, have appeared that tend to demonstrate that MSG does not have an interacting effect on the taste intensities of the four basic tastes. The work of Kurihara (1987) is typical of this conclusion. The same general conclusion can be drawn from the data shown in Table 7. It can be seen that the addition of MSG did not increase the absolute taste threshold of the four basic tastes over that of a pure water control.

Sugita (1990) has concluded that the taste quality of MSG is distinctly different from those resulting from the four basic tastes and that its taste properties are not duplicated by combining any of the four basic tastes. In addition, it is his conclusion that the taste receptor for MSG is different from that for the other basic tastes.

In early reports (Galvin, 1948; Dorn, 1949; Lockhart and Gainer, 1950; Foster, 1955) MSG was described as possessing a sweet-saline property, which could have been attributed to compound impurity. In addition, several groups (Mosel and Kantrowitz, 1952; Van Cott et al., 1954; Pilgrim et al., 1955) reported a potential interaction of MSG and certain of the basic tastes. It should be noted that most if not all of the later studies dismissed results obtained in the earlier studies, however, the latter groups may be only partially correct, especially if concentration is considered. Later studies, in general, utilized higher concentrations of MSG than were used in the early studies. However, in defense of the later studies utilizing the technique of multidimensional scaling (Yoshida and Sato, 1969; Yamaguchi, 1987), it was experimentally shown that the taste of MSG is composed of a dimension that is independent of the four basic tastes. In light of the conflicting data briefly presented above, Sugita (1990) has described MSG as enhancing flavor characteristics of continuity, mouth-fullness, impact, and mildness, all of which improve food acceptability.

The relationship between taste intensity and MSG concentration has been studied (Yamaguchi, 1979), and it was concluded that concentration and resulting taste intensity did follow a straight line, however, the slope was not as steep for MSG as for the other basic tastes.

Chi and Chen (1992) utilized response surface methodology to determine the effects of MSG and salt additions on the hedonic score of chicken broth. Varying combinations of MSG ranging from 0.0 to 0.50% and salt (0.4–1.2%) were added in a rotatable central composite design experiment to prepared chicken broth. However, it should be noted that the naturally occurring MSG level present in the

Table 7 Influence of Added MSG on Basic Taste Thresholds

	Pure water	Water plus 5×10^{-3} M MSG
Sweet	2.50×10^{-3} M	1.25×10^{-3} M
Salt	6.25×10^{-4} M	6.25×10^{-4} M
Sour	6.25×10^{-5} M	1.25×10^{-4} M
Bitter	6.25×10^{-7} M	6.25×10^{-7} M

Source: Yamaguchi and Kimizuka, 1979.

broth was not determined or considered. In any event, calculations via a second-order polynominal equation revealed that the maximum hedonic score was 7.28 on a 9-point hedonic scale. This was achieved with a combination of 0.33% added MSG and 0.83% salt. An increase in MSG and salt levels was found to have a quadratic effect on hedonic score. In addition, they found that it was possible to maintain hedonic score at the same level by actually reducing the amount of added salt by increasing the amount of added MSG. This approach may have some practical application in formulating reduced-salt foods with optimum flavor properties.

It can be concluded from various cross-cultural studies (Moskowitz et al., 1975; Lundgren, 1978; Druz and Baldwin, 1982; Cooper and Brown; 1990) that culture can influence responses to the common basic tastes. Recently, Prescott et al. (1992) evaluated potential differences among Japanese and Australians to various tastes, including umami compounds. Increasing concentrations of MSG ranging from 40 to 240 mM in water were presented to panel members who were asked to rate their liking for each sample using a 9-point hedonic scale. With both groups, preference ratings for MSG declined as concentration increased. However, divergences occurred between the groups at the lowest (40 mM) and highest (120 mM) concentrations evaluated. At low concentrations, MSG was more preferred by the Australians, while at high concentrations, MSG was most preferred by the Japanese. Thus, it was concluded that since the Japanese are more familiar with umami-type flavor, they were more tolerant of its flavor at high concentrations. However, they were quick to point out that this study was conducted as a non–food model system study, and thus it is not known if these results are directly transferable to food systems.

Several groups (Bellisle et al., 1989, 1991) have attempted to address an important concept that the addition of MSG to certain foods may serve as a means to increase palatability and thereby consumption. Certain disease states decrease food consumption, thereby impairing patient recovery. A group of young, healthy French men and women were fed familiar foods to which increasing levels of MSG (0–1.2%) were added. Initial tests demonstrated that MSG improved palatability ratings, with the optimum added MSG level being 0.6%. Weekly free food intake testing revealed that the foods with 0.6% added MSG had greater consumption levels and were eaten faster than corresponding control foods containing no added MSG. The study was repeated utilizing a group of 65 institutionalized elderly persons, and similar results were noted for most of the foods evaluated (Bellisle et al., 1991). However, it should be noted that no attempt was made to compare optimum MSG levels between the young and elderly groups.

Various groups have evaluated the relative taste intensity of MSG with various synthesized monosodium derivatives composed of other amino acids, and as seen in Table 8, few come close to the flavor intensity possessed by MSG.

The above presentation has centered on MSG taste-perception properties, but one could also ask if MSG can influence odor perception or intensity. Contradictory reports appear in the literature with some claiming that MSG does not influence odor perception (Yamaguchi, 1979), whereas others (Mage and Lorenz, 1972) have reported that the addition of MSG resulted in increased volatiles as detected by gas-liquid chromatography.

Table 8 Relative Flavor Intensity Among Various Amino Acid Derivatives

Compound	Intensity relative to MSG
MSG	1
Monosodium DL-threo-β hydroxyglutamate	0.86
Monosodium DL-homocystate	0.77
Monosodium L-α-amoniadipate	0.098
Monosodium L-aspartate	0.077

Source: Maga, 1983.

An interesting question that still requires complete resolution is what the mode of action is for observed MSG potentiation. This topic is compounded by the fact that basic taste perception mechanisms are not fully understood and since flavor potentiation represents a subset of flavor perception, relatively few researchers have attempted to specifically address the problem of understanding flavor potentiator perception.

One proposal (Strong, 1968) has suggested two possible mechanisms. The first would result in an increase in the amount of flavor compounds that actually reach the taste buds, while with the second mechanism there is an actual increase in the magnitude of the signal generated by a taste compound in the presence of MSG. Others (Woskow, 1969) have proposed that perhaps flavor potentiators do not actually enhance flavors but actually suppress undesirable flavors, thereby making the presence of the remaining flavors more noticeable. In turn, others have suggested that MSG acts as a neurotransmitter and is activated by the taste bud (Cagen, 1977; Nada and Hirata, 1975).

F. Stability

MSG is usually marketed as a white crystalline material that is readily soluble in water. The product is not hygroscopic and thus is quite stable during prolonged storage at room temperature. The compound is 100%, L-form, since the D-form does not exhibit flavor potentiation properties.

MSG is quite stable to normal food-processing conditions, with little or no degradation occurring. However, at high temperatures some degree of racemization can occur, resulting in the formation of DL-glutamate. Since structurally it is an amino acid containing a nitrogen source, it can react at high temperatures via the Maillard reaction with available reducing sugars to produce a wide range of compounds. With a combination of high heat and acidic conditions (pH 2.2–4.4), MSG can partially dehydrate to produce its lactam, pyrrolidone carboxylic acid, as shown in Figure 2.

Since MSG is an ampholyte, it can exist in various ionic forms when in solution dependent upon pH. As seen in Figure 3, its major dissociated forms are glutamic acid hydrochloride, free glutamic acid, neutral MSG, and disodium glutamate under alkaline conditions. It appears that MSG is most effective as a flavor potentiator in the pH range of 5.5–8.0; as can be seen in Table 9, the R_3 form is most prevalent.

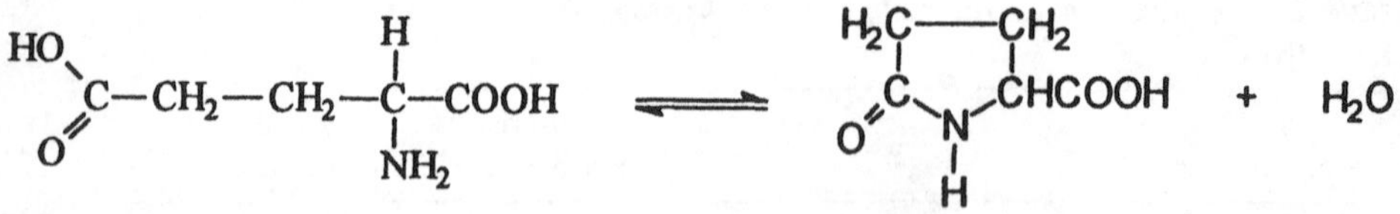

Fig. 2 MSG dehydration reaction.

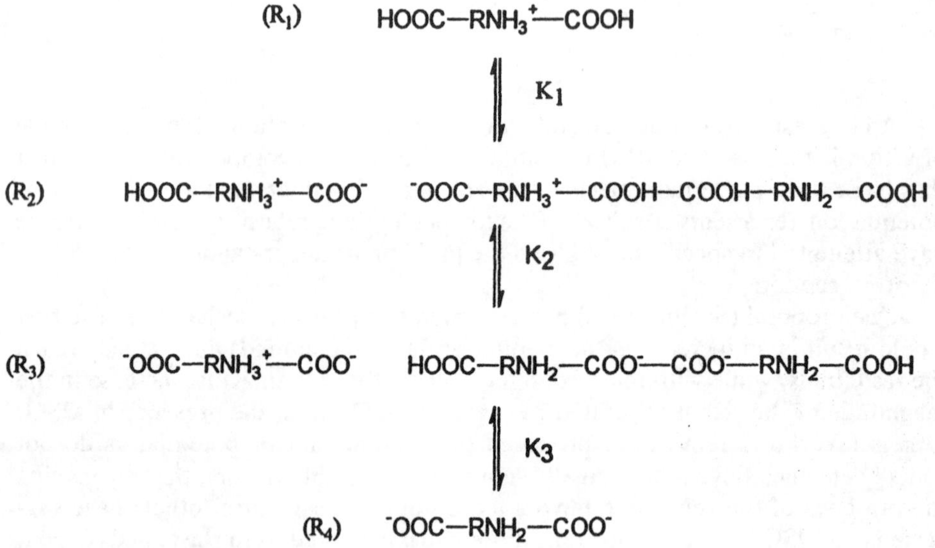

(R_1) $HOOC-RNH_3^+-COOH$

K_1

(R_2) $HOOC-RNH_3^+-COO^-$ $^-OOC-RNH_3^+-COOH-COOH-RNH_2-COOH$

K_2

(R_3) $^-OOC-RNH_3^+-COO^-$ $HOOC-RNH_2-COO^--COO^--RNH_2-COOH$

K_3

(R_4) $^-OOC-RNH_2-COO^-$

Fig. 3 MSG dissociation forms.

Table 9 Distribution (%) of MSG Ionic Forms as Influenced by pH

pH	R_1	R_2	R_3	R_4
3.0	13.4	81.3	5.3	0
3.5	4.0	80.9	15.1	0
4.0	0.9	63.1	36.0	0
4.5	0	36.0	64.0	0
5.0	0	15.1	84.9	0
5.5	0	5.3	94.7	0
6.0	0	1.8	98.2	0
7.0	0	0	99.8	0
8.0	0	0	96.9	3.1
9.0	0	0	76.9	24.0
10.0	0	0	24.6	75.4
11.0	0	0	3.1	96.9
12.0	0	0	0.3	99.7

Source: Fagerson, 1954.

Gayte-Sorbier et al. (1985) evaluated the roles of pH, temperature, time, and oxygen in glutamic acid and MSG stability and reported that the compounds at concentrations of 1 and 5 g/L in contact with the atmosphere were not decomposed at room temperature for 24 hours independent of pH. Under acidic conditions small changes began to occur after 3 days and increased between 3 and 5 days. In alkaline conditions no changes were noted for at least 10 days. They reported that compound disappearance resulted in the quantitative formation of pyroglutamic acid. The above study was repeated in the direct presence of either oxygen or nitrogen, and, as would be expected, the presence of oxygen caused a more rapid loss of glutamic acid than did the presence of nitrogen. Compounds were also stored at 4°C at varying pH, which resulted in less loss than storage at room temperature. In addition, compounds were boiled under reflux for up to 2 hours at varying pH, and they were found to be stable for up to approximately 60 minutes in very acidic, almost neutral and very alkaline conditions. Upon autoclaving, the compounds were found to be stable to very acidic and alkaline conditions, however, they were most unstable in the pH range of 2–3.5.

In the above study the only degradation product identified was pyroglutamic acid. A logical follow-up question would then be: What is the stability of pyroglutamic acid? This was addressed in a later study (Airaudo et al., 1987), where it was reported that pyroglutamic acid was stable in the pH range of 2.5–11 for at least 15 days of room temperature storage. Outside this pH range it was found to be unstable and was converted to glutamic acid. Similar results were obtained when pyroglutamic acid was boiled or autoclaved.

Thus, from the above studies it can be concluded that under normal food-processing conditions, MSG appears to be quite stable. However, it should be noted that the above studies were solely model systems involving only water and MSG, and thus one could postulate that the presence of numerous reactants and precursors can exist in a food system. Therefore, MSG stability in a true food system may not be the same as demonstrated in model systems.

G. Assay Techniques

Since flavor potentiators are usually used at relatively low concentrations, one has to adopt an analytical technique that is sensitive enough to detect the compound in question. In the case of MSG, this can present an interesting contradiction in that all of the analytical techniques involve measuring the amount of MSG parent compound, namely, glutamic acid, that is present in a food sample. This is compounded by the fact that in most if not all foods, a certain amount of naturally occurring glutamic acid exists, and thus one can be hard-pressed to conclude with a high degree of accuracy as to the exact amount of MSG that was intentionally added to a specific food system. Also, by the addition of appropriate precursors and subsequent processing, MSG can be formed, and thus, if not added directly to a food, it does not have to be declared on the food ingredient label.

Numerous analytical techniques are available, including paper (Bailey and Swift, 1970), thin-layer (Gayte-Sorbier et al., 1975), liquid column (Spackman et al., 1958), and gas-liquid chromatography (Conacher et al., 1979), as well as potentiometric titration (Coppola et al., 1975). Various enzymatic assays have also been reported (Gayte-Sorbier et al., 1975; Papic and Gruner, 1978) that involve the utilization of L-glutamate dehydrogenase. This enzyme specifically converts L-glutamate to α-ketoglutarate, which can then be specifically assayed.

H. Regulatory Status

Based on its wide natural occurrence in numerous foods, it is not surprising that numerous organizations and governments have not set restrictions for the use of MSG in food. Certain early literature reports, to be discussed later, have not provided enough significant evidence to limit MSG use. Previously these earlier reports had lead to restrictions relative to the establishment of acceptable daily intakes (ADI) for MSG as well as suggestions to limit MSG intake in humans under the age of 12 weeks. However, as of 1987, both the Joint Expert Committee on Food Additives (JECFA) of the Food and Agricultural Organization (FAO) of the United Nations and the World Health Organization (WHO) have removed these former restrictions, and currently the ADI for MSG is "not specified," thereby permitting its unlimited use.

In the United States, MSG is currently on the Generally Recognized as Safe (GRAS) list of food ingredients, which is administered by the U.S. Food and Drug Administration (FDA). However, since it is a food additive, various standards of purity exist for MSG, two of which are recorded in the U.S. Food Chemicals Codex and the Japanese Standard of Food Additives. In addition, the Scientific Committee on Foods of the European Community has given permission under additive number E621 for the use of MSG.

I. Dietary Aspects

The intentional addition of MSG to foods has been reported to influence diet in two distinct areas. The first is directly associated with dietary sodium intake. Obviously, since sodium is an inherent compound of MSG, it can be expected to be metabolically available as free sodium when ingested. Therefore, individuals on low or restricted sodium diets should pay attention to the levels of intentionally added and naturally occurring MSG in their food supply. However, it should be noted that MSG contains only 12% sodium, whereas the sodium content of salt is 40%. Since the normal usage level of MSG is approximately one-tenth that of salt, dietary sodium from MSG is usually one-twentieth to one-thirtieth that of salt. As mentioned earlier, it is possible with certain commercial food preparations to reduce salt addition by adding or increasing MSG levels. It has been estimated (Anonymous, 1987) that an average American diet containing commercially prepared foods with added MSG has a sodium contribution from MSG of approximately 0.5 g, however, the study did not report the sodium contribution from salt. In any event, MSG appears to make a relatively small contribution to the average diet versus the contribution of sodium from salt. In addition, nonsodium forms (calcium, potassium, ammonium) of glutamic acid are available to individuals where no added sodium to the diet is required.

The second, and perhaps more significant, influence of added MSG and diet is its reported idiosyncratic reactions. These first started to appear as a number of letters to the editor of a medical journal (Kwock, 1968; Anonymous, 1968; Schamburg, 1968; Kandall; 1968; Beron, 1968; Menken, 1968; McGaghren, 1968; Gordon, 1968; Schamburg and Byck, 1968; Ambos et al., 1968; Porter, 1968) wherein various individuals described unpleasant reactions associated with the ingestion of Chinese food. This phenomenon was quickly identified as Chinese Restaurant syndrome (CRS) and was attributed to the ingestion of MSG, which resulted in a tightness in the face or upper body, warmth or tingling, and a feeling of pressure (Schamburg et al., 1969).

Since these initial reports, various physiological and survey-type studies have been conducted in attempts to verify the initial observations (Kenney and Tidball, 1972; Go et al., 1973; Ichimura et al., 1974; Reif-Lehrer, 1976, 1977; Kerr et al., 1977, 1979; Nochaman and McPherson, 1986; Kenney, 1986). As might be expected, the studies utilizing surveys have most often been criticized due to their potential for bias and poor questionnaire design. Similar mixed results have been obtained from various objective studies (Rosenblum et al., 1971; Zanda et al., 1973; Kenney, 1980; Gore and Saimon, 1980; Allen and Baker, 1981a, 1981b; Garattini, 1982; Gore, 1982; Tanphaichitr et al., 1983; Wilken, 1986; Schwartzstein et al., 1987), probably due to the application of statistics when relatively small numbers of test subjects were involved, or the action/reaction of other unknown conditions existing in the subjects evaluated. In any event, it does appear that a certain relatively small portion of the population is provoked by MSG ingestion, but the exact mechanism(s) is not yet identified. However, several theories have been advanced as possible explanations for the mechanism of response among individuals where obvious reactions occur. These include a vitamin deficiency (Folkers et al., 1981, 1984), excessive sodium (Smith et al., 1982), and stimulation of esophageal receptors (Kenney, 1986).

J. Biochemical Aspects

The pathways for the absorption and metabolism of both free and protein-bound glutamate have been extensively studied and are well understood. In addition, glutamate can be synthesized in the body to meet demand if not supplied as an external source. It appears that glutamate plays an important role in nutrition and energy metabolism, as summarized in Figure 4. Normally, glutamate metabolism steps include oxidative deamination, transamination, decarboxylation, and amidation.

When ingested, a large portion of the α-amino nitrogen of both free and protein-bound glutamate appears in the portal blood as alanine. This results via the transamination of glutamate to pyruvate, with α-ketoglutarate being the other end product. However, when large amounts of glutamate are ingested, portal plasma glutamate levels increase until the liver can effectively metabolize glutamate into glucose and lactate. Therefore, under normal conditions, most mammals, including humans, have the metabolic ability to handle large external doses of MSG.

Since glutamic acid is the major amino acid of most protein sources, it is not surprising that glutamate levels can be at significant levels in various mammalian milk supplies, as seen in Table 10. Data of these type have often been cited to demonstrate the apparent safety of MSG ingestion in that if mother's milk can be effectively metabolized relative to glutamate, the addition of glutamate in the form of MSG should be of little consequences. It is interesting to note that cow's milk has only approximately one-tenth the amount of glutamate found in human milk.

The transfer of glutamate across the placenta has been studied in various animals, and it appears that humans have the ability to effectively metabolize MSG

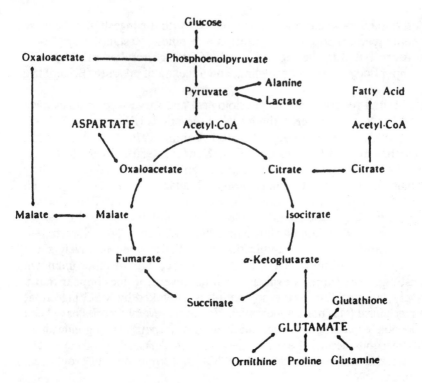

Fig. 4 Glutamate metabolism pathways.

Table 10 Glutamate Levels in Various Milks

Species	Glutamate (μM/dL)
Mouse	5.7
Guinea pig	11.1
Dog	15.1
Cat	17.7
Cow	12.8
Rhesus monkey	31.4
Baboon	43.9
Chimpanzee	264.0
Human	127.0

Source: Rassin et al., 1978.

so that little or no glutamate appears in the fetus. However, when high levels of MSG were infused, maternal glutamate levels increased to approximately 70 times normal, while fetal glutamate levels increased to approximately 10 times normal (Stegink et al., 1975).

The free glutamate level in the brain has been found to be large (Oldendorf, 1971) and is synthesized in brain cells at rates sufficient to support metabolic demand. It appears that blood-brain barriers are impermeable to glutamate except when large doses are administered (Liebschutz et al., 1977).

K. Pharmacological Aspects

As is true with any research involving animal models, one has to eventually be able to directly extrapolate experimental data to humans. This approach has been especially difficult relative to MSG since it has become quite evident that significant and dramatic species differences have been reported.

For example, a report (Lucas and Newhouse, 1957) appeared indicating that when infant mice were subjected to subcutaneous injections of MSG, a rapid degeneration of the neurones in the inner layers of the retina occurred. Other researchers confirmed the initial study (Potts et al., 1960; Cohen, 1967; Olney, 1969a), and since then similar results have been noted for rats and rabbits (Freedman and Potts, 1962, 1963; Hamatsu, 1964; Hannsson, 1970; Karlsen and Fonnum, 1976).

Without question, the area that has received the most attention is the effect of large amounts of glutamate on the modification and/or destruction of brain nerve cells in certain species. This phenomenon appears to be clearly species specific and has been noted to occur in mice (Olney, 1969a, 1971; Arees and Mayer, 1970, 1972; Olney and Ho, 1970; Abraham et al., 1971; Burde et al., 1971, 1972; Murakami and Inouye, 1971; Arees et al., 1971; Perez and Olney, 1972; Lemkey-Johnston and Reynolds, 1972, 1974; Paull and Lechan, 1974; Paull, 1975; Lemkey-Johnston et al., 1974; Holzwarth and Hurst, 1974; Lechan et al., 1976; Olney et al., 1977), rats (Redding and Schally, 1970; Everly, 1971; Berry et al., 1974; Nemeroff et al., 1975, 1977; Carson et al., 1977; Nikoletiseas, 1978), guinea pigs (Olney et al., 1973), hamsters (Lamperti and Blaha, 1976; Tafelski, 1976), fowl (Snapir et al., 1971, 1973), dogs (Oser et al., 1971), and some primates (Olney, 1974; Olney and Price, 1976; Olney and Sharpe, 1969; Olney et al., 1972), although it has not been found to occur in other primates (Reynolds et al., 1979). Interestingly, the earlier studies in rodents prompted the voluntary removal of added MSG from commercially processed baby foods.

Other adverse manifestations reported to occur with the administration of large amounts of glutamate include convulsions in rats (Bhagavan et al., 1971; Stewart et al., 1972; Johnson, 1973), cats (Goodman et al., 1946) and monkeys (Olney et al., 1972), as well as vomiting in dogs (Madden et al., 1945), monkeys (Olney et al., 1972) and humans (Levey et al., 1949). Several reports have appeared (Yu, 1970; Ahlawalia and Malik, 1989) demonstrating that elevated MSG intake apparently influenced lipid metabolism, in that elevated total serum cholesterol and triglyceride levels were noted. Early administration of MSG to mice and rats has clearly been shown to induce adulthood obesity (Olney, 1969b; Redding et al., 1971; Araujo and Mayer, 1973; Djazayery and Miller, 1973; Bunyan et al., 1976; Cameron et al., 1976; Pizzi and Barnhart, 1976; Poon and Cameron, 1976; Nikoletiseas, 1978) and diabetes (Poon and Cameron, 1976).

L. Toxicology

As can be seen from the data summarized in Table 11, the acute toxicity for MSG is rather low, with the LD_{50} values for the oral route being higher than the parenteral

Table 11 Acute Toxicity LD_{50} Values for MSG in Rodents

Species	Route	LD_{50} (g/kg body wt.)	
		Male	Female
Male	p.o.	17.7	15.4
	s.c.	8.2	8.4
	i.p.	6.6	5.7
	i.v.	3.7	3.3
Rats	p.o.	17.3	15.8
	s.c.	5.8	6.4
	i.p.	5.7	4.8
	i.v.	3.3	3.3

Source: Moriyuki and Ichimura, 1978.

routes. Based on these data, it can be calculated that a 70-kg human would have to consume in excess of 3 lb of MSG at one time to observe a toxic effect. In the case of a 22-kg child, the toxic dose would be close to 1 lb. Therefore, it is highly unlikely that human death resulting from direct one-time overconsumption of MSG will ever be recorded in healthy individuals.

Numerous long-term feeding trials involving various test animals have been conducted with MSG. For example, over 16 weeks of growth, chickens that ingested up to 1 mg/g body weight did not have significant differences in feed intake or body weight gain over a non-MSG control diet (Carew and Foss, 1971). Ebert (1979) fed both mice and rats 0, 0.4, and 4% MSG for 2 years and found no evidence of chronic toxicity or carcinogenicity. In another multigenerational study (Anantharaman, 1979) using male and female mice fed 0, 1, and 4% MSG, no differences in sterility, fertility, gestation, viability, lactation indices, and pre- and postweaning performances of the offspring were found. Levels of 0, 0.1, and 0.4% MSG were fed to Sprague-Dawley rats for 2 years (Owen et al., 1978a) with no significant differences noted in weight gain, food consumption, hematological values, tumor incidence, and survival rate. Incorporation of 4% MSG in rat diets for 2 years resulted in no significant changes in weight gain, food intake, hematology, or survival, but increased water consumption, urine volume, and sodium secretion were noted (Owen et al., 1978a).

Wen et al. (1973) fed ad libitum weaning rats levels of up to 35% MSG in the diet for 5 weeks. Growth depression was noted, probably due to high sodium intake. These animals had greater water consumption rates, large testes and kidneys, and high urinary pH as compared to a control group. Similar growth depression in both male and female rats was noted when rats were fed 35% MSG in their diet (J. A. Maga, unpublished data). In addition, the experimental group has increased heart weights, increased testes weight in males, and decreased ovary weights in females (J. A. Maga, unpublished data).

Male adult gerbils were fed MSG equivalent to 30 g/kg of body weight per day without apparent clinical pathological changes (Bazzano et al., 1970). Gestating rabbits were fed up to 8.5% of their diet with MSG with no apparent effects being noted on reproduction (Ebert, 1971). Beagle dogs fed up to 10% MSG for 2 years had no apparent changes in body weight gain, mortality, general behavior, blood chemistry, and organ weights (Owen et al., 1978b). Bazzano et al. (1970) fed 14 male human adults 25–147 g of MSG per day for 21–42 days with no apparent clinical changes being observed. Various glutamates have been evaluated utilizing the Ames test with and without metabolic activation to measure genotoxicity with no mutagenic activity being found (Ishidate et al., 1984).

The above studies demonstrate that at normal consumption levels, MSG does not appear to produce negative clinical changes. The interested reader is directed to the review of Heywood and Worden (1979), where toxicological MSG differences among species are discussed in detail.

IV. 5′-NUCLEOTIDES

A. Food Occurrences

The two nucleotides of commercial significance as flavor potentiators, IMP and GMP, can also be found in nature. Other nucleotides, such as AMP, are also naturally present, but they contribute little if any to umami flavor. As can be seen from Table 12, IMP is primarily associated with animal sources, whereas GMP is more prevalent in plant-based foods (Table 13). Most marine animals appear to be good sources of IMP, especially when the product is dried, while mushrooms are usually good sources for GMP.

In the case of animal tissues, IMP is derived from ATP, but the resulting IMP can be degraded due to the presence of phosphomonoesterase into inosine and eventually hypoxanthine. GMP is widely distributed at low levels as a component of RNA in all living organisms and can be found at high levels in yeast extracts, some of which are used for their flavor modification properties (Kojima, 1974).

Table 12 IMP and GMP Distribution in Animal Foods

Food	IMP (mg/100 g)	GMP (mg/100 g)
Beef	163	2.2
Pork	186	3.7
Chicken	115	2.2
Whale	326	5.3
Horse mackerel	323	0
Sweet fish	287	0
Sea bass	188	0
Pilchard	287	0
Black sea bream	421	0
Pike	227	0
Mackerel	286	0
Keta salmon	235	0
Tuna	286	0
Globefish	287	0
Eel	165	0
Dried bonito	630–1310	0

Source: Sugita, 1990.

Table 13 IMP and GMP Distribution in Plant Foods

Food	IMP (mg/100 g)	GMP (mg/100 g)
Asparagus	0	Trace
Head lettuce	Trace	Trace
Japanese radish	Trace	0
Onion	0	0
Mushroom, shiitake	0	103
Mushroom, dried shiitake	0	216
French mushroom	0	Trace
Mushroom, enokidake	0	32
Mushroom, matsutake	0	95
Mushroom, syoro	0	9
Mushroom, hatsutake	0	85

Source: Sugita, 1990.

Table 14 Foods to Which IMP and GMP Are Added

Food	IMP/GMP usage levels (%)
Canned soups	0.002–0.003
Canned asparagus	0.003–0.004
Canned crab	0.001–0.002
Canned fish	0.003–0.006
Canned poultry	0.006–0.010
Canned sausage	0.006–0.010
Canned ham	0.006–0.010
Dressings	0.010–0.150
Ketchup	0.010–0.020
Mayonnaise	0.012–0.018
Sausage	0.002–0.014
Snacks	0.003–0.007
Soy sauce	0.030–0.050
Vegetable juice	0.005–0.010
Processed cheese	0.005–0.010
Dehydrated soups	0.100–0.200
Sauces	0.010–0.030

Source: Sugita, 1990.

B. Food Applications

The intentional addition of IMP and GMP, usually in a 50:50 ratio, to a wide variety of processed foods can perhaps best be appreciated by viewing the data shown in Table 14. Major applications are in various canned foods, soups, condiments, and sauces.

C. Total Consumption

No published studies have specifically addressed the actual quantity of IMP and GMP consumed, however, based on the average purine content of various foods, it has been indirectly estimated (Kojima, 1974) that the Japanese consume 1875 mg/day of IMP, while the typical American diet contained approximately 2500 mg/day of IMP. No estimates have been made for GMP, nor has the amount of added versus naturally occurring IMP and GMP consumed been estimated.

D. Manufacturing Process

Currently there are two commercial procedures for the manufacture of IMP and GMP. The first involves the degradation of isolated RNA with 5'-phosphodiesterase to form 5'-nucleotides, while the second involves fermentation which produces nucleotides, which in turn are phosphorylated into 5'-nucleotides (Schwartz and Margalith, 1971).

E. Sensory Properties

The role of nucleotide structure and umami taste has been extensively studied and it is known that purine ribonucleotides that have a hydroxy group on the 6-carbon of the purine ring along with a phosphate ester on the 5'-carbon of the ribose portion of a molecule will possess a umami flavor. These structural combinations correspond to IMP and GMP, as shown in Figure 5.

Interestingly, purine ribonucleotides that are phosphorylated at either the C-2' or C-3' positions of ribose do not have a umami taste. In addition, purine deoxyribonucleotides possessing a hydroxy group on the C-6 position of the purine ring along with a phosphate ester on the C-5' position of the corresponding deoxyribose portion also possesses umami properties, however, their overall taste intensities are weaker than those of the corresponding ribonucleotides. Thus, the

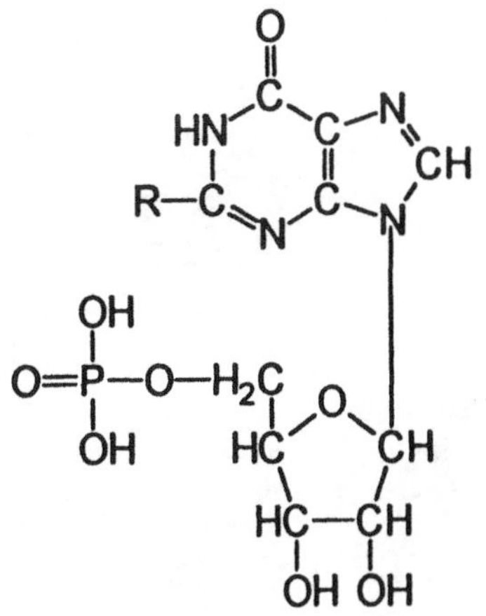

IMP: R=H

GMP: R=NH$_2$

Fig. 5 5'-Nucleotide structures.

phosphate ester linkage at the C-5' position in the ribose portion of the molecule is needed to impart a umami taste. In addition, the C-5' phosphate must possess both primary and secondary dissociation of the hydroxy group, since if it is esterified or amidified, no umami taste is apparent.

Knowing the above structural requirements, numerous researchers have synthesized various nucleotide derivatives that possess stronger taste properties than their natural counterparts. Some of these compounds are summarized in Table 15. It is interesting to note that GMP is approximately 2.3 times more potent than IMP.

The average taste thresholds for IMP and GMP have been reported (Sugita, 1990) to be 0.025 and 0.0125 g/100 ml, respectively. Interestingly, when the two compounds are combined in equal proportions, the taste threshold drops to 0.0063%. This phenomenon is referred to as taste synergism and has been the subject of numerous studies. Similar but less intense reactions occur when IMP and GMP are mixed with MSG. Therefore, most commercial food processors will use a combination of flavor potentiators so that a lower total amount of material will be used. For example, when IMP, GMP, and MSG are used in combination, taste threshold drops to 0.000031% (Sugita, 1990).

The mechanism for taste synergism has been studied extensively, and it appears that the presence of IMP and GMP induces a dramatic increase in the affinity of MSG to bind to taste receptor sites on the tongue. However, the total amount of glutamate bound does not appear to be increased.

Prescott et al. (1992) had groups of Japanese and Australians taste IMP at concentrations ranging from 30 to 105 mM and GMP ranging from 15 to 115 mM. Both groups showed similar decreases in preference ratings for both IMP and GMP. Although the Japanese gave higher overall ratings for both compounds, they were

Table 15 Umami Intensities of Synthesized Nucleotides

Compound	Relative potency
5'-Inosinate (IMP)	1.0
5'-Guanylate (GMP)	2.3
2-Methyl-5'-inosinate	2.3
2-Ethyl-5'-inosinate	2.3
2-Phenyl-5'-inosinate	3.6
2-Methylthio-5'-inosinate	8.0
2-Ethylthio-5'-inosinate	7.5
2-Ethoxyethylthio-5'-inosinate	13.0
2-Ethoxycarbonylethylthio-5'-inosinate	12.0
2-Furfurylthio-5'-inosinate	17.0
2-Tetrahydrofurfurylthio-5'-inosinate	8.0
2-Isopentylthio-5'-inosinate	11.0
2-Methoxy-5'-inosinate	4.2
2-Ethoxy-5'-inosinate	4.9
2-Allyloxy-5'-inosinate	6.5

Source: Sugita, 1990.

not significantly different from the Australian ratings. Thus, both culturally diverse groups seemed to respond in the same manner.

F. Stability

IMP and GMP are not nearly as stable as MSG in various food systems. For example, if IMP or GMP are added to various raw food systems, there is the potential for enzymatic destabilization. The key phosphomonoester linkage of IMP and GMP can rather easily be split by phosphomonoesterases, which are naturally present in many raw plant and animal products.

In addition, IMP and GMP can be somewhat unstable at high processing temperatures, typical of those encountered during canning. This thermal instability can also be influenced by pH. For example, it is a well-accepted fact that under acidic conditions, purine nucleotides hydrolyze at the glycosidic bond to their corresponding nucleosidic bases. Under alkaline conditions these compounds can be hydrolyzed to their corresponding base, and the base can then be destroyed. As a result, numerous reports have appeared (Nguyen and Sporns, 1984, 1985; Shaoul and Sporns, 1987; Matoba et al., 1988; Kuchiba et al., 1990; Kuchiba-Manabe et al., 1991a) reporting such findings with IMP and GMP.

One group has apparently taken advantage of the apparent instability at high temperature of IMP by intentionally reacting IMP with other reactive compounds to produce a series of compounds possessing meatlike flavor (Zhang and Ho, 1991).

Several reports have appeared (Kuchiba et al., 1989; Kuchiba-Manabe, 1991b) demonstrating that IMP and GMP have some limited antioxidative ability, probably due to their chelating action.

G. Assay Techniques

As is the case for the analysis of many compounds, one has to be especially concerned with the complete extraction and freedom from interference by other compounds when attempting to quantitate the nucleotide content of a complex food. For example, the use of anion-exchange chromatography has been the predominant method for the separation and quantitation of nucleotides from biological systems, however, results are usually rather disappointing when the technique is applied to foods where salt addition can interfere with accurate results. Therefore, the current method of choice for the analysis of nucleotides in food systems appears to be some form of high-performance liquid chromatography (HPLC). Most recently the merits of ion-pairing reversed-phase HPLC was reported to overcome the limitations of other techniques (Fish, 1991).

H. Regulatory Status

Since IMP and GMP are derived from natural sources, they are permitted for addition to foods internationally. As with MSG, they also possess the unique condition that they are naturally present in a wide range of foods and their addition levels, due to synergism, are quite low.

Currently the Scientific Committee on Foods of the European Community has an "ADI not specified" for the calcium and disodium salts of guanylic and inosinic acids (GMP and IMP), which can be liberally interpreted that, in light of current scientific evidence, numerical limitation is not deemed necessary.

I. Biochemical Aspects

Nucleotides are quite common in many locations in the body, thus demonstrating their various roles in metabolism. They can be either synthesized from nonpurine precursors or supplied in dietary form. They are most predominantly found in two general pathways. The first is in muscle and red blood cells, where they are associated with energy production, and the second is in organs such as the liver, brain, and spleen, where they are metabolism intermediates. As an example, adult human liver contains approximately 6.4 mg of free IMP and 8.3 mg of free GMP per 100 g fresh weight (Kojima, 1974).

GMP appears to be enzymatically degraded to uric acid in the rat intestine (Sugita, 1990). It appears that GMP and IMP are digested mainly in the duodenum and absorbed as a form of nucleotide (Kojima, 1974). At levels of 25 mg/kg rat body weight, 5′-nucleotides were primarily excreted in the urine, while when the same level was given orally to pregnant rats, 0.77% 5′-IMP and 0.01% 5′-GMP were found in the fetuses after 24 hours.

Since these compounds are metabolized to uric acid, some researchers have proposed that they contribute to gout. However, daily administration of 2.5 g of IMP only caused serum uric acid levels to rise from 3.6 to 6.9 mg%, while urinary levels increased from 506 to 1100 mg/day (Kojima, 1974). Since the daily intake of IMP is assumed to be much lower than 2.5 g, IMP does not appear to be directly related to gout.

J. Pharmacological Aspects

Little material has been published on the pharmacology of exogenously administered IMP and GMP. Kojima (1974) reported that 15 minutes after the intravenous administration of 500 mg/kg of GMP, mice had abnormal floor positions as well as slight respiratory depression along with depression of the avoidance response. Similar observations were noted with IMP. Both compounds at 500 mg/kg did not induce muscle relaxation or alter electroshock-induced convulsion rates. Also, oral administration of IMP and GMP did not affect the analgesic responses of mice to a thermal stimulus. No diuretic effect or change in gastric juice secretion were noted. Intravenous injection of 10 mg/kg of IMP in rats produced no significant changes in calcium, potassium, chloride, or sodium levels. Using an anesthetized rat, injection of up to 50 mg/kg of IMP did not affect blood pressure, heart rate, ECG, or blood flow (Kojima, 1974). Intestinal transport in mice that had been fasted for 18 hours before IMP or GMP was subcutaneously injected at 100 mg/kg was shown not to be affected (Kojima, 1974).

Diets containing 2% IMP/GMP were fed to rats or dogs for up to 2 years, and there was no reported evidence of chronic toxicity or carcinogenicity (Sugita, 1990). A three-generation study in rats fed up to 2% nucleotides produced no significant differences in growth and reproduction performances over controls (Kojima, 1974).

K. Toxicology

IMP and GMP appear to have low systemic toxicity due to their relatively high LD_{50} values in mice and rats (Table 16). In turn, near-lethal does of IMP and GMP produced signs of depression, clonic convulsion, and dyspnea (Kojima, 1974).

Table 16 LD$_{50}$ Values for IMP and GMP in Rats and Mice

Animal	IMP (mg/kg body wt)	GMP (mg/kg body wt)
Mouse	12,000–14,000	>14,000
Rat	>10,000	>10,000

Source: Kojima, 1974.

Up to 1000 mg/kg body weight of IMP and GMP were orally given to male rats for 90 days (Kojima, 1974). No significant changes in body weight gain, blood chemistry, weight or volume of cerebrum, cerebellum, thyroid, heart, stomach, liver, spleen, kidney, adrenal, testes, epididymis or urinary bladder, weight of lung, or length of tail in comparison to a control group were noted. In addition, no internal organ histological changes were noted by macroscopic or microscopic examination (Kojima, 1974).

Male and female beagle dogs were orally given up to 2% of their diets as IMP/GMP. No adverse changes were seen in erythrocyte sedimentation rate, packed cell volume, hemogloblin, reticulocyte count, mean corpuscular hemoglobin concentration, mean corpuscular volume, red cell count, white cell count and differential, platelet count, prothrombin time, plasma urea and glucose, serum proteins and electrophoresis, albumin/globulin ratio, serum alkaline phosphatase, serum glutamic-pyruvic transaminase, bilirubin, sodium, potassium, allantoin, uric acid, urine pH, volume, specific gravity, protein, total red substances, glucose, ketones, bile pigments, bile salts, urobilinogen, and microscopy of spleen deposit (Kojima, 1974). Typical of the above studies, it would appear that IMP and GMP at normal levels of consumption present little if any risk to the short- and long-term health of normal humans.

V. MISCELLANEOUS COMPOUNDS

Through the years, other naturally occurring compounds have been identified that possess flavor potentiation properties. For example, ibotenic and tricholomic acids (Fig. 6) have been identified in mushrooms. However, due to the effectiveness and availability of compounds such as MSG, IMP, and GMP, these compounds are not currently commercially utilized. Undoubtedly, other naturally occurring flavor potentiators exist, and the synthetic chemist can provide structural permutations well into the future.

VI. CONCLUSIONS

Flavor potentiator or umami compounds such as MSG, IMP, and GMP have the unique ability to modify certain food flavors, thereby increasing the palatability of our food supply. All of these compounds have been identified as being naturally occurring in a wide range of foods. However, since they are intentionally added to various foods, their safety aspects have to be considered. Based on their relatively high LD$_{50}$ values, it appears that their toxicological potential is rather low. However, concerns relative to long-term ingestion and consumption among infants have

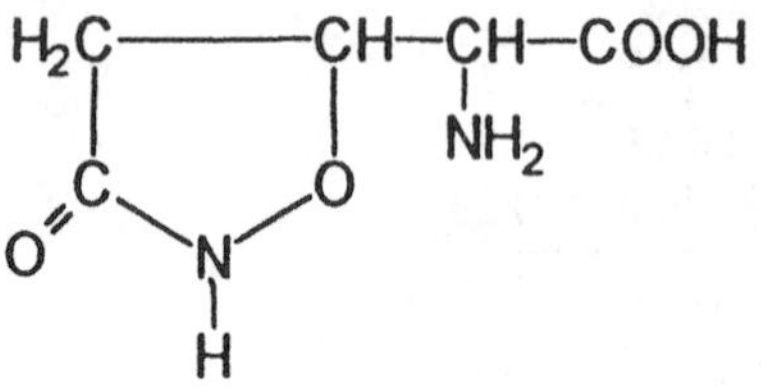

(a)

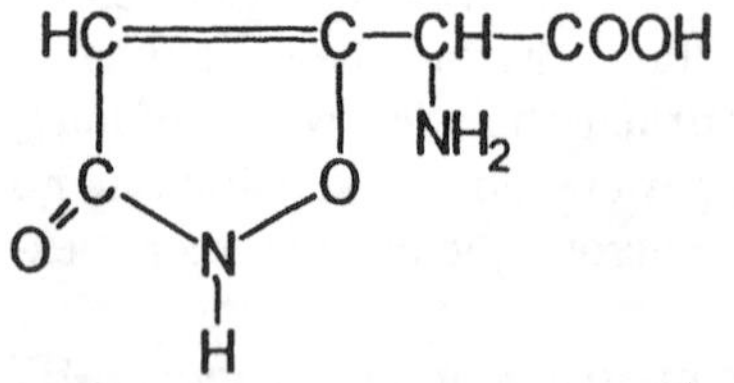

(b)

Fig. 6 Structures for (a) tricholomic acid and (b) ibotenic acid.

resulted in numerous studies. From these studies it would appear that the normal, healthy human is quite capable of metabolically dealing with the direct ingestion of all three compounds in question. However, certain individuals apparently do have a metabolic intolerance to MSG. Such intolerance to IMP and GMP has not been documented in the literature.

REFERENCES

Abraham, R., Dougherty, W., Goldberg, L., and Coulston, F. (1971). The response of the hypothalamus to high doses of monosodium glutamate in mice and monkeys: cysto-chemistry and ultrastructural study of lysomal changes. *Exp. Mol. Pathol. 15*:43–60.

Ahlawalia, P., and Malik, V. B. T. (1989). Effects of monosodium glutamate (MSG) on serum lipids, blood glucose and cholesterol in adult male mice. *Toxicol. Lett. 45*:195–198.

Airaudo, C. B., Gayte-Sorbier, A., and Armand, P. (1987). Stability of glutamine and pyroglutamic acid under model system conditions: influence of physical and technological factors. *J. Food Sci. 52*:1750–1752.

Allen, D. H., and Baker, G. J. (1981a). Asthma and MSG. *Med. J. Aust. 68*:576.

Allen, D. H., and Baker, G. J. (1981b). Chinese restaurant asthma. *N. Engl. J. Med. 305*:1154–1155.

Ambos, M., Leavitt, N. R., Marmorek, L., and Wolschina, S. B. (1968). Chinese restaurant syndrome. *N. Engl. J. Med. 279*:1005.

Anantharaman, K. (1979). In utero and dietary administration of monosodium L-glutamate to mice: reproductive performance and development in a multigeneration study. In *Glutamic Acid: Advances in Biochemistry and Physiology*, L. J. Filner (Ed.). Raven Press, New York, p. 231.

Anonymous. (1968). Post-sino-cibal syndrome. *N. Engl. J. Med. 278*:1122.

Anonymous. (1987). Monosodium glutamate (MSG). *Food Technol. 41*(5):144–154.

Araujo, P. E., and Mayer, J. (1975). Activity increase associated with obesity induced by monosodium glutamate in mice. *Am. J. Physiol. 225*:764–765.

Arees, E., and Mayer, J. (1970). Monosodium glutamate-induced brain lesions: electron microscopic examination. *Science 170*:549–550.

Arees, E., and Mayer, J. (1972). Monosodium glutamate-induced brain lesions in mice. *J. Neuropathol. Exp. Neurol. 31*:181.

Arees, E. A., Sandrew, B., and Mayer, J. (1971). Monosodium glutamate-induced optic pathway lesions in infant mice following subcutaneous injection. *Fed. Proc. 30*:521.

Bailey, B. W., and Swift, H. L. (1970). Note on a rapid paper chromatographic method for estimation of added monosodium glutamate in food. *J. Assoc. Off. Anal. Chem. 53*:1268–1270.

Bazzano, G., D'Ella, J. A., and Olson, R. E. (1970). Monosodium glutamate: feeding of large amounts in man and gerbils. *Science 169*:1208–1209.

Bellisle, F., Tournier, A., and Louis-Sylvestre, J. (1989). Monosodium glutamate and the acquisition of food preferences in a European context. *Food Qual. Pref. 1*:103–108.

Bellisle, F., Monneuse, M. O., Chabert, M., Larue-Achagiotis, C., Lanteaume, M. T., and Louis-Sylvestre, J. (1991). Monosodium glutamate as a palatability enhancer in the European diet. *Physiol. Behav. 49*:869–873.

Beron, E. L. (1968). Chinese restaurant syndrome. *N. Engl. J. Med. 278*:1123.

Berry, H. K., Butcher, R. E., Elliott, L. A., and Brunner, R. L. (1974). The effect of monosodium glutamate on the early biochemical and behavioral development of the rat. *Dev. Psychobiol. 7*:165–173.

Bhagavan, H. N., Coursin, D. B., and Stewart, C. N. (1971). Monosodium glutamate-induced convulsion disorders in rats. *Nature 232*:275–276.

Bunyan, J., Murrell, E. A., and Shah, P. P. (1976). The induction of obesity in rodents by means of monosodium glutamate. *Br. J. Nutr. 35*:25–39.

Burde, R. M., Schainker, B., and Kayes, J. (1971). Monosodium glutamate: acute effect of oral and subcutaneous administration on the arcuate nucleus of the hypothalamus in mice and rats. *Nature 233*:58–60.

Burde, R. M., Schainker, B., and Kayes, J. (1972). Monosodium glutamate: necrosis of hypothalamic neurons in infant rats and mice following either oral or subcutaneous administration. *J. Neuropathol. Exp. Neurol. 31*:181.

Cagen, R. H. (1977). A framework for the mechanism of action of special taste substances: the example of monosodium glutamate. In *The Chemical Senses and Nutrition*, M. R. Kare and O. Maller (Eds.). Academic Press, New York, p. 343.

Cairncross, S. E., and Sjostrom, L. B. (1948). What glutamate does in food. *Food Ind. 20*:982–984.

Cameron, D. P., Poon, T. K., and Smith, G. L. (1976). Effects of monosodium glutamate administration in the neonatal period on the diabetic syndrome in KK mice. *Diabetolog 12*:621–624.

Carew, L. B., and Foss, D. C. (1971). Monosodium glutamate in chicks. *Poult. Sci. 50*:1501–1505.

Carson, K. A., Nemeroff, C. B., Rone, M. S., Youngblood, W. M., Prange, A. J., Hanker, J. S., and Kizer, J. S. (1977). Biochemical and histochemical evidence for the existence of a tuberinfundibular cholinergic pathway in the rat. *Brain Res. 129*:169–173.

Chi, S. P., and Chen, T. C. (1992). Predicting optimum monosodium glutamate and sodium chloride concentrations in chicken broth as affected by spice addition. *J. Food Process. Preserv. 16*:313–326.

Cohen, A. I. (1967). An electron microscopic study of the modification by monosodium glutamate on the retinas of normal and "rodless" mice. *Am. J. Anat. 120*:319–356.

Conacher, H. B. S., Iyengar, J. R., Miles, W. F., and Botting, H. G. (1979). Gas-liquid chromatographic determination of monosodium glutamate in soups and soup bases. *J. Assoc. Off. Anal. Chem. 62*:604–606.

Cooper, H. R., and Brown, S. (1990). Trans-Tasman differences in consumer perceptions. *Food Aust. 42*:494–497.

Coppola, E. D., Christie, S. N., and Hanna, J. G. (1975). Fast, short-column separation and fluorametric determination of monosodium glutamate in foods. *J. Assoc. Off. Anal. Chem. 58*:58–63.

Crocker, E. C., and Henderson, L. (1932). The glutamate taste. *Am. Perfumer Essent. Oil. Rev. 27*:156–161.

Djazayery, A., and Miller, S. D. (1973). The use of gold thioglucose and monosodium glutamate to induce obesity in mice. *Proc. Nutr. Soc. 32*:30–35.

Dorn, H. W. (1949). Role of monosodium glutamate in seasoning. *Food Technol. 3*:74–76.

Druz, L. L., and Baldwin, R. E. (1982). Taste thresholds and hedonic responses of panels representing three nationalities. *J. Food Sci. 47*:561–563, 569.

Ebert, A. G. (1971). Chronic toxicology and teratology studies of L-monosodium glutamate and related compounds. *Toxicol. Appl. Pharmacol. 17*:274–278.

Ebert, A. G. (1979). Dietary administration of L-monosodium glutamate, DL-monosodium glutamate and L-glutamic acid to rats. *Toxicol. Lett. 3*:71–78.

Everly, J. L. (1971). Light microscopic examination of MSG-induced lesions in the brain of fetal and neonatal rats. *Anat. Rec. 169*:312.

Fagerson, I. S. (1954). Possible relationship between the ionic species of glutamate and flavor. *J. Agric. Food Chem. 2*:474–476.

Fish, W. W. (1991). A method for the quantitation of 5′-mononucleotides in foods and food ingredients. *J. Agric. Food Chem. 39*:1098–1101.

Folkers, K., Shizukuishi, S., Scudder, S. L., Willis, R., Takemura, K., and Longenecker, J. B. (1981). Biochemical evidence for a deficiency of vitamin B-6 in subjects reacting to monosodium L-glutamate by the Chinese restaurant syndrome. *Biochem. Biophys. Res. Comm. 100*:972–977.

Folkers, K., Shizukuishi, S., Willis, R., Scudder, S. L., Takemura, K., and Longenecker, J. B. (1984). The biochemistry of vitamin B-6 is basic to the cause of the Chinese restaurant syndrome. *Z. Physiol. Chem. 365*:405–414.

Foster, D. (1955). Taste testing methodology concerning glutamate. In *Monosodium glutamate—a Second Symposium*, The Quartermaster Food and Container Institute for the Armed Forces, p. 42.

Freedman, J. K., and Potts, A. M. (1962). Repression of glutaminase I in the rat retina by administration of sodium L-glutamate. *Invest. Ophthalmol. 1*:118–121.

Freedman, J. K., and Potts, A. M. (1963). Repression of glutaminase I in the rat retina by administration of sodium L-glutamate. II. *Invest. Ophthalmol. 2*:252.

Galvin, S. L. (1948). The taste of monosodium glutamate and other amino acid salts in dilute solutions. In *Symposium on Monosodium Glutamate*, The Quartermaster Food and Container Institute for the Armed Forces, p. 39.

Garattini, S. (1982). Chinese restaurant asthma. *N. Engl. J. Med. 306*:1181.

Gayte-Sorbier, A., Armand, P., and Abello, G. (1975). Methods for the determination of sodium glutamate. I. Soups and broth. *Ann. Chim. 68*:439–443.

Gayte-Sorbier, A., Airaudo, C. B., and Armand, P. (1985). Stability of glutamic acid and monosodium glutamate under model system conditions: influence of physical and technological factors. *J. Food Sci. 50*:350–352.

Go, G., Nakamura, F. H., Rhoads, G. G., and Dickinson, L. E. (1973). Long-term health effects of dietary mono-sodium glutamate. *Hawaii Med. J. 32*:13–17.

Goodman, L. S., Swinyard, E. A., and Thomas, J. E. P. (1946). Effects of L-glutamic acid and other agents in experimental seizures. *Arch. Neurol. Psychiatr. 56*:20–29.

Gore, M. (1982). The Chinese restaurant syndrome. In *Adverse Effects of Foods*, E. F. Jelliffe and D. B. Jelliffe (Eds.). Plenum Press, New York, p. 211.

Gore, M. E., and Saimon, P. R. (1980). Chinese restaurant syndrome: fact or fiction? *Lancet 1*:251–252.

Gordon, M. E. (1968). Chinese restaurant syndrome. *N. Engl. J. Med. 278*:1123.

Hamatsu, T. (1964). Effect of sodium iodate and sodium L-glutamate in ERG and histological structure of retina in adult rabbits. *Nippon Ganka Gakkei Zasshi. 68*:1621–1624.

Hannsson, H. A. (1970). Ultrastructure studies on long-term effects of MSG on rat retina. *Virchows Arch. 6*:1.

Hashimoto, Y. (1965). Paste-producing substances in marine products. In *The Technology of Fish Utilization*, R. Kreuzery (Ed.). Fishing News, London, p. 57.

Henkel, H. J., Johl, H. J., Trosch, W., and Chmiel, H. (1990). Continuous production of glutamic acid in a three phase fluidized bed with immobolized *Corynebacterium glutamicum. Food Biotech. 4*:149–154.

Heywood, R., and Worden, A. N. (1979). Glutamate toxicity in laboratory animals. In *Glutamic Acid: Advances in Biochemistry and Physiology*, L. J. Filner (Ed.). Raven Press, New York, p. 203.

Holzwarth, M. A., and Hurst, E. M. (1974). Manifestations of monosodium glutamate (MSG) induced lesions of the arcuate nucleus of the mouse. *Anat. Rec. 178*:378.

Ichimura, M., Tanaka, M., Tomita, K., Kirimura, J., and Ishizaki, T. (1974). *Epidemiological Investigations on the Chinese Restaurant Syndromes* (CRS), WHO Food Additives Series No. 5, World Health Organization, Rome, p. 449.

Ikeda, K. (1908). Japanese patent 14,805.

Ikeda, K. (1909). On a new seasoning. *J. Tokyo Chem. Soc. 30*:820–836.

Ishidate, M., Sofuni, T., Yoshikawa, K., Hayashi, M., and Nohmi, T. (1984). Primary mutagenicity screening of food additives currently used in Japan. *Food Chem. Toxicol. 22*:623–636.

Johnson, G. A. R. (1973). Convulsions induced in 10-day-old rats by intraperitoneal injection of monosodium glutamate and related excitant amino acids. *Biochem. Pharmacol. 22*:137–140.

Kandall, S. R. (1968). Chinese restaurant syndrome. *N. Engl. J. Med. 278*:1123.

Kanegae, Y., Nakatsui, I., Sugiyama, Y., and Kanzaki, T. (1991). Role of biotin in glutamate synthesis with a mixed substrate of glucose and acetate. *J. Agric. Chem. Soc.* (Japan) *65*:737–746.

Karlsen, R. L., and Fonnum, F. (1976). The toxic effect of sodium glutamate on rat retina: changes in putative transmitters and their corresponding enzymes. *J. Neurochem. 27*:1437–1441.

Kenney, R. A. (1980). Chinese restaurant syndrome. *Lancet 1*:311–312.

Kenney, R. A. (1986). The Chinese restaurant syndrome: an anecdote revisited. *Food Chem. Toxic. 24*:351–354.

Kenney, R. A., and Tidball, C. S. (1972). Human susceptibility to oral monosodium L-glutamate. *Am. J. Clin. Nutr. 25*:140–146.

Kerr, G. R., Wu-Lee, M., El-Lozy, M., McGandy, R., and Stare, F. J. (1977). Objectivity of food-symptomatology surveys. *J. Am. Diet. Assoc. 71*:263–268.

Kerr, G. R., Wu-Lee, M., El-Lozy, M., McGandy, R., and Stare, F. J. (1979). Prevalence of "Chinese restaurant syndrome." *J. Am. Diet. Assoc. 75*:29–33.

Kodama, A. S. (1913). Separation of inosinic acid. *J. Tokyo Chem. Soc. 34*:751–756.

Kojima, K. (1974). Safety evaluations of disodium 5'-inosinate, disodium 5'-guanylate and disodium 5'-ribonucleotide. *Toxicol. 2*:185–206.

Kuchiba, M., Mitsutomi, E., Matoba, T., and Hasegawa, K. (1989). Antioxidative ability of 5'-ribonucleotides in dehydrated model system. *Agric. Biol. Chem. 53*:3187–3191.

Kuchiba, M., Kaizaki, S., Matoba, T., and Hasegawa, K. (1990). Depressing effect of salts on thermal degradation of inosine-5'-monophosphate and guanosine-5'-monophosphate in aqueous solution. *J. Agric. Food Chem.* 38:593–598.

Kuchiba-Manabe, M., Matoba, T., and Hasegawa, K. (1991a). Sensory changes in umami taste of inosine-5'-monophosphate solution after heating. *J. Food Sci.* 56:1429–1432.

Kuchiba-Manabe, M., Shigekawa, K., Hirakawa, K., Nakazawa, T., Matoba, T., and Hasegawa, K. (1991b). Degradation of 5'-ribonucleotides caused by the peroxidation of methyllinoleate in dehydrated systems. *Agric. Biol. Chem.* 55:2273–2279.

Kuninaka, A. (1960). Studies on taste of ribonucleic acid derivatives. *Nippon Nogeikagaku Kaishi 34*:489–493.

Kurihara, K. (1987). Recent progress in the taste receptor mechanism. In *Umami: A Basic Taste*, Y. Kawamura and M. R. Kare (Eds.). Marcel Dekker, New York, p. 3.

Kwock, R. H. M. (1968). Chinese restaurant syndrome. *N. Engl. J. Med.* 278:796.

Lamperti, A., and Blaha, G. (1976). The effects of neonatally-administered monosodium glutamate on the reproductive system in adult hamsters. *Biol. Reprod. 14*:362–369.

Lechan, R. M., Alpert, L. C., and Jackson, I. M. D. (1976). Synthesis of luteinising hormone releasing factor and thyrotropin-releasing factor in glutamate-lesionel mice. *Nature 264*:465–467.

Lemkey-Johnston, N., and Reynolds, W. A. (1974). Nature and extent of brain lesions in mice related to ingestion of monosodium glutamate. A light and electron microscope study. *J. Neuropathol. Exp. Neurol. 33*:74–97.

Lemkey-Johnston, N., and Reynolds, W. A. (1972). Incidence and extent of brain lesions in mice following ingestion of monosodium glutamate. *Anat. Rec. 172*:354.

Lemkey-Johnston, N., Butler, V., and Reynolds, W. A. (1974). Brain damage in neonatal mice following high dosages of monosodium glutamate (MSG), salt and sucrose. *Anat. Rec. 178*:401–405.

Levey, S., Harroun, J. E., and Smyth, C. J. (1949). Serum glutamic acid levels and the occurrences of nausea and vomiting after the intravenous administration of amino acid mixtures. *J. Lab. Clin. Med. 34*:1238–1248.

Liebschutz, T., Airoldi, L., Brownstein, M. J., Chinn, N. G., and Wurtman, R. J. (1977). Regional distribution of endogenous and parenteral glutamate, aspartate and glutamine in rat brain. *Biochem. Pharmacol. 26*:443–449.

Lockhart, E. E., and Gainer, J. M. (1950). Effects of monosodium glutamate on the taste of pure sucrose and sodium chloride. *Food Res. 15*:459–463.

Lucas, D. R., and Newhouse, J. P. (1957). The toxic effect of sodium L-glutamate on the inner layer of the retina. *AMA Arch. Opthalmol. 58*:193–201.

Lundgren, B. (1978). Taste discrimination versus hedonic response to sucrose in coffee beverage. An inter-laboratory study. *Chem. Senses Flavor. 3*:249–265.

Madden, S. C., Woods, R. R., Schull, F. W., Remington, J. H., and Whipple, G. H. (1945). Tolerance to amino acid mixtures and casein digests given intravenously. Glutamic acid responsible for reactions. *J. Exp. Med. 81*:439–448.

Maga, J. A. (1983). Flavor potentiators. *CRC Crit. Rev. Food Sci. Nutr. 18*:231–312.

Maga, J. A., and Lorenz, K. (1972). The effect of flavor enhancers on direct headspace gas-liquid chromatography profiles of beef broth. *J. Food Sci. 37*:963–964.

Matoba, T., Kuchiba, M., Kimura, M., and Hasegawa, K. (1988). Thermal degradation of flavor enhancers inosine-5'-monophosphate and guanosine-5'-monophosphate in aqueous solution. *J. Food Sci. 53*:1156–1159, 1170.

Matsunaga, T., Takeyama, H., Sudo, H., Oyama, N., Ariura, S., Takano, H., Hirano, M., Burgess, J. G., Sode, K., and Nakamura, N. (1991). Glutamate production from CO_2 by marine cyanobacterium *synechococcus* sp. using a novel bisolar reactor employing light-diffusing optical fibers. *Appl. Biochem. Biotech. 28/29*:157–161.

McGaghren, T. J. (1968). Chinese restaurant syndrome. *N. Engl. J. Med.* 278:1123.

Menken, M. (1968). Chinese restaurant syndrome. *N. Engl. J. Med. 278*:1123.

Moriyuki, H., and Ichimura, M. (1978). Acute toxicity of monosodium L-glutamate in mice and rats. *Oyo Yakuri. 15*:433–437.

Mosel, J. N., and Kantrowitz, G. (1952). The effect of monosodium glutamate on acuity to the primary tastes. *Am. J. Psychol. 65*:573–576.

Moskowitz, H. W., Kumaraiah, V., Sharma, K. N., Jacobs, H. L., and Sharma, S. D. (1975). Cross-cultural differences in simple taste preference. *Science. 199*:1217–1218.

Murakami, U., and Inouye, M. (1971). Brain lesions in the mouse fetus caused by maternal administration of monosodium glutamate. *Congenital Anomalies. 11*:171–177.

Nada, O., and Hirata, K. (1975). The occurrence of cell type containing a specific monoamine in the taste bud of the rabbit's foliate papilla. *Histochem. 43*:237–243.

Nakadai, T., and Nasuno, S. (1989). Use of glutaminase for soy sauce made by koji for a preparation of proteases from *Aspergillus oryzae. J. Ferm. Bioeng. 67*:158, 162.

Nemeroff, C. B., Grant, L. D., Bissette, G., Ervin, G. N., Harrell, L. E., and Prange, A. J. (1977). Growth, endocrinological and behavioral defects after monosodium L-glutamate ingestion in the neonatal rat: possible involvement of arcuate dopamine neuron damage. *Psychoneuroendocrinology 2*:179–196.

Nemeroff, C. B., Grant, L. D., Harrell, L. E., Bissette, G., Ervin, G. N., and Prange, A. J. (1975). Histochemical evidence for the permanent destruction of arcuate dopamine neurons by monosodium L-glutamate in the neonatal rat. *Neurosci. Abstr. 1*:434.

Nikoletiseas, N. M. (1978). Obesity in exercising, hypophagic rats treated with monosodium glutamate. *Physiol. Behavior. 19*:767–773.

Nochaman, M. Z., and McPherson, S. R. (1986). Estimating prevalence of adverse reactions to foods: principles and constraints. *J. Allerg. Clin. Immunol. 78*:148–155.

Nguyen, T. T., and Sporns, P. (1984). Liquid chromatographic determination of flavor enhancers and chloride in food. *JAOAC 67*:747–752.

Nguyen, T. T., and Sporns, P. (1985). Decomposition of the flavor enhancers monosodium glutamate, inosine-5′-monophosphate and guanosine-5′-monophosphate during canning. *J. Food Sci. 50*:812–817.

Oldendorf, W. H. (1971). Brain uptake of radiolabeled amino acids, amines and hexoses after arterial injection. *Am J. Physiol. 221*:1629–1634.

Olney, J. W. (1969a). Glutamate-induced retinal degradation in neonatal mice: electron microscopy of the acutely evolving lesion. *J. Neuropathol. Exp. Neurol. 28*:455–459.

Olney, J. W. (1969b). Brain lesions, obesity, and other characteristics in mice treated with monosodium glutamate. *Science 164*:719–721.

Olney, J. W. (1971). Glutamate-induced neuronal necrosis in the infant mouse hypothalamus. *J. Neuropathol. Exp. Neurol. 30*:75–90.

Olney, J. W. (1974). Toxic effects of glutamate and related amino acids on the developing central nervous system. In *Heritable Disorders of Amino Acid Metabolism*, W. L. Nyhan (Ed.). John Wiley, New York, p. 501.

Olney, J. W., and Ho, O. L. (1970). Brain damage in infant mice following oral intake of glutamate, aspartate or cysteine. *Nature 227*:609–611.

Olney, J. W., and Price, M. T. (1976). Excitoxic amino acids as neuroendocrine probes. In *Kainic Acid as a Tool in Neurobiology*. E. G. McGeer, J. W. Olney and P. L. McGeer (Eds.). Raven Press, New York, p. 38.

Olney, J. W., and Sharpe, L. G. (1969). Brain lesions in an infant rhesus monkey treated with monosodium glutamate. *Science 16*:386–388.

Olney, J. W., Sharpe, L. G., and Feigin, R. D. (1972). Glutamate-induced brain damage in infant primates. *J. Neuropathol. Exp. Neurol. 31*:464–488.

Olney, J. W., Ho, O. L., Rhee, V., and De Gubareff, T. (1973). Neurotoxic effects of glutamate. *N. Engl. J. Med. 289*:1374–1375.

Olney, J. W., Rhee, V., and Gubareff, T. D. (1977). Neurotoxic effects of glutamate on mouse area postrerna. *Brain Res. 120*:151–157.

Oser, B. L., Carson, S., Vogin, E. E., and Cox, G. E. (1971). Oral and subcutaneous administration of monosodium glutamate to infant rodents and dogs. *Nature 229*:411–413.

Owen, G., Cherry, C. P., Prentice, D. E., and Worden, A. N. (1978a). The feeding of rats diets containing up to 4% monosodium glutamate for two years. *Toxicol. Lett. 1*:221–226.

Owen, G., Cherry, C. P., Prentice, D. E., and Worden, A. N. (1978b). The feeding of diets containing up to 10% monosodium glutamate to beagle dogs for two years. *Toxicol. Lett. 1*:217–219.

Papic, J., and Gruner, M. (1978). Determination of sodium glutamate. *Hrana Ishrana 19*:461–465.

Paull, W. K. (1975). Autoradiographic analysis of acruate neuron sensitivity of monosodium glutamate. *Anat. Rec. 181*:445–448.

Paull, W. K., and Lechan, R. (1974). The median eminence of mice with a MSG-induced acruate lesion. *Anat. Rec. 178*:436.

Perez, V. J., and Olney, J. W. (1972). Accumulation of glutamic acid in the arcuate nucleus of the hypothalamus of the infant mouse following subcutaneous administration of monosodium glutamate. *J. Neurochem. 19*:1777–1782.

Pilgrim, F. J., Schultz, H. G., and Peryam, D. R. (1955). Influence of monosodium glutamate on taste perception. *Food Res. 20*:310–315.

Pizzi, W. J., and Barnhart, J. E. (1976). Effects of monosodium glutamate on somatic development obesity in KK mice. *Pharmacol. Biochem. Behav. 5*:551–557.

Poon, T. K., and Cameron, D. P. (1976). Effects of monosodium glutamate (MSG) on diabetes and obesity in KK mice. *Aust. J. Ophthalmol. 50*:900–907.

Porter, W. C. (1968). Chinese restaurant syndrome. *N. Engl. J. Med. 279*:106.

Potts, A. M., Modrell, K. W., and Kingsbury, C. (1960). Permanent fractionation of the ERG by sodium glutamate. *Am. J. Ophthalmol. 50*:900–907.

Prescott, J., Laing, D., Bell, G., Yoshida, M., Gillmore, R., Allen, S., Yamazaki, K., and Ishii, R. (1992). Hedonic responses to taste solutions: a cross-cultural study of Japanese and Australians. *Chem. Senses. 17*:801–819.

Rassin, P. K., Sturman, J. A., and Gaull, G. E. (1978). Taurine and other free amino acids in milk of man and other mammals. *Early Human Dev. 2*:1–10.

Redding, T. W., and Schally, A. V. (1970). Effect of monosodium glutamate on the endocrine axis in rats. *Fed. Proc. 2*:754.

Redding, T. W., Schally, A. V., Arimura, A., and Wakabaysahi, I. (1971). Effect of monosodium glutamate on some endocrine functions. *Neuroendocrinol. 8*:245–255.

Reif-Lehrer, L. (1976). Possible significance of adverse reactions to glutamate in humans. *Fed. Proc. 35*:2205–2211.

Reif-Lehrer, L. (1977). A questionnaire study of the prevalence of Chinese restaurant syndrome. *Fed. Proc. 36*:1617–1623.

Reynolds, W. A., Lemkey-Johnston, N., and Stegink, L. D. (1979). Morphology of the fetal monkey hypothalamus after in utero exposure to monosodium glutamate. In *Glutamic Acid: Advances in Biochemistry and Physiology*, J. Filner (Ed.). Raven Press, New York, p. 217.

Rhodes, J., Titherley, A. C., Norman, J. A., Wood, R., and Lord, D. W. (1991). A survey of the monosodium glutamate content of foods and an estimation of the dietary intake of monosodium glutamate. *Food Add. Contam. 8*:663–672.

Rosenblum, I., Bradley, J. D., and Coulston, F. (1971). Single and double blind studies with oral monosodium glutamate in man. *Toxicol. Appl. Pharmacol. 18*:367–373.

Schamburg, H. (1968). Chinese restaurant syndrome. *N. Engl. J. Med. 278*:1122.

Schamburg, H. H., and Byck, R. (1968). Sin cib-syn: accent in glutamate. *N. Engl. J. Med.* *279*:105.

Schamburg, H. H., Byck, R., Gerstl, R., and Mashman, J. H. (1969). Monosodium glutamate: its pharmacology and role in the Chinese restaurant syndrome. *Science 163*:826–828.

Schwartz, J., and Margalith, P. (1971). Production of flavor-enhancing material by streptomycetes: screening for 5'-nucleotides. *J. Appl. Bact. 34*:347–353.

Schwartzstein, R., Kelleher, M., Weinberger, S., Weiss, J., and Drazen, J. (1987). Airway effects of monosodium glutamate in subjects with chronic stable asthma. *J. Asthma 24*:167–172.

Shaoul, O., and Sporns, P. (1987). Hydrolytic stability at intermediate ph of the common purine nucleotides in food, inosine-5'-monophosphate, guanosine-5'-monophosphate and adenosine-5'-monophosphate. *J. Food Sci. 52*:810–812.

Smith, S. J., Markandu, N. D., Rotellar, C., Elder, D. M., and MacGregor, G. A. (1982). A new or old Chinese restaurant syndrome. *Br. Med. J. 285*:1205.

Snapir, N., Robinzon, B., and Perek, M. (1971). Brain damage in the male domestic fowl treated with monosodium glutamate. *Poult. Sci. 50*:1511–1514.

Snapir, N., Robinzon, B., and Perek, M. (1973). Development of brain damage in the male domestic fowl injected with monosodium glutamate at five days of age. *Pathol. Eur. 8*:265–270.

Spackman, D. H., Stein, W. H., and Moore, S. (1958). Automatic recording apparatus for use in the chromatography of amino acids. *Anal. Chem. 30*:1190–1193.

Steginks, L. D., Reynolds, W. A., and Filer, L. J. (1975). Monosodium glutamate metabolism in the neonatal monkey. *Am. J. Physiol. 229*:246–250.

Stewart, C. N., Coursin, D. B., and Bhagavan, H. N. (1972). Electroencephalographic study of L glutamate-induced seizures in rats. *Toxicol. Appl. Pharmacol. 23*:635–642.

Strong, A. M. (1968). Flavours—their uses and abuses. Flavour enhancers. *Food Technol. Aust. 20*:574–583.

Sugita, Y. (1990). Flavor enhancers. In *Food Additives*, A. L. Branen, P. M. Davidson and S. Salminen (Eds.). Marcel Dekker, New York, p. 259.

Tafelski, T. J. (1976). Effects of monosodium glutamate on the neuroendocrine axis of the hamster. *Anat. Rec. 184*:543–544.

Tanphaichitr, V., Srianujata, S., Pothisiri, P., Sammasut, R., and Kulapongse, S. (1983). Postpandial response to Thai foods with and without added monosodium glutamate. *Nutr. Rept. Intl. 28*:783–792.

Van Cott, H., Hamilton, C. E., and Littell, A. (1954). *The Effects of Sub-threshold Concentrations of Monosodium Glutamate on Absolute Taste Thresholds.* Presented at the 75th Annual Meeting of the Eastern Psychological Association, New York, April 9–10.

Wen, C., Hayes, K. C., and Gershoff, S. N. (1973). Effect of dietary supplementation of monosodium glutamate in infant monkeys, weanling rats and suckling mice. *Am. J. Clin. Nutr. 26*:803–807.

Wilken, J. K. (1986). Does monosodium glutamate cause flushing (or merely "Glutamania")? *J. Am. Acad. Dermatol. 15*:225–230.

Woskow, M. H. (1969). Selectivity in flavor modification by 5'-ribonucleotides. *Food Technol. 23*:1364–1366.

Yamaguchi, S. (1979). The umami taste. In *Food Taste Chemistry*, J. C. Boudreau (Ed.). American Chemical Society, Washington, DC, p. 33.

Yamaguchi, S. (1987). Fundamental properties of umami in human taste perception. In *Umami: A Basic Taste*, Y. Kawamura and M. R. Kare (Eds.). Marcel Dekker, New York, p. 41.

Yamaguchi, S., and Kimizuka, A. (1979). Psychometric studies on the taste of monosodium glutamate. In *Glutamic Acid: Advances in Biochemistry and Physiology*, L. J. Filner, S. Garattini, M. R. Kare, W. A. Reynolds, and R. J. Wurtman (Eds.). Raven Press, New York, p. 35.

Yoshida, M., and Sato, S. (1969). Multidimensional sealing of the taste of amino acids. *Japan Psychol. Res. 11*:149–153.

Yu, K. W. (1970). Lipid metabolism in sodium cyclamate and sodium glutamate fed rats. *Korean J. Publ. Health. 7*:705–710.

Zanda, G., Franciosi, P., Tognoni, G., Rizzo, M., Standen, S. M., Morselli, P. L., and Garattini, S. (1973). A double blind study on the effects of monosodium glutamate in man. *Biomedicine 19*:202–204.

Zhang, Y., and Ho, C. T. (1991). Formation of meatlike aroma compounds from thermal reaction of inosine-5'-monophosphate with cysteine and glutathione. *J. Agric. Food Chem. 39*:1145–1148.

8
Salts

John N. Sofos and S. Raharjo*
Colorado State University
Fort Collins, Colorado

I. INTRODUCTION

Common salt, or sodium chloride, is not only the most frequently used salt, but is also the most common food additive in food processing. It has been used for centuries as a flavoring and preservative agent and can also serve several other functions in the preparation of various types of food products (Marsh, 1983; Sofos, 1984). It has an important role in the production of processed meats and sausages, where it solubilizes muscle proteins, which contribute to meat binding, moisture and fat retention, and the formation of a desirable gel texture upon cooking (Schmidt, 1988). In cheese production, salt is added to the milled curd or applied on the cheese surface to remove whey, to suppress the growth of unwanted microorganisms, to slow down acid development, and to develop flavor (Lindsay et al., 1982; Adda et al., 1988). In the processing of bread and bakery products, salt serves a variety of functions including enhancement of the overall flavor formation, control of the rate of fermentation of yeast-leavened products, and reduction of the water-absorption rate (Crocco, 1982). In the fermentation of sauerkraut and other fermented vegetables, salt not only imparts flavor, but also extracts water and nutrients from the plant tissue to form a brine in which the desirable organisms can grow while the undesirable ones are suppressed (Marsh, 1983).

In spite of the fact that both ions of NaCl, sodium and chloride, are essential elements for normal physiological function in the human body, the extent of NaCl consumption has become a major issue for consumers, primarily because sodium intake appears to be related to development of hypertension in certain individuals (Freis, 1976; Altschul and Grommet, 1980; Fregly and Kare, 1982; Langford, 1982; MacGregor, 1985; Kurtz et al., 1987; Law et al., 1991a), and second, because the

---

* *Current affiliation*: Gadjah Mada University, Yogya Karta, Indonesia

average consumption of sodium in modern societies is 10–20 times greater than the amount needed for physiological balance (NAS, 1980). Toxicological studies have also indicated that sodium chloride may have mutagenic, clastogenic, and cytotoxic effects in laboratory animals (Ashby, 1985; Galloway et al., 1987; Parker and von Borstel, 1987; Tuschy and Obe, 1988; Fujie et al., 1990).

In response to the growing concern about salt intake, food processors have developed a wide variety of low-salt/sodium-reduced food products. The reduction of sodium in foods can be achieved by: (1) lowering the level of sodium chloride (NaCl) added; (2) replacing part or all of the NaCl with other chloride salts (KCl, $CaCl_2$, and $MgCl_2$); (3) replacing part of the NaCl with nonchloride salts, such as phosphates, or with new processing techniques or process modifications; and (4) combinations of any of the above approaches (Terrell, 1983; Sofos, 1984, 1986, 1989).

Concern about NaCl and sodium consumption has led to a growing use of salt substitutes. Common salt (NaCl) is often replaced partially by KCl. Research on the taste of NaCl and KCl salt blends indicates that a 1:1 ratio by weight is the maximum that results in an acceptable combination from a sensory standpoint (Frank and Mickelsen, 1969; Olson and Terrell, 1981). Higher amounts of KCl contribute to bitter taste, depending on the type of product. Wyatt (1981) evaluated green beans and corn canned with either reduced NaCl content or with a 1:1 (by weight) NaCl/KCl mixture. At a level of 1.7%, the salt mixture rated well in desirability for green beans. The sodium level of this mixture is half that of the 1.5% NaCl, while the potassium level is almost tripled. For corn, however, the salt mixtures were less desirable at either the 1.0 or 1.5% level than NaCl used alone at the same levels. The products of this study were evaluated only immediately after canning, so the effects of storage was unknown. Lindsay et al. (1982) reduced the NaCl content of Cheddar cheese by replacing it with KCl. The samples made with the NaCl/KCl mixture (1.25% or 1.5%) were judged to be more bitter than the corresponding controls (1.25 or 1.5% NaCl). The off-flavor difference was statistically significant only with the 1.5% salt mixture. Wyatt (1983) tested cottage cheese made with 25, 50, and 75% reduction of NaCl from the normal 1% level. A significant difference in the texture, flavor, and overall acceptability was noted when the salt content was reduced by 50% or more. Wyatt and Ronan (1982) reduced the levels of NaCl (1.0, 0.75, and 0.50%) or replaced the NaCl in both white and wheat bread with a NaCl/KCl mixture (1.0, 0.75, and 0.50%). The white bread formulated with 0.75% NaCl had significantly higher desirability score than the white bread formulated with 1.0% NaCl. The reduction of NaCl levels in the wheat bread, however, had no significant effect on desirability scores. It was concluded that the use of a 1:1 NaCl/KCl mixture was a successful means of lowering the sodium/potassium ratio in white and wheat breads, while maintaining their desirability.

Since processed meat products contain relatively high levels of sodium, they have been targeted for lowering ingoing levels of NaCl (Sofos, 1984, 1986, 1989). Extensive reduction of sodium chloride levels, however, results in inadequate meat cohesion, water retention, product quality, and shelf life (Sofos, 1983a, b, 1984). This had led to the use of phosphates or chloride salts other than NaCl as partial substitutes for common salt (Madril and Sofos, 1985, 1986; Sofos, 1985, 1986, 1989). Bologna (Olson and Terrell, 1981) formulated with 2.25% NaCl had the highest flavor, texture, and acceptability scores compared to bologna formulated with NaCl/KCl mixtures (0.75%/1.0%, 0.75%/1.25%, and 0.75%/1.5%). Bitter aftertaste appeared to be a major drawback with inclusion of KCl in the formulation. Seman et al. (1980) conducted a study of bologna in which NaCl was partially replaced by $MgCl_2$ or KCl, with or without tripotassium phosphate. The results showed that a one-half reduction in sodium from the 2.5% NaCl level resulted in a bologna product that was not inferior to the control. A two-thirds reduction in sodium, however, adversely affected the flavor of the product. When a low level of NaCl (0.40%) was replaced with an equivalent ionic strength of KCl (0.51%) in restructured pork roasts, off-flavor intensity increased and overall palatability decreased significantly (Hand et al., 1982a). This suggested that in an unseasoned meat product, such as pork roast, extremely low levels of KCl may elicit undesirable sensory properties. Effects of NaCl (2.8%) replacement with KCl, $MgCl_2$, or LiCl on the physical and sensory properties of frankfurters were studied by Hand et al. (1982b). Initially, frankfurters in which 35% of the NaCl was replaced with KCl or $MgCl_2$ were not different in flavor or overall palatability from the control (2.8% NaCl). However, after 6 weeks of storage at 3°C, the flavor and overall palatability of the control frankfurters had not deteriorated, but those of frankfurters with partial NaCl replacement were significantly reduced. For product in which 100% of the NaCl was replaced with KCl or $MgCl_2$, the initial scores for flavor and overall palatability were significantly lower than the controls (Hand et al., 1982b).

The antimicrobial properties of NaCl in foods have been reviewed by Sofos (1984). Although NaCl reduces water activity and is an important inhibitor of microbial growth, the published research is too limited to provide answers to the questions that may be raised in relation to partial or total replacement of NaCl and antimicrobial activity in processed foods.

Reducing the salt content of foods in order to restrict sodium consumption and possibly reduce hypertension is an oversimplification. Many other factors related to product quality and shelf life should be considered before low–sodium chloride formulations are adopted in food processing (Sebranek et al., 1983; Camirand et al., 1983; Wekell et al., 1983; Anonymous, 1983; Weaver and Evans, 1986; Sofos, 1986, 1989). In addition, the use of potassium-containing salt substitutes to lower sodium intake may also contribute to life-threatening incidences of hyperkalemia (Swales, 1991).

II. FUNCTIONS, PROPERTIES, AND SAFETY PROFILE OF SALTS AND THEIR IONS

Both ions of NaCl are essential for normal physiological function in the human body. Sodium is the most abundant cation in the extracellular fluids, and it acts with other electrolytes, especially potassium in the intracellular fluid, to regulate the osmotic pressure and maintain proper water balance in the body (Anderson et al., 1982). Other functions of sodium include maintenance of acid-base balance, transmittance of nerve impulses, muscle relaxation, glucose absorption, and nutrient transport. Chloride is the most common anion found with sodium in the extracellular fluid, but also with potassium inside the cells, where it can pass freely through the cell membranes. It can enhance the capacity of erythrocytes to carry carbon dioxide, which aids in the maintenance of the acid-base equilibrium; and it is involved in digestion as hydrochloric acid. As indicated above, potassium is found mostly in the intracellular fluid, where it acts as a catalyst of energy metabolism and is involved in the synthesis of proteins and glycogen. It also maintains osmotic equilibrium with sodium, which is present in the extracellular fluid, but a small amount of potassium in the extracellular fluid is needed for proper muscle function. Approximately 50–60% of magnesium in the body is combined with calcium and phosphorus in the bones, while the remaining is present in body cells, such as muscle and red blood cells. Only about 1% of the total body magnesium is found in extracellular fluids. Magnesium is involved in basically all major biochemical pathways of the human body, where it activates enzymes. It also is involved in binding of RNA to ribosomes during protein synthesis, in the maintenance of membrane, DNA and RNA integrity, and in neuromuscular activity. Calcium comprises approximately 2% of the adult human body, with most (99%) of it found in the bones and teeth, where it is found together with phosphorus. In addition to their importance in bones and teeth, the small amounts of calcium and phosphorus found in the blood are essential for normal body function (Anderson et al., 1982).

Sodium chloride is a colorless substance forming transparent crystals or white crystalline powder and has a molecular weight of 58.44. It is also known as common salt, rock salt, saline, salt, sea salt or table salt, and is soluble in water and glycerin. Sodium chloride is classified as GRAS (Generally Recognized as Safe) when used in accordance with good manufacturing practices. It is used in baked goods, cheeses, butter, meat and poultry products, and nuts as a curing agent, dough conditioner, flavoring agent, preservative, and to reduce the freezing point in brines. Direct contact with NaCl can cause skin or eye irritations. When bulk sodium chloride is heated to high temperatures, a vapor is emitted that is irritating, particularly to the eyes. When heated to decomposition, it emits toxic fumes of Cl^- and Na_2O. Ingestion of large amounts of sodium chloride can cause irritation of the stomach (Lewis, 1989). Other toxicological effects listed in the *Food Additives Handbook* (Lewis, 1989) include: "poison by intraperitoneal and intracervical routes; moderately toxic by ingestion, or administration through intravenous and subcutaneous routes; experimental teratogen; having human systemic effects when taken by ingestion; blood pressure increase; human reproductive effects when administered by intraplacental route: terminates pregnancy." Toxicity data include mild rabbit skin irritation at 50 mg/24 h; moderate rabbit eye irritation at 100 mg/24 h; inhibition of DNA synthesis in human fibroblasts at 125 mmol/L; TDLo (Toxic Dose Low) by intraplacental administration in 15-week pregnant women for reproductive effects, 27 mg/kg; TDLo by intraperitoneal injection in 13-day pregnant rats for teratogenic effects at 1710 mg/kg; TDLo by intrauterine administration in 4-day pregnant rats for reproductive effects at 500 mg/kg; TDLo by oral administration for cardiomuscular effects in humans at 12,357 mg/kg/23 days; and lethal dose-50 (LD_{50}) by oral administration in rats at 3000 mg/kg (Lewis, 1989).

Potassium chloride is in the form of colorless or white crystals or powder and is odorless, with a salty taste and a 74.55 molecular weight. It is soluble in water and insoluble in absolute alcohol. It is also known as chloropotassuril, potassium monochloride, dipotassium dichloride, tripotassium trichloride, enseal, kalitabs, and kaochlorand slow-K (Lewis, 1989). Potassium chloride is classified as GRAS when used in accordance with good manufacturing practices, but when in the form of tablets containing ≥100 mg of potassium it is considered a drug. It is used in meat, poultry, jellies, and preserves as a flavoring agent and flavor enhancer, gelling agent, pH control agent, salt substitute, tissue softening agent, yeast nutrient, and dietary supplement. It is an eye irritant, and its ingestion can result in nausea, blood clotting changes, and cardiac arrythmias. It results in explosive reactions when mixed with BrF_3 or with a mixture of sulfuric acid and potassium perman-ganate. When heated to decomposition, it emits toxic fumes of K_2O and Cl^- (Lewis, 1989). Other toxicological effects listed in the *Food Additives Handbook* (Lewis, 1989) are: "human poison by ingestion, or when administered through intravenous and intraperitoneal routes; moderately toxic when taken by subcutaneous route; and mutagen." Toxicity data include mild rabbit eye irritant at 500 mg/24 h; mi-crobial mutations at 100 mg/plate; cytotoxic to hamster lung tissue at 12 g/L; TDLo by oral route causing gastrointestinal and blood effects in women at 60 mg/kg/d; lethal dose low (LDLo) by oral route in infants at 938 mg/kg/2 days; LDLo by oral route causing cardiovascular, gastrointestinal and blood effects in man at 20 mg/kg; and LD_{50} by oral route in rats at 2600 mg/kg (Lewis, 1989).

Calcium chloride forms cubic, colorless, and deliquescent crystals, has a mo-lecular weight of 110.98, and is soluble in water and alcohol. It is also known as calcium chloride anhydrous, calplus, caltac, dowflake, snowmelt, and superflake anhydrous. Calcium chloride is classified as GRAS with a limitation of 0.3% in baked goods and dairy product analogs; 0.22% in nonalcoholic beverages and beverage bases; 0.2% in cheese and processed fruit and fruit juices; 0.32% in coffee and tea; 0.4% in condiments and relishes; 0.2% in gravies and sauces; 0.1% in commercial jams and jellies; 0.25% in meat products; 0.2% in plant protein prod-ucts; 0.4% in processed vegetable juices; 0.05% in all other foods when used in accordance with good manufacturing practices. It can be used as an anticaking, antimicrobial, curing and firming agent, as well as a flavor enhancer, humectant, nutrient supplement, pH control agent, processing aid, sequestrant, stabilizer, sur-face active agent, texturizer and thickener in food products. Products in which it can be used include baked goods, beverages, cheeses, fruit and vegetable products, meat and poultry products. Reaction with zinc releases explosive hydrogen gas. Calcium chloride catalyzes exothermic polymerization of methyl vinyl ether and exothermic reaction with water. When heated to decomposition it emits toxic fumes of Cl^- (Lewis, 1989). The compound is a "poison when administered by intrave-nous, intramuscular, intraperitoneal and subcutaneous routes; moderately toxic by ingestion; an experimental tumorigen; and mutagen." Toxicity data include: TDLo by oral route as a tumorigen in rats at 112 g/kg/20 weeks; LD_{50} by oral route in rats at 1000 mg/kg; LD_{50} by intraperitoneal route in rats at 264 mg/kg; and LD_{50} by subcutaneous route in rats at 2630 mg/kg (Lewis, 1989).

Magnesium chloride is thin, white to opaque, gray granules and/or flakes with a molecular weight of 95.21. It is classified as GRAS when used in accordance with good manufacturing practices. It may be used in meat and poultry products as a firming, color retention, tissue softening, and flavoring agent. Solutions consisting of water and approved proteolytic enzymes applied or injected into raw meat cuts shall not result in a gain of more than 3% above the weight of the untreated product. It is also a common food additive as a constituent of a coagulating agent for tofu (i.e., soybean curd) (Kurata et al., 1989). In humid environments it causes steel to rust very rapidly. When heated to decomposition it emits toxic fumes of Cl^- (Lewis, 1989). Magnesium chloride is a "poison by intraperitoneal and intravenous routes; moderately toxic by ingestion and subcutaneous administration; and a mutagen." Its oral LD_{50} in rats is 2800 mg/kg (Lewis, 1989).

III. SALT INTAKE AND HYPERTENSION

The intake of NaCl by humans is controlled by (1) the salt content of foods as purchased or served, (2) the preference of individual consumers for salt or their desire for salty taste, and (3) their salty taste threshold (Langford, 1982). Bartoshuk et al. (1974) indicated that the tongue adapts rapidly to the ambient concentration of salt. Therefore, if the amount of salt in a food is lower than the salt concentration in the saliva, the individual will be unable to experience the salty sensation. Increased salt intake depresses aldosterone production and increases salivary sodium, which consequently increases the difficulty of detection (salty taste) in food.

Modern societies consuming high amounts of processed foods have been exposed to consumption of high levels of NaCl. In general, there is evidence indicating that there is a correlation between salt intake and prevalence of hypertension among certain cultures (Altschul and Grommet, 1980). Several local tribes in different parts of the world consume low-salt foods, and they are characterized by absence of hypertension and lack of rise in arterial pressure with age (Prior et al., 1968; Page et al., 1974). Other studies have also indicated that blood pressure rises with age in societies where salt is added to food (Fregly and Kare, 1982). It appears, however, that in populations that do not add salt to their food, blood pressure does not rise with age (Freis, 1976).

Several studies in which salt intake has been altered demonstrate that salt intake may play an important role in determining blood pressure levels within a community (Altschul and Grommet, 1980). When a group of soldiers in Kenya were given a daily 16-g salt ration, their blood pressure rose (Shaper et al., 1969). Consumer education efforts by the government of Belgium resulted in a reduction in daily salt consumption in that country from 15 to 9 g from 1968 to 1981. During this time, stroke mortality also declined (Joossens and Geboers, 1983). In some individuals with "essential hypertension" (i.e., a term used to describe the 90% of hypertension cases for which the cause is unknown), blood pressure decreases with restriction of dietary salt and increases with its subsequent supplementation (Dole et al., 1950). This response is now said to characterize "salt-sensitive" hypertension (Fujita et al., 1980).

The issue of the association of sodium consumption and high blood pressure has been controversial. Studies indicate that not all individuals will have their blood pressure increase by high sodium intakes, nor will all individuals with high blood pressure undergo a decrease when sodium is restricted in their diet (Weinberger et al., 1986). Authorities, however, tend to agree that low sodium intakes result in lower blood pressure in most hypertensive patients, while there is evidence that high sodium intake becomes a burden for individuals having a physiological deficiency in handling sodium (Altschul and Grommet, 1980). In addition, low sodium intakes appear to enhance the activity of hypertensive drugs. Genetics is also a factor that needs to be recognized as playing a role in development of hypertension, while potassium intake confounds the effects of sodium intake on blood pressure. Law et al. (1991a) concluded, however, that the association of blood pressure with sodium intake is substantially larger than thought and that it increases with age and initial blood pressure.

The hypertensive effects of sodium have also been examined in animals. Ball and Meneely (1957) demonstrated that blood pressure in ordinary 9-month-old laboratory rats increased with the amount of NaCl in the diet. Blood pressure in baboons (Cherchovich et al., 1976) and sheep (Whitworth et al., 1979) also rose with an increase in NaCl intake. Grollman and Grollman (1962) demonstrated that an increase in NaCl intake in pregnant rats resulted in offspring with higher blood pressure than was found in offspring of pregnant rats given less salt.

By selectively inbreeding rats for five to seven generations, Knudsen and Dahl (1966) produced strains that were either highly susceptible or resistant to the effect of NaCl. They found that the young sodium-sensitive rats go through a phase in which they are more susceptible to the effects of salt. They also showed that feeding salt-sensitive rats with commercial baby food induced hypertension and increased their death rate (Dahl et al., 1970). Parabiotic experiments between two strains of rats demonstrated that the rise in blood pressure was due, at least in part, to a bloodborne factor (Dahl et al., 1969). Kidney cross-transplantation between the two strains of rats before high blood pressure had developed indicated clearly that the kidney carried the underlying genetic message for the high blood pressure (Dahl and Heine, 1975). Tobian et al. (1978) subsequently demonstrated in isolated kidneys of the normotensive, salt-sensitive, and salt-resistant rats that the salt-sensitive kidneys excreted less sodium than the salt-resistant kidneys. Other studies indicated that salt-induced hypertension in salt-sensitive rats could have been attributed to a reduction in the natriuretic capacity of the kidneys (Takeshita and Mark, 1978; Fink et al., 1980; Mueller, 1983). A study by Azar et al. (1978) found that hypertensive salt-sensitive rats had fewer glomeruli and fewer functioning nephrons than the salt-resistant rats. Although this salt-induced hypertension in salt-sensitive or salt-resistant rats has been attributed to a humoral factor, the mechanism by which salt-sensitive rats become hypertensive remains to be elucidated (Simchon et al., 1989).

Elevations in blood pressure induced by ingestion of NaCl with the diet have been associated with changes in hormonal levels, sodium excretion and body fluid compartments in various experimental models (Kurtz et al., 1987; Simchon et al., 1989). Limited work has been done on investigating long-term effects of dietary chloride in normotensive animals. Kaup et al. (1991) studied the effect of various levels and types of dietary chloride salts on blood pressure in rats, which were fed with semipurified diet containing moderate (1.9 mg Cl/g diet) and supplemental (15.6 mg Cl/g diet) chloride levels as NaCl, KCl, lysine monohydrochloride with or without $CaCO_3$ or $MgCl_2$ for 56 or 119 days. Rats fed diets with excess chloride excreted more than 84% of the chloride in urine, excreted more urine volume, consumed more fluid (especially when NaCl was fed), had increased blood pressure, had hypertrophied kidneys, and had altered levels of sodium and potassium in their kidneys; but they did not experience any changes in the size of fluid compartments, such as plasma volume or bromine space (Kaup et al., 1991).

The sequence of events that results in hypertension begins with an increase in extracellular fluid volume (ECFV). An increased sodium intake results in an expanded ECFV in order to maintain osmotic balance. The resulting increase in blood pressure allows for greater renal filtration and removal of both sodium and water via the urine (Frohlich and Messerli, 1982). In individuals with essential hypertension, the ECFV, cardiac output, and sodium concentration may return to near-normal levels, but increased vascular resistance and blood pressure remain high, perhaps to maintain the necessary renal filtration efficiency. It has been suggested that in hypertensive individuals, their kidneys have higher pressure requirements that must be reached in order to adequately remove excess sodium and water (Freis, 1976).

Thus, a hypothesis advanced to explain development of hypertension indicates that high sodium levels in the diet may overload the renal capacity to excrete sodium and result in fluid retention, which may promote secretion of natriuretic hormone, which inhibits the sodium pumps of the kidneys, promoting fluid and sodium excretion. Inhibition of the sodium-potassium pumps by the natriuretic hormone, however, increases intracellular sodium concentration in the vascular smooth muscles, which leads to an accumulation of intracellular calcium through the sodium-calcium exchange. This then results in an increase in peripheral vascular resistance, which frequently underlies hypertension (Weaver and Evans, 1986). High-salt diet was found to induce renal growth in salt-sensitive and -resistant rats, but the extent of the enlargement and its mechanism differed between strains. These differences could be an important factor reflecting variations between salt-sensitive and -resistant individuals (McCormick et al., 1989).

The association between dietary NaCl and blood pressure has been assumed to be related primarily to the sodium content of salt (MacGregor, 1985). Several investigators, however, observed that the ingestion of nonchloride sodium salts, such as sodium bicarbonate, sodium ascorbate, sodium phosphate, sodium glutamate, sodium aspartate, sodium glycinate, and sodium citrate, did not cause an elevation in blood pressure and concomitant depressed plasma renin activity in animal models and human subjects (Kurtz and Morris, 1983, 1985; Kotchen et al., 1983; Whitescarver et al., 1984; Kurtz et al., 1987). Ingestion of chloride salts, such as calcium chloride, potassium chloride, choline chloride, and lysine hydrochloride, has been associated with elevated blood pressure and suppressed plasma renin activity in animals (Kirchner et al., 1978; Kotchen et al., 1980, 1983). Some investigators noted that the hypertensive effect of sodium chloride is dependent on the concomitant presence of both chloride and sodium ions by inhibiting plasma renin activity (Koletsky et al., 1981; Whitescarver et al., 1986).

Dietary calcium levels have been found to have an inverse relationship with systolic blood pressure, especially in combination with sodium, while magnesium levels in the diet had no effect on blood pressure or the effect of calcium (Weaver and Evans, 1986; McCarron et al., 1991). There is also evidence of interactive effects of sodium and calcium on the regulation of hypertension. Increased sodium intake resulted in higher urinary excretion of calcium, calcium supplementation reversed hypertension induced by salt (0.5%) in the drinking water of rats, increased dietary sodium (1%) and calcium (2%) prevented development of hypertension, and restriction of both dietary calcium and sodium resulted in the highest blood pressures. Therefore, the antihypertensive activity of calcium in rats is expressed fully in the presence of sodium, indicating that sodium may be important for intestinal absorption of calcium and for the membrane stabilizing effects of calcium (Weaver and Evans, 1986). Epidemiological findings have indicated that there may be a threshold of a potential protective effect of adequate calcium intake (700–

800 mg/d), below which the risk of hypertension increases at a greater rate (Wegener and McCarron, 1986; McCarron et al., 1991). Oparil et al. (1991) reported that sensitivity to pressor effects of dietary NaCl and depressor effects of dietary calcium appear to be inherited in hypertensive rats. Activation of central nervous system pathways that result in enhanced sympathetic outflow is an important effective mechanism of NaCl sensitivity, as is impairment in the ability of the kidneys to excrete an acute sodium and water load. It was also reported that dietary calcium supplementation prevents or reverses these changes, and that the genetic defect in NaCl or calcium sensitivity of blood pressure is not identified, but probably involves cation transport at the cellular level (Oparil et al., 1991).

Advising the public to reduce NaCl consumption is important, but its widespread use in food processing limits what individuals can readily achieve (James et al., 1987). Labeling of foods with their salt content and reduction in the amount of salt added to processed foods are important requirements for individuals to make informed choices in their sodium intakes. In addition, however, sodium-sensitive individuals should avoid adding salt to food by themselves. These activities could reduce sodium intake by an average of 100 mmol/24 h, which could reduce the incidence of stroke by 39% and that of ischemic heart disease by 30% (Law et al., 1991b). When such recommendations or choices are made, however, their effects on the total health of the individual should be considered (Weaver and Evans, 1986).

IV. HYPERKALEMIA

The ratio of sodium to potassium may be more important than the absolute level of NaCl in the diet (Weaver and Evans, 1986). The safe and adequate daily dietary ranges of sodium and potassium are 1100–3300 mg and 1875–5625 mg, respectively, and yield ratios of 0.2 to 1.8. In the U.S. diet, however, the average daily intakes of 3.9–4.7 g sodium and 1.2–3.1 g potassium yield sodium-to-potassium ratios of 1.3 to 3.9—higher than those considered to have a beneficial effect on blood pressure. Thus, it has been recommended to lower the sodium-to-potassium ratio in the diet by using potassium-based salt substitutes and increasing the consumption of fruits and vegetables (Weaver and Evans, 1986).

Some salt substitutes for table seasoning of foods contain 38–72 mmol potassium per teaspoon (Hoyt, 1986). One-half teaspoon of a commercial NaCl/KCl mixture was reported to contain approximately 550 mg sodium and 733 mg potassium (Snyder et al., 1975). Replacing NaCl intake with such a salt substitute would therefore increase human daily potassium intake. There are three possible health benefits from such a change: (1) protection against hypokalemia, (2) lowering of blood pressure, and (3) protection against stroke (Swales, 1991). However, several life-threatening incidences or fatalities from misuse of potassium-containing salt substitutes have been reported (Haddad and Strong, 1975; Snyder et al., 1975; Kallen et al., 1976; Wetli and Davis, 1978; Messerli and Pappas, 1980; Hoyt, 1986). A 75-year-old woman with a history of myocardial infarction developed ankle edema, shortness of breath, and congestive heart failure after consuming a potassium-containing salt substitute ad lib for over a period of approximately 6 weeks (Snyder et al., 1975). In individuals with chronic renal failure, the use of a few grams of potassium-containing salt substitute may be hazardous (Haddad and Strong, 1975).

Kallen et al. (1976) reported the occurrence of near-fatal hyperkalemia in an 8-month-old infant without renal disease who was accidentally given a large dose of commercially available potassium-containing salt substitute. This infant ingested up to 17.2 g of salt substitute, which contained 90% KCl. The infant became "stiff" with "rolling back" eyes and diarrhea and was anorectic (Kallen et al., 1976).

A 32-year-old hypokalemic female was given slow-release KCl for her treatment. She died after ingestion of 47 tablets of KCl (Wetli and Davis, 1978). A 2-month-old, 4.8-kg boy had colic and subsequently was given a mixture of 3 g KCl and human breast milk. A few hours later the baby became cyanotic, stopped breathing, and died 28 hours later (Wetli and Davis, 1978). Three patients (65–77 years of age) had life-threatening cardiovascular complications immediately after, or during, ingestion of 15–20 mL of 10% KCl solution for at least 3 days. Two of these patients died with fresh embolus obstructing the left pulmonary artery or massive embolus in the right kidney (Messerli and Pappas, 1980). A near-fatal case of hyperkalemia, caused by repeated ingestion of soup heavily seasoned with a potassium-containing salt substitute, was reported by Hoyt (1986). The individual (a 70-year-old female) developed transient severe muscle weakness following dinner. She had consumed large quantities of homemade soup. Analysis of her soup revealed its potassium concentration to be 94 mmol/L. The fatal dose of intravenously administered potassium in dogs varied from 5.6 to 8.5 mmol/kg body weight (Taylor et al., 1965).

At least 98% of the body's potassium is contained within the intracellular fluid compartment, and the high concentration of potassium within cells (approximately 160 mmol/L) is maintained by an active transport process with rate-limited characteristics. In view of the limited rate of cellular uptake, the sudden accession into extracellular fluid of a large load of potassium may cause hyperkalemia even in persons with healthy kidneys (Kallen et al., 1976).

Excessive use of salt substitutes that contain potassium may lower blood pressure slightly and may conceivably lower the incidence of stroke, but they can cause some deaths among vulnerable individuals (Swales, 1991). Labels on commercial salt substitutes often have not included contraindications or dosage information. This could lead the consumers to believe that the salt substitutes are harmless (Wetli and Davis, 1978). The best policy is probably to ensure that those who are vulnerable by reasons of disease, age, or medical treatment are warned both by their doctors and by the manufacturers. Salt substitutes that contain potassium should be used only for adding to food to taste, and not for cooking (Swales, 1991). Haddad and Strong (1975) proposed that the term "salt substitute" should be changed to a more informative name, such as "medical salt," to inform the patient that what he or she is taking is a drug and not an inert substitute for common salt.

V. MUTAGENIC AND CARCINOGENIC EFFECTS OF SALTS

A review of the toxicology of NaCl reveals a profile of genotoxic activities almost identical to those of sodium saccharin (Ashby, 1985). It is suggested that the recorded genotoxic and cancer-promoting activities of these chemicals will only become apparent at elevated levels (Ashby, 1985). Ashby and Ishidate (1986) attempted to explain the action of simple salts on the basis of enhanced osmolality, which could act upon the tertiary structure of mitotic chromosomes. They suggested that the high concentration of salt (8–16 mg/mL) would cause perturbation of the ionic interactions that presumably occur between histones and metal ions to maintain the condensed structure of chromatin during metaphase and anaphase. The condensed structure protects the chromosomes from breakage. Sodium chloride and KCl are both capable of inducing lethality and mutations when each is administered at a level of 2 M for different lengths of time (up to 6 hours) to logarithmic phase cells of the yeast *Saccharomyces cerevisiae* (Parker and von Borstel, 1987). Furthermore, the revertants indicated that the reversions can be base substitutions of both the transition and the transversion type, as well as frameshift mutations. It was concluded that NaCl and KCl were equally efficient in inducing all types of mutations (Parker and von Borstel, 1987).

Galloway et al. (1987) indicated that substantial increases in chromosome aberrations were induced in Chinese hamster ovary cells by a medium made hypertonic with NaCl (250 mM) or KCl (160 mM). Weak increases in DNA single-strand and double-strand breaks were also detectable, especially when NaCl was used. Galloway et al. (1987) also demonstrated that simply increasing the osmotic strength of the medium was not sufficient to induce chromosome aberrations, but the solute molecule was more important. Wheatley et al. (1984) showed that cells treated with 600 mM glycerol rapidly shrank but recovered their full volume within 5 minutes. In contrast, there was severe shrinkage within 2 seconds of addition of 600 mM NaCl, and during 3 hours in hyperosmotic medium there was very limited recovery of cell volume. Administration of 40 mmol NaCl/kg body weight positively caused in vivo chromosome aberration in rat bone marrow cells (Fujie et al., 1990).

Tuschy and Obe (1988) reported that restriction endonuclease Alu I (recognition site AG/CT) induced chromosome aberrations in Chinese hamster ovary cells whose frequencies were considerably elevated with the presence of $MgCl_2$ (3.2 M), $CaCl_2$ (1.6 M), or NaCl (3.2 M). The most plausible explanation for these findings is that salts lead to partial dehistonization of the chromatin, which makes more recognition sites available for Alu I (Tuschy and Obe, 1988).

NaCl has been found to increase in vivo stomach carcinogenesis in rats induced by *N*-methyl-*N*-nitro-*N*-nitrosoguanadine. A single oral dose of saturated NaCl solution was followed by inductions of 200-fold increase in ornithine decarboxylase activity within 6 hours and 9-fold increase in DNA synthesis within 3 hours in rat stomach mucosa. Also, NaCl caused dose-dependent induction of ornithine decarboxylase activity at doses of 0.25 to 1.5 g/kg body weight and of DNA synthesis at doses of 0.5 g to 1.5 g/kg body weight (Furihata et al., 1984). Administration of 1 mL of 3.3 M NaCl by gastric intubation induced a maximal 15-fold increase in replicative DNA synthesis in the pyloric mucosa of male Fischer 344 rats by 17 hours; this had returned to the control level by 48 hours (Furihata et al., 1989). Administration of 1 mL of 20–400 mM $CaCl_2$ 1 hour before the administration of NaCl resulted in 60–100% inhibition of the increase in replicative DNA synthesis within 4–48 hours. These results suggest that the calcium ion may act as an antitumor promoter in stomach carcinogenesis (Furihata et al., 1989).

Kurata et al. (1989) examined the potential of carcinogenicity of $MgCl_2 \cdot 6H_2O$ in B6C3F$_1$ mice. The male and female mice were given $MgCl_2 \cdot 6H_2O$ at levels of 0, 0.5, and 2% in the diet for 96 weeks. Survival rates did not differ between the treatment and control groups for males or females. Hematological, urinary, and other clinical parameters showed no treatment-related effects. No differences were noted in the tumor incidence between the treated and control animals. Thus, the study clearly showed a lack of carcinogenicity of $MgCl_2 \cdot 6H_2O$ in mice. Urinary bladder carcinogenesis in rats initiated with N-butyl-N-C_4-hydroxybutyl nitrosamine was promoted with $NaHCO_3$ in their diet, but not with NaCl. Dietary $NaHCO_3$ increased urinary pH and sodium concentration, while NaCl increased sodium concentration, but not urinary pH (Fukushima et al., 1988). Administration of deoxycorticosterone acetate (DOCA) and NaCl to hypertensive rats increased norepinephrine concentrations in the gastric wall and promoted gastric carcinogenesis, while potassium supplementation decreased norepinephrine concentration in the gastric wall and suppressed gastric carcinogenesis (Tatsuta et al., 1991).

VI. OTHER BIOLOGICAL EFFECTS OF SALTS

It has been demonstrated that extraamniotic injection of hypertonic saline (20%) is followed by (1) damage to decidual cells and (2) release of prostaglandin $F_{2\alpha}$ into the amniotic fluid (Gustavii and Green, 1972). As prostaglandin $F_{2\alpha}$ has been found in a high concentration in the decidua, but not in the placenta, it has been proposed that hypertonic saline exerts its abortifacient activity by liberation of prostaglandins from damaged decidual cells (Gustavii and Brunk, 1974). Gustavii (1974) reported that replacement of amniotic fluid by 5% saline solution injected intraamniotically in five pregnant women did not result in abortion, while the extraamniotic injection of 20% saline solution induced abortion in 16 of 19 pregnant women despite the fact that the salinity of their amniotic fluid did not rise above 4.4%. Furthermore, physiological saline (0.9%) injected extraamniotically provoked abortion in 3 of 6 pregnant women. Gustavii (1974) concluded that saline does not exert its effect by acting on tissues within the amniotic sac or in the fetal part of the placenta, but rather by acting on extraamniotic tissues. Calcium supplementation during pregnancy lowers blood pressure, which may reduce the incidence of prematurity, possibly by affecting circulatory concentrations of parathyroid hormone and renin, resulting in smooth muscle relaxation (Pepke and Villar, 1991).

Balnave and Scott (1986) indicated that adding any one of a range of mineral salts including NaCl (250 mg/L) to the drinking water of laying hens for 6 weeks increased the incidence of broken and cracked eggs. The chloride salts of sodium and potassium were particularly effective when given for 6 weeks, and the numbers of defective shells laid by commercial pullets approximately doubled during this period. In addition, the birds continued to produce large numbers of damaged shells over a subsequent 4-week period when the salt supplements were excluded from the drinking water (Balnave and Scott, 1986). Similar studies were also performed by Balnave and Yoselewitz (1987) by adding 0, 200, 400, or 600 mg NaCl/L in drinking water of laying hens for 5 weeks. They found a significant increase in eggshell defects and significant decreases in various eggshell-quality measurements during the period of the study. The incidence of damaged egg shells was increased up to threefold by including 600 mg NaCl/L in the drinking water compared to the control, where no NaCl was added in the drinking water. Shell defects remained twice as high as the control values when the treated birds were placed back on normal drinking water for 5 weeks. Results from these studies suggest that the NaCl intake with drinking water was influencing calcium metabolism in such a way as to affect permanently the ability of some birds to produce normal egg shells (Balnave and Yoselewitz, 1987). If so, the supply of NaCl-contaminated drinking water to young laying pullets, even for short periods of time, could have long-term economic consequences for poultry producers.

VII. SUMMARY

Most average consumers are not willing to sacrifice the taste or flavor that salt adds to a food product. Only individuals on a medically prescribed low-sodium diet, or those individuals highly motivated to reduce their sodium intake, will purchase low- or reduced-sodium food products (Dunaif and Khoo, 1986). There is evidence that NaCl consumption is a major factor in causing hypertension, and at least is not conclusive. For a certain group of populations who are genetically predisposed to hypertension, however, high intake of sodium chloride could increase the risk of developing hypertension. The involvement of nutrient interactions in the development of hypertension should also be considered, because the urinary excretion of potassium, magnesium, calcium, and chloride is linked to excretion of sodium (Weaver and Evans, 1986). It was indicated in animal studies that neither sodium nor chloride intake alone produced hypertension, but the combination of sodium and chloride was responsible for the development of hypertension (Whitescarver et al., 1986).

It has been demonstrated that extraamniotic injection of hypertonic saline (5–20%) in pregnant women could result in abortion. It has been proposed that the hypertonic saline exerts its abortifacient activity by liberation of prostaglandins from damaged decidual cells (Gustavii and Brunk, 1974). Sodium chloride intake from drinking water (up to 600 mg/L) may also affect calcium metabolism in such a way that permanently affects the ability of some laying hens to produce normal eggshells (Balnave and Yoselewitz, 1987). It was also suggested that salts (2 M NaCl or KCl) can break chromosomes and induce mutations in yeasts (Parker and van Borstel, 1987).

The public needs to be more aware of the potential danger of potassium-containing salt substitutes. Although moderate use of potassium-containing salt substitutes may lower blood pressure, they may also cause some deaths among vulnerable individuals. Therefore, potassium-containing salt substitutes should not be used to increase potassium intake without proper care of physicians.

REFERENCES

Anderson, L., Dibble, M. V., Turkki, P. R., Mitchell, H. S., and Rynbergen, H. J. (1982). *Nutrition in Health and Disease*. J. B. Lippincot Company, Philadelphia.

Anonymous (1983). Sodium in processed foods. *J. Am. Med. Assoc. 249*:784–789.

Adda, J., Czulak, J., Mocquot, G., and Vassal, L. (1988). Cheese. In *World Animal Science*: *Meat science, milk science and technology*, Part B, Vol. 3, H. R. Cross and A. J. Overby (eds.). Elsevier Science Publishers, New York, pp. 373–392.

Altschul, A. M., and Grommet, J. K. (1980). Sodium intake and sodium sensitivity. *Nutr. Rev. 38*:393–402.

Ashby, J. (1985). The genotoxicity of sodium saccharin and sodium chloride in relation to their cancer-promoting properties. *Food Chem. Toxicol. 23*:507–519.

Ashby, J., and Ishidate, M., Jr. (1986). Clastogenicity in vitri of the Na, K, Ca and Mg salts of saccharin; and of magnesium chloride; consideration of significance. *Mutation Res. 163*:63–73.

Azar, S., Johnson, M. A., Iwai, J., Bruno, L., and Tobian, L. (1978). Single nephron dynamic in "post-salt" rats with chronic hypertension. *J. Lab. Clin. Med. 91*:156–166.

Ball, C. O. T., and Meneely, G. R. (1957). Observation on dietary sodium chloride. *J. Am. Diet. Assoc. 33*:366–370.

Balnave, D., and Scott, T. (1986). The influence of minerals in drinking water on eggs shell quality. *Nutr. Report Int. 34*:29–34.

Balnave, D., and Yoselewitz, I. (1987). The relation between sodium chloride concentration in drinking water and egg-shell damage. *Br. J. Nutr. 58*:503–509.

Bartoshuk, L. M., McBurney, D. H., and Pfaffman, C. (1974). NaCl thresholds in man: thresholds for water taste or NaCl taste. *J. Comp. Physiol. Psychol. 87*:310–325.

Camirand, W., Randall, J., Popper, K., and Andich, B. (1983). Low-sodium/high-potassium fermented sauces. *Food Technol. 37*(4):81–85.

Cherchovich, G. M., Capek, K., Jefremova, Z., Pohlova, I., and Jelinek, J. (1976). High salt intake and blood pressure in lower primates. *J. Appl. Physiol. 40*:601–604.

Crocco, S. C. (1982). The role of sodium in food processing. *J. Am. Diet. Assoc. 80*:36–39.

Dahl, L. K., and Heine, N. (1975). Primary role of renal homographs in setting chronic blood pressure levels in rats. *Circulation Res. 36*:692–696.

Dahl, L. K., Heine, N., Leitl, G., and Tassinari, L. (1970). Hypertension and death from consumption of processed baby foods in rats. *Proc. Soc. Exp. Biol. Med. 133*:1405–1408.

Dahl, L. K., Knudsen, K. D., and Iwai, J. (1969). Humoral transmission of hypertension: evidence from parabiosis. *Circulation Res. 24&25*(Suppl. I):21–33.

Dole, V. P., Dahl, L. K., Cotzias, G. C., Eder, H. A., and Krebs, M. E. (1950). Dietary treatment of hypertension: clinical and metabolic studies of patients on the rice-fruit diet. *J. Clin. Invest. 29*:1189–1206.

Dunaif, G. E., and Khoo, C.-S. (1986). Developing low- and reduced-sodium products: an industrial perspective. *Food Technol. 40*(12):105–107.

Fink, G. D., Takeshita, A., Mark, A. L., and Brody, M. J. (1980). Determinants of renal vascular resistance in the Dahl strain of genetically hypertensive rat. *Hypertension 2*:274–280.

Frank, R. L., and Mickelsen, O. (1969). Sodium-potassium chloride mixtures as table salt. *Am. J. Clin. Nutr. 22*:464–470.

Fregly, M. J., and Kare, M. R. (Eds.). (1982). *The Role of Salt in Cardiovascular Hypertension*. Academic Press, New York.

Freis, E. D. (1976). Salt, volume and the prevention of hypertension. *Circulation 53*:589–595.

Frohlich, E. D., and Messerli, F. H. (1982). Sodium and hypertension. In *Sodium: Its Biologic Significance*, S. Papper (Ed.). CRC Press, Boca Raton, FL, pp. 143–174.

Fujie, K., Nishi, J., Wada, M., Maeda, S., and Sugiyama, T. (1990). Acute cytogenic effects of tyramine, MTCAs, NaCl and soy sauce on rat bone marrow cells in vivo. *Mutation Res. 240*:281–288.

Fujita, T., Henry, W. L., Bartter, F. C., Lake, C. R., and Delea, C. S. (1980). Factors influencing blood pressure in salt-sensitive patients with hypertension. *Am. J. Med. 69*:334–344.

Fukushima, S., Tamano, S., Shibata, M. A., Kurata, Y., Hirose, M. and Ito, N. (1988). The role of urinary pH and sodium ion concentration in the promotion stage of two-stage caranogenesis of the rat urinary bladder. *Carcinogenesis 9*:1203–1206.

Furihata, C., Sato, Y., Hosaka, M., Matsushima, T., Furukawa, F., and Takahashi, M. (1984). NaCl induced ornithine decarboxylase and DNA synthesis in rat stomach mucosa. *Biochem. Biophys. Res. Commun. 121*:1027–1032.

Furihata, C., Sudo, K., and Matsushima, T. (1989). Calcium chloride inhibits stimulation of replicative DNA synthesis by sodium chloride in the pyloric mucosa of rat stomach. *Carcinogenesis 10*:2135–2137.

Galloway, M. M., Deasy, D. A., Bean, C. L., Kraynak, A. R., Armstrong, M. J., and Bradley, M. O. (1987). Effects of high osmotic strength on chromosome aberrations, sister-chromatid exchanges and DNA strand breaks, and the relation to toxicity. *Mutation Res. 189*:15–25.

Grollman, A., and Grollman, E. F. (1962). The teratogenic induction of hypertension. *J. Clin. Invest. 41*:710–714.

Gustavii, B. (1974). Intra-amniotic and extra-amniotic injection of sodium chloride solution: amniotic fluid salinity and abortifacient effect. *Am. J. Obstet. Gynecol. 118*:218–219.

Gustavii, B., and Brunk, U. (1974). Lability of human decidual cells. In vivo effects of hypertonic saline. *Acad. Obstet. Gynec. Scand. 53*:271–274.

Gustavii, B., and Green, K. (1972). Release of prostaglandin $F_{2\alpha}$ following injection of hypertonic saline for therapeutic abortion: a preliminary study. *Am. J. Obstet. Gynecol. 114*:1099–1100.

Haddad, A., and Strong, E. (1975). Potassium in salt substitutes. *N. Engl. J. Med. 292*:1082.

Hand, L. W., Terrell, R. N., and Smith, G. C. (1982a). Effects of chloride salt, method of manufacturing and frozen storage on sensory properties of restructured pork roasts. *J. Food Sci. 47*:1771–1772.

Hand, L. W., Terrell, R. N., and Smith, G. C. (1982b). Effects of chloride salts on physical, chemical and sensory properties of frankfurters. *J. Food Sci. 47*:1800–1802, 1817.

Hoyt, R. E. (1986). Hyperkalemia due to salt substitutes. *J. Am. Med. Assoc. 256*:1726.

James, W. P. T., Ralph, A., and Sanchez-Castillo, C. P. (1987). The dominance of salt in manufactured food in the sodium intake of affluent societies. *Lancet i*:426–429.

Joossens, J. V., and Geboers, J. (1983). Salt and hypertension. *Prev. Med. 12*:53–59.

Kallen, R. J., Rieger, C. H. L., Cohen, H. S., Sutter, M. A., and Ong, R. T. (1976). Near-fatal hyperkalemia due to ingestion of salt substitute by an infant. *J. Am. Med. Assoc. 235*:2125–2126.

Kaup, S. M., Greger, J. L., Marcus, M. S. K., and Lewis, N. M. (1991). Blood pressure, fluid compartments and utilization of chloride in rats fed various chloride diets. *J. Nutr. 121*:330–337.

Kirchner, K. A., Kotchen, T. A., Galla, J., and Luke, R. G. (1978). Importance of chloride for acute inhibition of renin by sodium chloride. *Am. J. Physiol. 235*:F 444–450.

Koletsky, R. J., Dluhy, R. G., Cheron, R. G., and Williams, G. H. (1981). Dietary chloride modifies renin release in normal humans. *Am. J. Physiol. 241*:F 361–363.

Kotchen, T. A., Krzyzaniak, K. E., Anderson, J. E., Ernst, C. B., Galla, J. H., and Luke, R. (1980). Inhibition of renin secretion by HCl is related to chloride in both dog and rat. *Am. J. Physiol. 239*:F 44–49.

Kotchen, T. A., Luke, R. G., Ott, C. E., Galla, J. H., and Whitescarver, S. A. (1983). Effect of chloride on renin and blood pressure responses to sodium chloride. *Ann. Intern. Med. 98*:817–822.

Knudsen, K. D., and Dahl, L. K. (1966). Essential hypertension: inborn error of sodium metabolism. *Postgrad. Med. J. 42*:148–152.

Kurata, Y., Tamano, S., Shibata, M.-A., Hagiwara, A., Fukushima, S., and Ito, N. (1989). Lack of carcinogenicity of magnesium chloride in a long-term feeding study in B6C3F$_1$ mice. *Food Chem. Toxicol. 27*:559–563.

Kurtz, T. W., and Morris, R. C., Jr. (1983). Dietary chloride as a determinant of "sodium-dependent" hypertension. *Science 222*:1139–1141.

Kurtz, T. W., and Morris, R. C., Jr. (1985). Hypertension and sodium salts. *Science 228*:359–360.

Kurtz, T. W., Al-Bander, H. A., and Morris, R. C., Jr. (1987). Salt-sensitive essential hypertension in men. Is the sodium ion alone important? *N. Engl. J. Med. 317*:1043–1048.

Langford, H. G. (1982). Sodium, potassium and arterial pressure in human beings. In *Salt and hypertension*. J. Iwai. (Ed.). Igaku-Shoin, New York, NY, pp. 57–65.

Law, M. R., Frost, C. D., and Wald, N. J. (1991a). By how much does dietary salt reduction lower blood pressure? I. Analysis of observational data among populations. *Br. Med. J. 302*:811–815.

Law, M. R., Frost, C. D., and Wald, N. J. (1991b). III. Analysis of data from trials of salt reduction. *Br. Med. J. 302*:819–824.

Lewis, R. J., Sr. (1989). *Food Additives Handbook*. Van Nostrand Reinhold, New York.

Lindsay, R. C., Hargett, S. M., and Bush, C. S. (1982). Effect of sodium/potassium (1:1) chloride and low sodium chloride concentrations on quality of Cheddar cheese. *J. Dairy Sci. 65*:360–370.

MacGregor, G. A. (1985). Sodium is more important than calcium in essential hypertension. *Hypertension 7*:628–637.

Madril, M. T., and Sofos, J. N. (1985). Antimicrobial and functional effects of six polyphosphates in reduced NaCl comminuted meat products. *Lebensm. Wissensch. Technol. 18*:316–322.

Madril, M. T., and Sofos, J. N. (1986). Interaction of reduced NaCl, sodium and pyrophosphate and pH on the antimicrobial activity of comminuted meat products. *J. Food Sci. 52*:252–256, 262.

Marsh, A. C. (1983). Processes and formulations that affect the sodium content of foods. *Food Technol. 37(7)*:45–49.

McCarron, D. A., Morris, C. D., Young, E., Roullet, C., and Drüzke, T. (1991). Dietary calcium and blood pressure: modifying factors in specific populations. *Am. J. Clin. Nutr. 54*:2155–2195.

McCormick, C. P., Rauch, A. L., and Buckalew, V. M., Jr. (1989). Differential effect of dietary salt on renal growth in Dahl salt-sensitive and salt-resistant rats. *Hypertension 13*:122–127.

Messerli, F. H., and Pappas, N. D. (1980). Potassium chloride and thromboembolic complications: a hypothesis. *Lancet 2*:919–920.

Mueller, S. A. (1983). Longitudinal study of hindquarter vasculature during development in spontaneously hypertensive and Dahl salt sensitive rats. *Hypertension 5*:489–497.

NAS (National Academy of Science). (1980). *Toward Healthful Diets*. National Research Council, National Academy of Science, Washington, D.C.

Olson, D. G., and Terrell, R. N. (1981). Sensory properties of processed meats using various sodium salt substitutes. In *Proceedings of the Meat Industry Research Conference*. American Meat Institute Foundation, Arlington, VA, pp. 59–66.

Oparil, S., Chen, Y. F., Jin, H., Yang, R. H., and Wyss, J. M. (1991). Dietary Ca^{2+} prevents NaCl-sensitive hypertension in spontaneously hypertensive rats via sympatholytic and renal effects. *Am. J. Clin. Nutr. 54*:2275–2365.

Page, L. B., Daman, H., and Moellering, R. C. (1974). Antecedents of cardiovascular disease in six Solomon Islands societies. *Circulation 49*:1132–1140.

Parker, K. R., and van Borstel, R. C. (1987). Base-substitution and frameshift mutagenesis by sodium chloride and potassium chloride in *Saccharomyces cerevisiae*. *Mutation Res. 189*:11–14.

Pepke, J. T., and Villar, J. (1991). Pregnancy-induced hypertension and low birth weight: the role of calcium. *Am. J. Clin Nutr. 54*:2375–2415.

Prior, I. A. M., Grimley Evans, J., Harvey, H. P. B., Davidson, F., and Lindsey, M. (1968). Sodium intake and blood pressure in two Polynesian populations. *N. Engl. J. Med. 279*:515–520.

Schmidt, G. R. (1988). Processing. In *World Animal Science: Meat Science, Milk Science and Technology*, Part B, Vol. 3, H. R. Cross and A. J. Overby (Eds.). Elsevier Science Publishers, New York, pp. 83–114.

Sebranek, J. G., Olson, D. G., Whiting, R. C., Benedict, R. C., Rust, R. E., Kraft, A. A., and Woychik, J. H. (1983). Physiological role of dietary sodium in human health and implications of sodium reduction in muscle foods. *Food Technol. 37*(7):51–59.

Seman, D. L., Olson, D. G., and Mandigo, R. W. (1980). Effect of reduction and partial substitution of sodium on bologna characteristics and acceptability. *J. Food Sci. 45*:1116–1121.

Shaper, A. G., Leonard, P. J., Jones, K. W., and Jones, M. (1969). Environmental effects on the body build, blood pressure and blood chemistry of nomadic warriors serving in the army of Kenya. *East Afr. Med. J. 46*:282–289.

Simchon, S., Manger, W. M., Carlin, R. D., Peeters, L. L., Rodriguez, J., Batista, D., Brown, T., and Merchant, N. B. (1989). Salt-induced hypertension in Dahl salt-sensitive rats. *Hypertension 13*:612–621.

Snyder, E. L., Dixon, T., and Bresnitz, E. (1975). Abuse of a salt "substitute." *N. Engl. J. Med. 292*:320.

Sofos, J. N. (1983a). Effects of reduced salt (NaCl) levels on the stability of frankfurters. *J. Food Sci. 48*:1684–1688, 1691.

Sofos, J. N. (1983b). Effects of reduced salt (NaCl) levels on sensory and instrumental evaluation of frankfurters. *J. Food Sci. 48*:1692–1695, 1699. 1684–1688, 1691.

Sofos, J. N. (1984). Antimicrobial effects of sodium and other ions in foods: a review. *J. Food Safety 6*:45–78.

Sofos, J. N. (1985). Influence of sodium tripolyphosphate on the binding and antimicrobial properties of reduced NaCl comminuted meat products. *J. Food Sci. 50*:1379–1383, 1391.

Sofos, J. N. (1986). Use of phosphates in low-sodium meat products. *Food Technol. 40*(9):52, 54–58, 60, 62, 64, 66, 68–69.

Sofos, J. N. (1989). Phosphates in meat products. In *Developments in Food Preservation—5*, S. Thorne (Ed.). Elsevier Applied Science, New York, pp. 207–252.

Swales, J. D. (1991). Salt substitutes and potassium intake. *Br. Med. J. 303*:1084–1085.

Takeshita, A., and Mark, A. L. (1978). Neurogenic contribution to hindquarters vasoconstriction during high sodium intake in Dahl strain of genetically hypertensive rat. *Circulation Res. 43*(Suppl. I):86–91.

Tatsuta, M., Iishi, H., Baka, M., and Tanigachi, H. (1991). Enhanced induction of gastric carcinogenesis by *N*-methyl-*N*-nitro-*N*-nitrosoguanadine in deoxycorticosterone acetate-NaCl hypertensive rats and its inhibition by potassium chloride. *Canc. Res. 51*:3863–3866.

Taylor, P. M., Seder, H. B., Mering, J., and Watson, D. W. (1965). Comparison of the tolerances of anesthetized adult dogs and pups to KCl infusion. *Pediatrics 36*:905–910.

Terrell, R. N. (1983). Reducing the sodium content of processed meats. *Food Technol. 37*(7):66–71.

Tobian, L., Lange, J., Azar, S., Iwai, J., Koop, D., Coffee, K., and Johnson, M. A. (1978). Reduction of natriuretic capacity and renin release in isolated, blood-perfused kidneys of Dahl hypertension-prone rats. *Circulation Res. 43*(Suppl. I):92–97.

Tuschy, S., and Obe, G. (1988). Potentiation of Alu I-induced chromosome aberrations by high salt concentrations in Chinese hamster ovary cells. *Mutation Res. 207*:83–87.

Weaver, C. M., and Evans, G. H. (1986). Nutrient interactions and hypertension. *Food Technol. 40*(12):99–101.

Wegener, L. L., and McCarron, D. A. (1986). Dietary calcium: an assessment of its protective action in human and experimental hypertension. *Food Technol. 40*(12):93–95.

Weinberger, M. H., Miller, J. Z., Luft, F. C., Grim, C. E., and Fineberg, N. S. (1986). Sodium sensitivity and resistance of blood pressure in humans. *Food Technol. 40*(12):96–98.

Wekell, J. C., Teeny, F. M., Gauglitz, E. J., Jr., Hathorn, L., and Spinelli, J. (1983). Implications of reduced sodium usage and problems in fish and shellfish. *Food Technol. 37*(9):51–58.

Wetli, C. V., and Davis, J. H. (1978). Fatal hyperkalemia from accidental overdose of potassium chloride. *J. Am. Med. Assoc. 240*:1339.

Wheatley, D. N., Inglis, M. S., and Clegg, J. S. (1984). Dehydration of HeLa S-3 cells by osmosis. I. Kinetics of cellular responses to hypertonic levels of sorbitol, amino acids and other selected agents. *Molecular Physiol. 6*:163–182.

Whitescarver, S. A., Ott, C. E., Jackson, B. A, Guthrie, G. P., Jr., and Kotchen, T. A. (1984). Salt-sensitive hypertension: contribution of chloride. *Science 223*:1430–1432.

Whitescarver, S. A., Holtzclaw, B. J., Downs, J. H., Ott, C. E., Sowers, J. R., and Kotchen, T. A. (1986). Effect of dietary chloride on salt-sensitive and renin-dependent hypertension. *Hypertension 8*:56–61.

Whitworth, J. A., Coghlan, J. P., Denton, D. A., Hardy, K., and Scoggins, B. A. (1979). Effect of sodium loading and ACTH on blood pressure of sheep with reduced renal mass. *Cardiovascular Res. 13*:9–15.

Wyatt, C. J. (1981). Comparison of sodium and sodium/potassium salt mixtures in processed vegetables. *J. Food Sci. 46*:302–303.

Wyatt, C. J. (1983). Acceptability of reduced sodium in breads, cottage cheese and pickles. *J. Food Sci. 48*:1300–1302.

Wyatt, C. J., and Ronan, K. (1982). Evaluation of potassium chloride as a salt substitute in bread. *J. Food Sci. 47*:672–673.

9
Modified Food Starches

Otto B. Wurzburg*
National Starch and Chemical Company
Bridgewater, New Jersey

I. STARCH TECHNOLOGY: BACKGROUND

Starch is a polymer consisting of anhydroglucose units linked together primarily through α-D-(1–4) anhydroglucose bonds to form either a linear polymer known as amylose or a branched polymer known as amylopectin. The latter comprises, in addition to the α-D-(1 → 4) glucosidic linkages, α-D-(1 → 6) linkages at which points branches are introduced (Fig. 1).

In general amylose molecules tend to be considerably lower in molecular weight than amylopectin molecules. Depending upon the plant source, amylose may consist of about 200–2000 anhydroglucose units compared to thousands for amylopectin, which may have molecular weights of several million.

Except for the terminal anhydroglucose units and those at which branching occurs, each of the remaining units has one primary and two secondary hydroxyls. As a result there is an abundance of hydroxyls, which impart hydrophilic or water-loving properties to the molecule. At the same time the hydroxyls may also have an affinity for any other nearby hydroxyls and form hydrogen bonds, reducing their affinity for water. This takes place when the mobility and geometry of the molecules permit them to align closely enough to permit hydrogen bonding to occur. The size and linearity of amylose makes it particularly prone to this type of association, which results in the formation of aggregates. At dilute concentrations the aggregates will precipitate from solution. If the concentration is high the molecules will be able to align only in limited segments where hydrogen bonds may form to create a three-dimensional network in whose interstices water can be entrapped forming a gel structure like that formed when cooked cornstarch is cooled. This phenomenon

---

* Retired, currently consultant.

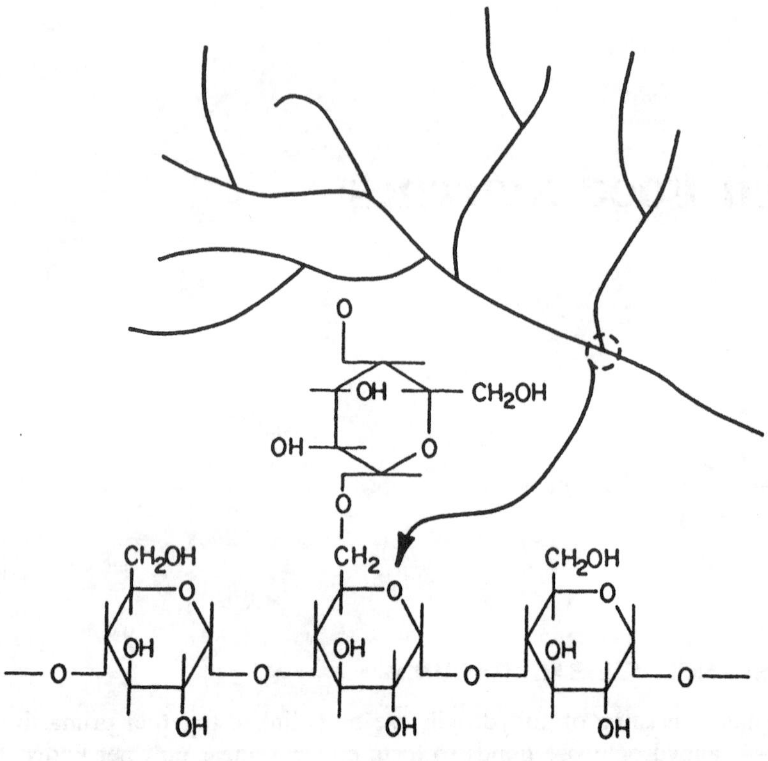

Fig. 1 Amylopectin linkages. Circled section represents alpha-D-(1→6) linkages at which points branches are introduced.

involving the intermolecular association of amylose is known as *retrogradation*. Figure 2 shows a schematic of retrogradation.

The large size and highly branched nature of amylopectin prevent its molecules from aligning with each other. As a result amylopectin does not retrograde like amylose. However, if dispersions of amylopectin are stored at low temperatures or are frozen, segments of its branches may align closely enough for some hydrogen bonds to form resulting in loss of water-holding capacity, clarity, and viscosity. Gelling or setback may also result. Unlike retrogradation, this phenomenon may be reversed by reheating.

Starches from most plant sources such as regular maize, cassava or tapioca, wheat, potato, etc., contain about 17–27% amylose. The exceptions are starches from waxy grains such as waxy corn or maize, waxy rice, etc., which are nearly pure amylopectin, and high-amylose grains like high-amylose corn, which may contain up to 55–80% amylose depending upon the genetic background.

The starch in plants normally occurs in the form of minute granules, which are insoluble in cold water. The size and shape of the granules vary depending upon the plant source. Rice starch has very small polygonal granules 3–5 μ in diameter, cornstarch granules are polygonal or rounded and average about 15 μ in diameter, and potato starch granules are oyster shaped and large running up to 100 μ in diameter.

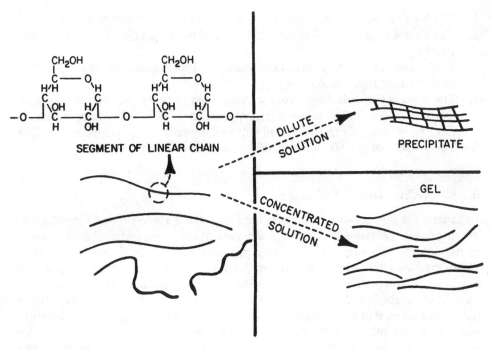

SEGMENT OF LINEAR CHAIN

DILUTE SOLUTION

CONCENTRATED SOLUTION

PRECIPITATE

GEL

Fig. 2 Schematic of retrogradation.

The granules owe their integrity and insolubility in cold water to intermolecular hydrogen bonds between segments of amylopectin branches. When an aqueous suspension of starch is heated beyond a critical temperature, which varies with the starch type, the hydrogen bonds weaken and the granules imbibe water, swelling to many times their original size and undergoing an irreversible change. As the process proceeds the viscosity increases dramatically, and as the hydrogen bonds break the swollen granules rupture into molecular dispersions and aggregates, the viscosity decreases, with the extent varying with the type of starch.

During the initial stage of swelling before the swollen granules start rupturing, the cook develops a salvelike texture, which is quite palatable from a food standpoint. However, it is in a very tenuous state, which disappears quickly as the granules rupture and the sol develops an elastic, cohesive texture. On cooling, dispersions of regular cereal starches will lose their clarity and form opaque gels. Waxy starches and starches such as tapioca and potato tend to form cohesive, elastic sols under similar conditions.

Unmodified starch is a food. It has a long history of use in the food industry: as a fermentation medium in the brewing industry, in sugar grinding, as a bulking agent in dry mixes, as a dusting agent, a molding medium in candy making, etc. However, in many applications where a cooked starch is used to thicken or provide texture to food systems, unmodified starch has serious limitations. Modified starches were developed to overcome one or more of the following shortcomings associated with native starches.

1. The high viscosity of their sols when dispersed at low concentrations
2. The undesirable cohesive or elastic texture of the dispersions of some types of starches
3. The tendency of cooked sols to lose clarity and form gels at room temperature because of retrogradation
4. The tendency of sols made from starches such as waxy corn, tapioca, etc. to lose clarity, gel, and synerese after exposure to storage at low temperature or freezing because of the association between segments of amylopectin branches
5. The absence of specific functionality such as hydrophobicity

II. MODIFIED FOOD STARCHES

In general the modification processes used in making these products involve relatively minimal alteration of the chemical nature of the starch but significant changes in its physical behavior. The resulting products perform more effectively than unmodified starch or impart unique properties that are unattainable with native starches. There are five types of modified starches: bleached, converted, cross-linked, monosubstituted, and cross-linked monosubstituted. In the United States the treatments used in bleaching or conversion with acid may be used in combination with any of the others. With the exception of dextrins (made by means of dry heat), the other modifications are classified as food additives by the FDA and regulated under the Code of Federal Regulations—21CFR172.892 (CFR, 1990). This specifies the types of approved treatments, level of treatment, and certain critical specifications. Dextrins, which are not classified as food additives, are considered GRAS (generally recognized as safe).

A. Bleached Starch

The treatments for bleaching starch are covered under 21CRF172.892(b). Normally they involve treating suspensions of ungelatinized starch granules with minimal amounts of oxidizing agents such as hydrogen peroxide or peracetic acid (active oxygen 0.45% max.); ammonium persulfate (0.075% max.) and 0.05% max. sulfur dioxide; chlorine as sodium hypochlorite (0.0082 lb of chlorine per lb of starch max.); potassium permanganate (0.2% max. with a limit of 50 ppm manganese residue on the starch); and 0.5% max. sodium chlorite. In addition, a 0.36% max. instance of calcium hypochlorite may only be used in batter for use in processed foods. Except for this, the objective of bleaching treatments is to whiten starch. This is particularly true with cornstarch, which has a yellowish cast caused by traces of xanthophyll, carotene, and related pigments associated with the corn gluten (Kerr, 1950; Wurzburg, 1978). These impurities are then solubilized and removed by washing.

Starch bleaching agents are also used as sterilizers, lowering levels of undesired microorganisms such as thermophiles in order to meet the requirements of the canning industry (Wurzburg, 1962). While oxidants are capable of introducing carboxyl groups onto the starch at higher concentrations, few such groups are introduced in the starch at the levels of oxidant used in bleaching or sterilization. The treatment is no more than might occur in food or in the gut as evidenced by the absence of viscosity changes (FAO/WHO, 1974). The residues, i.e., reduced forms, of the bleaching agents are water, acetic acid, ammonium sulfate, sodium chloride, and manganous sulfate. These are largely removed during the washing and dewatering processes. In addition where there might be concern over traces of manganese, as noted above, a specification of 50 ppm max. manganese has been placed on the starch bleached with permanganate.

B. Converted Starches

Conversions, the processes for making converted starches, involve reducing the viscosity of native starches by weakening the starch granule and decreasing the size of its molecules through scission of some of the glucosidic linkages. By weakening the granule strength and decreasing the size of the molecules, conversions reduce the tendency of the granules to swell and absorb water and decrease the water-binding capacity of the dispersed molecules and aggregates. As a result, converted starches can be dispersed in water at higher concentrations than can native starches. Most of the conversion processes used to make converted starches involve treating granular starch in water suspensions or in the dry powdered form. There are three classes of converted starches: acid-modified or fluidity (reciprocal of viscosity) starches, oxidized or chlorinated starches, and dextrinized starches.

Acid-Modified Starches

These are made by hydrolyzing aqueous suspensions of starch granules using hydrochloric and/or sulfuric acid as catalysts with mild heat, keeping the temperature well below the gelatinization temperature of the starch. When the conversion reaches the desired level, as determined by checking the viscosity or fluidity, the acid is neutralized and the granules are recovered by washing, dewatering, and drying. Since these treatments are normally run on aqueous suspensions, the extent of conversion is limited to avoid degrading the starch to the point where it starts to swell due to solubilization. The basic reaction is hydrolysis of the α-D-$(1\rightarrow 4)$ or -$(1\rightarrow 6)$ linkages. As a result acid-modified starch is chemically identical to unmodified starch except for the lower molecular weight.

Acid-modified wheat starch fed at 63.7% dietary level to weanling rats over 25 days was comparable to unmodified wheat starch based on weight gains (Booher, 1951). Since acid-modified starches are, from a chemical standpoint, identical to unmodified starch except for a lower molecular weight, they are considered equivalent to unmodified starch and as such have been used as controls in feeding studies, such as the use of acid-modified waxy starch in a control diet where it contributed 25% of the calories in a 28-day feeding study on Pitman-Moore miniature pigs (Anderson et al., 1973, 1974). All organs, including the ceca, appeared grossly normal on autopsy. The liver weight as a percentage of body weight was slightly less than that of sow-reared pigs, but the weights of the other organs as percent of body weight were comparable.

Dextrins

Dextrins or pyroconversions are produced by roasting powdered starch, usually in the presence of traces of mineral acid such as hydrochloric acid and moisture. Depending upon conditions such as temperature, rate of heating, air flow, etc., white dextrins, yellow dextrins, or British gums may be produced. Since these are made by a dry treatment, there is no limit to the extent of conversion because of solubilization. As in acid modification, hydrolysis of the glucosidic linkages predominates. In addition, particularly with yellow dextrins and British gums, transglucosidations involving molecular rearrangements will occur.

Dextrins were fed to groups of six weanling male rats each at 60 g/kg body weight for 21–28 days. The digestibility of wheat dextrin was somewhat lower than that of wheat starch, but rats fed potato dextrin had better weight gains than those fed potato starch (Booher, 1951). Since dextrins have had a long history of use, not only as specific products but as products formed during food preparation, as in baking and the toasting of bread, and they are regarded as being similar to intermediates in the normal digestion of food, they have been given GRAS status by the FDA.

Oxidized Starches

These, like acid-modified starches, are made by treating aqueous suspensions of starch granules with sodium hypochlorite. They are covered under 21CFR172.892(g). Chlorine, usually as sodium hypochlorite, is used at levels up to 5.5% max. on the weight of the starch as the converting agent. Chlorine oxidizes starch randomly, introducing carboxyl or carbonyl groups in place of both primary and secondary hydroxyls. At the same time it ruptures some of the glucosidic bonds. The carboxyl groups introduced in place of some of the hydroxyls are bulkier and more hydrophilic than the hydroxyls they replace. As a result, they exert a stabilizing effect on the molecules, reducing their tendency to retrograde or associate. Dispersions of oxidized starches consequently generally are more stable than those of acid-modified starch. Depending upon the conditions and extent of oxidation, they may contain up to 1.0% carboxyl groups.

Digestion and Metabolism

In vitro digestibility by pancreatin or saliva of slightly and highly oxidized starch showed that they were 10–15% less digested by pancreatin than unmodified starch, but digestibility with saliva was comparable to that obtained with unmodified starch (Shuman and Mertz, 1959). Rat feeding studies with groups of three rats each in which cornstarch oxidized with 3.9, 4.5, or 5.5% available chlorine on dry starch weight (which contained 0.57, 0.8, or 0.9% carboxyls, respectively) were fed at 1-, 2-, or 4-g levels with 5 g of a basal diet (White, 1963). There was a very slight in vitro digestibility decrease with increasing levels of oxidation, but this was not reflected in the caloric values.

Rat studies involving feeding groups of six male and six females fed a series of oxidized cornstarches treated with 2.5, 6.0, or 43.2% chlorine on the starch and containing 0.32, 0.9, and 1.46% carboxyls were run over a 21-day period. The animals were given a 5 g per day basal diet for 7 days and then were given either 1 or 2 g per day supplements of the control or test starches (Whistler and Belfort, 1961). Rats fed the starches containing 0.32 or 0.9% carboxyls appeared normal. However, those fed starch with 1.46% carboxyls had poor weight gains at both dietary levels. They also had marked cecal enlargement. It should be noted that the level of oxidation in this starch was far above the maximum used in making oxidized modified food starches.

Short-Term Study

Cornstarch treated with 5.5% available chlorine (0.4% carboxyl) was fed to groups
of 15 male and 15 female weanling albino rats at dietary levels of 0.5, 10, or 25%
for 90 days. A cornstarch control was used, the test starches replacing an equal
amount of control in the diets (Til et al., 1973). No differences in hematological
indices, biochemical blood values, and urine composition could be attributed to
the starch treatment. There were no significant differences in growth and food
intake. Organ–to–body weight ratios of the heart, kidneys, liver, brain, gonad,
thymus, and thyroid of test animals and controls were similar. No differences were
noted in the histological examinations that could be attributed to treatments. The
relative weight of the cecum in females fed the test starch at 25% dietary level was
slightly higher than in the control females. Nephrocalcinosis in the corticomedullary
region was noted in 7 of 15 female controls and 10 of 15 females fed the test starch.

C. Cross-Linked Starches

These are the third major class of modified food starches, covered under
21CFR172.892(d) with limitations on the type and amount of cross-linking agent
used and residues in the starch. As noted previously, when unmodified starch is
heated in water the hydrogen bonds responsible for the integrity of the granules
weaken, the granules start to swell imbibing water, and on continued cooking the
hydrogen bonds break and the swollen granules rupture and collapse. When this
occurs the viscosity drops and the texture of the sol changes from a short salvelike
nature to an elastic unpalatable texture. The short salvelike quality of the swollen
granules is highly desirable in food systems. However, it is very tenuous and is
quickly destroyed by minor variations in cooking time, temperature, acidity, shear,
and ingredients. The objective of cross-linking is to reenforce the hydrogen bonds
in the granule with chemical bonds linking together nearby molecules within the
granule (Wurzburg, 1986). These chemical bridges are much stronger than hydrogen bonds and will help retain the integrity of the swollen granules after the
hydrogen bonds have been destroyed. Cross-links may be introduced in the granules
by reacting glucosidic hydroxyls on nearby molecules with bifunctional chemicals
capable of adding adipate or phosphate cross-links. Mixed adipic-acetic anhydride
is used to introduce adipate cross-links and phosphorous oxychloride or sodium
trimetaphosphate used to add phosphate cross-links. 21CFR172.892(d) covers these
treatments allowing the use of 0.12% max. adipic anhydride, 0.1% max. phosphorous oxychloride, or enough sodium trimetaphosphate to introduce no more
than 0.04% phosphorous. Since cross-linking reactions are run on aqueous suspensions of starch granules, it takes relatively few cross-links to have a major impact
since each granule contains millions of anhydroglucose units. Adipic-acetic mixed
anhydride is very unstable in water, so any that doesn't react with starch rapidly
hydrolyzes to the sodium salts of adipic or acetic acid. Phosphorous oxychloride is
also very unstable in water, either reacting rapidly with starch or hydrolyzing to
the salts of hydrochloric and phosphoric acids. Trimetaphosphate hydrolyzes to
pyrophosphate and then phosphate salts. All residues are water soluble and largely
removed during the subsequent washing and dewatering processes. The extent of
cross-linking varies depending upon the food system in which they will be used.
Starch cross-linked for a given application will provide greater thickening power

or viscosity and resistance to acidic conditions than unmodified starch, as shown in Figure 3. This permits them to be used at significantly lower use levels than native starch. For example, in retorted cream soups, 3.5% cross-linked starch can replace 5% unmodified starch.

(While the U.S. and European starch industries have voluntarily withdrawn the use of epichlorohydrin as a cross-linking agent to make distarch glycerol, reference will be made to studies on distarch glycerol in which the starch is bridged with ether links which are far more resistant to attack by enzymes in digestion than either adipate or phosphate cross-links. For this reason studies on it should reflect the maximum changes that might occur in the digestion and metabolism of cross-linked starch.)

In vitro digestibility by amyloglucosidase of distarch glycerol made by treating cornstarch with 0.3% epichlorohydrin was 98.3% that of unmodified cornstarch. Both starches were cooked 20 minutes in a boiling water bath before digestion (Kruger, 1970). Caloric value of distarch glycerols made by treating waxy maize starch with 0.07 or 0.5% epichlorohydrin were run using unmodified waxy cornstarch as a control. Groups of 10 male weanling rats were fed a basal diet supplemented with 3 g of each starch against feeding daily sucrose supplements of 0, 1.5, 3, 4.5, and 6 g equivalent to 0, 6, 12, 18, and 24 calories (Oser, 1961a). The caloric values of the test starches were slightly less than that of the control, but the differences were not statistically significant.

Short-term [90 day] Study

Groups of 10 male and 10 female weanling FDRL rats were fed diets comprising 71% [about 60 g/kg body weight] of unmodified waxy maize starch or waxy maize starch treated with 0.5% epichlorohydrin (Oser, 1961a). Food intake and weight gains of the test groups were similar to those of the controls. No adverse effects from feeding the test starch were noted in the hematology, blood nonprotein nitrogen levels, urinary parameters, or organ:body weight ratios of liver, kidneys, or adrenals. There were no gross pathological differences between animals fed the

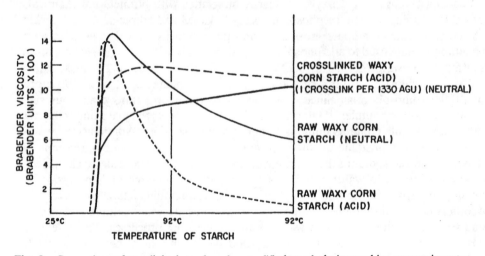

Fig. 3 Comparison of crosslinked starch and unmodified starch during cooking process in water.

test starch and those fed the control. It should be noted that the treatment level was 0.2% above the maximum set in 21CFR172.892(e).

Distarch Adipate:Digestibility and Metabolism

In vitro digestibility of modification made by treating waxy maize starch with 0.15% adipic acid as a 1:3 adipic-acetic mixed anhydride with amyloglucosidase was 98% that of the control (Kruger, 1970b). In vitro studies of the hydrolysis with pancreatin showed that the adipate unit was not hydrolyzed by the pancreatin. In vivo studies were conducted involving administering acetylated distarch adipate containing adipate tagged with ^{14}C to one group of young male rats and a physical mixture of unmodified starch with ^{14}C adipic acid to another group (Morgareidge, 1959). Within 4 hours 70% of the radioactivity administered as the free acid was recovered in the respired air compared to 12% with the tagged acetylated distarch adipate. After 25 hours 99.3% of the activity was recovered in the respired air from animals given the mixture compared to 70.5% of the activity in the acetylated distarch adipate. Activity levels recovered in urine and feces were 7.2 and 24.5%, respectively. None was found in the carcass (see also Sec. II.E).

Distarch Phosphate

Digestibility and Metabolism

In vitro digestibility of waxy maize starch cross-linked with 0, 0.035, 0.070, or 0.10% phosphorous oxychloride by amyloglucosidase ranged from 96 to 98% that of unmodified waxy maize starch (Kruger, 1970b). The starches were gelatinized in water and digested with amyloglucosidase (Diazyme L 30-Miles Chemical) for 16 hours at 50–55°C. In vitro pancreatin digestibility of potato starch cross-linked with 0.05 or 0.1% phosphorous oxychloride was the same as that of unmodified starch (Janzen, 1969). Potato starch treated with 0.5 or 1.5% phosphorous oxychloride, far above the 0.1% limit in 21CFR172.892(d), was not readily digested by pancreatin because the granules were too cross-linked to swell under normal cooking conditions (Janzen, 1969). In vitro digestibility of gelatinized milo distarch phosphate with salivary, pancreatic, or intestinal enzymes was similar to that of gelatinized unmodified milo. The starch was cross-linked with sodium trimetaphosphate (Rosner, 1960). In vitro α-amylase digestion of potato distarch phosphate for 3 hours at 95°C at 10% concentration showed the same distribution of sugars, ranging from DP 1 to DP 6, as unmodified potato starch treated similarly (Heyns et al., 1977). Caloric studies on milo distarch phosphate and unmodified milo starch were run on groups of 10 rats fed over a period of 7 days on a 4 g/day basal diet supplemented with 0.9 or 3.6 g of distarch phosphate (Hixson, 1960). There were no significant differences between the test animals and the control as regards caloric value and organ weights.

Caloric evaluation on weanling Wister-Purdue rats of distarch phosphate made by treating cornstarch with sodium trimetaphosphate showed a caloric value similar to that of unmodified starch after 21 days (Whistler and Belfort, 1961). Caloric studies in which groups of six male and six female weanling FDRL rats were fed waxy maize starches treated with 0.03 or 0.1% phosphorous oxychloride and unmodified waxy maize starch as a control at 52% dietary level for 6 weeks showed that the rats fed the test starches had caloric values comparable to those of the control (Oser, 1954). Metabolic tests on male Wistar rats over a 5-day period with pregelatinized potato distarch phosphate and pregelatinized potato starch with and without an added antibiotic to reduce the activity of hind gut microorganisms showed that the test starch was equal to the control in digestibility (Bjorck et al., 1989). The acetyl groups appeared to be removed in the upper gastrointestinal tract.

Acute Toxicity

LD_{50}s determined by feeding 50% aqueous suspensions of distarch phosphate made from waxy milo as a single dose exceeded the following (Hodge, 1956):

10 female mice: 19,000 mg/kg body weight
10 female rats: 35,000 mg/kg body weight
2 guinea pigs: 18,000 mg/kg body weight
2 rabbits: 10,000 mg/kg body weight
2 cats: 9,000 mg/kg body weight

Short-Term Studies

In a 90-day study, groups of 10 male and 10 female rats were fed distarch phosphates containing 0.085 or 0.128% phosphorous as esterified phosphate at 0, 5, 15, and 45% dietary levels (5% corresponded to about 4 g/kg body weight, 15% to about 12 g/kg body weight, and 45% to about 36 g/kg body weight) (Til et al., 1970). No abnormalities were seen in test animals' general appearance, behavior, mortality, food consumption, hematology, serum chemistry, or urinalyses. Gross and histo-pathological examinations showed no treatment-related abnormalities. Weanling male Wistar albino rats (initial body weights 45–55 g) from the University of Surrey colony were fed diets comprising 71% maize starch and 55% maize starch plus 16% unmodified waxy maize or 16% distarch phosphates made from waxy maize starch having DS levels of 0.0025, 0.006, and 0.01 for 21 days. The animals fed the test starches showed the same efficiency of food utilization as those fed the unmodified waxy starch. There was no significant evidence of cecal enlargement (Walker and El Harith, 1978).

Groups of eight 3-day-old Pitman-Moore miniature pigs were fed dietary formulas containing acid-modified waxy cornstarch or distarch phosphate made from it. The distarch phosphate contained 0.08% phosphorous in the ester form (Anderson, 1973). The starches provided 24% of the dietary calories. They were fed over a 25-day period. The organ weights as a percent of the body weight, serum cholesterol, triglycerides, calcium, phosphorous, alkaline phosphatase, urea nitrogen, total protein, albumin, and globulin levels in the pigs fed the test starch were similar to those fed the control.

Summary

The number of cross-links introduced into starch for food applications is so low that it has minimal effect on in vitro enzymatic digestion and has no apparent effect on the caloric value and acute toxicity.

D. Starches Stabilized by Monofunctional Chemicals

These are modified starches that have been reacted with monofunctional chemicals to introduce substituent groups in place of some of the hydroxyls on the starch molecules. By replacing hydroxyls with bulkier substituents such as acetate, phosphate, hydroxypropyl groups, etc., the amylose fraction and segments of the amylopectin are made more resistant to intermolecular association. In addition, some of the substituents introduce new functionality into the starch, such as increased hydrophilicity or hydrophobicity. In general the level of substitution (DS) is relatively low, running from one substituent for roughly 80 or more anhydroglucose units to a high of one for about 5 anhydroglucose units.

Acetylated Starches

These are prepared by reacting water suspensions of starch granules with acetic anhydride or vinylacetate in the presence of alkali in accordance with 21CFR172.892(d), which specifies a maximum substitution of 2.5% acetyl. After the reaction is completed, the slurry of starch is neutralized, washed, and dewatered to remove most of the byproducts. Since acetic anhydride is extremely unstable in water, any that doesn't react with starch is hydrolyzed to acetic acid and water. The vinylacetate also hydrolyzes readily.

Digestibility and Metabolism

In vitro amyloglucosidase digestion of cornstarches containing 1.50, and 2.41% acetyl was 84 and 69%, respectively, that of unmodified starch (Kruger, 1970). In vitro digestion of starch acetate with 1.98% acetyl by pancreatin and porcine nucosal enzyme was 90% that of unmodified starch (Leegwater, 1971). Starch acetate (1.98% acetyl) was fed to groups of 10 male and 10 female weanling rats in a semi-purified diet at dietary levels of 25 or 50% (about 50 or 100 g/kg body weight). After 7 days 4% cellulose was included in the basal diet to decrease diarrhea noted at the higher feeding level, but it did not help. The study was continued for 3 days for a total of 10 days (de Groot and Spanjers, 1970). Body weights were slightly reduced in both sexes fed the test starch.

Groups of 10 male Sprague-Dawley rats were fed diets containing 60% (about 50 g/kg body weight) of starches acetylated with vinylacetate to 1.24, 2.0, 2.56, or 3.25% acetyl. Weight gains were lowered compared to the control animals with those fed starches containing 2.56 or 3.25% acetyl. The ones fed starches having 2.0% or higher acetyl content developed diarrhea and enlarged ceca. However, there was no evidence of tissue damage or inflammation in these animals (Turner, 1961).

Short-Term Studies

Groups of 10 male and 10 female rats were fed acetylated potato starch having 1.36% acetyl at 15 and 45% dietary levels (about 10 and 30 g/kg body weight) for 13 weeks (Feron et al., 1967a). Growth and hematological values were not significantly different in the test animals and those fed unmodified starch. The relative weights of the liver, kidney, adrenals, and pituitary of the test animals were generally lower than those of the controls. Male rats fed the acetylated starches had enlarged and heavier ceca at both feeding levels. There were no histopathological changes attributable to the acetylated potato starch.

Twelve human volunteers were fed 60 g (about 1 g/kg body weight) of starch acetate (1.98% acetyl) on each of 4 consecutive days (Pieters, 1971). No effect was seen in the frequency of defecation or in the amount of feces, fecal water, or lactic acid content. There was no indication of any adverse effects.

Reproduction Study

A three-generation study involving feeding at 10% dietary level acetylated starch having a DS of 0.079 was run on 10 male and 10 female rats to produce successive generations by mating at weeks 12 and 20 after weaning. The F_{3b} generation was kept for 3 weeks after weaning and then sacrificed for histological study. The P, F_{1b}, and F_{2b} parents were used to determine implantation sites (de Groot et al., 1974). No adverse effects were noted in the animals fed the acetylated starch in regard to health, behavior, mortality, body weights, fertility, litter size, resorption quotient, weaning weight of pups, or mortality of young. An increase in cecal weight was noted. Gross and microscopic examination of the F_{3b} generation did not reveal any deleterious effects.

Long-Term Studies

Potato starch acetate having 1.98% acetyl and unmodified potato starch were fed to groups of 30 male and 30 female rats at 5, 10, and 30% dietary levels (about 2.5, 5, and 15 g/kg body weight) over a 2-year period (de Groot et al., 1974). The modified starch replaced an equal amount of pregelatinized potato starch. Body weight of males at the 30% diet level was significantly lower at 76 weeks but not at 104 weeks. There was no diarrhea even at the 30% level. At no time were the number of deaths in the test group significantly different than those of the controls. Hematological parameters, urine composition, and organ weights were not affected in rats fed the test starch except for the enlarged and heavier ceca in animals fed the test starch at 10 and 30% dietary levels. This did not result in any relevant microscopic changes in the tissues. Histopathology indicated that in rats fed the test starch at the highest dietary level there were slightly more frequent occurrences of suburothelial deposits of calcium accompanied by hyperplasia of the epithelium lining of the renal pelvis (subsequently called pelvic nephrocalcinosis, or PN). It was noted that there was evidence of a parasite, *Trichosomoides crassicauda*, in the males, which might be related to the incidence of PN.

In an 89-week study potato starches acetylated with vinyl acetate to 1.6–2.5% acetyl levels were fed to groups of 75 male and 75 female specific pathogen-free random-bred albino Swiss strain mice along with pregelatinized potato starch as a control. The dietary level was 55% (about 80 g/kg body weight). As reference, other groups were fed 55% lactose or 25% sodium alginate (Feron et al., 1978). Average body weight of mice fed starch acetate did not differ significantly from those fed the control except for a significant decrease in body weight of the males at weeks 16, 20, 40, and 72 and for the females at week 84. There was no evidence of any more loose stools in mice fed the acetylated starch than in those fed the control starch. Mortality was normal for mice fed the test starch. Death rate of the control mice was abnormally high between 39 and 65 weeks. Fifty percent of the control mice who died had hemorrhagic mycocarditis. Hematology, fasting glucose, and blood urea nitrogen were within normal limits for mice receiving the test starch. There was more amorphous material in the urine of males fed the test starch than in the controls. Analyses of the urine sediment showed about 95% protein with small amounts of phosphates, carbohydrates, and possibly silica. Sodium, calcium, magnesium, and potassium were identified. Organ–to–body weight ratios in mice fed the acetylated starch were not significantly different from the controls except for the cecum and colon of both sexes, which were higher than for controls. There was also a slight but significant increase in this ratio for the kidneys of females. The overall incidence of very slight to slight calcareous deposits in the renal pelvis of the males (9/74) was greater than in the controls (0/73). However, the findings could not be tested for statistical significance because of the early deaths in the control males. In mice that survived for at least 79 weeks, the frequencies were 7 of 49 against 0 of 28, respectively. Incidence of intratubular calcareous deposits was greater in males fed the test starch who survived at 74 weeks (25/49) compared to the control males (5/28). Incidence in the females receiving the test starch was 13 of 56 against 11 of 58 for the control females. There was no evidence of hyperplasia of the epithelium. It was concluded that the urinary and renal changes, which were similar to those in mice fed lactose, had little if any toxicological significance. Overall this study indicated that PN is not prevalent in mice and is apparently unique in rats.

Hydroxypropylated Starch

This modification is made by reacting a water suspension of starch at high pH with propylene oxide to introduce hydroxypropyl groups on the starch. Since strongly alkaline conditions are required for the reaction, care must be exercised to avoid swelling the starch either through the use of salt such as sodium sulfate to repress starch swelling or the use of lime as a catalyst in place of a highly soluble alkali such as sodium hydroxide. Care must be exercised to minimize chloride ions since these can react with propylene oxide to form propylene chlorohydrins, which are potentially mutagenic and must be largely removed. This type of modified starch is covered under 21CFR172.892(e), which allows the use of 25% propylene oxide. However, the Joint Experts Committee on Food Additives of the FAO/WHO only allows the use of 10% maximum propylene oxide. A limit of 1 mg/kg max. propylene chlorohydrin residuals has also been set as well as 7.0% max. hydroxypropyl groups on the starch, which is approximately 0.2 DS (FAO, 1990).

Digestibility and Metabolism

In vitro digestion of hydroxypropyl potato starches ranging from DS 0.020 to 0.45 with pancreatin ran 89 to 3.8% that of unmodified starch (Leegwater and Luten, 1971). In vitro digestion of hydroxypropyl wheat starch (DS 0.06) by porcine α-amylase was 76.6% that of unmodified wheat starch (Wootton and Chaudhry, 1979).

The hydrolysates obtained by the partial digestion of starch ranging from DS 0 to 0.17 were separated into oligosaccharides and polysaccharides. With increasing DS of the modified starch there was an increase in the degree of polymerization of the oligosaccharides in the hydrolysates (Wootton and Chaudhry, 1981). The oligosaccharide fractions contained most of the modifying groups in the total digest.

Hydroxypropyl cornstarch (DS 0.12) prepared by reacting cornstarch with propyleneoxide tagged with ^{14}C carbon in the 2 position was administered by stomach tube to a rat (Leegwater, 1971b). During the ensuing 50 hours 92% of the radioactivity was excreted in the feces and 3.6% in the urine. To further clarify the metabolic fate of the tagged starch, Leegwater repeated these experiments with unlabeled hydroxypropyl starches and mixtures of these with unmodified starch to provide samples having DS values of 0.025, 0.047, and 0.106.

Ten male rats (2 months old, weighing 180–230 g) of inbred Wistar strain were fed on diets of 56% pregelatinized unmodified potato starch or the samples having the above-noted DS values (Leegwater and Speek, 1972). The rats received each of the diets for 3–5 days. The feces were collected quantitatively and stored under refrigeration until analyzed. The digestibility of the starches decreased with increasing substitution. The major components in the fecal carbohydrates were tentatively identified as hydroxypropyl maltose, dihydroxypropyl maltose, and dihydroxypropyl maltotetrose. The major metabolite isolated from the feces of the rats fed hydroxypropylated starch with DSs up to 0.106 were subsequently identified as 4-O-{2-O-[<RS>-2-hydroxypropyl]-α-D-glucopyranosyl}-D gluco-pyranose. In addition, O-[hydroxypropyl]-D-glucosyl-D glucose was also present (Leegwater and Ten Noever de Brauw, 1972; Leegwater and Marsman, 1973).

Short-Term Study

Groups of 10 male and 10 female rats were fed diets containing 5, 15, or 45% (about 4, 12, or 35 g/kg body weight) hydroxypropylated acid-modified potato starch (DS 0.042) and acid-modified potato starch as a control for 90 days. Weight gains of males fed the test starch at the 15 and 45% dietary levels were less but not significantly less than those fed a control diet. Diarrhea occurred in the 45% diet level group but the intensity diminished in the later stages of the feeding. Male rats fed the two higher dietary levels of the hydroxypropylated starch had enlarged ceca, but only the females fed the highest level had enlarged ceca. There was no evidence of inflammation or histological abnormalities in the enlarged ceca. Hematological values were comparable in the test animals and the controls. No pathological changes were noted on microscopic examination of the major organs (Feron et al., 1967b).

Sensitivity Tests

Mild irritation was noted in eyes of rabbits when hydroxypropyl starches (DS 0.1 and 0.41) was applied in powder form or as an aqueous solution of the DS 0.1 product (Pallota, 1959). Patch tests on 210 human volunteers with moistened patches of hydroxypropyl wheat starch (DS 0.1) in which the patch was in contact with the skin for 72 hours followed by a challenge exposure 2 weeks later showed that there was no more irritation from the hydroxypropyl starch than from unmodified wheat starch. In another test 23 humans were subjected to the Repeat Insult Patch Test involving 24-hour exposure at intervals of 2–3 days with hydroxypropyl starch (DS 0.1). There was no evidence of irritation, and a challenge exposure 1 week after the last exposure gave no evidence of sensitization (Majors and Rubenkoenig, 1959; Rubenkoenig, 1959).

Long-Term Feeding Studies

See Section II.E on hydroxypropyl distarch phosphate.

Starch Phosphate Monoester

The monostarch phosphate esters are prepared by reacting dry starch with sodium orthophosphate or sodium tripolyphosphate in the presence of heat (Solarek, 1986). A typical approach is to impregnate a slurry of starch with salts, dewatering the starch and heating the recovered impregnated starch to form the monophosphate starch. These products are regulated under 21CFR172.892(d), which specifies a maximum substitution of 0.4% phosphorus calculated as phosphorus. The added phosphate moiety not only stabilizes the starch, but also increases its hydrophilicity and viscosity.

Monostarch phosphates contain phosphoric ester linkages attached primarily to the 6-carbon of an anhydroglucose unit. In addition, some substitution may take place at the 2- and 3-carbons. Native potato starch also contains phosphate ester groups at a level as high as 0.1% phosphorus. Gramera et al. (1966) found that the phosphate is present in the dibasic form.

Digestion and Metabolism

Wheat monostarch phosphate is hydrolyzed by α-amylase at a faster rate than unmodified wheat starch (International Minerals, 1955). Starch phosphate labeled with ^{32}P disodium phosphate, and sodium pyrophosphate were administered by gavage to female Sprague-Dawley rats. The amount of ^{32}P recovered in the liver, kidneys, blood plasma, and bone as well as the amount excreted in the feces and urine were similar to those for animals receiving disodium phosphate. It was concluded that phosphorus in the form of starch phosphate is metabolized in a manner similar to that of inorganic phosphate.

Short-Term Study

Groups of 6 and 20 weanling Sprague-Dawley rats were fed starch phosphate for 4 weeks at 1, 5, and 10% dietary levels (about 1, 5, and 10 g/kg body weight) on a semi-purified diet (International Minerals, 1955). The growth and feed efficiency of animals fed the starch phosphate was similar to those fed the unmodified starch. The weights of the testes, liver, thymus, adrenal, spleen, and kidney were not affected by the test starch in the 6-animal group. Autopsies in all animals in all rat groups revealed no abnormalities.

Long-Term Study

See Section II.E on acetylated distarch phosphate.

Starch Sodium Octenylsuccinate

This type of modification is prepared by reacting suspensions of starch granules in water with octenyl succinic anhydride under mildly alkaline conditions (Caldwell and Wurzburg, 1953). The sodium salt of the starch half-ester of octenylsuccinate is formed. It is covered under 21CFR172.892(d), which places a maximum of 3.0% on the treatment level. This results in a product having a DS of about 0.02. The unreacted octenyl succinic anhydride hydrolyzes to the sodium salt of the acid, which is partially removed by washing. The resulting modified starch has the ability to stabilize oil in water emulsions. These are largely used at low levels to stabilize food emulsions, for the encapsulation of flavors and clouding agents, and in beverage emulsions.

Digestibility and Metabolism

In vitro digestibility studies with pancreatic amylase from pigs, human salivary amylase, β-amylase from barley, and glucoamylase from *Aspergillus niger* were run on starch sodium octenylsuccinate made from waxy maize starch and acid-modified waxy maize starch as well as dextrinized starch octenylsuccinate (Kruger et al., 1980). The results are summarized below:

Enzyme type	% Digestion		
	Starch sodium octenylsuccinate	Acid-modified	Dextrinized
Pancreatic	82.9	91.3	135
Salivary	87.3	98.6	147
β-Amylase	91.6	86.5	115
Glucoamylase	88.3	87.5	113

Groups of 10 weanling male albino rats were fed 2.74 g of a basal diet and 1.5 or 3.0 g (about 20 or 40 g/kg body weight) unmodified cornstarch or starch sodium octenylsuccinate made from cornstarch daily for 4 weeks (Carson, 1960a). Growth rates of the test starch and control did not differ significantly, and caloric values were not lowered in animals fed the test starch. All animals were normally active and appeared in good health throughout the experiment.

90-Day Subchronic In Utero Feeding Study

One hundred and forty female (110 g) and 50 male (135 g) Fisher rats from the Charles River Breeding Labs (56 days old) were fed laboratory chow for 5 days, then randomly divided into four dietary groups. One group was fed acid-modified waxy cornstarch as the control. The second was fed 6% starch sodium octenylsuccinate (SSOS), the next 12% SSOS, and the last 30% SSOS until the animals were of breeding age. The first group was fed 30% of the control starch, the second 6% SSOS and 24% control, the third 12% SSOS and 18% control, and the last 30% SSOS and no control. The first litters were discarded and the females rebred. At weaning, two male and two female rats were randomly selected from each litter and assigned to the same dietary groups as their parents (Buttolph and Newberne, 1980). A total of 440 weanling rats participated in a 90-day feeding study. Diets were fed ad libitum. There was no difference in growth between rats on the test diets and those fed the control diet. Interim sacrifices were performed after 30 days on 10 rats of each sex from the control group and the group fed 30% SSOS. Complete autopsies and histopathological evaluation showed that growth and hematology were unaffected but that the liver, kidney, and cecal weights tended to increase with increasing SSOS intake. Female rats had higher levels of urinary magnesium and calcium than did the male rats. The higher concentrations correlated with an increased incidence of renal cortico-medullary mineralization. These changes occurred in females on the control as well as on the test diets. There was no evidence of pelvic nephrocalcinosis. It was concluded that no adverse effects were associated with feeding SSOS under the conditions of this study.

90-Day Feeding Study in Rats

Three test diets containing variations in the mineral composition of the diets were used in combination with 30% SSOS or unmodified starch as a control to assess the effect of purified diets containing SSOS on nephrocalcinosis and hepatic lipidoses. The variations in the mineral composition were:

1. Colworth House developed "in-house diet" containing 10% fat; 25% protein; and a magnesium content of 0.05%.

2. The American Institute of Nutrition (AIN-76) diet containing 5% fat and 20% protein but modified by the Environmental Safety Laboratory (Unilever Research Center) using maize starch to replace cariogenic sucrose and raising the magnesium content from 0.04% to 0.2%.
3. Same as AIN-76 but supplemented with a trace element mixture present in commercial rodent diets but not present in the refined materials used to formulate the purified diet.

Each test and control diet was fed to 10 male and 10 female Colworth-Wistar rats for 90 days. Observations made during the study included daily checks for clinical signs of ill health, weekly body weight measurements, twice-weekly measures of food intake, and analysis of 24-hour urine samples from each rat during the 12th week. At terminal sacrifice the plasma chemistry was thoroughly studied and organ weights of the liver, kidney, and empty cecum checked as percent of body weight. Liver composition was analyzed for fat, protein, and moisture (Parish et al., 1984). Overall, the rats fed diets containing SSOS gained slightly less than those fed the control starch. Food utilization tended to be slightly poorer. However, the differences were not statistically significant except for the male rats fed the "in-house purified diet." No differences of biological significance in plasma chemistry were observed between animals fed the test starch and those fed the control starch. Any differences noted were reflected in the mineral compositions. Plasma magnesium levels were elevated in rats fed AIN-76 type diets, plasma urea levels were down in males fed AIN-76 type diets, and plasma triglycerides were higher in rats fed this diet. There also appeared to be a trend toward higher plasma levels of inorganic phosphate and total protein in rats fed AIN-76 type diets compared to those fed the ESL "in-house" purified diet. The differences were not all statistically significant. The urine chemistry results were similar regardless of the type of starch. There were differences in the types of dietary minerals. Urine magnesium was greatest in rats fed the AIN-76 type diet, reflecting its high magnesium content. The 24-hour urine volumes, as well as total urea, inorganic phosphate, and creatinine excreted, were less in rats whose diets contained the trace mineral supplement. The observation of Buttolph and Newberne (1980) concerning heavier livers and kidneys in rats fed 12 and 30% SSOS was not confirmed. There was no difference in liver, kidney, and cecal weights between those rats fed SSOS and those fed the control. However, differences in the basic diet types had an influence. There was a trend toward heavier livers and lighter kidneys, especially relative to body weight, in rats fed on AIN-76 type diets compared to those fed the ESL "in-house" purified diet. Heavier kidneys in females fed this diet were noted. It would appear that they reflect the incidence of cortico-medullary nephrocalcinosis found in rats fed this diet.

Mutagenicity Studies

SSOS did not cause any dose-related reversion to occur in any of the five tester strains of *Salmonella typhimurium* up to a limit of solubility (5 mg/plate). It did not increase the sister chromatid exchange frequency in cultured Chinese hamster V 79 cells at concentrations up to 50 mg/ml tissue culture fluid (Parish et al., 1984).

Long-Term Chronic Toxicity and Carcinogenicity Study

SSOS prepared by treatment of acid-modified waxy maize starch with 3.0% octenylsuccinic anhydride was fed along with acid-modified waxy maize as a control
to four groups of 52 male and 52 female rats for 120–122 weeks (males) and 116–
119 weeks (females) by incorporating in the diet 0, 5, 12.5, and 30% SSOS. Acid-
modified waxy maize starch was used as the control and supplement in the test
diets to maintain the total carbohydrate level constant (Parish et al., 1987).

Clinical Signs.   No clinical feature was noted in rats of either sex that could
be related to the treatment.

Survival.   Survival up to 2 years was good in both sexes, but death rate after
that increased, especially in males, and resulted in early terminal sacrifices. SSOS
did not have an adverse effect on the mortality rate.

Body Weight and Weight Gain.   No treatment-related differences in body
weights were seen in males fed SSOS. Those fed 5% SSOS had slightly higher
mean body weight at the end of the study, but it was not statistically significant.
The body weights of female rats fed 5 and 12.5% SSOS were significantly greater
than controls at week 114. Body weight gain was significantly greater than the
controls in females fed 5% SSOS in weeks 54–78 and for overall body weight gain
(weeks 0–114) in the groups fed 5 and 12.5% SSOS.

Food Efficiency.   During the period when food intake and body weight were
measured on a weekly basis, there were no treatment-related differences.

Urine Biochemistry.   Calcium and magnesium levels in the urine rose in a
dose-related manner in male rats fed SSOS, but the rise was not statistically significant except in the 30% group. In female rats urinary magnesium and urea were
significantly higher in those fed SSOS at the 30% level than in the controls, but a
dose-response relationship was not seen at the lower feeding levels. Urinary calcium
and phosphate levels were higher in the test females than in the controls in a dose-
related, but not statistically significant, manner.

Ophthalmoscopy.   No treatment-related effects were observed.

Serum Electphoresis.   Total protein in the serum was significantly increased
in males fed 30% SSOS. α-1-Globulin was significantly higher in males fed 12.5
and 30% SSOS, however, the increases were small and within the normal range.
Female rats fed 5% SSOS showed reduced serum albumin, raised α-1-globulin,
and a reduced albumin:globulin ratio.

Plasma Biochemistry.   Total cholesterol, log lactate dehydrogenase, and pseu-
docholinesterase were significantly raised relative to control values in male rats fed
30% SSOS. However, the increases were small and within the normal range.

Hematology.   There were no treatment-related significant differences for red
cell count and red cell indices in male or female rats. The white cell count in male
rats was significantly higher in the group fed 5% SSOS, but this was caused by one
animal who had a very high count. When the result from this one animal was
removed there was no statistically significant differences for the white cell count.
There was no statistically significant treatment-related differences in female rats
fed the test starches or those fed the control.

Organ Weights.   Variations were observed, but they appeared to be chance
observations not specifically related to treatment.

Pathology.   There were no variations in tissue morphology specifically related
to dietary groups. Severe dental disease was noted, but the incidence was greater
in the control group than in the subjects fed SSOS.

Histology. A low level of nephrocalcinosis was seen in the control rats. It was no higher in rats fed 30% SSOS. Neither the incidence nor the severity of any of the histological observations was considered to be modified by the inclusion of 30% SSOS in the diet. The tumor types identified in this study were similar to those seen in previous long-term studies with the Colworth-Wistar rat in this laboratory and elsewhere. The control group had a higher incidence of fatal tumors. When fatal and incidental tumors were combined, there were no significant differences between the control and treatment groups.

Conclusion

Under the conditions of this study there was no evidence for either carcinogenicity or chronic toxicity of SSOS when fed to male or female rats at levels of up to 30% in their diet for a period in excess of 2 years. This is equivalent to an approximate intake of 17 g SSOS/kg body weight/day for male rats and 21 g SSOS/kg body weight/day for female rats.

Starch Aluminum Octenylsuccinate

This modification is prepared by treating SSOS that has been made by treatment with only 2% octenylsuccinic acid anhydride and aluminum sulfate (2% max.) to form an aluminum salt of starch octenylsuccinate. It is covered under 21CFR172.892(d), which specifies 2% maximum treatment for the anhydride and 2% maximum for aluminum sulfate. The powdered product is a free-flowing water-repellent powder used as a dusting agent and processing aid in the pharmaceutical industry. It has not been cleared as a modified food starch with the JECFA of the FAO/WHO.

Digestion and Metabolism

Groups of 10 weanling male albino rats were fed for 4 weeks on a 2.74-g basal diet supplemented with 1.5 or 3.0 g (about 20 or 40 g/kg body weight) daily of either acid-modified starch or its aluminum octenylsuccinate derivative. The caloric value of the starch aluminum octenylsuccinate was comparable to that of the control. Growth was continuous, and there were no deaths during the study. All the rats were normally active throughout the 4-week period (Carson, 1961).

Short-Term Study

Groups of 6 male and 6 female weanling albino rats were fed over 8 weeks on a basal diet containing 35% corn starch or diets in which 1, 10, or 25% (about 1, 10, or 25 g/kg body weight) starch aluminum octenylsuccinate replaced an equal amount of cornstarch (Oser, 1950). There was no evidence of any adverse effects associated with the test starch at any level on the growth, food consumption, efficiency of food utilization, blood cell count, hemoglobin, sugar, or nonprotein nitrogen.

Starch Sodium Succinate

This type is prepared by reacting starch in water suspension with succinic anhydride under mildly alkaline conditions. It is covered under 21CFR172.892(d), which sets a treatment level maximum of 4% succinic anhydride. The resulting product is characterized by high viscosities and stable sols. It has not been cleared with the FAO/WHO.

Digestibility and Metabolism

Groups of 10 weanling male albino rats were fed over a 4-week period a basal diet
to which 1.5 or 3.0 g/day (about 20 or 40 g/kg body weight) of cornstarch sodium
succinate or cornstarch were added. Sucrose was also fed at levels of 0, 0.75, 1.5,
3.0, and 4.5 g/day to provide a baseline for determining the caloric values (Carson,
1960b). The results were 378 calories/100 g for starch sodium succinate and 382
calories/100 g for unmodified cornstarch.

Short-Term Study

Weanling albino rats in groups of 3 males and 3 females were each fed ad libitum
for 10 weeks on diets containing 70% (about 60 g/kg body weight) starch sodium
succinate or unmodified cornstarch (Oser, 1945). There were no significant differences in average weight gains and feed efficiencies between the test starch and
unmodified starch. It should be noted that this starch was not cleared with JECFA
of the FAO/WHO.

E. Stabilized Cross-Linked Starches

This last group covers those modifications that are cross-linked as well as stabilized
with substituent groups such as acetyl, hydroxypropyl, or phosphoryl. They represent a very important segment of modified food starches, combining the strength-
ening of the swollen granule with the stabilizing action and/or functionality of the
substituent groups. These types of modified starches are widely used in the food
industry as stabilizers and thickeners for retorted foods, frozen foods, bakery fillings, and numerous other foods such as instant puddings and convenience foods.

Acetylated Distarch Adipate

This category comprises modifications made by reacting starch with adipic-acetic
mixed anhydride with or without additional reaction with acetic anhydride. This
type is covered under 21CFR172.892(d), with treatment limitations of 0.12% adipic
anhydride and a maximum of 2.5% acetyl substitution.

Digestion and Metabolism

In vitro digestibility (see Sec. II.C) is high (98% with amyloglucosidase). As the acetyl
level rises, the in vitro digestibility decreases (Kruger, 1970a; Leegwater, 1971a).

Caloric value of acetylated distarch adipate prepared by treating acid-modified
waxy maize starch with 0.2% adipic acid in adipic-acetic mixed anhydride and a
total of 5.5% acetic anhydride was determined in a 26-day feeding study (Oser,
1961b). Acid-modified waxy maize starch was used as the control. Groups of 10
weanling male albino rats were fed 2.74 g of a basal diet to which 1.5 or 3.0 g/day
of test starch or control were added. Various levels of sugar were fed separately
to establish a base curve for calculating the caloric value. The caloric value of the
modified starch was equal to that of the control.

Short-Term Study

Acetylated distarch adipate made by treating acid modified waxy maize starch with
a mixed anhydride of 0.12% adipic acid and a total of 10.5% acetic anhydride and
acid modified waxy maize starch as control were fed to groups of 15 male and 15
female FDRL rats at a dietary level of 50% (about 40 g/kg body weight) for 90
days (Oser, 1964). Weight gain of males in the test group was moderately but

significantly lower (15%) than for males in the control group. Food intake and food efficiency were also lower. Cecal weights both full and empty were significantly greater for both sexes than in the controls. No differences were observed between groups in regard to hematology, blood chemistry, urinalysis, liver, or kidney weights. No differences were seen in gross and histopathological evaluations. No renal pelvic nephrocalcinosis was reported, but corticomedullary nephrocalcinosis was present in both the test and control animals. It was randomly distributed. It should be noted that the extent of acetylation of the starch was roughly one-third greater than the level covered by regulation.

Long-Term Study

Groups of 30 male and 30 female Sprague-Dawley rats were fed over a 2-year period diets containing 62% (about 30 g/kg body weight) of acetylated distarch adipate (2.5% acetyl) or unmodified starch. The rats were bred under specified pathogen-free conditions and aged 4–5 weeks at the start of the study (Truhaut et al., 1979). Ten additional rats of each sex were added to the study, but they were necropsied at 90 days. Weight gains for the control and test groups were similar for the first 90 days, but by the sixth month the animals fed the test starch tended to show less weight gain (about 3% less for the males and 12.5% for the females). At the end of the study the mean body weight of the males was 12.7% below the control, and the adjusted mean for the females was 17.4% below the controls. However, femur measurements indicated no accompanying difference in skeletal growth, and at autopsy control rats contained markedly greater adipose deposits than found in the rats fed the test starch. These findings limit the significance of the body weight differences. Hematology, serum biochemical analyses, bacteriological examinations, and organ-weight checks showed no significant differences of pathological interest between control and animals fed the test starch. Over the 2-year period the mortality of the animals fed the control was slightly higher than that of the animals fed the acetylated distarch adipate. Histological examination of the main organs showed no significant differences between rats fed the test starch and those fed the control. All the lesions and tumors were distributed randomly. Hyperplasia of the kidney urothelium sometimes accompanied by calcification was observed in all groups and was not considered to be related to the administration of the modified starch. However, in an appendix further examination indicated that for the females there was a statistically significant greater incidence of hyperplasia in those fed the modified starch than the control.

Multigeneration Study

The above study was multigenerational (three generations over about 2 years). The parent animals, F_0, were 10 males and 10 females from each group participating in the oral study. After two matings the parents were returned to the oral study. The first generation was sacrificed and autopsied, and the second generation was killed except for 10 male and 10 female rats taken at random from each group. These were mated twice to produce the F_{2a} and F_{2b} generations and were then killed and autopsied. The procedure followed with the F_2 generation was the same as that for the first-generation groups. The resulting F_{3a} and F_{3b} generations were killed and autopsied at weaning and 6 weeks after weaning, respectively. The F_{3b} generation was also examined histopathologically (Truhaut et al., 1979). The study showed no effects on fertility, litter size, or embryonic or preweaning mortality.

Histological examination of the F_{3b} generation showed no treatment-related abnormalities.

Acetylated Distarch Phosphate

This is made by a combination of cross-linking with phosphorus oxychloride and acetylating with acetic anhydride or vinylacetate. It is covered under 21CFR172.892(d) with limits of 0.1% max. phosphorus oxychloride and 8% acetic anhydride or 7.5% max. vinyl acetate with a 2.5% max. acetyl content on the final product.

Digestibility

In vitro digestibility of acetylated distarch phosphates prepared from potato starch containing 1.6 and 2.3% acetyl was 93 and 69%, respectively (Leegwater, 1971a).

Short-Term Study

Groups of 10 male and 10 female weanling Wistar rats were fed over 8 weeks 25 or 50% acetylated distarch phosphate (about 30 or 60 g/kg body weight) made by cross-linking potato starch with 0.02% phosphorus oxychloride and acetylating with 8% acetic anhydride to 2.3% acetyl substitution (de Groot and Spanjers, 1970). Weight gains were similar to the control animals fed pregelatinized potato starch. Slight diarrhea was noted during the fifth week in males receiving the test starch at 50% dietary level. At termination the cecal weights of both male and female rats were greater than those of the control rats. Microscopic examination indicated that there was no difference in the ceca of the test animals and those of the controls. In another experiment, in which the same dietary levels were used in a semipurified diet over 10 days, moderate diarrhea occurred at the 50% level. On the seventh day 4% cellulose was added, but it failed to reduce the diarrhea.

Groups of four male and four female pigs were fed diets containing 0, 35, or 70% acetylated distarch phosphate for 14.5 weeks (Shillam, 1971). Growth rate and food consumption in animals fed the test starch were comparable to those in animals fed the control starch. Three animals in the higher dietary group died of unknown causes. One pig in each of the test groups showed evidence of neurological malfunction. One in the lower group recovered, but one in the 70% group died. Hematology, blood chemistry, urinalysis, organ weights, and gross and histopathology of the pigs showed no treatment-related abnormalities. There was no evidence of nervous system abnormality in any of the animals.

In a subsequent study, groups of eight pigs were fed 0, 5, 15, or 25% acetylated distarch phosphate for 14 weeks (Shillam, 1973). No effect of the test starch was noted on the growth, food consumption, hematology, or biochemistry. One pig died of an unknown cause. No significant abnormalities postmortem were found.

Long-Term Study

Acetylated potato distarch phosphate made by treating starch with 0.02% phosphorus oxychloride and acetylating with 8% acetic anhydride (2.33% acetyl) was included in a long-term feeding and multigeneration rat studies run on five chemically modified starches by de Groot et al. (1974). These included, in addition to the acetylated distarch phosphate, the following: acetylated diamylopectin phosphate (treatment of amylopectin with 1.2% phosphorus oxychloride to introduce 0.043% phosphorus and 4.5% vinyl acetate to add 1.6% acetyl), starch acetate (1.98% acetyl content), hydroxypropyl distarch glycerol (made with 0.1% epichlorohydrin and 5% propylene oxide), and phosphated distarch phosphate (made by treating white milo maize starch with sodium trimetaphosphate to introduce up to 0.04% phosphorus and sodium tripolyphosphate to give a total of 0.35% bound phosphorus). In the 2-year study no adverse effects were observed on mortality, food intake, hematology, blood biochemistry, or urine composition. With the exception of phosphated distarch phosphate, each caused a slight reduction of body weight at the 30% dietary level. Cecal enlargement occurred at the 10 and 30% levels, but the microscopic structure of the cecum was normal. All males fed the modified starches at the 30% feeding level showed a slightly increased incidence of focal hyperplasia of the renal papillary and pelvic epithelium along with calcified patches in underlying tissue (subsequently labeled as PN or pelvic nephrocalcinosis).

Multigeneration Study

There was no effect of any of the starches on fertility, lactation performance, or embryonic or preweaning mortality. Microscopic examination of the F_{3b} rats failed to indicate any changes attributable to modified starch treatments (de Groot et al., 1974).

Hydroxypropyl Distarch Phosphate

This modification, made by cross-linking hydroxypropyl starch with phosphorus oxychloride, is covered under 21CFR172.892(f), which sets maximum treatment levels of 10% propylene oxide and 0.1% phosphorus oxychloride. In addition, a limit of 1 part per million (1 mg/kg) propylene chlorohydrin residue has been set by the U.S. and European starch industries. The EEC Scientific Committee on Food Additives is pushing to lower this to 0.1 mg/kg.

Digestion and Metabolism

In vitro digestion of hydroxypropyl distarch phosphate, prepared from tapioca having a molar substitution of 0.045 hydroxypropyl groups and cross-linked with phosphorus oxychloride, by hog pancreatic α-amylase or by fungal amylase, ran about 80% that of gelatinized tapioca starch (Hood and Arneson, 1976).

Hydroxypropyl distarch phosphate prepared by treating tapioca starch with 8% propylene oxide and 0.1% phosphorus oxychloride was fed to five weanling male Sprague-Dawley rats at 1- or 3-g levels in a 5 g/day basal diet (Prier, 1961). The caloric value as measured by 7-day weight gains was equal to that of unmodified starch.

Groups of 10 weanling male albino rats were fed for 10 days, 5 g/day, of a basal diet to which 1, 2, or 4 g (about 20, 40, or 80 g/kg body weight) of maize starch treated with 0.0123% phosphorus oxychloride and 3, 6, or 8% propylene oxide (DS.0.085, 0.173 and 0.23, respectively) were added (Porter, 1971). Calorie values relative to the control decreased slightly with increasing DS. The value for DS 0.23 starch was 93% that of unmodified starch. Diarrhea occurred when this starch was fed at the two higher dietary levels and when the lower DS starches were consumed at the highest dietary level.

Short-Term Studies

Groups of 15 male and 15 female weanling FDRL Wistar rats were fed over a 90-day period diets containing 5, 10, or 25% (about 4, 8, and 20 g/kg body weight) hydroxypropyl distarch phosphate, replacing an equal amount of unmodified starch in the diet. The test starch was made by reacting maize starch with 10% propylene oxide and 0.1% phosphorus oxychloride (Bailey et al., 1973). There was a slight decrease in feed efficiency in males fed the treated starch at 25% level. Otherwise there were no deviations from control values in regard to growth, body weight gains, food intake, or feed efficiency. No treatment-related response was noted in any organ weight except the cecum, which showed a marked enlargement when full. However, only the males on the 25% diet had empty ceca significantly heavier than those of the controls. Hematological, biochemical values and urinalyses were similar to those in the control animals. The only pathological finding of any significance was calcareous deposits in the renal pelvis and/or epithelium in rats fed the modified starch. Focal renal tubular calcification was noted in both the test animals as well as the controls.

Another 90-day study on groups of 15 male and 15 female weanling Wistar rats involved feeding pregelatinized maize hydroxypropyl distarch phosphate (treated with 0.1% phosphorus oxychloride and 5% propylene oxide—DS 0.07) at 0, 5, 10, or 25% dietary levels (about 0, 4.8, and 20 g/kg body weight) (Til et al., 1974). Growth, food intake, efficiency of food utilization, hematology, blood chemistry, and urinalysis of test animals were similar to those of the controls. Diarrhea did not occur, but the water content of the feces from the test animals at the 10 and 25% levels was slightly greater than that from the controls. Organ:body weight ratios of the adrenals and testicles of males in the 25% test group were slightly decreased compared to the controls ($p = 0.05$). The relative cecum weight both full and empty was higher in test animals at the 25% dietary level. Very slight to slight calcareous deposits were identified in the intercortico-medullary area of the kidneys in 11 of 15 test females at the highest dietary level compared with 0 of 15 test males and 2 of 15 female controls. These were not considered to be of toxicological significance in female Wistar rats.

Long-Term Study

An 89-week·study on hydroxypropylated potato starch cross-linked with 0.1% phosphorus oxychloride and having a hydroxypropyl DS of 0.075 (4.3 mg/kg propylene chlorohydrin) was run on groups of 75 male and 75 female weanling SPF mice (Swiss random strain) fed at 55% dietary level (about 80 g/kg body weight). Other test materials included were acetylated starch at 55%, lactose at 55%, and alginate at 25%. During week 80, 10 mice of each sex and group were sacrificed, necropsied, and the tissues examined microscopically. A similar examination was made on all survivors at termination (Feron et al., 1978). Death rate in the group fed modified starch was normal for this strain of mice. However, it was abnormally high for males in the control group between weeks 39 and 65. About 50% of the controls that died had hemorrhagic myocarditis. About 12% of the males and 5% of the females fed hydroxypropyl distarch phosphate had loose stools compared to about 4% of males and 3% of females receiving the control diet. The body weights of males fed the hydroxypropyl distarch phosphate were significantly reduced from weeks 16–48 and of females from week 40 to the end as compared to the controls. Hematological indices and levels of fasting blood glucose and urea nitrogen were within normal ranges. The males, but not females, had more amorphous material in the urine than did the controls. There was a greater incidence of very slight calcareous material and thickened submucosa and epithelium in the urinary bladder of males receiving this modified starch. There was no evidence for hyperplasia in the urinary bladder or treatment-related neoplastic changes.

Effect on Iron Retention

Hydroxypropylated distarch phosphate made from tapioca starch (DS 0.045) along with unmodified tapioca starch were fed in semipurified diets at a 35% dietary level (about 50 g/kg body weight) to groups of 6–11 weanling Holtzman rats for 25–28 days. The starches were added to the diets in cooked and uncooked forms. On days 16–19, iron retention was measured by whole-body counter assay after administering ^{59}Fe-tagged ferric chloride in varying amounts (Hood et al., 1976). Weight gains, hemoglobin levels, and ^{59}Fe retention in rats fed iron-adequate diets were not affected by the modification. Cooking the starch tended to reduce the iron retention. Rats fed low-iron diets showed no difference in hemoglobin level that could be attributed to the type of starch that was fed. When uncooked starch was used, the iron retention was unaffected by the type of starch fed. When cooked starches were used, iron retention was 36% of the dose for the modified starch compared to 74% for cooked unmodified starch.

Phosphated Distarch Phosphate

This modification made by treatment of starch with the sodium salts of trimetaphosphate and tripolyphosphate is covered under 21CFR172.892(d) with a max. limit of 0.4% phosphorus.

Digestibility and Metabolism

In vitro digestibility of phosphated distarch phosphate made from potato starch by pancreatin and porcine intestinal amylase was lower than that of unmodified starch (Leegwater, 1971a). In vitro digestibility by pancreatin of phosphated distarch phosphate made from maize starch was about 80% that of unmodified maize starch (Kohn and Kay, 1963a). In vivo digestibility and utilization of phosphated distarch phosphate made from milo starch as measured by weight gain of weanling rats fed a basal diet supplemented with 1, 2, or 4 g/day of modified or unmodified starch for 10 days was similar to that of unmodified starch (Kohn and Kay, 1963b).

Short-Term Studies

Groups of 10 male and 10 female weanling rats were fed a diet containing initially 10% (about 30 g/kg body weight) of phosphated distarch phosphate but increasing to 35% (about 70 g/kg) on the 13th day (Kohn et al., 1964a). On the 60th day urine and blood samples were taken and the animals sacrificed and necropsied. The average weight gain of female test animals was slightly but significantly lower ($p = 0.05$) than for the controls. No treatment-related effects were noted in the urine or the hematological parameters. Kidney: and liver:body weight ratios were significantly lower for males in the test group. These were believed to be coincidental and not related to the ingestion of the test starch. Histopathological findings in the test animals were comparable to those for the controls.

Groups of 25 female Sprague-Dawley weanling rats were fed diets containing 0.2, 1.0, or 5.0% (about 0.2, 0.8, or 4 g/kg body weight) of phosphated distarch phosphate made from white milo starch over a 90-day period (Kohn et al., 1964b). Body weight gains were not significantly different from those of the controls. Urinalyses, hematological parameters, organ:body weight ratios, gross pathology, and histopathological observations were normal.

Groups of 10 male and 10 female weanling Wistar rats were fed potato phosphated distarch phosphate (0.3% phosphorus) at dietary levels of 25 or 50% (about 25 or 50 g/kg body weight) for 8 weeks. Body weight gains were similar to those of the controls. No diarrhea occurred. Cecal weight was slightly raised in the male rats, but no consistent effect was seen in the females (de Groot and Spanjers, 1970). Dogs (beagle) participated in a 90-day acute toxicity test. Groups of three male and three female beagles were fed standard dog chow supplemented daily with 0.05, 0.25, or 1.25 g/kg body weight phosphated distarch phosphate administered in capsules. The modified starch was made from white milo starch (Cervenka and Kay, 1963). Body weight gains and organ:body weight ratios of the test animals did not differ significantly from the controls. No abnormalities were seen in the gross and histopathological examinations.

Groups of eight 3-day-old Pitman-Moore miniature pigs were fed formula diets containing phosphated distarch phosphate made from acid-modified waxy maize starch (treated with 4.8% sodium tripolyphosphate and 0.59% sodium trimetaphosphate) or acid-modified waxy maize starch as a control. The starch provided 24% of the calories in the diet, which was fed over a 25-day period (Anderson et al., 1973). Weight gains, organ:body weight ratios, clinical blood chemistry, as well as liver and carcass composition of the test animals were similar to those of the controls.

Twelve human volunteers ingesting on each of 4 consecutive days 60 g (about 1 g/kg body weight) phosphate distarch phosphate containing 0.35% phosphorus (Pieters, 1971) showed no adverse effects as regards frequency of defecation, amount of fecal water or feces, or lactic content of feces.

Long-Term and Multigeneration Studies
See Section II.E and de Groot et al. (1974).

III. GENERAL SAFETY ASPECTS

Modified food starches are chemically very closely related to native starches. They contain low to relatively low levels of substituent groups. Bleached and converted starches with the exception of oxidized starches either involve no significant change in the chemical structure or produce changes similar to those that starch undergoes in human digestion or in well-accepted food processes such as baking. Oxidized starches contain minimal amounts of carboxyl groups. For these reasons scientists, toxicologists, and regulatory groups have readily accepted their use in foods.

Cross-linked starches contain very low levels of substituents ranging in the order of only one cross-link in hundreds to a few thousand anhydroglucose units. They are present at such low levels that they have minimal effect on in vitro digestibility and no effect on in vivo digestibility as well as acute toxicity. The cross-linking moieties are esters of acids found in natural foods. Chronic and multigeneration studies on cross-linked monosubstituted starches have also provided evidence of their safety.

Evidence for the safety of monosubstituted and monosubstituted cross-linked food starches has been presented. In general it has been accepted as an indication of the safety and nontoxicity of such products. Two phenomena observed in feeding studies that appear to be related to the level of monosubstituent groups in the starch are cecal enlargement and pelvic nephrocalcinosis. Reviews and further studies have been made to clarify their nature and etiology.

A. Cecal Enlargement

This is observed not only in rats fed certain modified starches containing mono-substituent groups, but also natural foods including some raw starches such as ungelatinized potato starch, lactose, maltitol, high molecular weight fractions of glucose syrup, etc. (Reussner et al., 1963; Hosoya, 1972; Birch et al., 1973). It has also been observed in feeding synthetics such as polyethylene glycol (Loeschke et al., 1973). Leegwater et al. (1974) studied the phenomenon by investigating the effect of hydroxypropyl starches ranging in DS from 0.025 to 0.106, lactose, raw potato starch, polyethylene glycol 1000, and magnesium sulfate on cecal size and some of the constituents of the cecum in male rats varying in age from 4 weeks to 3 months. The experiments lasted from 10 days to 3 months.

Under the conditions, all the materials caused cecal enlargement. Those rats fed hydroxypropyl starch (DS 0.047), lactose, or raw potato starch returned to normal size within 4 weeks after going back to the control diet consisting of pre-gelatinized potato or cornstarch. The hydroxypropyl starch was chosen over the other modifications because it tended to cause more cecal enlargement than any of the other modifications. The data did not show a consistent relationship between the cecal size and amount of dry matter, sodium, potassium, chloride, or volatile fatty acids in the cecal contents. The osmotic value of the cecal contents of animals fed the control or test diets were all of the same order of magnitude. The cecal enlargement of animals fed hydroxypropyl starches varied with the dietary dose level and roughly with the level of substitution: the higher the substitution the greater the chance for enlargement. Leegwater et al. (1974) hypothesized that dietary components that are not completely digested and/or absorbed in the small intestine increase the amount of osmotically active material in the intestine. This results in increased water retention, causing the cecum to distend. The osmotic activity in the cecum varies with the composition of the diet, but the osmotic pressure is kept relatively constant by the inflow of water accompanied by enlargement of the cecum. It is concluded that the enlargement is a process of physiological adaption. The significance of cecal enlargement in rats has little relevance to humans. It appears that the rat can derive a substantial part of its energy supply from the biological processes taking place in the cecum. In humans the cecum is certainly less important in size and physiological function, so it is unlikely that observations based on the rat cecum have any relevance to humans. Moreover, the dietary level (>2.5 g/kg body weight per day) where cecal enlargement is observed in rats is far higher than the likely consumption of modified starch by humans, which at maximum is estimated at 0.5 g/kg body weight.

B. Pelvic Nephrocalcinosis

The term pelvic nephrocalcinosis (PN) covers those mineral deposits, presumably calcium salts, within the lumen of the renal pelvis attached to or situated beneath the pelvic epithelium, which in some cases is associated with hyperplasia of the epithelium. Observations of this phenomenon have been confined to rats fed mono-substituted or monosubstituted cross-linked starches. With one exception (Bailey et al., 1973), it usually occurs in long-term feeding studies on rats. It appears that rats are particularly sensitive to the development of PN. There was much less evidence of PN in mice fed modified food starch in a 89-week study (Feron et al., 1978). PN is not a specific lesion. Many other substances cause PN including whole milk, lactose, various polyols, etc. (Roe, 1979; Roe, 1989; Lord and Newberne, 1990). Phosphate urolithiasis in rats was shown to be related to dietary mineral imbalance and did not occur in diets where the levels of calcium, phosphorus, and magnesium were properly controlled (Chow et al., 1980).

Metabolism Studies on Hamsters

The effect of modified food starch on Syrian Golden hamsters was studied by Newberne and Buttolph at the Massachusetts Institute of Technology. Groups of 12 female and 8 male Syrian Golden hamsters were fed diets containing 40% unmodified starch as a control and a series of diets in which hamsters were fed 10% unmodified starch and 30% of acetylated distarch adipate (0.08 DS), hydroxypropyl distarch phosphate (0.13 DS), or hydroxypropyl distarch phosphate (0.19 DS). In all cases 0.51% calcium and 0.40% phosphorus were added and the effect of magnesium levels of 0.017, 0.060, 0.090, 0.120, or 0.210% were checked. Four males and six females from each group were sacrificed at 30 days and the remainder at 60 days (Newberne and Buttolph, 1979). There were wide variations in food efficiency, but average daily intake was similar in all groups. Hamsters receiving diets containing only 0.017% magnesium and hydroxypropyl distarch phosphate showed marked growth retardation. This appears to be the result of an interaction between the starch and magnesium in the diet. This level of magnesium was only 28% of the NRC minimal recommendation. In groups receiving hydroxypropyl distarch phosphate (0.23 DS) there was a direct correlation between body weight gain and level of magnesium. When sufficient magnesium was in the diet, the weight gains approached those of the control and renal lesions (cortical scarring and tubular dilation) were eliminated. The study demonstrated the importance of supplying adequate dietary magnesium in animal studies on hamsters. Neutron activation analyses of kidneys suggested a correlation between the severity of the lesion and calcium level but not the magnesium level (Buttolph et al., 1979). It was hypothesized that the role of magnesium in preventing lesions might be to prevent the precipitation of the calcium complexes that otherwise accumulate in the kidney.

Metabolism Studies on Rats

The short-term (30- and 90-day) effects of 40% unmodified maize starch and diets in which 10% unmodified starch was used with 30% acetylated distarch adipate (2.14% acetyl) or 30% hydroxypropyl distarch phosphate (4.7% hydroxypropyl groups) were studied with special attention to the influence of the dietary levels of calcium, phosphorus, and magnesium. Groups of six male and six female or twice this number of Charles River Sprague-Dawley rats were fed on various modifications in the mineral levels of a basic semisynthetic diet. Metabolism measurements were made during the fourth week routinely and at some other times in special cases. Autopsies and histopathological evaluations were run after 30 or 88 days (Newberne and Buttolph, 1980; Wurzburg and Vogel, 1983).

The following conclusions were drawn:

1. Only lesions in the corticomedullary junction of the kidney consisting of mineralized tubules were observed. No PN was noted.
2. There was no indication that modified starch contributed to the lesions.
3. Lowering the phosphorus content and increasing the Ca/P ratio dramatically reduced the severity and incidence of the renal lesion.
4. Increasing the dietary magnesium concentration from 0.02 to 0.2% tended to decrease the severity of the lesion.
5. There is a consistently higher concentration of Mg, Ca, and phosphate in the urine of rats fed hydroxypropyl distarch phosphate than in rats given the same mineral composition and the control or acetylated distarch adipate.
6. These studies indicate that many diets used in rat studies contain too high phosphorus levels and too low Ca/P ratios. In addition many of the diets are deficient in magnesium.

Long-Term Metabolism Studies on Rats

Long-term mineral metabolism studies of diets containing waxy maize starch, acetylated distarch adipate, acetylated distarch phosphate, and lactose were investigated (Hodgkinson et al., 1982). In one experiment, groups of 25 weanling SPF Sprague-Dawley rats were fed on a basic diet containing 30% unmodified pregelatinized waxy maize starch or 30% pregelatinized acetylated distarch adipate (2.1% acetyl) or 30% pregelatinized acetylated distarch phosphate (1.2% acetyl) or 30% lactose. Subgroups were studied using metabolism cages at 1- and 3-month intervals to compare the effect of different diets on food consumption; urinary volume, Ca, P, and Mg levels; fecal Ca, P, and Mg; and other parameters. The basic diet used was the same as that used by de Groot et al. (1974). After a year the animals were killed and examined postmortem for changes in the kidneys, lower urinary tract, and other organs. Samples of kidney tissue were examined chemically for residual calcium. A second experiment was similar to the first except that the animals were about 9 months old at the start of the experiment, which lasted 34 weeks before termination (Hodgkinson et al., 1982).

At the end of the study with 9-month-old rats, the mean body weight of the rats fed lactose was significantly lower than that of the controls fed starch. The animals fed modified starch were slightly but not significantly heavier than those fed unmodified starch in both experiments. The main treatment-related changes in the three test diets were enlarged ceca, increased urinary excretion of calcium, increased renal calcification as measured at autopsy, and increased medullary and pelvic nephrocalcinosis assessed histopathologically. The animals fed lactose showed these changes to a greater extent than either modified starches. As might be expected because of the higher acetyl level, the acetylated distarch adipate had a slightly greater effect than the acetylated distarch phosphate. The calcium content in the kidneys of all animals, including the controls, increased with age. The deposits found in the kidneys were identical to those found by de Groot's group (1974) and were identified as calcium phosphate. The relative absence of cortico-medullary deposits was a reflection of adequate magnesium levels in the diet.

Summary

These findings, along with the literature search by F. J. C. Roe (1979) and subsequent examination of the matter not only in regard to modified starches but also lactose and polyols (Roe, 1989), have put the matter in perspective (Roe, 1984). [See also Lord and Newberne (1990).] The observations and findings are as follows:

1. PN is a relatively common occurrence in untreated rats particularly in the older animals. It is an aging phenomenon rarely observed in young rats.
2. Many substances, including milk, lactose, as well as modified starches containing significant amounts of substituent groups, may aggravate the incidence of PN.
3. The above substances increase calcium absorption from the gut and into the urine, thus increasing chances for the development of PN.
4. The levels of Ca, P, and Mg are controlling factors. High P levels, low Ca:P ratios, and insufficient Mg all favor the development of PN.
5. Recommended dietary levels for Ca, P, and Mg apparently are based on overt evidence of diet deficiencies with little attention to their effect on histopathology. Shah and Belonie (1991) have taken steps to correct this problem.

IV. CONCLUSIONS

After reviewing the background data, the Joint FAO/WHO Expert Committee on Food Additives (1982) concluded that

> there is now experimental evidence that pelvic nephrocalcinosis may arise as a consequence of increased absorption of calcium. This occurs, inter alia, with the increased availability of monosaccharides for absorption within the lower bowel. Such increased availability may occur because of dietary overloading, particularly with the more poorly absorbed monosaccharides, or because more complex carbohydrates are not degraded to monosaccharides before the food bolus reaches the cecum. Cecal enlargement commonly accompanies increased calcium absorption in either case.

The Committee went on to confirm that the acceptable daily intakes (ADIs) of the modified (food) starches were confirmed as "not specified." This, along with past reviews by the FDA as reflected in 21CFR172.892 and an extensive review by the Life Sciences Research Office—Federation of American Societies for Experimental Biology (1979) commissioned by the FDA, provides assurances of the safety of modified food starches. In addition, the usage of modified food starches in foods for infants and young children has been subjected to an in-depth review by a Subcommittee of the National Academy of Sciences (1971) and by a Committee on Nutrition, American Academy of Pediatrics (1978). On the basis of the review the modified food starches used in infant foods were generally approved for use in infant foods with the exception of hydroxypropylated starches. In 1988, L. J. Filer, Jr., presented an update reaffirming the value of modified starch for use in baby foods (1988).

REFERENCES*

Anderson, T. A. et al. (1973). Effect of waxy corn starn modification on growth, serum biochemical values and body composition of Pitman-Moore miniature pigs. *Food Cosmet. Toxicol.* 11:747–754.

---

* Unpublished reports dated prior to 1979 are cited in Life Sciences, 1979. Those dated 1979 or later have been submitted to the FDA and are available through the Freedom of Information Act.

Anderson, T. A. et al. (1974). Digestibility of acetylated distarch glycerol-effect on growth, serum biochemical values and body composition of Pitman-Moore miniature pigs. *Food Cosmet. Toxicol. 12*:201–207.

Bailey, D. E., Cox, G. E., and Morgareidge, K. (1973). Subacute feeding studies in rats with hydroxypropyl distarch phosphate. Report 1420. Food and Drug Research Laboratories Inc., Maspeth, NY.

Birch, G. G., Etheridge, I. J., and Green, L. F. (1973). Short term effects of feeding rats with glucose syrup fractions and dextrose. *Br. J. Nutr. 29*:87–93.

Bjorck, I., Gunnarsson, A., and Ostergard, K. (1989). A study of native and chemically modified potato starch. *Die Starke 41*:128–134.

Booher, L. E. (1951). Toxicological evaluation of unmodified and modified starches. *J. Nutr. 45*:75–95.

Buttolph, M. L., and Newberne, P. M. (1980). Subchronic studies in rats fed octenylsuccinate modified food starch. *Food Cosmetic Toxicol. 18*:357–362.

Buttolph, M. L., Newberne, P. M., and Janghorbani, M. (1979). Effect of modified and unmodified starch diet on mineral composition of kidneys and renal lesions. *Trace Substances in Environmental Health.* D. D. Hemphill, ed. pp. 217–223. U. of Missouri, Columbia, MO.

Caldwell, C. G., and Wurzburg, O. B. (1953). U.S. Patent 2,661,349.

Carson, S. (1960a). Caloric evaluation of RX12K1 [corn starch sodium octenylsuccinate] and corn starch. Report No. 80878b-c, Food and Drug Research Laboratory, Inc., Maspeth, NY.

Carson, S. (1960b). Caloric evaluation of starch succinate and corn starch. Report No. 80878c-e, Food and Drug Research Laboratories, Inc., Maspeth, NY, for National Starch and Chemical Corp., NJ.

Carson, S. (1961). The calorie value of RX615-9. Report Food and Drug Research Laboratory Inc. Maspethy, NY, for National Starch and Chemical Corp., Bridgewater, NJ.

Cervenka, H., and Kay, J. H. (1963). Subacute oral toxicity of phosphate starch 4822. Report by Industrial Bio-Test Laboratories, Inc. Northbrook, IL, for Corn Products Co., Argo, IL.

CRF.21CFR892.172 (1990). Code of Federal Regulations, Office of the Federal Register—National Archives and Records Adm. Washington, DC.

Chow, F. C., Taton, G. F., Boulay, J. P., Lewis, L. D., Remmenga, E. E., and Hamar, D. W. (1980). Effect of dietary calcium, magnesium, and phosphorus on phosphate urolithiasis in rats. *Invest. Urol. 17*:273–276.

Committee on Nutrition, American Academy of Pediatrics (1978). Review of safety and suitability of modified food starches in infant foods. Under FDA contract 223-76-2091.

de Groot, A. P., and Spanjers, M. T. (1970). Observations on rats fed on diets containing 5 different chemically modified starches. Report 3096, Centraal Instituut voor Voedingsonderzoek, Zeist, Holland.

de Groot, A. P., Til, H. P., Feron, V. J., Dreef-van der Meulen, H. C., and Willems, M. I. (1974). Two-year feeding and multi-generation studies in rats on five chemically modified starches. *Food Cosmet. Toxicol. 12*:651–663.

FAO Food and Nutrition Paper No. 49 (1990). Food and Agriculture Organization of the United Nations, Rome, Italy.

Feron, V. J., Til, H. P., and de Groot, A. P. (1967a). Report No. 2329. Centraal Instituut voor Voedingsonderzoek, Zeist, Holland.

Feron, V. J., Til, H. P., and de Groot, A. P. (1967b). Sub-chronic toxicity test with modified potato starch [propylene oxide] and an alginate in albino rats. Report No. R2456, Centraal Instituut voor Voedingsonderzoeg, Zeist, Holland.

Feron, V. J., Til, H. P., and Immel, H. R. (1978). Chronic (89 week) feeding study with hydroxypropyl distarch phosphate, starch acetate, and sodium alginate in mice. Report No. R5690, Centraal Instituut voor Voedingsonderzoek. Zeist, Holland.

Filer, Jr., L. J. (1971). Modified food starches for use in infant foods. (Major findings of Subcommittee on Safety and Suitability of MSG and Other Substances in Baby Foods of the Food Protection Committee, Food and Nutrition Board, NAS-NRC by the Chairman.) *Nutrition Rev. 29*:55–59.

Filer, Jr., L. J. (1988). Modified food starch—an update. *Perspect. Pract. 88*:342–344.

Gramera, R. E., Heerma, J., and Parrish, F. W. (1966). Distribution and structural form of phosphate ester groups in commercial starch phosphates. *Cereal Chem. 43*:104–111.

Heyns, K., Graefe, G., and Mahlmann, H. (1977). On the matter of modified starches in the industrial production of prepared food products. Submission to Hearing Clerk, FDA, by CPC Int. Inc. See *Life Sciences* (1979), Ref. 112.

Hixson, O. F. (1960). Laboratory Report No. M-1004 of Rosner-Hixson Laboratory, Chicago, Ill. Submitted to Corn Products Co., Argo, IL. See *Life Sciences* (1979), Ref. 115.

Hodge, H. C. (1956). Acute oral screening toxicity test of S823 white milo (distarch phosphate). Report of Division of Pharmacology and Toxicology—U. of Rochester School of Medicine and Dentistry, Rochester, NY, submitted by Corn Products Co., Argo, IL. See *Life Sciences* (1979), Ref. 117.

Hodgkinson, A., Davis, D., Fourman, J., Robertson, W. G., and Roe, F. J. C. (1982). A comparison of the effects of lactose and of two chemically modified waxy maize starches on mineral metabolism in the rat. *Fd. Chem. Toxicol. 20*:371–382.

Hood, L. F., and Arneson, V. G. (1976). In vitro digestibility of hydroxypropyl distarch phosphate and unmodified tapioca starch. *Cereal Chem. 53*:282–290.

Hood, L. F., Vancampen, D. R., House, W. A., and Szatkowski, E. (1976). Effect of modified and unmodified tapioca starches on ^{59}Fe retention in rats. *J. Nutr. 106*:1768–1772.

Hosoya, N. (1972). Effect of sugar alcohol in the intestine. Ninth International Congress of Nutrition, Mexico City, pp. 164–168.

International Minerals and Chemical Corp. (1955). Report submitted by American Maize Products Co., Roby, Ind. to JECFA. See *Life Sciences* (1979), Ref. 109.

Janzen, G. J. (1969). Digestibility of starches and phosphatized starches with pancreatin. *Die Starke 9*(21):231–237.

Joint FAO/WHO Expert Committee on Food Additives (1974). Toxicological evaluation of certain food additives. Food Additive Series No. 5. World Health Organization, Geneva, Swit.

Kerr, R. W. (1950). Manufacture of modified corn starches. In *Chemistry and Industry of Starch*, 2nd ed. R. W. Kerr, ed. Academic Press Inc., New York, pp. 63.

Kohn, F. E., and Kay, J. H. (1963a). The digestion of various starches by pancreatic amylase. Report by Industrial Bio-Test Laboratory, Inc., Northbrook, IL, to Corn Products Co., Argo, IL.

Kohn, F. E., and Kay, J. H. (1963b). Nutritional Assay of starch 4822. Report of Industrial Bio-Test Laboratories, Inc., Northbrook, IL, for Corn Products Co., Argo, IL.

Kohn, F. E., Kay, J. H., and Calandra, J. C. (1964a). 60-day target organ study on phosphate starch number 4822. Report by Industrial Bio-Test Laboratories, Inc., Northbrook, IL, for Corn Products Co., Argo, IL.

Kohn, F. E., Kay, J. H., and Calandra, J. C. (1964b). Subacute oral toxicity of phosphate starch 4822. Report by Industrial Bio-Test Laboratories, Inc., Northbrook, IL, for Corn Products Co., Argo, IL.

Kruger, L. H. (1970a). In vitro digestibility of acetylated and crosslinked acetylated starch. Laboratory Report 406, National Starch and Chemical Corp., Bridgewater, NJ.

Kruger, L. H. (1970b). In vitro digestibility of crosslinked starches. Laboratory Report 405 of National Starch and Chemical Corp., Bridgewater, NJ.

Kruger, L. H., Chiu, C., and Smith, A. L. (1980). In vitro enzyme digestibility of starch sodium octenyl succinate. Report 1508. National Starch and Chemical Corp., Bridge-water, NJ.

Leegwater, D. C. (1971a). Report No. R3431. Centraal Instituut voor Voedingsonderzoek, Zeist, Holland.

Leegwater, D. C. (1971b). Report No. 3441. Centraal Instituut voor Voedingsonderzoek, Zeist, Holland.

Leegwater, D. C., and Luten, J. B. (1971). A study on the in vitro digestibility of hydroxy-propyl starches by pancreatin. *Die Starke 23*:430–432.

Leegwater, D. C., and Marsman, J. W. (1973). Identification of a {6-*O*-[hydroxypropyl]-D-glucosyl}-D-glucose as a fecal metabolite of *O*-[hydroxypropyl] starch in the rat. *Car-bohydr. Res. 29*:271–273.

Leegwater, D. C., and Speek, A. J. (1972). Study of the faecal metabolites of hydroxypropyl starch in the rat. *Die Starke 24*:373–374.

Leegwater, D. C., and Ten Noever de Brauw, M. C. (1972). Isolation and identification of an *O*-[2-hydroxypropyl] maltose from the feces of rats fed with *O*-hydroxypropyl starch. *Carbohydr. Res. 25*:411–418.

Leegwater, D. C., de Groot, A. P., and van Kalmthout-Kuyper, M. (1974). The aetiology of cecal enlargement in the rat. *Food Cosmet. Toxicol. 12*:687–697.

Life Sciences Research Office Federation of American Societies for Experimental Biology (1979). Evaluation of the health aspects of starch and modified starches as food ingre-dients. SCOGS-115 prepared for Bureau of Foods, FDA, Washington, DC. Contract No. FDA 223-75-2004 Natl. Technical Information Service, U.S. Dept. Commerce.

Loeschke, K., Uhlich, E., and Halbach, R. (1973). Cecal enlargement combined with sodium transport stimulation in rats fed polyethylene glycol. *Proc. Soc. Exp. Biol. Med. 142*:96–102.

Lord, G. H., and Newberne, P. M. (1990). Renal mineralization—a ubiquitous lesion in chronic rat studies. *Food Chem. Toxic. 28*:449–455.

Majors, P. A., and Rubenkoenig, H. L. (1959). Schwarz prophetic patch test of Ceron N and starch. Report of Hill Top Research Institute, Inc., Miamiville, OH, to Hercules Powder Co., Wilmington, DE.

Morgareidge, K. (1959). Further studies on 78-1087 starch rate of metabolism in albino rats. Report No. 79408 of Food and Drug Research Laboratories, Inc., Maspeth, NY, sub-mitted to National Starch and Chemical Corp.

Newberne, P. M., and Buttolph, M. L. (1979). Final report—Review and conclusions of hamster studies. Study #78-4 by Dept. of Nutrition and Food Science—Massachusetts Institute of Technology, Cambridge, Massachusetts.

Newberne, P. M., and Buttolph, M. L. (1980). Metabolism studies in rats fed modified starches. Final Report on Study 79-2. Dept. of Nutrition and Food Science, Massa-chusetts Institute of Technology, Cambridge, Massachusetts.

Oser, B. L. (1945). The examination of starch samples for non-toxicity. Report No. 39989-92, Food and Drug Research Laboratories, Inc., Maspeth, NY.

Oser, B. L. (1950). Toxicological studies of certain products Report No. 58380-1, Food and Drug Research Laboratories Inc., Maspeth, NY, for National Starch and Chemical Corp., Bridgewater, NJ.

Oser, B. L. (1954). Estimation of the physiologically available calories in nine samples of starch. Report No. 69190a-1 of Food and Drug Research Laboratories, Inc., Maspeth, NY.

Oser, B. L. (1961a). Biological evaluation of modified starches. Report No. 78400, Food and Drug Research Laboratories Inc., Maspeth, NY, submitted to National Starch and Chemical Corp., Bridgewater, NJ.

Oser, M. (1961b). Caloric evaluation of an adipic-acetic (mixed) anhydride treated starch.

Report 81776, Food and Drug Research Laboratories, Inc., Maspeth, NY, for National Starch and Chemical Corp., Bridgewater, NJ.

Oser, B. L. (1964). Subacute (90 days) feeding studies with Amioca (waxy maize starch) treated with adipic-acetic mixed anhydride. Report 85555, Food and Drug Research Laboratories, Inc., Maspeth, NY, for National Starch and Chemical Corp., Bridgewater, NJ.

Pallota, A. J. (1959). Ceron N: acute eye application. Report of Hazelton Laboratories, Inc., to Hercules Powder Co., Wilmington, DE.

Parish, W. E., Chamberlain, M., Beard, R. J., and Leftwich, D. J. (1984). Mutagenicity studies with starch sodium octenylsuccinate Report CC/31/84 Ames test and CC/32/84 Sister chromatid exchange assay, Environmental Safety Laboratory, Unilever Research—Colworth House, UK.

Parish, W. E., Wilson, R., and Willson, G. A. (1984). 90-day feeding study in rats to assess the effect of purified diets containing starch sodium octenylsuccinate on nephrocalcinosis and hepatic lipidosis. Report 46240/Study No. 1327, Environmental Safety Laboratory, Unilever Research—Colworth, UK.

Parish, W. E., Wilson, R., and Willson, G. A. (1987). Combined chronic toxicity and carcinogenicity study in rats fed starch sodium octenylsuccinate for 130 weeks. Study Reference 1369, Environmental Safety Laboratory, Unilever Research—Colworth House, Sharnbrook, UK.

Pieters, J. J. L. (1971). Digestibility studies with chemically modified starches in man. Report No. R3433, Centraal Instituut voor Voedingsonderzoek, Zeist, Holland.

Porter, M. W. (1971). Nutritional and toxicological properties of hydroxypropyl distarch phosphates when fed to weanling rats as part of the carbohydrate source. Report, A. E. Staley Mfg. Co., Decatur, IL.

Prier, R. F. (1961). Assay report (hydroxypropyl distarch phosphate). Report, Wisconsin Alumni Research Foundation, Madison, Wisconsin. See *Life Sciences*, Ref. 125.

Reussner, G. Jr., Andros, J., and Thissen, R., Jr. (1963). The utilization of various starches and sugars in the rat. *J. Nutr.* 80:291–298.

Roe, F. J. C. (1979). Mineral deposition in the renal pelvis of rats: a brief review. Document submitted to the JECFA of FAO/WHO by Starch Experts Committee of the European Starch Producers. Brussels, Belgium.

Roe, F. J. C. (1984). Modified starches and nephrocalcinosis in rats: Implications for the ADI principle for food ingredients. European Toxicology Forum, Vol. II, Sept. 18–21, 1984, pp. 308–324.

Roe, F. J. C. (1989). Relevance for man of the effects of lactose, polyols, and other carbohydrates on calcium metabolism seen in rats: a review. *Human Toxicol.* 8:87–98.

Rosner, L. (1960). Laboratory Report No. M-1004-1, Rosner-Hixon Laboratories, Inc., Chicago, IL, submitted to Corn Products Co., Argo, IL.

Rubenkoenig, H. L. (1959). Repeat Insult Patch Test of Ceron N and starch. Hill Top Research Institute, Inc., Miamiville, OH, to Hercules Powder Co., Wilmington, DE.

Shah, B. G., and Belonie, B. (1991). Different dietary calcium levels required to prevent nephrocalcinosis in male and female rats. *Nutr. Res.* 11:385–390.

Shillam, K. W. G. (1971). Report No. 3978/71/136, Huntingdon Research Centre. See *Joint FAO/WHO Report* (1974).

Shillam, K. W. G. (1973). Report No. CRN5/73/254, Huntingdon Research Centre. See *Joint FAO/WHO Report* pp. 334–337.

Shuman, A. C., and Mertz, E. T. (1959). Unpublished Report No. 4 of Shuman Chemical Lab. Inc. to Corn Industries Research Foundation, Washington, DC.

Solarek, D. B. (1986). Phosphorylated starch and miscellaneous inorganic esters. In *Modified Starches: Properties and Uses*, Wurzburg, O. B. (ed.). CRC Press Inc., Boca Raton, FL.

Til, H. P., Spanjers, M. Th., Reuzel, P. G. J., and de Groot, A. P. (1974). Subchronic (90-day) toxicity study with hydroxypropyl distarch phosphate in rats. Report No. R 4082, Centraal Instituut voor Voedingzonderzoek, Zeist, Holland.

Til, H. P., Spanjers, M. Th., van der Heijden, C. A., and de Groot, A. P. (1973). Subchronic (90-day) toxicity study with oxidized starch in rats. Report No. 4081 of Centraal Instituut voor Voedingsonderzoek, Zeist, Holland.

Til, H. P., van der Meulen, H. C., and de Groot, A. P. (1970). Report No. R 3303 of the Centraal Instituut voor Voedingsonderzoek, Zeist, Holland.

Truhaut, R., Coquet, B., Fouillet, X., Galland, D., Guyot, D., Long, D., and Rouaud, J. L. (1979). Two-year oral toxicity and multigeneration studies in rats on two chemically modified maize starches. *Food Cosmet. Toxicol. 17*:11–17.

Turner, A. W. (1961). The safety of Mira-clear and other acetylated types of starches. Report from A. E. Staley Co., Decatur, IL.

Twenty-sixth Report of the Joint FAO/WHO Expert Committee on Food Additives. (1982). Evaluation of certain food additives and contaminants. World Health Organization Technical Report Series 683, World Health Organization, Geneva, pp. 11–12.

Walker, R., and El Harith, E. A. (1978). Nutritional and toxicological properties of some raw and unmodified starches. *Ann. Nutr. Alim. 32*:671–679.

Whistler, R. L., and Belfort, A. M. (1961). Nutritional value of chemically modified starch. *Science 133*:1599–1600.

White, T. A. (1963). Food starch modified. *Cereal Science Today 8*(48):54–55.

Wootton, M., and Chaudhry, M. A. (1979). Enzymic digestibility of modified starches. *Die Stärke 31*:224–228.

Wootton, M., and Chaudhry, M. A. (1981). In vitro digestion of hydroxypropyl derivatives of wheat starch II. Effect of substitution on the products of partial digestion by porcine pancreatic alpha amylase. *Die Stärke 33*:168–170.

Wurzburg, O. B. (1978). Starch, modified starch and dextrin *Seminar Proceedings, Products of the Corn Refining Industry*, Corn Refiners Association, Washington, DC.

Wurzburg, O. B. (1986). Crosslinked starches. In *Modified Starches: Properties and Uses*, O. B. Wurzburg (ed.). CRC Press Inc., Boca Raton, FL, pp. 41–54.

Wurzburg, O. B., and Kruger, L. H. (1962). U.S. Patent 3,058,853.

Wurzburg, O. B., and Vogel, W. F. (1983). Modified food starch—safety and regulatory aspects. In *Gums and Stabilizers for the Food Industry 2*, Phillips, G. O., Wedlock, D. J., and Williams, P. A. (eds.). pp. 405–415. Pergamon Press, Oxford, U.K.

10
Incidental Food Additives

S. S. Deshpande* and D. K. Salunkhe
Utah State University
Logan, Utah

I. INTRODUCTION

Incidental or unintentional food additives are substances present in our food that can alter its properties but have not been added on purpose. This group of food chemicals can be broadly classified under the general heading of contaminants and residues. These substances end up in our food supply by indirectly entering our food chain. Some of these chemicals are extremely hazardous to human health, while others are responsible for inducing plasmid-mediated drug resistance in several human pathogens. Still others may interact with natural food constituents, particularly the lipids, to generate free radicals with carcinogenic potency. Generally, most of these chemicals are broken down naturally or washed away. Nevertheless, residual amounts do remain in our food supply. Such unintentional addition is unfortunate but unavoidable.

Incidental food additives come from three major sources:

1. Contamination of soil and water supplies with heavy metals, radioisotopes, pesticides, and other toxic industrial chemicals
2. Manufacturing processes, which may contribute packaging contaminants, particles of the equipment used, and the remains of errant animals
3. Chemicals applied to crops and livestock to maintain or improve their health (e.g., insecticides, herbicides, fungicides, drugs, and antibiotics)

These various sources of incidental food additives, their properties, and toxicological aspects are briefly described below.

Current affiliation: Idetek, Inc., Sunnyvale, California.

II. TOXIC METALS

It is difficult to draw a clear distinction between essential—especially the trace elements in human nutrition—and toxic metals. Nearly all metals are toxic to humans if ingested in abnormal amounts. Moreover, the physiological effects of some metals, such as cadmium, are closely related to the amount of other essential nutrients in the human diet (Reilly, 1991). Similarly, all metals are capable of interacting in the body with other cellular constituents. Nevertheless, it is possible to differentiate among elements that are known with certainty to be essential and those that display severe toxicological symptoms at extremely low levels and have no known beneficial physiological functions. The heavy metals, most noticeably mercury, lead, and cadmium, probably constitute the single largest group of elements that contaminate agricultural soils, water supplies, and the environment and eventually find their way into the human food chain. Other toxic metals include arsenic, beryllium, boron, selenium, and other metals and metalloids. The possible sources of contamination of our food and the physiologically adverse and toxic effects of these metals are described below.

A. Sources of Contamination

Soil

Soil is the primary source of toxic metals found in food crops. Although most nutrients are absorbed from the top 10–30 cm of soil, plants that are capable of developing extensive deep root systems can effectively penetrate the soils to a depth of more than 6–10 meters. Hence, the toxic metal content of agricultural soils needs to be considered from the viewpoint of both surface contamination as well as the nature of the underlying soil and the surrounding area (Hall et al., 1953).

Although most toxic metal contamination of soils occurs because of environmental pollution, natural factors also play an important role in this regard. For example, the volcanic soils that are intensively cultivated in Java and Sumatra contain inherently high levels of mercury and other toxic metals. Recently, Reilly et al. (1989) reported the mercury and arsenic contents in soil, water, and foods grown in the Dieng Plateau area of Java. They found a significant accumulation of mercury in locally grown vegetables. It was estimated that the consumption of as little as 100 g of potato each day would contain almost twice the World Health Organization's (WHO) tolerable level of mercury intake.

Accumulation by Pasture Plants and Crops

Plants are capable of absorbing toxic metals from contaminated soils and accumulating them in various tissues. Selenium toxicity was first noticed in livestock grazing on pastures and herbage grown in selenium-rich soils (Knott and McCray, 1959; Gardiner et al., 1962). Cadmium poisoning of humans was reported in Japan when rice paddy fields were irrigated with water contaminated by effluent from a local zinc-cadmium-lead mine (Reilly, 1991). Similar incidences of cadmium, copper, and zinc toxicity were also reported in England and Zambia (Reilly and Reilly, 1971; Morgan, 1988).

Some plants are also capable of absorbing and accumulating certain toxic metals in large amounts. The shrub *Camellia sinesis* absorbs large quantities of both aluminum and manganese from the soil and concentrates them in its leaves (Pennington, 1987). The dried leaves of this shrub are used to make tea. In the United Kingdom, tea drinking alone appears to contribute a significant dietary intake of manganese in the elderly population (Wenlock et al., 1979). Metal accumulation in foods thus is a natural occurrence, with benefits as well as possible disadvantages for those who consume the foods.

Sewage Sludge

The application of sewage sludge to agricultural lands constitutes a significant source of food contamination by toxic metals. Although it contains more than 40% organic matter and is a rich source of both nitrogen and phosphorus, sewage sludge, especially from heavily populated urban and industrial areas, can contain relatively high levels of several toxic metals. Incidents of crop failures from soils where such sludge is applied are not uncommon (Mackenzie and Purves, 1975).

Normal concentrations of several metals in typical sludge samples are presented in Table 1. The metals are usually industrial in origin, although domestic waste also makes a substantial contribution. Mercury, zinc, lead, and cadmium have been reported to occur at high levels in household dust as well as in domestic garbage (Harrison, 1978; Price, 1988). The levels of toxic metals found in sewage sludge are considerably higher than those found in typical agricultural land, with more than 300 times as much zinc and 100 times as much boron and copper as would occur in the normal arable rural soils (Berrow and Webber, 1972). Significant accumulation of these metals in food crops may result in potential health problems for the consumers. Of the different metals found in sewage sludge, lead, cadmium,

Table 1 Normal Ranges of Metals in Dry Matter of Sewage Sludge

Metal	Content (mg/kg)
Boron	15–1000
Cadmium	60–1500
Chromium	40–8800
Cobalt	2–260
Copper	200–8000
Iron	6000–62000
Lead	120–3000
Manganese	150–2500
Mercury	3–77
Molybdenum	2–30
Nickel	20–5300
Scandium	2–15
Silver	5–150
Titanium	1000–4500
Vanadium	20–400
Zinc	700–49000

Source: Pike et al., 1975; Capon, 1981.

and mercury pose more serious problems than metals such as copper and zinc (Strenstrom and Vahter, 1974).

Agricultural Chemicals and Fertilizers

Some of the widely used commercial fertilizers are capable of introducing significant levels of cadmium to the soil. Such incidences have been reported from Sweden and Australia (Williams and David, 1973; Strenstrom and Vahter, 1974). The acid rain phenomenon observed in both Europe and North America further enhances the mobilization of toxic metals in agricultural soils, thereby facilitating a greater uptake by the food crops (Reilly, 1991).

Certain toxic metals, e.g., mercury and arsenic, have also been used in both inorganic and organic forms in fungicides and other agrochemicals. The use of organomercurial compounds has been the cause of far more serious and better documented cases of food poisoning in Iraq, Pakistan, and Guatemala (Bakir et al., 1973; Reilly, 1991). Mercurial compounds are no longer common in agricultural practices and have been largely replaced by less persistent fungicides. The use of arsenic pesticides in horticulture has similarly declined appreciably (MAFF, 1982).

Metal-Containing Water

Contamination of both surface and ground water by industrial wastes is a prime source of heavy metal toxicity in human and animal nutrition. The contamination and subsequent consumption of seafood is particularly serious in this regard. The water used for food production and drinking, however, is often treated to remove excessive levels of toxic metals. Besides cadmium and mercury, large-scale pollution of water by other metals is quite common in several industrial countries (Prater, 1975; Reilly, 1991).

Food Processing

Metal contamination may occur at several stages during food processing. Contamination sources include:

1. The factory door
2. Plant and equipment
3. Catering operations
4. Ceramic and enameled utensils
5. Metal containers.

Generally, only high-quality stainless steel, plastics, and other structural materials approved for contact with foods are used in food-processing plants. The use of ceramics and enameled utensils is a significant source of metal poisoning, particularly aluminum, copper, lead, and cadmium, in the less-developed countries. Wrapping paper, cardboard containers, as well as the print and color applied to plastic containers are also capable of contaminating food (Klein et al., 1970; Watanabe, 1974; Heichel et al., 1974; Gramiccioni, 1984).

B. Occurrence and Toxicity

The occurrence and toxicity of some of the more common metal pollutants in the human food chain are briefly described below.

Lead

The presence of lead in the human food chain continues to be a major health problem worldwide. It is used on a very wide and increasing scale in the modern world, with production totaling in the Western world alone 2.131 million tons in the first 6 months of 1988 (ALDA, 1988). It is present in practically every organ and tissue of the human body, with amounts ranging from 100 to 400 mg or about 1.7 $\mu g/g$ tissue (Barry, 1975). Over 90% of the lead in the human body occurs in the bone. Lead is also a normal ingredient of the human diet (Table 2). The daily intake of lead via food in human nutrition was estimated to be 100–300 μg, with considerably higher levels occurring as a result of increasing environmental pollution (WHO, 1976).

The absorption of lead from food is estimated to be 10% in adults and 40% in children (Reilly, 1991). Several dietary factors influence the level of absorption. A low body-calcium status, iron deficiency, and diets rich in carbohydrates but lacking protein and those containing high levels of vitamin D result in increased absorption of lead. In the normal adult, about 90% of the ingested lead is generally excreted in the urine and feces.

The symptoms of acute lead poisoning in humans are well documented. The major effects are related to hemopoietic, nervous, gastrointestinal, and renal functions (Reilly, 1991). Generally, anorexia, dyspepsia, and constipation are followed by an attack of colic with intense paroxysmal abdominal pain. Lead encephalopathy is also observed in young children (NAS, 1972; Reilly and Reilly, 1972). However, little is known about chronic lead poisoning over a long period of time. Mild anemia, mental deterioration and hyperkinetic or aggressive behavior, peripheral neuropathy, lead palsy, and kidney damage are some of the clinical symptoms of chronic lead poisoning (WHO, 1976).

Mercury

Its persistent presence in the environment, bioaccumulation and transport in the aquatic chain, and levels in a variety of foods make mercury among the most dangerous of all metals in the human food chain. It occurs in three different forms:

Table 2 Lead Content of Some Foods and Drinks

Food	Mean (mg/kg)	Range (mg/kg)
Cereals	0.17	<0.01–0.81
Meat and fish	0.17	<0.01–0.70
Fruit (fresh)	0.12	<0.01–0.76
Fruit (canned)	0.40	0.04–10.0
Vegetables (fresh)	0.22	<0.01–1.5
Vegetables (canned)	0.24	0.01–1.5
Milk	0.03	<0.01–0.08
Drinking water	5[a]	1–50[a]
Alcoholic beverages		50–100[a]

[a]$\mu g/L$.
Source: WHO, 1976; Reilly, 1991.

elemental mercury, mercuric mercury, and alkyl mercury. The chemical form greatly influences absorption, distribution in body tissues, and the biological half-life. Normal human diets generally contain less than 50 μg mercury/kg food (Bouquiaux, 1974). In the absence of gross contamination of soil or irrigation water, the following levels (μg/kg wet weight) generally occur in different food groups: meat, 10; fish, 200; dairy products, 5; vegetables, 10; cereals, 10; other foods, 5 (Oehme, 1978). Thus seafood appears to be a prime source of mercury in the human diet.

Mercury is a cumulative poison and is stored mainly in the liver and kidney. The level of accumulation depends on the type of organism and the chemical form of mercury. Mercury in its pure metallic form is poorly absorbed, readily excreted from the body, and thus unlikely to cause poisoning. In contrast, the inorganic and organic compounds of mercury are highly toxic to humans. Methyl mercury has been listed as one of the six most dangerous chemicals in the environment (Bennet, 1984). It is efficiently absorbed from the food in the intestine, rapidly enters the blood stream, and is bound to plasma proteins. Methyl mercury also accumulates in the human brain. It is thus neurotoxic to both adults and the fetus (Berlin et al., 1963).

The clinical signs of methyl mercury poisoning generally manifest in sensory disturbances in the limbs, the tongue, and around the lips; irreversible damage to the central nervous system resulting in ataxia, tremor, slurred speech; tunnel vision blindness; loss of hearing; and finally death (Reilly, 1991). Selenium appears to counteract both inorganic and organic mercury poisoning in several animal species (Stoewsand et al., 1974).

Cadmium

Because of its high solubility in organic acids, cadmium contamination of the human food chain is quite common. Being highly toxic, it is recognized as one of the most dangerous trace elements in food and the environment (Vos et al., 1987). Therefore, similar to lead and mercury, cadmium levels are often monitored in the food supply and in drinking water by the health authorities, and the permitted levels are regulated by legislation in several countries.

Unless contamination has occurred, the levels of cadmium in most foods are normally very low (Table 3). The overall range appears to be 0.095–0.987 mg/kg, with a mean of 0.469 mg/kg. Generally, meat and seafoods tend to contain higher levels of cadmium than any other food groups. The dietary intake of cadmium in several countries was estimated to be 10–80 μg/day (Dabeka et al., 1987). The WHO standard for cadmium levels in the drinking water was established at 10 μg/L (WHO, 1963). Most well-documented cases of cadmium contamination of foods and subsequent human poisoning are reported from Japan and Australia (Asami, 1984; Rayment et al., 1989).

Under normal dietary conditions, about 6% of the cadmium ingested in food and beverages is believed to be absorbed by the human body (Reilly, 1991). Higher dietary levels of calcium and protein tend to increase cadmium absorption. Most of the absorbed cadmium is retained in the kidneys. Thus long-term chronic ingestion of cadmium often results in serious renal damage, as well as bone disease leading to brittleness and even collapse of the skeleton (Frieberg et al., 1974). Cadmium toxicity is the prime cause of itai-itai disease observed in certain population segments of Japan (Asami, 1984). Abnormally high levels of cadmium in

Table 3 Cadmium Content of Selected Foods

Food	Cadmium (µg/kg)
Bread	<2–43
Potatoes	<2–51
Cabbage	<2–26
Apples	<2–19
Poultry	<2–69
Minced beef	<2–28
Kidney (sheep)	13–2,000
Prawns	17–913
Seafoods	50–3,660
Drinking water	<1–21 µg/L

Source: WHO, 1963; Dabeka et al., 1987; Reilly, 1991.

the diet also enhance the rates of several cancers in humans (Browning, 1969). In human and animal nutrition, cadmium toxicity is counteracted by the presence of cobalt, selenium, and zinc.

Arsenic

Arsenic has been traditionally associated with homicide and the forensic scientist. Its toxicity is related to the chemical form of the element. Its inorganic compounds are the most toxic, followed by the organic arsenicals and finally arsine gas (Buck, 1978). In the past, arsenic-based herbicides, fungicides, wood preservatives of several kinds, insecticides, rodenticides, and sheep dips were in common usage. Because of their toxicity and the persistent nature of arsenic poison, their use at present has been severely restricted in many countries.

Because of its wide distribution in the environment and its past uses in agriculture, arsenic is present in most human foods. With the exception of seafood, it is generally present in very low levels of less than 0.5 mg/kg. A recent Canadian survey (Dabeka et al., 1987) has reported the following levels (µg/kg with ranges in the parentheses) in different food groups: cereal 8.6 (0.71–61); dairy products 2.58 (0.6–11.3); starchy vegetables 13.69 (4–81.9); other vegetables 2.60 (0.6–8.3); and meat and fish 60.1 (4–625). Cereals, starchy vegetables, and meat and seafood thus together accounted for over 65% of the daily intake of 2.6–101 µg of arsenic in the Canadian diet.

The average daily intake of arsenic was reported to be 62 µg in the United States (Gartrell et al., 1985); 55 µg in New Zealand (Dick et al., 1978); 89 µg in the United Kingdom (FACC, 1984), 15–45 µg in Sweden (Slorach et al., 1983), and 12 µg in Belgium (Buchet et al., 1983). The FAO/WHO maximum allowable daily intake of arsenic in the human diet is restricted to 2 µg/kg body weight (CAC, 1984).

Arsenic is also present in almost all potable waters with levels ranging from 0 to 0.2 mg/L. The U.S. Federal Regulations for drinking water set a maximum limit of 0.01 mg arsenic/L (Drinking Water Standards, 1962).

Both tri- and pentavalent arsenic are easily absorbed from food in the gastrointestinal tract. It is then rapidly transported to all organs and tissues. Arsenic is primarily accumulated in skins, nails, and hair and, to some extent, in bone and muscle. Total body levels of arsenic in humans have been estimated at 14–20 mg (Schroeder and Balassa, 1966).

Arsenic is a general protoplasmic poison with its pentavalent form being less toxic than the trivalent one. It binds to organic sulfhydral groups and thus inhibits the action of several enzymes, especially those involved in cellular metabolism and respiration (Reilly, 1991). Its clinical symptoms are manifested in the dilation and increased permeability of capillaries, especially in the intestine. Chronic arsenic poisoning generally results in loss of appetite leading to weight loss, gastrointestinal disturbances, peripheral neuritis, conjunctivitis, hyperkeratosis, and skin melanosis. Arsenic is also a suspected carcinogen (IARC, 1973). Arsenic is believed to counteract the toxicity of an excessive intake of selenium in the animal feeds (Rhian and Moxon, 1943).

Selenium

Although selenium is an essential trace element in both human and animal nutrition, its excessive intake often results in the manifestation of toxic syndromes. Selenosis of livestock has been widely reported from several parts of the world, including China, the United States, Australia, Mexico, Canada, Colombia, Israel, and Ireland (Reilly, 1991).

The presence of selenium in the human food chain is primarily influenced by its levels in agricultural soils. Its daily dietary intake, therefore, varies greatly with geographical region. Selenium consumption (μg/day) in the different parts of the world was estimated to be as follows: New Zealand, 28; the United States, 132; Canada, 98–224; Japan, 88; Venezuela, 326; the United Kingdom, 60; Italy, 13; China, 4.99 mg in a selenosis region, 750 μg in a high-selenium but nonselenosis region, and 11 μg in a selenium-deficient region (Thomson and Robinson, 1980; Reilly, 1991). The Food and Nutrition Board of the U.S. National Research Council recommends a range of 50–200 μg/day, with 10–40 for infants and 20–120 for children under the age of six.

Selenium occurs in food mainly in the form of seleno-amino acids, especially as selenomethionine and selenocysteine. About 80% of organic selenium ingested from foods appears to be absorbed, absorption generally being greater from plant foods than from meat or other animal products (Young et al., 1982). Metabolically, selenium occurs as a prosthetic group of glutathione peroxidase enzyme (Combs and Combs, 1984). The enzyme plays an important role as a free radical scavenger in human metabolism. Through its interactions, selenium also appears to counteract the toxicity of several heavy metals including cadmium, mercury, and silver.

Excessive intake of selenium in the human diet result in dermatitis, dizziness, brittle nails, gastric disturbances, hair loss, and a garlic odor on the breath. The margin of safety between essential trace levels of selenium in the human diet and for the manifestation of its toxic symptoms appears to be quite small.

Antimony

Antimony is toxic and occurs widely in many foods. Its levels are restricted by food regulations in several countries. High levels of antimony in the food are generally attributed to contamination from containers glazed with antimony-containing enamel in which the food is cooked or stored.

Very little is known about the dietary intake of antimony. The daily intake is believed to be 0.25–1.25 mg for children in the United States (Murthy et al., 1971). The U.S. Environmental Protection Agency (EPA) has recommended a limit, normally not exceeding 0.1 mg/L, for antimony in drinking water.

Prolonged exposure to antimony results in dermatitis, conjunctivitis, and nasal septum ulceration. Ingested antimony has apparently a low inherent toxicity (Nielsen, 1986). It is primarily stored in the liver, kidney, and skin. Symptoms of antimony poisoning include colic, nausea, weakness, and collapse with slow or irregular respiration and a lowered body temperature (Reilly, 1991).

Aluminum

Aluminum is widely used in several industrial applications. Its compounds are used in the food industry as food additives, in baking powder, processed cheese, manufactured meats and other products, cooking and storage utensils, and foil and takeout food containers. Aluminum is also widely used in the pharmaceutical and cosmetic industries, toothpaste, antiperspirants, and a variety of therapeutic agents and related products. Aluminum sulfate and other compounds are also used for particle sedimentation in water treatment (ALCOA, 1969). In recent years, high aluminum levels associated with short-term memory loss, dementia, parkinsonism, motor neuron disease, amyotrophic lateral sclerosis (ALS), and the brain tissue of Alzheimer's disease patients have generated a great deal of interest in its presence in the human food chain.

Intakes of aluminum in the U.S. diet were estimated to be 9 mg/d for teenage and adult females and 12–14 mg/d for teenage and adult males (Pennington, 1987). Pennington and Jones (1988) have reported the following aluminum levels (mg/kg) in 234 foods sampled in FDA's Total Diet Survey in 1984:

Cow's milk, 0.6; cheddar cheese, 0.19; American (processed) cheese, 0.411; infant
    formula (milk-based), 0.05
Meat: beef, 0.28; meat loaf, 1.26; bacon, 3.63; sausage, 1.82; roast chicken, 0.22
Fish: cod, 0.47; fish sticks, 51.4; canned tuna, 0.67
Fruit: apples, 0.14; cherries, 0.19; grapes, 1.81
Vegetables: brocolli, 0.98; canned beets, 0.26; carrots, 0.19
Cereals: corn grits, 0.2; oatmeal, 0.68; rice, 1.42
Cereal products: biscuits, 16.3; white bread, 2.33, rye bread, 4.07; pancakes from
    mix, 69.0, tortilla flour, 129.0, chocolate cake, 86.0
Others: milk chocolate, 6.84; chocolate chip cookies, 5.61
Tea from bag, 4.46
Domestic water (eastern United States), 0.12

With the exception of certain spices and tea leaves, natural levels of aluminum in foods tend to be quite low. In contrast, most dietary aluminum primarily comes from the use of food additives such as sodium aluminum phosphates and aluminum silicates. These compounds are widely used as acidifying agents, emulsifiers, binders, anticaking agents, stabilizers, thickeners, bleaching agents, and texturizers. Contamination may also occur from the use of aluminum utensils and cans in the food industry. Water generally is not an important source of dietary aluminum.

The chemical form of the element is an important factor controlling the absorption of aluminum in the human nutrition. In one study, about 7% of ingested aluminum was absorbed by healthy young men consuming a diet containing 10–33 mg of the element over a 28-day period (Gormican and Catli, 1971). As compared to its phosphate salts, aluminum citrates appear to be readily absorbed from the gut. Vitamin D, parathyroid hormone, and iron levels appear to influence the absorption of aluminum (Reilly, 1991). In the human body, aluminum is primarily stored in liver, kidney, spleen, bone, and brain and heart tissue.

Under certain conditions, aluminum is known to be toxic to plants and fish. Accumulation of aluminum in the human brain has been associated with Alzheimer's disease (Crapper et al., 1973). The use of aluminum-containing water in kidney dialysis and the ingestion of aluminum-containing phosphate binding gels by renal patients were reported to cause dialysis dementia (Platts et al., 1977). Excessive intakes of aluminum in the human diets are also associated with osteomalacia and bone fractures (Boyce et al., 1982). Aluminum has also been implicated in metabolic alkalosis, parkinsonism-dementia, and bowel obstruction (Pennington and Jones, 1988).

Tin

Tin is widely distributed in small amounts in most soils. It occurs at <1.0 mg/kg levels in all major food groups except for canned vegetables (9–80 mg/kg) and fruit products (12–129 mg/kg) (Sherlock and Smart, 1984). A primary source of tin contamination is the use of lacquered cans in the canning industry.

Tin in foods appears to be poorly absorbed and is excreted mainly in feces (WHO, 1973). Small amounts of absorbed tin may be retained in kidney, liver, and bone. High levels of tin in food can cause acute poisoning, the fatal toxic dose for humans being 5–7 mg/kg body weight. Chronic tin poisoning is manifested in growth retardation, anemia, and histopathological changes in the liver. Tin also influences iron absorption and hemoglobin formation (Reilly, 1991).

III. PESTICIDES

Pesticides, in general, refer to a group of chemicals used worldwide in agricultural production to control, destroy, or inhibit weeds, insects, fungi, and other pests. Approximately 320 active pesticide ingredients are available in a few thousand different registered formulations (Hotchkiss, 1992). However, not all compounds or formulations are used. Some formulations may have only limited use, some none at all, while others are used in large quantities.

Fewer than 1% of all 500,000 estimated species of plants, animals, and microorganisms are known pests. The remaining greatly benefit agriculture and other sectors of world economy by degrading organic wastes, removing pollutants from water and soil, recycling vital chemicals within the ecosystem, buffering air pollutants, moderating climatic changes, conserving soil and water, providing medicines, pigments, and spices, preserving genetic diversity, and supplying food via the harvest of fish and other animal life (Pimentel, 1991). Nevertheless, the 1% pest component is extremely costly. Insects, plant pathogens, and weeds destroy about 37% of U.S. agricultural production, with losses being 50–60% in the developing world.

According to Pimentel (1991), approximately 500 million kg of pesticides are applied annually in an effort to control pests in the United States alone at a cost of about $4 billion. This figure, however, does not consider the indirect costs related to the destruction of beneficial organisms, the disturbance of ecological systems, and human poisoning and illness. Such indirect costs are estimated to be at least one billion dollars and could be twice that amount (Pimentel, 1991).

Of the estimated total pesticide uses in the United States, 60% are herbicides, 24% insecticides and 16% are fungicides applied to about 61% of the U.S. cropland (Pimentel, 1981). The application of agricultural pesticides, however, is not evenly distributed. Pimentel (1981) estimates that 93% of all food crops are treated with some type of pesticide as compared to less than 10% of forage crops. Nearly 75% of the total herbicides used are applied to corn and soybeans, with corn alone accounting for about 52% of the total usage. Of the total insecticides used, nearly 40% are applied to cotton and another 20% to corn. In contrast, fungicides and soil fumigants are used primarily on fruit and vegetable crops, which account for a relatively small percentage of agricultural land. These compounds are, however, important residues in the human diet.

A. Classification

There are three major chemical groups of insecticides: organochlorines, organophosphates, and carbamates. A fourth group includes synthetic pyrethroids such as permethrin, bioresmethrin, tetramethrin, allethrin, phenothrin, and deltamethrin. These are artificially synthesized chemicals related to natural pyrethrins found in chrysanthemums. These substances have generally low toxicity in mammals, including humans, and most are biodegradable.

The most commonly used herbicides are also organochlorine compounds (e.g., 2,4-D, 2,4,5-T, MCPA, PCP Picloram, Dicamba, and sodium trichloroacetate), but include others such as paraquat, diquat, MSMA, simazine, amitrole, DSMA, and glycerophosphates. The commonly used fungicides are pentachlorophenol, copper arsenate, Benomyl, cadmium chloride, captan, Maneb, mancozeb, Thiram, and Zineb. Most are based on transition and heavy metals as one of the active ingredients. Warfarin, thallium sulfate, bromadiolone, and coumatretralyl are generally used as rodenticides to control rats and mice, while ethylene dibromide is the most widely used fumigant in the world.

B. Toxicology

Most pesticides are extremely potent carcinogenic, teratogenic, and fetotoxic chemicals. Some also adversely affect the central nervous system. The organochlorines in the human tissue are bioactivated by liver enzymes, rather than being detoxified and excreted. The resulting epoxides and peroxides cause membrane damage and lead to the formation of free radicals. These free radicals in turn can interact with DNA to act as mutagens (Pryor, 1980). Organochlorines also restrict the transport of minerals across cell membranes and inhibit cellular respiration. Lindane specifically inhibits the energy generating center of cells.

Organophosphates inhibit acetyl cholinesterase, a key enzyme involved in the nerve transmission process. These pesticides are often highly toxic and, being volatile, can be easily inhaled. They are more biodegradable than organochlorines but are still suspected of chronic and delayed effects.

Carbamates also act as nerve poisons, but their toxicities are variable. The most toxic carbamate is carbaryl, which is believed to be converted into a potent carcinogen in the stomach. It may also cause sterility. The toxicology of heavy metals in human nutrition was described earlier.

C. Associated Risks

When pesticides are applied improperly, resulting residues in foods can pose significant health risks to consumers. The use of pesticides in agricultural production represents three related but distinct risks defined as the quantifiable probability that harm or injury will occur (Hotchkiss, 1992):

1. The environmental risks associated with adverse effects on nontarget organisms and ground water contamination
2. Occupational risks associated with agricultural workers, which are considerably higher than other sources of human exposures and pose the foremost human health concern related to pesticides
3. The occurrence of pesticides as residues on or in edible foods

The occupational risks can be reduced by strict controls and use of appropriate protective technology. The environmental effects are associated with some pesticides, especially heavy metal compounds and organochlorines. These are extremely toxic and are resistant to biodegradation. They can last for decades in the soil and, being fat soluble, can be stored in human and animal fat tissues, liver, and the central nervous system to produce suspected chronic and delayed effects. In lactating animals, residues are removed more quickly and end up in the animal's milk. The use of fat-soluble stable pesticides, or disposal of their wastes where they might volatilize or be washed from soil or foliar surfaces into water, can also lead to the accumulation of residues in plants and animals. It is now a well-known fact that residual levels of DDT, an organochlorine pesticide widely used in the 1950s and 1960s, occur in every living form on the planet, while heptachlor, a toxic metabolite of chlordane, is now found in over 90% of the population.

Organochlorines have become most hazardous to human health through a process called biomagnification. Spray drifts and drain-offs from treated fields contaminate water bodies. Small plankton and other organisms living in the water absorb the pesticides and store them in their tissues. The next animal feeding on the plankton in the food chain takes in a diet enriched with the pesticides and their metabolites. After a period of time, the concentration of these residues rises in the animal. There is thus a stepwise increase in pesticide concentration along the food chain. Eventually, they all accumulate in human adipose tissue with increasing age.

D. Residues in Food

Public concern over pesticide residues in food has been increasing during the last decade. A recent national survey by the Food Marketing Institute (1988) showed that approximately 75% of consumers are very concerned about pesticide residues in their food—a higher percentage than that of consumers worried about cholesterol, fat, salt, additives, or any other components. Contributing to such concerns have been the discovery of hazardous effects from certain pesticides, such as ethylene dibromide and chlordane, that were once deemed safe and publicized acute food poisoning from improperly used pesticides. Such was the case with aldicarb contamination of watermelon in the western United States and Canada in 1985 (OTA, 1988). The high level of uncertainty concerning the health effects of pesticide residues has further heightened consumer concern.

To address the public's concern, the U.S. EPA requested the Board on Agriculture of the National Research Council (NRC) in 1985 to study the EPA's methods for setting tolerances for pesticide residues in food. The Committee on Scientific and Regulatory Uses Underlying Pesticide Use Patterns and Agricultural Innovation that was subsequently formed undertook three principal tasks. First, it examined the statutory framework for setting tolerances for pesticide residues in food and the operation of the tolerance-setting process at the EPA. Second, it developed a computerized data base for estimating the impacts of the current standards for setting tolerances on dietary cancer risks as well as on pesticide use and development. Finally, it analyzed the impacts of different standards for establishing pesticide tolerances on dietary cancer risk and pesticide use and development. The following information is largely based on this committee's report.

The NRC (1987) study used a Q^* rating to express quantitatively a pesticide's oncogenic potency. The Q^* value was the slope of the dose-response curve (namely, tumor incidence vs. changes in dose) from animal tests yielding a positive response. The potency factor was expressed as tumors/mg of pesticide/kg body weight/d, and it estimated tumor incidence expected to occur at the relatively low doses of pesticides in the U.S. diet. A high Q^* indicates a strong oncogenic response (i.e., more tumors) to the administered dose; a low number indicates a weak response. These ratings for different pesticides were averages derived from several positive oncogenicity studies in animals. Based on this, the dietary oncogenic risk was calculated by multiplying the Q^* value by the exposure, i.e., food consumption × pesticide residues.

The NRC (1987) study found that, among the 28 pesticide residues commonly occurring in the U.S. diet, fungicides accounted for about 60% of all estimated dietary oncogenic risk, 27% from crop uses of herbicides, and 13% from insecticides. Similarly, about 55% of the total estimated dietary oncogenic risk occurs from residues on crops that have raw (35%) and processed (20%) food forms, while the remaining 45% risk was from foods that the EPA considers to have no processed form. These foods include several fruits and vegetables and *all* meat, milk, and poultry products.

When estimated risks from individual foods were ranked, 15 crops and animal products contributed nearly 80% of all estimated dietary oncogenic risk from pesticide residues, the remaining 20% coming from 186 other food products studied (Table 4). Tomatoes and beef were the two food crops posing the greatest risks. The data on estimated crop risks broken down among fungicides, herbicides, and insecticides are summarized in Table 5. Fungicide residues on just 10 crops represented 42% of the total estimated dietary risk.

The NRC (1987) study indicates that relatively few pesticides account for high percentages of total estimated risks in selected high-risk foods. The herbicide, linuron, and the two pesticides, chlordimeform and permethrin, represented more than 99% of the total estimated herbicide and insecticide risk associated with most crops, while no single fungicide accounted for more than 43% of the total fungicide

Table 4 Foods with the Greatest Estimated Oncogenic Risk

Food	Total dietary oncogenic risk estimates	
	Number	Percentage
Tomatoes	8.75×10^{-4}	14.9
Beef	6.49×10^{-4}	11.1
Potatoes	5.21×10^{-4}	8.9
Oranges	3.76×10^{-4}	6.4
Lettuce	3.44×10^{-4}	5.8
Apples	3.23×10^{-4}	5.5
Peaches	3.23×10^{-4}	5.5
Pork	2.67×10^{-4}	4.5
Wheat	1.92×10^{-4}	3.3
Soybeans	1.28×10^{-4}	2.2
Beans	1.23×10^{-4}	2.1
Carrots	1.22×10^{-4}	2.1
Chicken	1.12×10^{-4}	1.9
Corn (bran, grain)	1.09×10^{-4}	1.9
Grapes	1.09×10^{-4}	1.9
Total[a]		78.0

[a]Percentage of the 15 crops based on a total of 201 foods analyzed
Source: NRC, 1987.

risk from any crop. Similarly, the study also reveals that about 99% of the herbicide risk from estimated residues in beef is from one herbicide, while 72% of the estimated tomato risk was from five fungicides, which were close analogs of each other.

As a reference, the WHO guidelines on acceptable daily intakes and maximum residue limits of different pesticides are presented in Table 6.

E. Residue-Monitoring Program

The federal regulations governing pesticide use were first enacted as the Federal Insecticide Act (FIA) in 1910. The FIA was later replaced by the Federal Insecticide, Fungicide and Rodenticide Act (FIFRA) of 1947, which, as amended, remains the basis for regulating the use of pesticides today. Currently, federal jurisdiction over pesticide residues in foods is divided among four bodies: the EPA, the Food and Drug Administration (FDA) of the U.S. Department of Health and Human Services, and the Food Safety and Inspection Service (FSIS) and Agricultural Marketing Service (AMS) of the U.S. Department of Agriculture (USDA). Their authority for this work comes primarily from five laws: FIFRA, Federal Food, Drug and Cosmetic Act (FFDCA), Federal Meat Inspection Act (FMIA), the Poultry Products Inspection Act (PPIA), and the Egg Products Inspection Act (EPIA).

The EPA, under FIFRA, must register a pesticide before it can be distributed or sold in the United States. All pesticides that are legally sold and used on domestically grown or imported food crops, therefore, must be registered with EPA *for that crop* prior to use. Compounds that may be deemed safe by the EPA

Table 5 Estimated Oncogenic Risk from Fungicides, Herbicides, and Insecticides in Major Foods

Pesticide and Crop	Estimated risk	
	Number	Percentage
Fungicides		
Tomatoes	8.23×10^{-4}	14.1
Oranges	3.72×10^{-4}	6.3
Apples	3.18×10^{-4}	5.4
Peaches	2.86×10^{-4}	4.9
Lettuce	1.81×10^{-4}	0.1
Potatoes	1.29×10^{-4}	2.2
Beans	1.17×10^{-4}	2.0
Grapes	1.08×10^{-4}	1.8
Wheat	6.65×10^{-5}	1.1
Celery	6.04×10^{-5}	1.1
% of Total Risk		42.0
Herbicides		
Beef	5.38×10^{-4}	10.0
Potatoes	3.89×10^{-4}	6.7
Pork	2.17×10^{-4}	3.7
Soybeans	1.22×10^{-4}	2.1
Wheat	1.22×10^{-4}	2.1
Carrots	5.95×10^{-5}	1.0
Corn	4.98×10^{-5}	0.9
Asparagus	1.48×10^{-5}	0.3
Celery	1.04×10^{-5}	0.2
Milk	7.87×10^{-6}	0.1
% of Total Risk		27.1
Insecticides		
Lettuce	1.59×10^{-4}	2.5
Chicken	1.11×10^{-4}	1.9
Beef	1.10×10^{-4}	1.9
Cottonseed	9.95×10^{-5}	1.7
Milk	5.19×10^{-5}	0.9
Tomatoes	5.17×10^{-5}	0.9
Pork	5.02×10^{-5}	0.9
Peaches	3.50×10^{-5}	0.6
Spinach	2.80×50^{-5}	0.5
Cabbage	1.82×10^{-5}	0.3
% of Total Risk		12.1

Source: NRC, 1987.

but are not registered for a specific crop cannot be used legally on that crop, except under special state-approved circumstances. The most important health-related provision of the registration process is the requirement that pesticide manufacturers submit scientific data to the EPA demonstrating both effectiveness and lack of significant health risks for each crop use.

Table 6 FAO/WHO Guidelines for Acceptable Daily Intake (ADI),
Maximum Residue Limit (MRL), and Extraneous Residue Limit
(ERL) for Pesticide Residues in Human Foods

Pesticide	ADI (mg/kg body weight)	MRL or ERL (mg/kg)
sec-Butylamine	0.1	
Captan	0.1	0.1
Cartap	0.1	20
Chlordimeform	0.0001	2
Chlorothalonil	0.03	0.2
Coumaphos	0.0005	0.02
Cyanofenphos	0.005	
Cyhexatin	0.008	0.05–2
DDT	0.005	0.05–5
Dimethoate	0.02	0.05–3
Diquat	0.008	0.2–5
Ethiofencarb	0.1	
Fenamiphos	0.0006	0.2
Fenthion	0.0005	
Formothion	0.02	0.2
Guazatine	0.03	0.1–5
Lindane	0.01	0.01–1
Omethoate	0.0005	
Paraquat	0.002	0.05–2
Parathion-methyl	0.001	
Phosmet	0.005	0.01–10
Primicarb	0.01	0.05–50
Propargite	0.08	0.5–5
Tecnazene	0.01	0.1–2
Thiophanate-methyl	0.08	
Trichlorfon	0.01	0.05–2
Triforine	0.02	0.02–5

Source: WHO, 1979.

The EPA also establishes tolerances for pesticide residues on raw commodities under section 408 of the FFDCA. Enacted in 1954, this law stipulates that tolerances are to be set at levels deemed necessary to protect the public health, while taking into account the need for "an adequate, wholesome, and economical food supply." Section 408 thus explicitly recognizes that pesticides confer benefits and risks and that both should be taken into account in setting raw commodity tolerances.

Pesticide residues that concentrate in processed foods above the levels authorized to be present in or on their parent raw commodities are governed by FFDCA section 409, the law governing food additives. Under section 409, such residues must be proven safe, i.e., showing a "reasonable certainty" that "no harm" to consumers will result when the additive is put to its intended use. Consideration of benefits, however, is not authorized. Moreover, section 409 contains the Delaney Clause, which prohibits the approval of a food additive that has been found to "induce cancer" (or, under the EPA's interpretation, to induce either benign or malignant tumors, i.e., is oncogenic) in humans or animals. Thus, if any portion of a crop to which an oncogenic pesticide has been applied is processed in a way that will concentrate residues, the EPA's current policy is to deny not only a section 409 tolerance for the processed food but also a section 408 tolerance for residues of the pesticide in or on the raw commodity. Further, if the required section 408 tolerances cannot be granted for a food-use pesticide, the EPA must also deny registration of the pesticide under the FIFRA. A list of all current oncogenic pesticides with section 409 food or feed additive tolerances is presented in Table 7.

A large and complex system has been established for controlling the occurrence of pesticides as residues in foods. Nearly all elements of the agricultural system are actively involved in controlling the use of pesticides. Regulation thus takes the form of both premarket federal and state government controls, as well as post-market "policing." The private sector also plays an effective role in regulation. Growers, food processors, and food manufacturers all have an economic interest in the safe use of pesticides.

However, the use of pesticides in agriculture is not without serious health and environmental risks or costs. Nevertheless, their residues in the human food chain are monitored by numerous agencies. The adequacy of testing of pesticides, however, still remains questionable. Carcinogenic effects in humans may take 20–30 years to appear after exposure to the carcinogen. Similarly, mutagenic effects may surface generations after the initial exposure. Nor have the possible adverse effects of pesticide residues on behavior been examined. Surprisingly, very few studies examine the possible adverse interactions among different pesticides and among pesticides and other components used during crop production. The cumulative effect of chronic low-dose exposure to a single pesticide and the additive effect

Table 7 Presumed Oncogenic Pesticides with Section 409 Tolerances

Food-additive tolerances	Feed-additive tolerances
Benomyl	Acephate
Captan	Amitraz
Chlordimeform	Benomyl
Daminozide	Captan
Glyphosate	Chlordimeform
Azinphos-methyl	Cyromazine
Dicofol	Daminozide
Maleic hydrazide	Glyphosate
Mancozeb	Azinphos-methyl
Oryzalin	Linuron
Paraquat	Mancozeb
Toxaphene	Methanearsonic acid
Trifluralin	Paraquat
	Tetrachlorvinphos
	Thiodicarb
	Thiophanate-methyl

of small quantities of many different pesticides have also not been thoroughly examined.

IV. DRUG RESIDUE CONTAMINATION

The use of drugs as additives in animal feeds has been approved since the early 1950's. Among these nonnutritive additives are hormones, antibiotics, sulfonamides, nitrofurans, and arsenicals. These additives have had a major impact in increasing the efficiency of livestock production for human food purposes. For example, the hormone diethylstilbestrol (DES) reduced the amount of feed required 10–20% by stimulating the growth of cattle, thereby saving approximately 8 billion pounds of cattle feed annually in the United States alone (ACS, 1980). Without its use, retail expenditures for beef would have increased by about $480 million per year. However, because residues that remain in edible tissues of animals may cause cancer in humans, the U.S. FDA banned its use in livestock feed. The action was enlarged by the approval of other drugs that could replace DES for similar end uses.

Antibiotics and other drugs are administered to livestock at therapeutic, prophylactic, or subtherapeutic concentrations (Moorman and Koening, 1992). Therapeutic administration (200–1000 g drug/ton of feed, 220–1100 ppm) is used for disease treatment. Prophylactic doses (100–400 g/ton, 110–440 ppm) are used to prevent infectious diseases caused by bacteria or protozoa, whereas subtherapeutic administration is often used to increase feed efficiency and growth promotion. The FDA defines a subtherapeutic dose as ≥200 g (2.2–220 ppm) of the drug per ton of feed for 2 weeks or longer (NAS, 1980).

Although the mechanisms of action by which such drugs cause growth and feed enhancement are not well understood, the following are frequently cited (Franco et al., 1990; Moorman and Koening, 1992):

1. Microorganisms responsible for mild but unrecognized infections are suppressed.
2. Microbial production of growth-depressing toxins is reduced.
3. Antimicrobial agents reduce microbial destruction of essential nutrients in the gastrointestinal tract, or there is increased synthesis of vitamins or other growth factors.
4. The efficiency of absorption and utilization of nutrients is enhanced.

It is estimated that more than 45% of the 2.1–2.5 million kg of antimicrobial drugs used in the United States annually are utilized for animal feed supplementation (DuPont and Steele, 1987; Moorman and Koenig, 1992). Nearly 80% of poultry, 75% of swine, 60% of feedlot cattle, and 75% of dairy calves marketed or raised in the United States are estimated to have been fed an antimicrobial drug at some time during life. One survey estimated that the use of antibiotics in livestock production saved the consumers more than $2 billion in 1973 (NAS, 1980). The possible routes by which drug residues contaminate various milk and meat products are listed in Table 8.

According to Brady and Katz (1988), drug residues in human foods should be avoided for the following reasons:

Table 8 Possible Sources of Drug Residues in Milk and Meat Products

---

Extended usage or excessive dosage of approved drugs
Poor records of treatment
Increased frequency of intramammary antibiotic treatment on farms
Failure to observe recommended label withdrawal time
Prolonged drug clearance
Treated animal identification problems
Errors due to hired help
Large herd size
Increased frequency of use of medicated feed
Contaminated milking equipment
Multiple dosing
Milker or producer mistakes: accidental transfer in bulk tank
Products not used according to label directions
Lack of advice on withdrawal period
Withholding milk from treated quarters only
Early calving or short dry periods
Purchase of treated cows
Use of dry cow therapy to lactating cows

Source: Booth and Harding, 1986; Jones and Seymour, 1988; McEwen et al., 1991.

1. Some residues can cause idiosyncratic reactions in ultrasensitive consumers, which could be extremely serious.
2. Generally, drug residues above the prescribed tolerance limits are illegal.
3. Some drug residues in fluid dairy products are capable of interfering with starter cultures used in processed milk products and cheese.
4. Residues are generally indicative of the fact that the food may have come from animals that had a serious infection.
5. Public awareness and concern regarding the natural wholesomeness of our food supply is increasing.
6. Most importantly, drug residue contamination of human foods generally encourages the selection and spread of transferable multiple-resistance plasmids. This in turn leads to development of drug-resistant microorganisms that are pathogenic to humans.

The plasmid-mediated resistance was first recognized from studies on clinical bacterial isolates resistant to several gram-negative antimicrobial drugs that were able to transfer the genetic information encoding these resistances to other bacteria (Gustafson, 1991). Since the two most widely used families of antibiotics in animal feeds, the tetracyclines and the penicillins (beta-lactam group), are also used for the treatment of microbial infections in humans, this became the central point of focus on feed antibiotics and human health risks. The two greatest concerns were that (1) the use of certain antibiotics in animal feeds could generate large numbers of resistance plasmids in the enteric flora of livestock and the genetic material might eventually encode antibiotic resistance in human pathogens, and (2) the use of antibiotics in livestock feeds, particularly subtherapeutic or prophylactic, could ultimately induce a significant loss of antibiotic efficacy in human medicine.

The evidence for both these concerns largely comes from epidemiological studies of disease outbreaks. The Centers for Disease Control (CDC) estimated that 16% of the cases reported in the 1985 salmonellosis milk outbreak in Illinois were attributable to human consumption of antimicrobials (Ryan et al., 1987). The illness would not have occurred had the milk been contaminated with an antimicrobial-sensitive strain. The outbreak affected an estimated 200,000 people, making it the largest recorded outbreak of salmonellosis ever identified in the United States. The causative organism was *Salmonella typhimurium*, which contained an antibiotic resistance plasmid for ampicillin, tetracycline, carbenicillin, streptomycin, sulfisoxazole, erythromycin, sulfadiazine, penicillin, and a mixture of sulfabenzamide, sulfacetamide, and sulfathiazole. Ryan et al. (1987) also found through patient surveys that ill persons who had been taking antimicrobials that the *Salmonella* was resistant to consumed less milk than other ill persons, suggesting the antimicrobials lowered the infectious dose of *Salmonella*.

Similar outbreaks of salmonellosis in Great Britain in the mid-1960s were also traced to dairy calves that were exposed to low levels of antibiotics in feeds (*Federal Register*, 1977). The Swann Committee that was formed to study antibiotic resistance transfer and human health implications recommended that antibiotics used to treat human disease should not be used as feed additives for growth promotion. The British law banning such drug uses was subsequently enacted in 1970.

According to Moorman and Koening (1992), if salmonellosis in livestock takes a septic form, several antibiotics that are currently available to the veterinarian may be rendered useless. Their conclusions were based on the practice of the nonjudicious exposure of livestock to subtherapeutic doses of antibiotics in feeds commonly used in the livestock industry in the United States. It may also further reduce the effectiveness of antibiotic treatment of infectious diseases in humans. Indeed the CDC estimates that 25% of the *Salmonella* isolated from human infections are resistant to antibiotics and that antibiotic therapy of human salmonellosis is rarely the prescribed treatment (Linton, 1984; Holmberg et al., 1984).

Apart from the selection of plasmid-mediated resistant human pathogens, a direct consequence of the use of these drugs in the livestock industry, drug residue contamination of human foods is also undesirable from a public health viewpoint. It is estimated that 10% of the U.S. population is sensitive to penicillin (Jones and Seymour, 1988). Its residues, therefore, may cause hypersensitivity reactions. However, it should also be noted that, with the exception of the penicillins, such immunological reactions by humans to antimicrobial drugs used in animals are generally uncommon. In fact, such reactions from eating food contaminated with antibiotic residues have never been observed to cause anaphylactic reactions (Hewitt, 1975). The only adverse reaction of the hypersensitivity type has been associated with penicillin in milk, resulting in allergic reactions such as skin rashes, hives, asthma, and anaphylactic shock at concentrations as low as 0.003 IU penicillin/mL (Hewitt, 1975; Lindemayr et al., 1981). Allison (1985) later contradicted these arguments, suggesting that there is no evidence of an effect of oral administration (e.g., food consumption) on hypersensitivity. It was postulated that this was only a risk to extremely sensitive individuals and that hypersensitivity usually followed parenteral administration.

After reviewing data on drug-resistant plasmid transfer, the FDA published its intent to ban the subtherapeutic use of penicillin in 1977 (*Federal Register*, 1977). It also called for a restriction on the use of tetracycline and tetracycline-combination drugs. After much deliberation, the U.S. Congress requested the FDA to further study the relationship between antibiotic use and human health. As of July 1991, 23 antimicrobial agents were approved by the FDA for one or more uses as additives in poultry and livestock feeds (Anonymous, 1991). The regulations also call for specific withdrawal times after treatment of antibiotics for livestock prior to lactation or slaughter. For example, FDA regulations require the discarding of milk from treated cows for 96 hours following the last administration of the antibiotic.

In addition to withholding requirements, the FDA establishes tolerance limits for antibiotic residues in milk and meat tissues. The "safe levels" used by the FDA are only used as guides for prosecutorial purposes. They do not legalize residues found in milk that are below the safe level (Moorman and Koenig, 1992). For some drugs, no tolerance and/or safe level of the residue is allowed. The tolerance or safe levels for the current 23 FDA-approved drug residues in milk are summarized in Table 9.

Residues persist in the milk supply, but the magnitude of the problem is not clear. Two studies, co-sponsored by the *Wall Street Journal* and the Center for Science in the Public Interest (CSPI), were reviewed by Moorman and Koening

Table 9 Tolerances and/or Safe Levels of Animal Drug Residues in Milk Established by the Milk Safety Branch of FDA Center for Food Safety and Applied Nutrition

Drug	Tolerance and/or safe levels (ppb)[a]
Ampicillin	10
Amoxicillin	10
Cloxacillin	10
Cephapirin	20
Neomycin	150
Novobiocin	100
Tylosin	50
Erythromycin	50
Gentamicin	50
Dihydrostreptomycin	125
Tetracycline	80
Oxytetracycline	30
Chlortetracycline	30
Sulfachloropyridazine	10
Sulfadimethoxine	10
Sulfadiazine	10
Sulfamerazine	10
Sulfamethazine	10
Sulfamethiozole	10
Sulfanilamide	10
Sulfapyridine	10
Sulfaquinoxaline	10
Sulfathiazole	10

[a]Parts per billion = μg antimicrobial/L fluid milk.

(1992). They revealed the presence of antibiotics and sulfonamide residues in milk samples. Of the samples collected in 10 major U.S. cities, 38% were contaminated with sulfamethazine (a suspected carcinogen), sulfa drugs, and other antibiotics. These findings were in contrast with results from an earlier FDA-sponsored survey, which found a 1.5% sulfamethazine incidence level for samples collected from 23 states.

The issue of drug residues in foods has encouraged the development of numerous analytical test methods. The increasing use of drug-specific and rapid enzyme immunoassays by the livestock industry and a stricter control by the regulatory agencies have resulted in a significant decrease in the amount of drug-contaminated food sold in the retail market. The recent data reported by the FDA Milk Safety Branch on drug residue test results from January to June 1992 confirm these findings (FDA, 1992). During this period, 1,828,020 farm trucks containing 59.5 billion lb of milk from 38 states were screened by the industry for beta-lactam drug residues in accordance with the new requirements in Appendix N of the Pasteurized Milk Ordinance. Drug residues were found in 1,505 farm trucks containing 45,610,408 lb of milk (0.08%). Based on the average milk price ($11.64/cwt), the milk with drug residues was worth more than $5.2 million.

Additional drug residue testing results reported by 50 of the 51 state regulatory agencies included: sulfonamides, 12 positives of 26,818 samples from 20 states; tetracyclines, 7 positives out of 9,196 samples from 10 states; gentamicin, 1 positive of 1,556 samples from six states; and ivermectin, 2 positives out of 23 samples from one state.

During the same period, state regulatory agencies reported that four of 52,618 (0.008%) Grade A finished product samples were positive for drug residues. This compared to 0.02% (24 out of 107,381 samples) that were positive in 1991 (FDA, 1992).

Thus the development and more widespread use of increasingly sensitive and reliable analytical test methods as well as increased surveillance and regulatory activity in the areas of antibiotic residue testing have resulted in significantly lowering the drug residue contamination of food in the retail market. Drugs certainly have an important role in safeguarding both animal and human health. The health consequence of chronic subtherapeutic use of broad-spectrum antibiotics for growth promotion in animals leading to the selection of multidrug-resistant pathogens, however, appears to be of far greater significance than the actual drug residues themselves in our food supply. Subtherapeutic uses of drugs, therefore, should be discontinued in light of these consequences and the availability of alternative measures. Thus it is toward a more defined therapeutic use of these agents that the present-day livestock industry should strive.

V. FOOD-PACKAGING CONTAMINANTS

Unintentional additives that enter our food during processing derive mainly from materials in prolonged contact with the food. Certain substances migrate from the packaging materials: metals from cans, unpolymerized chemicals and polymerizing agents from plastic wrappings and coatings, inks and pigments from labels.

A. Food-Packaging Materials

The materials widely used for food packaging or in food contact applications include paper and coated-paper products, cellulose products, cellophane, metals such as tinplate, aluminum, stainless steel, and pewter, ceramics, glass, rubber, plastics, and miscellaneous materials such as wood, fabric, etc. Most of these materials have been in use for many years and have given rise to very few problems. Plastics, in contrast, while offering many advantages as a new range of packaging materials at the same time involve contact between food and a whole new range of chemical components not previously used in the food industry and for which no previous experience was available. Migration of additives used in their manufacture causes the greatest concern relating to food safety issues.

All plastics, in addition to the basic polymer derived from the petroleum industry, contain a number of other substances added either deliberately during manufacturing and processing or, unavoidably, as residues from polymerization reactions. Polymers themselves, being of very high molecular weight, inert, and of limited solubility in aqueous and fatty systems, are unlikely to be transferred into food to any significant extent (Crosby, 1981). Even if fragments were accidentally swallowed, they would not react with body fluids present in the digestive system. Concern over the safety-in-use of plastics as food-packaging materials arises principally from the possible toxicity of other low molecular weight components that may be present in the product and, hence, leached into the foodstuff during storage.

B. Sources of Contamination

Packaging contaminants from plastics primarily arise from two sources:

1. Polymerization residues including monomers, oligomers (with a molecular weight of up to 200), catalysts (mainly metallic salts and organic peroxides), solvents, emulsifiers and wetting agents, raw material impurities, plant contaminants, inhibitors, decomposition and side reaction products
2. Processing aids such as antioxidants, antiblocking agents, antistatic agents, heat and light stabilizers, plasticizers, lubricants and slip agents, pigments, fillers, mould release agents, and fungicides

The more volatile gaseous monomers, e.g., ethylene, propylene, vinyl chloride, usually decrease in concentration with time, but very low levels may persist in the finished product almost indefinitely (Crompton, 1979; Crosby, 1981). Styrene and acrylonitrile residues are generally the most difficult to remove.

Since compounds of the first group are present inadvertently, not much can be done to remove them. However, the efforts made by the industry to reduce vinyl chloride monomer levels in particular illustrate the effects of optimum manufacturing processes on the purity of the final product. In contrast, chemicals added deliberately during formulation to alter the processing, mechanical, or other properties of the polymer are likely to be present in greater amounts than polymerization residues and should be subject to strict quality control. Additives in the second group listed above are normally restricted to compounds appearing on an approved list for food contact use. Most legislative authorities now require extraction and migration tests on the finished product for the protection of the consumer. Analytical methods for the determination of a number of individual additives in extractants, in food simulants, and in polymers have been reviewed by Crompton (1979).

C. Toxicological Aspects

The toxicological aspects of most additives mentioned in group 2 above are described elsewhere in this book. The carcinogenic risk of some monomers to humans is briefly described below.

Vinyl Chloride

IARC (1973) has reviewed the relevant biological data and epidemiological studies on humans on the safety of vinyl chloride. Rats, mice, and hamsters have all been exposed to varying levels of vinyl chloride monomer (VCM), either by inhalation or by oral administration. Maltoni et al. (1974) showed that inhalation of levels of VCM in the range of 50–10,000 ppm in air for 4 h/d, 5 d/wk for 12 months resulted in the production of a number of tumors at different sites, including angiosarcomas of the liver. Oral administration of doses as low as 3.33 mg/kg body weight were also shown to be carcinogenic. VCM has also been shown to be mutagenic in Ames test, and metabolic studies provide some evidence of alkylation of nucleic acids (Crosby, 1981). The principal products formed during metabolism are chloroethylene oxide and chloroacetaldehyde.

In the IARC (1973) study, the principal toxic effects of VCM in humans included lesions of the bones in the terminal joints of the fingers and toes as well as histopathological changes in the liver and spleen. Long-term exposure gave rise to a rare form of liver cancer (angiosarcoma). VCM also has a long latent period for tumor development, requiring as many as 20 years for the symptoms to appear. The IARC (1973) study concluded that VCM causes angiosarcomas of the liver as well as tumors of the brain, lung, and hematolymphopoietic systems in humans.

Acrylonitrile

Acrylonitrile (AN) is considerably more toxic than the chlorinated monomers and has LD_{50} values of 80–90 mg/kg body weight in rats and 27 mg/kg in mice (Crosby, 1981). It converts to a mutagen after metabolic activation by the liver enzymes. In animals, AN is metabolized to cyanide, which is subsequently converted to thiocyanate and excreted in the urine. There is also some evidence of carcinogenicity in animals and possibly humans (IARC, 1973).

Vinylidene Chloride

Little toxicilogical information is available regarding the safety of vinylidene chloride (VDC). The LD_{50} values for rats and mice are around 1500 and 200 mg/kg body weight, respectively (Crosby, 1981). VDC affects the activity of several rat liver enzymes and decreases the store of glutathione. Some tumors have been observed after prolonged exposure but no teratogenic effects were seen in rats or rabbits. The main pathway of excretion is via the lungs, with other metabolites being discharged by the kidneys.

Styrene

Liebman (1975) has extensively reviewed the biological properties of styrene. The LD_{50} value for rats is 5 g/kg body weight. It is metabolized to styrene oxide, which is a potent mutagen in a number of test systems. Both styrene and its oxide have been shown to produce chromosomal aberrations under certain conditions.

Although little is known about the toxicity and carcinogenicity of monomers used in the production of food-grade plastics, there is clear evidence of the need for concern in the case of VCM and AN. Further studies are required to elucidate the interactions of various monomers with body components, their biotransformation and metabolism in the humans.

D. Regulatory Aspects

Although the majority of packaging contaminants are nontoxic in the small amounts in which they are present, food/package and package/process compatibility are food safety issues from FDA's viewpoint. The packaging materials are thus legally considered to be food additives, requiring premarket safety evaluation by the FDA. FDA requirements include conducting extraction tests to measure the amount of migration and providing appropriate toxicological data for the migrants by the manufacturers and processors (FDA, 1976). Adjuvant use, level of migration (or the lack thereof) under various conditions of use for foods, and consumption of these foods in the diet must be evaluated with regard to safety.

The potential toxicological hazards of foods contained in polymeric packages have received a great deal of attention since the passage of the 1958 amendment to the FFDCA. The determination of whether substances in food-contact materials may migrate into food and, if so, which substances and at what levels, is usually made on the basis of extraction experiments. Prior to the 1958 amendment, this determination was government's responsibility. Since then, it has been industry's responsibility.

Basically, a petition for use of an unregulated material should include the following information (FDA, 1976):

Identity, composition, properties, and specifications of the additive
Amount used and the type of food contact proposed
Intended physical or technical effect and efficacy data
Description of practicable extraction methods for estimating migration of the additive to food
Details of analytical methodology applicable to the additive and to extractive determination
Safety of the food additive
Proposed tolerance
Amendments for later use
Environmental impact analysis report

While no specific harm has been verified for any specific packaged food, at least three cases involving the additive polychlorinated biphenyl (PCB) and the monomers acrylonitrile (AN) and vinyl chloride (VCM) have been of major economic consequence. The PCB situation was primarily from contamination in recycled paper, while the AN case has resulted in multimillion dollar losses in the beverage container market (FDA, 1977). The VCM problem threatened to ban the usage of PVC for food packaging, but the ability of the industry to reduce the residues of VCM to the low ppb range has delayed the proposed ban.

A more practical concern is the presence of compounds in toxicologically in-significant amounts but at levels affecting quality by taste and/or odor changes in the packaged food. These residues can arise from a variety of origins, including AN and VCM monomers; reaction aids, such as catalysts or solvents; manufac-turing-related decompositions, such as from thermal oxidation in extrusion; coating resin components and solvents from inks and adhesives; and complex interactions, such as transesterification and hydrolysis to produce volatile or transferable prod-ucts. The formation of stilbene from the antioxidant BHT is another example of a detrimental chemical reaction (Gilbert, 1985).

The development of aseptic processing and packaging systems, especially those employing chemical sterilization of the container and the use of ionizing radiation, raised a number of safety issues. With regard to the use of a chemical sterilant, FDA's concerns were twofold: (1) to assure that the residue levels of the sterilant in food were kept within safe limits and (2) to assure that sterilization did not substantially alter the quality and nature of the migrants from the package. Con-sequently, the regulation for the use of hydrogen perioxide to sterilize food-contact surfaces, 21 CFR 178.1005, contains both a limit on residual hydrogen peroxide (0.1 ppm in food measured immediately after packaging) and a list of permitted materials.

The effects of ionizing radiation on packaging materials are of concern to FDA whether the irradiation is done as part of the manufacturing process for the food-contact material or the food is irradiated after packaging. Polymeric materials used to package food are irradiated during manufacturing for various purposes. These include cross-linking a polymer, curing an adhesive or promoting adhesion prior to lamination, and controlling microorganisms. Only three regulations for food-contact polymers in 21 CFR 177 specifically address irradiation: 21 CFR 177.1350 covers ethylene–vinyl acetate polymers, 21 CFR 177.1520 olefin polymers, and 21 CFR 177.1550 perfluorocarbon resins. In each case, the regulation is specific as to the technical effect to be achieved, as well as the maximum permitted intensity of the source and/or maximum allowed absorbed dose.

During the last decade, the development of more sensitive and accurate ana-lytical methods has greatly facilitated the control of packaging residues as well as identification of their origins. These methods also have aided in developing the theory of migration in very low concentration gradients to elucidate the mechanisms involved. Thus a better scientific data base has been developed to enable a more rational approach to packaging design for optimal retention of food quality in packaged foods. Considerable improvements in design effectiveness have also arisen from the introduction of new materials and processes for food packaging.

VI. MISCELLANEOUS CONTAMINANTS

Several chemicals other than those described above may also find their way into our food supplies. Some of the important miscellaneous contaminants are described below briefly.

Heavy nitrogen fertilizer applications can cause accumulation of potentially hazardous concentrations of nitrates, thereby adversely affecting the nutritional quality of vegetables (Maynard et al., 1976). The average nitrate concentrations (ppm fresh weight) in edible portions of selected fresh vegetables are as follows:

cabbage, 165; lettuce, 170; spinach, 534; celery, 535; beet, 600; radish, 402; rhubarb, 91; potato 42; asparagus, 25; snap bean, 35; and carrot, 32. Other factors that affect the nitrate content of plants include species, variety, plant part, stage of maturity, drought, high temperature, shading or cloudiness, time of day, deficiencies in certain nutrients, excessive soil nitrogen from manure, legume residues, and plant damage from insect and weed control chemicals (Keeney, 1970). Herbicides such as alachlor, linuron, lenacil, prometryne, and chloropropham also tend to increase the nitrate content of vegetables.

The toxic effects of excessive amounts of naturally occurring nitrates in foods and feeds were first reported by Mayo (1895). In three cases of fatal poisoning in cattle, the animals showed tremors, diuresis, collapse, and cyanosis after feeding of cornstalks that were later shown to contain 25% by dry weight potassium nitrate. The corn had apparently absorbed large amounts of nitrate from the accumulated soil manure. The symptoms were also experimentally reproduced by oral dosing of cattle with doses of potassium nitrate at about 1.3 g/kg body weight.

The occurrence of inorganic nitrate in vegetables has, at times, given rise to serious toxic effects, especially those resulting from methemoglobin formation. Holscher and Natzschka (1964) reported two cases of methemoglobinemia in infants after eating spinach puree. The spinach contained large amounts of nitrite (about 218 mg/100 g wet weight) and only small amounts of nitrate.

Sodium and potassium salts of nitrates and nitrites are also approved by the FDA for certain applications in foods. They are restricted for use as curing agents in meats such as salami, frankfurters, bacon, and bologna to prevent the growth of *Clostridium botulinum* responsible for the outbreaks of botulism poisoning in humans. They react with myoglobin in the meats, thus maintaining their red color. Their presence in foods, however, is also associated with the formation of nitrosamines, which are potent carcinogens in humans. Their use in foods thus is strictly regulated by federal and state agencies.

Other chemicals used in agriculture and livestock production include plant hormones such as indole-3-acetic acid, nitrated and chlorinated phenols, and giberellins for inhibition of sprouting of potatoes and onions, for deblossoming of fruit trees to thin the fruits and thus increase the size of fruits per cluster; ripening enhancers such as ethylene for uniform ripening of green fruits; estrogens to enhance animal growth; and bovine somatotropin to increase milk production. The chronic, long-term health risks associated with residual levels of these chemicals in our food supply are not well understood.

Smoke curing of meat products by traditional smoking process or by liquefied smoke is also commonly practiced in several countries. These processes impart unique flavor and color effects, which cannot be duplicated by any other method. More than 200 individual chemical compounds have been identified in curing smoke (Gilbert and Knowles, 1975). In general, the chemicals most commonly present in wood smoke are carbonyls, organic acids, phenols, organic bases, alcohols, and hydrocarbons (including polycyclic aromatics).

Depending on the chemical nature of wood smoke components, their interaction with food ranges from physical penetration to complex chemical reactions. In addition to beneficial effects such as characteristic color and flavor development as well as bactericidal and antioxidative properties, contamination with potentially toxic substances may also occur. At least two groups of chemical compounds, namely, polycyclic aromatic hydrocarbons and nitrosamines, known to be carcinogenic have been identified in smoked foods.

The levels of polycyclic aromatic hydrocarbons in smoked meats range between 1 and 58 ppm, with benzo[a]pyrene levels higher in fish than in meat. These compounds are formed in the smoke from thermally generated methylene radicals. Smoking may introduce the hazard of nitrosamine formation either directly by interaction of nitrogen oxide with secondary amines on the food surface or indirectly by formation of nitrites or nitrates on the food surface.

Excess presence of fluoride in drinking water is known to cause fluorosis or mottled teeth in children. Fluoride is also present in nearly every food, with the highest concentrations found in tea, seafood, bonemeal, spinach, and gelatin. Fluoride is taken up by vegetables and plants when fluoridated water supplies are used for irrigation and when superphosphate fertilizers and agricultural sprays containing fluoride are applied to fruits and vegetables. It is estimated that widespread use of fluoridated water (1 ppm) in food processing and preparation probably means a food fluoride intake of approximately 1.0–1.2 mg/person/d (Buist, 1986). Because of the health risks associated with fluoride consumption, several countries are now banning the fluoridation of drinking water supplies.

VII. SUMMARY

Incidental additives occur in our food chain inadvertently during crop production, food processing, and storage. While some of these are hazardous to human health directly or indirectly, others may affect both the sensory and nutritional quality of food. Generally, most of thse chemicals are broken down naturally or washed away. Nevertheless, residual amounts do remain in our food supply, and they continue to be a human health concern. Such unintentional addition is unfortunate but unavoidable.

Of the four major groups of incidental additives described here, namely, toxic metals, pesticide residues, drugs used in the livestock industry, and packaging contaminants, only the presence of heavy metals (especially lead, mercury, and cadmium) and the persistent occurrence of pesticide residues, particularly the non-biodegradable chlorinated hydrocarbons, pose significant human health risks. In contrast, the presence of drug contaminants in our food supply has far-reaching consequences, leading to transfer and selection of plasmid-mediated drug resistance in microorganisms that are pathogenic to humans. Packaging contaminants, especially those derived from plastics, are also of concern, since several of these have been shown to be carcinogenic in animal studies.

The residual levels of all four groups of indirect additives in the human food chain are monitored by both federal and state regulatory agencies in several countries, and tolerance levels have been established. In most cases, such levels are used only as guidelines for prosecutorial reasons, and they do not generally imply that the presence of such contaminants at lower levels is safe and without any risks associated with human health. Similarly, although most have been examined individually for their toxicological and adverse effects on human health, surprisingly few studies have been conducted thus far on the possible adverse interactions between different incidental contaminants. Nor have the cumulative effect of chronic low-dose exposure of individual contaminants or the additive effect of small quantities of several of these chemicals in combination been throughly examined. We should, therefore, continue to monitor the presence of these contaminants in our food supply for years to come.

REFERENCES

ACS (1980). *Chemistry and the Food System*. American Chemical Society, Washington, DC.

ALCOA. (1969). *Aluminum*. Aluminum Co. of American, Pittsburgh, PA.

ALDA (1988). Metals review. Australian Lead Development Association. *Elements 16*:7.

Allison, J. R. D. (1985). Antibiotic residues in milk. *Br. Vet. J. 141*:9–17.

Anonymous (1991). FDA revises program for finding drug residues in milk. *Food Chem. News 33*(22):51–52.

Asami, M. O. (1984). Pollution of soils by cadmium. In *Changing Metal Cycles and Human Health*, J. O. Nriagu (ed.). Springer-Verlag, Berlin, pp. 95–111.

Bakir, F., Damluji, S. F., and Amin-Zaki, L. (1973). Methylmercury poisoning in Iraq. *Science 181*:230–241.

Barry, P. S. (1975). Lead concentration in human tissues. *Br. J. Indust. Med. 32*:119–139.

Bennet, B. G. (1984). Six most dangerous chemicals named. Monitoring and Assessment Research Center, London, on behalf of UNEP/ILO/WHO International Program on Chemical Safety. *Sentinel 1*:3.

Berlin, M. H., Clarkson, T. W., and Frieberg, L. T. (1963). Maximum allowable concentrations of mercury compounds. *Arch. Environ. Health 6*:27–39.

Berrow, M. L., and Webber, J. (1972). The use of sewage sludge in agriculture. *J. Sci. Food Agric. 23*:93–100.

Booth, J. M., and Harding, F. (1986). Testing for antibiotic residues in milk. *Vet. Rec. 119*:565–570.

Bouquiaux, J. (1974). *CEC European Symposium on the Problems of Contamination of Man and His Environment by Mercury and Cadmium*. CID, Luxemborg.

Boyce, B. F., Elder, H. Y., and Ellio, H. L. (1982). Hypercalcaemic osteomalacia due to aluminum toxicity. *Lancet 2*:1009–1013.

Brady, M. S., and Katz, S. E. (1988). Antibiotic/antimicrobial residues in milk. *J. Food Protect. 51*:8–11.

Browning, E. (1969). *Toxicity of Industrial Metals*. Butterworths, London.

Buchet, J. P., Lauwerys, R., Vandevoorde, A., and Pycke, J. M. (1983). Oral daily intake of cadmium, lead, manganese, copper, chromium, mercury, calcium, zinc and arsenic in Belgium. A duplicate meal study. *Food Chem. Toxicol. 21*:19–24.

Buck, W. B. (1978). Toxicity of inorganic and aliphatic organic arsenicals. In *Toxicity of Heavy Metals in the Environment*, F. W. Oehme (ed.). Marcel Dekker, New York, pp. 357–369.

Buist, R. (1986). *Food Chemical Sensitivity*. Prism Press, San Leandro, CA.

CAC (1984). *Contaminants. Joint FAO/WHO Food Standards Program. Codex Alimentaritus*. Vol. XVII. World Health Organization, Geneva.

Capon, C. J. (1981). Mercury and selenium content and chemical form in vegetable crops grown on sludge-amended soil. *Arch. Environ. Contam. Toxicol. 10*:673–689.

Combs, G. F., and Combs, S. B. (1984). The nutritional biochemistry of selenium. In *Annual Reviews of Nutrition*, W. J. Darby, H. P. Broquist, and R. E. Olson (eds.). Annual Reviews, Inc., Palo Alto, CA, pp. 257–280.

Crapper, D. R., Krishnan, S. S., and Dalton, A. J. (1973). Brain aluminum distribution in Alzheimer's disease and experimental neurofibrillary degeneration. *Science 180*:511–513.

Crompton, T. R. (1979). *Additive Migration from Plastics into Food.* Pergamon Press, Oxford.

Crosby, N. T. (1981). *Food Packaging Materials.* Applied Science Publ., London.

Dabeka, R. W., McKenzie, A. D., and Lacroix, G. M. A. (1987). Dietary intakes of lead, cadmium, arsenic and fluoride by Canadian adults. A 24-hour duplicate diet study. *Food Add. Contam. 4*:89–102.

Dick, G. L., Hughes, J. T., Mitchell, J. W., and Davidson, F. (1978). Survey of trace elements and pesticide residues in the New Zealand diet. *NZ J. Sci. 21*:57–69.

Drinking Water Standards (1962). *Public Health Service Pub. No. 956.* U.S. Government Printers, Washington, DC.

DuPont, H. L., and Steele, J. H. (1987). Use of antimicrobial agents in animal feeds: implications for human health. *Rev. Infect. Dis. 9*:447–460.

FACC (1984). *Report on the Review of Arsenic in Food Regulations.* Food Additives and Contaminants Committee, Ministry of Agriculture, Fisheries and Food, FAC/REP/39, HMSO, London.

FDA (1976). *FDA Guidelines for Chemistry and Technology Requirements of Indirect Food Additive Petitions.* Bureau of Foods, Food and Drug Administration, Dept. of Health, Education and Welfare, Washington, DC.

FDA (1977). Indirect additives, polymers, acrylonitrile copolymers used to fabricate beverage containers. Final decision. *Fed. Reg. 42*:48528.

FDA (1992). Memorandum M-I-92-7, September 25, 1992.

Federal Register (1977). New animal drugs for use in animal feeds. Part 558. *Fed. Reg. 42*(168):43770–43792.

Food Marketing Institute. (1988). *Trends: Consumer Attitudes and the Supermarket.* Food Marketing Institute, Washington, DC.

Franco, D. A., Webb, J., and Taylor, C. E. (1990). Antibiotic and sulfonamide residues in meat: implications for human health. *J. Food Protect. 53*:178–185.

Frieberg, L., Piscator, M., Norberg, G., and Kjellstrom, T. (1974). *Cadmium in the Environment*, 2nd ed., CRC Press, Boca Raton, FL.

Gardiner, M. R., Armstrong, J., Fels, H., and Glenros, R. N. (1962). A preliminary report on selenium and animal health in Western Australia. *Aust. J. Exp. Ad. Anim. Husb. 2*:261–269.

Gartrell, M. J., Craun, J. C., Podrebarac, D. S., and Gunderson, E. L. (1985). Pesticides, selected elements and other chemicals in adult total diet samples, October 1978–September 1979. *J. Assoc. Off. Anal. Chem. 68*:862–875.

Gilbert, J., and Knowles, M. E. (1975). The chemistry of smoked foods. A review. *J. Food Technol. 10*:245–253.

Gilbert, S. G. (1985). Food/package compatibility. *Food Technol. 39*(12):54–56, 63.

Gormican, A., and Catli, E. (1971). Mineral balance in young men fed a fortified milk-base formula. *Nutr. Metabol. 13*:364–377.

Gramiccioni, L. (1984). Migration of metals into food from containers. *Rass. Chim. 36*:271–273.

Gustafson, R. H. (1991). Use of antibiotics in livestock and human health concerns. *J. Dairy Sci. 74*:1428–1432.

Hall, N. S., Chandler, W. F., and Van Bavel, C. H. M. (1953). *A Tracer Technique to Measure Growth and Activity of Plant Root Systems.* North Carolina Agric. Exp. Sta. Tech. Bull. No. 101, Raleigh, NC.

Harrison, R. M. (1978). Metals in household dust. *Sci. Total Environ. 8*:89–97.

Heichel, G. H., Hankin, L., and Botsford, R. A. (1974). Lead in colored wrapping paper. *J. Milk Food Technol. 37*:499–503.

Hewitt, W. L. (1975). Clinical implications of the presence of drug residues in food. *Fed. Proc. 34*:202–209.

Holmberg, S. D., Osterholm, M. T., Senger, K. A., and Cohen, M. L. (1984). Drug resistant *Salmonella* from animals fed antimicrobials. *N. Engl. J. Med. 311*:617–622.

Holscher, P. M., and Natzschka, J. (1964). Methemoglobinamine bei jungen Säuglingen durch nitrithaltigen Spinat. *Deut. Med. Wochschr. 89*:1751–1755.

Hotchkiss, J. H. (1992). Pesticide residue controls to ensure food safety. *Crit. Rev. Food Sci. Nutr. 31*:191–203.

IARC (1973). *Evaluation of Carcinogenic Risk of Chemicals to Man. Some Inorganic and Organometallic Compounds*, Vol. 2. International Agency for Research on Cancer, Lyon.

Jones, G. M., and Seymour, E. H. (1988). Cowside antibiotic residue testing. *J. Dairy Sci. 71*:1691–1699.

Keeney, O. R. (1970). Nitrates in plants and waters. *J. Milk Food Technol. 33*:425–428.

Klein, M., Namer, R., Harpur, E., and Corbin, R. (1970). Earthenware containers as a source of fatal lead poisoning. *N. Eng. J. Med. 283*:669–672.

Knott, S. G., and McCray, C. W. R. (1959). Two naturally occurring outbreaks of selenosis in Queensland. *Aust. Vet. J. 35*:161–165.

Liebman, K. C. (1975). Metabolism and toxicity of styrene. *Environ. Health Perspect. 11*:115–121.

Lindemayr, H., Knobler, R., Kraft, D., and Baumgartner, W. (1981). Challenge of penicillin-allergic volunteers with penicillin-contaminated meat. *Allergy 36*:471–479.

Linton, A. H. (1984). Antibiotic-resistant bacteria in animal husbandry. *Br. Med. Bull. 40*(1):91–95.

Mackenzie, E. J., and Purves, D. (1975). Toxic metals in sewage sludge. *Chem. Ind.* (Jan. 4):12–13.

MAFF (1982). *Survey of Arsenic in Food: The 8th Report of the Steering Group on Food Surveillance; the Working Party on the Monitoring of Foodstuffs for Heavy Metals*. Ministry of Agriculture, Fisheries and Food, London, England.

Maltoni, C., Lefemine, G., Chieco, P., and Carretti, D. (1974). Vinyl chloride carcinogenesis: current results and perspectives. *Med. Lav. 65*:421–430.

Maynard, D. N., Barker, A. V., Minotti, P. D., and Peck, N. H. (1976). Nitrate accumulation in vegetables. *Adv. Agron. 28*:71–118.

Mayo, N. S. (1895). *Cattle Poisoning by Potassium Nitrate*. Kansas Agric. Expt. Stn. Bull. No. 49, Manhattan, KS.

McEwen, S. A., Black, W. D., and Meek, A. H. (1991). Antibiotic residue prevention methods, farm management, and occurrence of antibiotic residues in milk. *J. Dairy Sci. 74*:2128–2137.

Moorman, M. A., and Koenig, E. (1992). Antibiotic residues and their implications in foods. *Scope 7*:4–7.

Morgan, H. (1988). *The Shipham Report. An Investigation into Cadmium Contamination and Its Implications for Human Health*. Elsevier, London.

Murthy, G. K., Rhea, U., and Peeler, J. R. (1971). Antimony in the diet of children. *Environ. Sci. Technol. 5*:436–442.

NAS (1972). *Airborne Lead in Perspective*. National Academy of Sciences, Washington, DC.

NAS (1980). *The Effects on Human Health of Subtherapeutic Use of Antimicrobials in Animal Feeds*. National Academy of Sciences, Washington, DC.

Nielsen, F. H. (1986). Other elements: antimony. In *Trace Elements in Human and Animal Nutrition*, W. Mertz (ed.). Academic Press, New York.

NRC (1987). *Regulating Pesticides in Food. The Delaney Paradox*. National Academy Press, Washington, DC.

Oehme, F. W. (1978). *Toxicity of Heavy Metals in the Environment*. Marcel Dekker, New York.

OTA (1988). *Pesticide Residues in Food: Technologies for Detection*, *OTA-F-398*. U.S. Congress, Office of Technology Assessment, U.S. Government Printing Office, Washington, DC.

Pennington, J. A. T. (1987). Aluminum content of food and diets. *Food Add. Contam.* *5*:161–232.

Pennington, J. A. T., and Jones, J. W. (1988). Aluminum in American diets. In *Aluminum in Health, A Critical Review*, H. J. Gitelman (ed.). Marcel Dekker, New York, pp. 67–100.

Pike, E. R., Graham, L. C., and Fogden, M. W. (1975). Metals in crops grown on sewage-enriched soil. *JAPA 13*:19–33.

Pimentel, D. (1981). *Handbook of Pest Management in Agriculture*, Vol. 1. CRC Press, Boca Raton, FL.

Pimentel, D. (1991). The dimensions of the pesticide question. In *Ecology, Economics, Ethics: The Broken Circle*, F. H. Bormann and S. R. Kellert (eds.). Yale University Press, New Haven, CT, pp. 59–69.

Platts, A. M., Goode, G. C., and Hislop, J. S. (1977). Composition of the domestic water supply and the incidence of fractures and encephalopathy in patients on home dialysis. *Br. Med. J. 2*:657–660.

Prater, B. E. (1975). Water pollution in the river Tees. *Water Pollut. Control 74*:63–76.

Price, B. (1988). Cleaner solutions from rubbish tips. *New Scientist 114*:47–50.

Pryor, W. A. (1980). *Free Radicals in Biology*, Vol. IV. Academic Press, New York.

Rayment, G. E., Best, E. K., and Hamilton, D. J. (1989). Cadmium in fertilizers and soil amendments. *Chemistry International Conference*, Brisbane, Aug. 28–Sept. 2, Royal Australian Chemical Institute, Brisbane, Australia.

Reilly, A., and Reilly, C. (1972). Patterns of lead pollution in the Zambian environment. *Med. J. Zambia 6*:125–127.

Reilly, C. (1991). *Metal Contamination of Food*, 2nd ed. Elsevier Applied Science, London.

Reilly, C., Sudarmadji, S., and Sugiharto, E. (1989). Mercury and arsenic in soil, water and foods of the Dieng Plateau, Java. *Proc. Nutr. Soc. Aust. 14*:118.

Rhian, M., and Moxon, A. L. (1943). Interaction of arsenic and selenium. *J. Pharmacol. Exp. Ther. 78*:249–264.

Ryan, C. A., Nickels, M. K., Hargett-Bean, N. T., Potter, M. E. et al. (1987). Massive outbreak of antimicrobial resistant salmonellosis traced to pasteurized milk. *JAMA 258*:3269–3274.

Schroeder, H. A., and Balassa, J. J. (1966). Abnormal trace metals in man: arsenic. *J. Chron. Dis. 19*:85–106.

Sherlock, J. C., and Smart, G. A. (1984). Tin in foods and the diet. *Food Add. Contam. 1*:277–282.

Slorach, S., Gustafsson, I. B., Jorhem, L., and Mattsson, P. (1983). Intake of lead, cadmium and certain other metals via a typical Swedish weekly diet. *Var Foda 35*:1–16.

Stoewsand, G. S., Bache, C. A., and Lisk, D. J. (1974). Dietary selenium protection of methylmercury intoxication of Japanese quail. *Bull. Environ. Contam. Toxicol. 11*:152–156.

Strenstrom, T., and Vahter, M. (1974). Heavy metals in sewage sludge for use on agricultural soil. *Ambio 3*:91–92.

Thomson, C. D., and Robinson, M. F. (1980). Selenium in human health and disease with emphasis on those aspects peculiar to New Zealand. *Am. J. Clin Nutr. 33*:303–323.

Vos, G., Hovens, J. P. C., and Delft, W. V. (1987). Arsenic, cadmium, lead and mercury in meat, livers and kidneys of cattle slaughtered in The Netherlands during 1980–1985. *Food Add. Contam. 4*:73–88.

Watanabe, Y. (1974). Cadmium and lead on decorated glass drinking glasses. *Ann. Rep. Tokyo Metropol. Lab. Pub. Health 25*:293–296.

Wenlock, R. W., Buss, D. H., and Dixon, E. J. (1979). Trace nutrients. 2. Manganese in the British diet. *Br. J. Nutr. 41*:253–261.

WHO (1963). *International Standards for Drinking Waters*, 2nd ed. World Health Organization, Geneva.

WHO (1973). *Trace Elements in Human Nutrition. Tech. Rep. Ser. No. 532.* World Health Organization, Geneva.

WHO (1976). *Environmental Health Criteria 3: Lead.* World Health Organization, Geneva.

WHO (1979). *Pesticide Residues in Food—1978.* A report of the joint meeting of the FAO panel of experts on pesticide residues and environment and the WHO expert group on pesticide residues. World Health Organization, Geneva.

Williams, C. H., and David, D. J. (1973). Heavy metals in Australian agricultural soil. *Aust. J. Soil Res. 11*:43–50.

Young, V. R., Nahapetian, A., and Janghorbani, M. (1982). Selenium bioavailability with reference to human nutrition. *Am. J. Clin. Nutr. 35*:1076–1088.

11
Antimicrobial Agents

John N. Sofos
Colorado State University
Fort Collins, Colorado

I. INTRODUCTION

The widespread occurrence and multiplication of microorganisms in the environment and the associated chemical/enzymatic reactions result in decomposition of materials, including foods and other items useful to humans. These effects modify the appearance, flavor, texture, color, consistency, and nutritional quality of the product. In addition, certain microorganisms are toxic to humans, causing infections or intoxications through formation of toxins when they proliferate in foods. Thus, except for useful microbial fermentations, growth of microorganisms in foods is undesirable, and there is a need for its avoidance or inhibition. Therefore, since prehistoric times, humans have developed procedures to inhibit undesirable microorganisms in order to preserve their food supply and ensure safety from pathogens. Preservation of foods is achieved through application of physical and/or chemical methods (Sofos and Busta, 1992). Physical methods of microbial inhibition or destruction include modification of temperature through the application of heat (e.g., cooking, pasteurization, sterilization) or cold temperatures (e.g., refrigeration, freezing), use of ionizing radiations, and removal of water (e.g., evaporation, drying). Chemical methods of food preservation involve use of desirable microorganisms in fermentations or direct application of chemical additives, which act as antimicrobial agents. In addition to chemicals added directly with the objective of acting as antimicrobial agents, other chemical additives (e.g., salts, curing agents, antioxidants, phosphates) may also exert direct or indirect antimicrobial activity. The objective of this chapter, however, is to discuss only the chemicals used with the specific objective of acting as antimicrobial agents in foods, feeds, pharmaceuticals, or other materials (Sofos and Busta, 1992, 1993).

Some chemicals have been used traditionally as direct or indirect inhibitors of microbial growth, but the antimicrobial agents that are the subject of this chapter were developed, tested, approved, and used only during the past 20–100 years. Major reasons for this development include the increase in human population, the development of highly populated urban areas, and the associated changes in life-styles of modern consumers. These developments of the past 50 years have led to changes in the marketing system for food products and in the development of products to meet consumer demands for convenience, quality, variety, availability, and safety. The needs for long-term storage, long-distance shipment, availability throughout the year and in adverse climates, and maintenance of eating, nutritional, and microbiological qualities have led to wider use of chemical antimicrobial agents in our food supply and in other consumer products. Overall, the modern food-marketing system is highly dependent on the use of chemical antimicrobial agents.

All the approved antimicrobial agents have limitations, and no single one can be employed in all potential applications. Antimicrobial action is dictated by several factors, including (1) physical and chemical properties (e.g., solubility, pKa, reactivity, toxicity), (2) the types of microorganisms of concern, and (3) the type and properties of the product to be preserved. Based on these factors, the most appropriate antimicrobial agent for a specific application is selected. In certain instances, combinations of more than one antimicrobial agent are the most beneficial for use in a product. In other applications, chemical antimicrobial agents may be combined with physical processes (e.g., heat, dehydration, refrigeration) in order to maximize preservation and to optimize product quality. Use of combinations of inhibitory factors is known (Leistner, 1985) as the "hurdle concept." Of the various properties of a product, pH is probably the most influential on the extent of the antimicrobial activity of a chemical antimicrobial agent. Acidity has a direct antimicrobial effect, but it also affects the antimicrobial properties of physical and chemical methods of preservation. Reduced pH potentiates the antimicrobial activity of weak mineral acids (e.g., nitrite, sulfite) and weak lipophilic acids (e.g., sorbic, benzoic, propionic). The antimicrobial activity of weak lipophilic acids is increased as the pH is reduced and approaches the dissociation constant (pKa value).

In conjunction with the increased need and use of chemical antimicrobial agents in the preservation of consumer goods, there has been an increase in consumer concern about the toxicological properties and safety of these compounds. In addition to the increased consumer awareness about safety, there have been developments and advances in methodologies used to detect chemicals in our food supply and in testing their toxicological properties. This has led to the discontinuation of the use of certain antimicrobials, to the questioning of the safety of certain others, and to the great scrutiny and difficulty in gaining approval for use of new compounds or expanded use of previously approved ones in new or additional food products.

Use of antimicrobial agents, as well as other food additives, is regulated and approved by the appropriate authorities of each country, while internationally the Food and Agriculture Organization (FAO) and the World Health Organization (WHO) deal with such matters. Before approval for a specific use in the United States, an antimicrobial agent has to be proven safe by its manufacturer or user, as required by the Food, Drug and Cosmetic Act and its amendments, which are administered by the U.S. Food and Drug Administration (FDA). Some of the chemical antimicrobial agents are designated as generally recognized as safe (GRAS) by the FDA and are exempted from food additive regulation. GRAS compounds, however, must be applied within a certain spectrum of activity and must be approved for a specific use. Their use should always be under good manufacturing practices and must be listed on the label of the product.

An antimicrobial agent is generally approved when the following conditions are met: (1) there is a need for antimicrobial activity; (2) the compound is effective in fulfilling that need; (3) the compound is nontoxic; (4) the compound is safe and noncarcinogenic; (5) the compound does not alter the identity and quality of the product; (6) the total consumption of the compound does not exceed safe limits; (7) the application of the compound is practical and compatible with product processing; and (8) the compound is available and cost-effective. These strict requirements have limited the number of new or additional uses approved in the past several years (Sofos and Busta, 1992).

The list of approved chemicals acting as direct antimicrobial agents includes (1) lipophilic acids (e.g., sorbic, benzoic, propionic), (2) esters (e.g., esters of *para*-hydroxybenzoic acid), (3) gases (e.g., sulfites, carbon dioxide, epoxides, ozone), (4) microbial metabolites (e.g., antibiotics, bacteriocins, ethyl alcohol, hydrogen peroxide), and (5) miscellaneous antimicrobials. This chapter discusses their chemical and antimicrobial properties, applications, and toxicological properties. Other chemical substances used in foods for other objectives (e.g., acidulants) may also have antimicrobial activity, but they are discussed in other chapters of this book.

II. SORBIC ACID AND ITS SALTS

A. Chemical Properties and Uses

Sorbic acid is a naturally occurring compound, which is also produced synthetically for application as an antimicrobial agent. It was first isolated from the oil of unripened rowan berries in the 1850s, while its antimicrobial properties were discovered in the 1930s and 1940s, with the first patent for use as an antimicrobial agent being awarded in 1945 (Sofos and Busta, 1981, 1993; Sofos, 1989).

The compound, 2,4-hexadienoic, is a straight-chain, *trans-trans*, unsaturated fatty acid ($CH_3 - CH = CH - CH = CH - COOH$) with a molecular weight of 112.13 and a highly reactive carboxyl group. Its conjugated double bonds are also reactive. Its solubility in water is only 0.15% at room temperature, which increases with increasing temperature and pH. In contrast, the water solubility of its potassium salt is high (58.2% at room temperature), which makes it a more frequently used form of the compound in antimicrobial applications. The solubility of the calcium and sodium salts in water is 1.2% and 32%, respectively. Solutions of sorbates in water are degraded through oxidation, but the compounds remain stable in the pure dry form. Oxidation can be inhibited by antioxidants and anaerobic packaging, but when it occurs, its products include crotonaldehyde, malonaldehyde, acetaldehyde, and β-carboxylactolein (Arya and Thakur, 1988). Oxidation rates are increased with reduced pH, acids, and light and increased temperatures. The extent of sorbic acid losses in stored materials depends on the concentration, type of food, pH, moisture content, storage temperature, and length of time (Sofos, 1989; Sofos and Busta, 1993).

In addition to its salts, other derivatives of sorbic acid evaluated for antimicrobial activity include alcohols, aldehydes, esters, salts, and amide derivatives, including sorbohydroxamic acid, sorboyl palmitate, sorbamide, methyl sorbate, ethyl sorbate, and sorbic anhydride. Sorbic acid is commercially available as a white, free-flowing powder or as granules and has a weak acrid odor and acid taste. The potassium salt is available as a powder or granules, sodium sorbate is a white, fluffy powder available commercially as an aqueous solution, and the calcium salt forms a white odorless and tasteless powder (Lück, 1980; Sofos and Busta, 1993).

Sorbates are widely used as antimicrobial agents throughout the world, especially the acid and the highly soluble potassium form. Materials preserved with sorbates include food products, animal feeds, pharmaceuticals, and cosmetics. Food groups preserved with 0.02–0.3% sorbate include dairy products, fruits and vegetables, bakery products, fat-emulsion products, meat, fish, and confectionery products (Sofos, 1989).

B. Antimicrobial Properties

Sorbic acid and its salts are effective antimicrobial agents against many yeasts and molds, as well as bacteria. As yeast inhibitors, the compounds are useful in fermented vegetable products, fruit juices, wines, dried fruits, meat, and fish products. Specific products protected from yeasts by sorbates include carbonated beverages, salad dressings, tomato products, syrups, jams, jellies, candy, and chocolate syrup (Lück, 1976, 1980; Sofos and Busta, 1981, 1993; Liewen and Marth, 1985; Sofos, 1989). As mold inhibitors, sorbates are effective against many molds, especially in cheese, butter, sausages, smoked fish, fruits, juices, grains, bread, and cakes, where they inhibit growth and mycotoxin formation. Subinhibitory concentrations of sorbate, however, may stimulate production of mycotoxins, depending on strain of mold, storage temperature, and other factors (Sofos, 1989). Although their antimicrobial activity is variable, sorbates inhibit many bacteria, including gram-positive and gram-negative, catalase-positive and catalase-negative, aerobic and anaerobic, and mesophilic and psychrotrophic species (Sofos et al., 1986).

Certain microorganisms, such as lactic acid bacteria, as well as certain yeasts and molds are resistant to inhibition by sorbate. In addition, being a fatty acid, sorbate is metabolized by certain microorganisms, such as lactic acid bacteria and molds. Decomposition of sorbate by molds (e.g., *Penicillium, Aspergillus, Mucor* spp.) has been observed in cheese and fruit products and depends on species and strains, prior exposure to subinhibitory levels of sorbate, microbial loads, concentration of sorbate, and type of food. Metabolism of sorbate by molds in cheese results in kerosene or plastic paint–type odors due to formation of 1,3-pentadiene (Liewen and Marth, 1985; Sofos, 1989). Degradation of sorbate by lactic acid bacteria may occur in wines and fermented vegetables resulting in geranium-type off-odors, through production of ethyl sorbate, 4-hexanoic acid, 1-ethoxyhexa-2,4-diene and 2-ethoxyhexa-3,5-diene (Edinger and Splittstoesser, 1986a,b; Sofos, 1989; Sofos and Busta, 1993).

The activity of sorbic acid against microorganisms is a function of synergistic or antagonistic interactions with product composition, pH, water activity, microbial flora, chemical additives, storage temperature, gas atmosphere, and packaging (Sofos and Busta, 1981). A major factor affecting the antimicrobial action of sorbate is pH of the substrate. As with other lipophilic acid antimicrobial agents, the activity of sorbate is increased as the pH approaches its dissociation constant (pKa = 4.76).

The maximum pH for activity is 6.5, while measurable inhibition of microbial growth has been detected even at pH 7.0. These values are higher than those for benzoate and propionate, which makes sorbate a more effective antimicrobial agent at higher pH values (Sofos and Busta, 1992; 1993). In addition to antimicrobial activity from the undissociated acid, the dissociated molecule is also inhibitory, but its activity is 10–600 times less than that of the undissociated acid (Eklund, 1983; Statham and McMeekin, 1988).

The concentrations (<0.3%) of sorbic acid applicable to food products only inhibit, and do not inactivate, microorganisms. Higher concentrations may inactivate microorganisms, but they are not used or permitted in foods because of their adverse effects on product flavor. The mechanisms, at the molecular level, involved in inhibition of cell growth and multiplication or bacterial spore germination and outgrowth by sorbate are not well defined (Sofos et al., 1986; Sofos, 1989). There is evidence indicating, however, that inhibition of bacterial spore germination involves inhibition of an undefined postgerminant binding step in the process of germination through inhibition of sporeolytic enzymes involved in germination or through sorbate interactions with spore membranes (Sofos et al., 1979a,b; 1986; Blocher and Busta, 1985).

Inhibition of metabolic function by sorbate may be variable with microbial species, substrate, food processing, and environmental conditions. Specific effects attributed to sorbate activity in inhibition of metabolic function include (1) alterations in morphology and appearance of microbial cells, (2) alterations in morphology, integrity, and function of cell membranes, (3) inhibition of transport functions and nutrient uptake, and (4) inhibition of enzymes and metabolic activity (Sofos et al., 1986; Sofos, 1989; Sofos and Busta, 1993). Specific effects observed include generation of holes in the cell membrane, inhibition of enzyme systems such as dehydrogenases and catalase, inhibition of the electron transport system, and inhibition of the proton-motive force that exists across cell membranes (Salmond et al., 1984; Eklund, 1985; Ronning and Frank, 1987, 1988; Sofos, 1989; Sofos and Busta, 1993).

C. Toxicological Properties

According to the *Food Additives Handbook* (Lewis, 1989), sorbic acid is "moderately toxic by intraperitoneal and subcutaneous administration; an experimental tumorigen; cause of experimental reproductive effects; and a severe human and experimental skin irritant." Similar descriptions have been given to its potassium, calcium, and sodium salts. It is combustible when exposed to heat, can react with oxidizing materials, and when heated to decomposition it emits acrid smoke and irritating fumes (Lewis, 1989).

In the United States, sorbic acid is characterized as GRAS when used under good manufacturing practices. Extensive studies on the toxicology of sorbates have involved feeding various species of animals (e.g., mice, rats, rabbits, dogs) to determine acute, short-term, and chronic toxicity levels and effects involving metabolic function, mutagenicity, carcinogenicity, teratogenicity, and reproduction (Sofos, 1989). Overall, the concentrations of sorbate used in food preservation have been found as nontoxic. Even when higher doses are evaluated, sorbate appears to be a safer compound than other commonly used food additives (Walker, 1990).

The oral lethal dose (LD_{50}) in rats for sorbic acid, potassium sorbate, and sodium sorbate has been reported to be in the range of 7.4–10.5, 4.2–6.2, and 5.9–7.2 g/kg body weight, respectively, while the mouse sorbic acid intraperitoneal LD_{50} is 1.3–2.5 mg/kg body weight (Lück, 1980; Guest et al., 1982; Sofos, 1989; Sofos and Busta, 1993). For comparison, the oral LD_{50} in rats for sodium chloride (i.e., common table salt) is 3 g/kg body weight (Lewis, 1989). Based on this, WHO has set the acceptable daily intake (ADI) for sorbate at 25 mg/kg body weight per day.

Exposure of mice for 2 months to 40 mg sorbic acid per kilogram body weight per day by oral intubation had no effect on food consumption, rate of weight gain, or survival, but a dose of 80 mg for 3 months restricted growth compared to controls (Shtenberg and Ignat'ev, 1970). Growth of rats was also not affected when they were fed diets with 1–10% added sorbic acid for periods of 42–90 days. More extended feeding, however, increased growth rate and liver weight, which was probably due to caloric utilization of metabolizable sorbic acid (Deuel et al., 1954a; Gaunt et al., 1975; Hendy et al., 1976; Lück, 1980; Sofos, 1989). Studies have also indicated that extensive feeding of sorbic acid is tolerated well by dogs and rabbits. Increased potassium intakes from studies involving testing of high levels (5–10%) of potassium sorbate may also result in increased kidney weights (Sofos, 1989).

Chronic toxicity has been evaluated through feeding mice or rats the life span of one or more generations with sorbic acid concentrations of 10% in the diet or as high as 90 mg/kg body weight for periods of up to 2 years. Presence of 10% sorbic acid in the diet of rats, which corresponds to an approximate daily intake of 150–200 g of sorbic acid by human adults, resulted in lower body weights and increased kidney, small intestine, and ovary weights. The concentration of 5% sorbic acid in the diet of rats for their entire lives caused no damage or modification in bodily functions, with the exception of accelerated growth and an increased life span in the males. This was also attributed to the increased caloric intake and the decrease in premature mortality rate caused by improved resistance to infection (Lück, 1976, 1980; Sofos and Busta, 1993). Increased amounts (10%) of sorbate in the diets of rats and mice had no adverse effects on their reproduction (Sofos, 1989). Subcutaneous injection of sorbic acid, but not potassium sorbate, resulted in local sarcomas in rats, while levels as high as 460 mg/kg body weight in the diet or in the drinking water of mice for 10 days or up to 2 years produced no teratogenic effects or tumors (Dickens et al., 1968; Sofos, 1989). Thus, sorbate in the diet has not been considered as a potential contributor to carcinogenicity or teratogenicity.

Levels of up to 1% sorbic acid had no effect on metabolism or blood cholesterol levels, but levels of 5–10% may be toxic because they increase fat deposition in the internal organs and blood cholesterol levels. Levels of less than 1.5% in the diet of rats and mice had no effects on hematological characteristics or renal function (Mason et al., 1976). Other studies found that sorbic acid increased immunobiological activity and the detoxifying function of the liver (Sofos, 1989).

As an aliphatic carboxylic acid, sorbic acid can be metabolized by microorganisms and animals similar to other fatty acids through β-oxidation (Deuel et al., 1954b). Final products of sorbic acid degradation in presence of carbohydrates include energy, carbon dioxide, and water. While in the absence of metabolizable carbohydrates, products of sorbic acid metabolism include acetone and acetoacetone (Deuel et al., 1954a,b). Dietary sorbic acid is almost entirely absorbed from the intestine and up to 85% is oxidized, while 3% was found in internal organs, 3% in skeletal muscle, 2% in the urine as urea and carbon dioxide, 0.4% in the feces, and 6.6% in other parts of the body (Sofos, 1989).

High levels of sorbate may cause allergic-type responses in sensitive individuals by irritating mucous membranes and the skin (Lück, 1980; NAS, 1982; Sofos, 1989). This, of course, may happen only to highly sensitive individuals using pharmaceuticals or cosmetic products preserved with sorbate. However, no allergenic activity from commercial foods preserved with sorbate has been documented (NAS, 1982).

When sorbate was tested as an alternative to the antimicrobial activity of nitrite in cured meat products in order to reduce formation of nitrosamines, while maintaining safety from botulism, concern was expressed relative to potential reactions of nitrite with sorbate and development of toxic effects (Sofos et al., 1979b; Sofos, 1981, 1989; NAS, 1982; Sofos and Busta, 1993). Results of a study evaluating the sensory quality of bacon treated with potassium sorbate (0.26%) and sodium nitrite (0.004%) indicated that some panelists experienced a "prickly" mouth sensation and "sweet aromatic" odors from some of their sorbate-nitrite bacon samples. Similar tests of bacon in other studies, however, failed to detect these effects (NAS, 1982; Sofos, 1989). A follow-up study (Hinton et al., 1981) tested commercially produced experimental bacon with a hamster cheek pouch test to evaluate irritation effects on mucus membranes. The results indicated that solutions of nitrite were more irritating than sorbate, sorbate-nitrite combinations, or nitrosamines. Both nitrite and sorbate were membrane irritants. Bacon processed only with nitrite (0.012%) or with a nitrite/sorbate (0.004/0.26%) combination was irritating. It was postulated that a potential nitrite-sorbate reaction involved addition of nitrite to either of the double bonds of sorbate, which might generate mutagenic and potentially harmful products (Sofos, 1989).

Studies on the mutagenic activity of sorbates have shown mixed results. Several studies have found no mutagenic or teratogenic activity, while others found activity by the bacterial "rec" assay or the chromosome test (Sofos, 1981, 1989). Use of mammalian test systems has indicated that potassium sorbate caused chromosomal breaks, sister chromatid exchanges, and translocations in Chinese hamster cells.

The genotoxic activity of potassium sorbate and sodium sorbate was studied using several tests, including the *Salmonella*/mammalian-microsome test, HGPRT and sister chromatid exchange test with Chinese hamster ovary cells, with no sign of genotoxicity in all in vitro tests (Münzner et al., 1990). A study (Mukherjee et al., 1988) reported a synergistic sorbic acid and sodium nitrite effect on the formation of compounds genotoxic to bone marrow cells of mice. Another study (Jung et al., 1992) found, however, that oral administration of sorbic acid at levels up to 5000 mg/kg body weight did not induce sister chromatid exchanges or the formation of micronuclei in bone marrow cells of mice. Intraperitoneal treatment of rats with 400–12,000 mg potassium sorbate/kg body weight did not alter the elution profile of DNA from isolated liver cells in an in vivo alkaline elution assay. In general, this study supported the conclusion that sorbic acid and its potassium salt are not genotoxic in vivo or in vitro. The oxidation product (i.e., 4,5-oxohexanoate) of sodium sorbate, however, was mutagenic in the Ames test (Jung et al., 1992).

Concern was also raised about potential mutagenic activity by reaction products of nitrite with sorbic acid. As an unsaturated fatty acid, sorbic acid may react with nitrite to form antimicrobial compounds with genotoxic activity against bacteria. Products with genotoxic activity produced by the reaction of nitrite with sorbate include ethylnitrolic acid and 1,4-dinitro-2-methyl pyrrole. Ethylnitrolic acid is highly mutagenic in the "rec" assay and the *Salmonella* forward-mutation assay, but has less activity in the *Salmonella*/microsome test. The compound has also strong antibacterial activity in culture media, but not in food; it is volatile by steam distillation; and it is degraded to form dinitrogen oxide and acetic acid (Sofos, 1981, 1989).

The pyrrole derivative formed is the most mutagenic of the compounds produced, and it is believed to be derived through nitration or nitrosation of sorbic acid, followed by decarboxylation. Other substances detected in the reaction mixture of nitrite and sorbate, such as a furoxan derivatives of sorbic acid, were not found to be genotoxic (Sofos, 1981, 1989).

Mutagenic activity from the reaction mixture of sorbic acid with sodium nitrite reached a maximum at pH values of 3.5–4.2 and molar ratios of 1:8. Maximum mutagenic activity was detected at 160 mM sodium nitrite. Heat (100°C) and a pH of 6.0 deactivated the mutagenic products. Mutagenic activity was also detected in a sorbate/nitrite molar ratio of 1:0.2, in mixtures of 0.1:0.01–0.04%, and at pH values approaching 6.0 (Robach et al., 1980a; Sofos, 1981, 1989; Hartman, 1983).

Formation of mutagenic products was inhibited or the mutagens were inactivated by food constituents such as ascorbic acid, cysteine, and vegetable juices. Evidence also exists indicating that the mutagenic products should not be expected to be formed in bacon curing brines or under simulated gastric conditions (Sofos, 1989).

It appears that the conjugated dienoic carbonyl structure is essential for the reaction of sorbic acid with nitrite to form mutagens, which are C-nitro and C-nitroso compounds. Thus, nitrite should also form mutagens with compounds other than sorbic acid, such as its analogs, as well as piperine and piperic acid and other fatty acids containing conjugated C-C double bonds. Certainly such products could be formed even in foods without added nitrite or sorbic acid, since certain vegetable products are good sources of nitrate and nitrite, and the acidic pH of the stomach should favor their reaction with C-C compounds. Degradation of these products by natural food constituents, however, may be a human defense mechanism against their toxic effects (Sofos, 1989).

Sorbate has been reported to be an indirect, as well as direct, inhibitor of nitrosamine formation (Sofos, 1989). When used in bacon-curing brines to control growth of pathogenic *Clostridium botulinum* in combination with reduced concentrations of sodium nitrite, formation of nitrosamines in the resulting product was reduced compared to bacon with regularly used nitrite levels (Sofos et al., 1980; Robach et al., 1980b). It was also reported that in its reaction with nitrite in acidic substrates, sorbic acid inhibited in vitro and in human saliva formation of *N*-nitrosodimethylamine from dimethylamine and nitrite (Tanaka et al., 1978). In addition, sorbic acid was found to inhibit formation of *N*-nitrosodiethanolamine, *N*-methyl-*N*-nitrosoamiline, and *N*-nitrosomorpholine. Inhibition was less pronounced in an anionic oil-water emulsion and nonexistent in animal stomachs with aminopyrine and sodium nitrite (Sofos, 1989). Overall, however, and under the conditions of commercial application, sorbic acid and its salts are considered to be one of the safest antimicrobial agents used in foods.

III. BENZOIC ACID AND ITS SALTS

A. Chemical Properties and Uses

Benzoic, also known as phenylformic or benzenecarboxylic, acid (C_6H_5COOH) is widely used as an antimicrobial agent in foods, especially as sodium benzoate. The compound is available as a white granular or crystalline powder with a sweet or a somewhat astringent taste, with a molecular weight of 122.13. Benzoic acid is found naturally in prunes, cranberries, geengage plums, cinnamon, apples, and ripe olives (Chipley, 1993). Its solubility in water of ambient temperature is 0.35%, but it is more soluble in alcohol, ether, chloroform, and oil. The commonly used sodium salt, available as a white powder or flakes, is highly soluble in water (50%), but it is insoluble in ether (Chichester and Tanner, 1972; Kimble, 1977; Sofos and Busta, 1992).

Benzoates are used widely for the preservation of foods with pH below 4.5 because of the low cost and ease of incorporation into the products. Limitations in their use include their narrow pH range of effectiveness, their undesirable flavor, and their toxicological profile, which is less desirable than that of other common antimicrobial agents (Lück, 1980; Chipley, 1993). Food products preserved with benzoates include fruit products, beverages, bakery items, and margarine. Specifically, benzoates are used in fruit juices and drinks, fruit salads and cocktails, salads and salad dressings, pickles and relishes, olives and sauerkraut, dried fruits and preserves, jams and jellies, margarine, and animal feeds. In addition, benzoic acid has a long history of use in the preservation of pharmaceuticals and cosmetic products. Concentrations used in preservation are in the range of 0.05–0.1%, but when flavor problems develop, it may be used at lower levels and in combination with other antimicrobial agents, such as sorbate and parabens (Jermini and Schmidt-Lorenz, 1987; Sofos and Busta, 1992).

B. Antimicrobial Properties

As an antimicrobial agent, benzoate is more effective against yeasts and bacteria than molds (Chichester and Tanner, 1972; Sofos and Busta, 1992). The antimicrobial activity varies, however, with food, its pH and water activity, and with types and species of microorganisms. Osmotolerant species of yeasts, which spoil intermediate moisture foods, appear to be resistant to inhibition by benzoate (Warth, 1977, 1985, 1988, 1989; Jermini and Schmidt-Lorenz, 1987; Chipley, 1993). Resistance to benzoate or sorbate in yeasts such as *Zygosaccharmyces bailii* appears to be due to an inducible, energy-requiring mechanism, which transports the compound out of the cell.

Certain microorganisms are capable of metabolizing benzoic acid. Bacteria metabolizing the compound include certain species of Enterobacteriaceae, *Pseudomonas, Corynebacterium glutamicum*, and thermophilic *Bacillus*. Metabolism appears to involve the β-ketoapidate pathway (Chipley, 1993). Pathogenic bacteria may be inhibited by concentrations of 0.01–0.02% undissociated benzoic acid (El-Shenawy and Marth, 1988; Sofos and Busta, 1992). As an antimicrobial agent, benzoate acts synergistically with sodium chloride, sucrose, boric acid, heat, carbon dioxide, and sulfur dioxide (Chichester and Tanner, 1972; Lück, 1980; Beuchat,

1981). In addition, antagonistic effects have been observed, since the antimicrobial activity of benzoic acid was reduced by nonionic surfactants (Chipley, 1993).

Similar to other lipophilic acid antimicrobial agents, the activity of the compound is due to its undissociated molecule. Therefore, its antimicrobial activity increases as the pH of the substrate approaches its dissociation constant (pKa) of 4.2 (Sofos and Busta, 1992). The maximum pH for significant antimicrobial activity is 4.5, and maximum activity occurs at pH values of 2.5–4.0. At pH 6.0, the antimicrobial activity is only 1% of that at pH 4.0. Therefore, the compound is more effective in acid foods or in products acidified with an acidulant. Proposed mechanisms of antimicrobial activity are the same as those described for sorbic acid.

C. Toxicological Properties

Benzoic acid and sodium benzoate are considered GRAS when used in accordance with good manufacturing practices. The *Food Additives Handbook* (Lewis, 1989) describes benzoic acid as "poison by subcutaneous route; moderately toxic by ingestion and intraperitoneal routes; causing human systemic effects by inhalation, such as dyspnea and allergic dermatitis; severe eye and skin irritant; combustible when exposed to heat or flame; reacting with oxidizing materials; the powder burning rapidly in oxygen; when heated to decomposition, it emits acrid smoke and irritating fumes." Sodium benzoate is described as "poison by intravenous and intraperitoneal routes; moderately toxic by ingestion; a corrosive irritant to skin, eyes and mucous membranes; mutagen; allergen; when heated to decomposition it emits toxic fumes of SO_x and Na_2O." The oral LD_{50} for rats is 2530 mg/kg for benzoic acid and 2000 mg/kg for sodium benzoate. Other toxicity data for benzoic acid include: moderate irritant to human skin at 22 mg/3 days of intermittent exposure; human skin toxic dose low (TDL_o) at 6 mg/kg; mild skin irritant in rabbits at 500 mg/24 hours of exposure; severe rabbit eye irritant at 100 mg; inhibitor of human lymphocyte DNA at 5 mmol/L; mutagen of *Escherichia coli* at 10 mmol/L; and oral lethal dose low (LDL_o) for humans at 500 mg/kg. Toxicity data for sodium benzoate include mutagen for *Salmonella typhimurium* at 1 mmol/L and for *Escherichia coli* at 1 mol/L (Lewis, 1989; Sax and Lewis, 1989).

Several studies have examined the toxicity of benzoic acid and sodium benzoate in animals and humans (Lück, 1980; Concon, 1988; Chipley, 1993). Acute toxicity data for several animals (cat, dog, rabbit, guinea pig) include doses for 100% mortality in the range of 1.4–2.0 g/kg body weight. Subchronic toxicity data include (1) exposure of mice to 3% benzoate in their diet for 5 days resulted in 50% mortality, while 4% in the diet for 3 months had no effect; (2) doses of 1 g/day for 3 months, 12 g/14 days, 0.3–0.4 g/60–100 days, and 5–10 g/several days had no effect in humans. In chronic toxicity studies, exposure of mice or rats to 40 mg/kg body weight per day for 17–18 months resulted in growth disturbance (Lück, 1980; Chipley, 1993).

Extensive human feeding studies at the beginning of benzoate use as an antimicrobial agent indicated that the compound causes no adverse effects on human health (Chichester and Tanner, 1972; Lück, 1980; Sofos and Busta, 1992; Chipley, 1993). Due to a detoxifying mechanism, benzoate does not accumulate in the human body. Detoxification involves absorbance of benzoate by the intestine, activation through linkage with coenzyme A to form benzoyl coenzyme A, which is catalyzed by a synthetase enzyme, and synthesis of hippuric acid in the liver from benzoyl coenzyme A and glycine, which is catalyzed by an acyltransferase enzyme. The hippuric acid is then excreted in the urine (Chichester and Tanner, 1972; Lück, 1980; Sofos and Busta, 1992; Chipley, 1993). It has been estimated that 60–99% of benzoic acid is excreted as hippuric acid, while there are indications that the remaining is excreted in the urine through conjugation with glucuronic acid (Thabrew et al., 1980; Chipley, 1993). Metabolism of benzoic acid, however, is variable with animal species, depending on their ability to carry out glycine and glucuronic acid conjugation (Kao et al., 1978).

Elimination of benzoic acid through the hippuric acid route was inhibited, while glucuronide formation was enhanced in male rats with thiamine deficiency, while the opposite occurred when thiamine levels were elevated (Chipley, 1993). Elimination of benzoic acid in channel catfish was reported to be through the renal route (Plakas and James, 1990). More than 80% of the radiolabeled compound was recovered in the urine within 24 hours, with more than 90% of this being unchanged benzoic acid. Of the metabolized compound, the major metabolite detected was benzoyltaurine (Chipley, 1993). Sodium benzoate has been reported to inhibit fatty acid oxidation in the liver of rats, and it has been prescribed for oral administration in patients with inherent problems in urea synthesis (Kalbag and Palekar, 1988; Kubota et al., 1988).

No mutagenic, teratogenic, and carcinogenic effects, or other adverse clinical signs due to benzoic acid, have been reported from animal feeding studies (Chipley, 1993). There is some evidence, however, that under certain conditions sodium benzoate may be an experimental mutagen and teratogen (Sax and Lewis, 1989), but in general benzoate is considered as a safe food preservative.

IV. PROPIONIC ACID AND ITS SALTS

A. Chemical Properties and Uses

Propionic acid (CH_3CH_2COOH) is also known as carboxyethane, ethane carboxylic acid, ethylformic acid, metacetonic acid, and methyl acetic acid. It is an aliphatic, monocarboxylic acid of 74.09 molecular weight, and is an oily liquid with a pungent, disagreeable, rancid odor. It is miscible in water, alcohol, ether, and chloroform, and it is somewhat corrosive. Its salts are white, free-flowing powders, having a slight cheeselike flavor, and the sodium (150%) salt is more soluble than the calcium (55.8%) salt (Chichester and Tanner, 1972; Lewis, 1989; Sofos and Busta, 1992; Doores, 1993).

Propionic acid occurs naturally in Swiss-type cheeses at levels as high as 1%, where it is formed by *Propionibacterium bacteria*, which are involved in the ripening of these cheeses. It is also found as a bacterial metabolite in the gastrointestinal tract of ruminants. The compound acts as an antimycotic agent in cheeses.

In addition to mold inhibition in cheeses, use of propionic acid and its salts involves preservation of baked goods, where they inhibit molds and rope-forming bacteria (*Bacillus mesentericus*). Other reasons for their usefulness in the preservation of baked products is their low cost and inactivity against the yeast involved in leavening of yeast-raised products. However, sodium propionate is a more suitable preservative in yeast-leavened products because the calcium ion of calcium propionate interferes with the leavening action. In products where calcium propionate is used, it contributes to their enrichment with calcium. Levels of propionate used as antimicrobial agents are in the range of 0.1–0.38%. Specific bakery products preserved with propionates include breads, cakes, pie crusts, and pie fillings. Other applications involve inhibition of mold growth on the surface of cheeses, processed cheese products, fruits, vegetables, jams, jellies, preserves, malt extract, and tobacco (Chichester and Tanner, 1972; Lück, 1980; Robach, 1980; Sofos and Busta, 1992; Doores, 1993).

B. Antimicrobial Properties

As indicated above, propionates are active inhibitors of molds and rope-forming bacteria, but have very little activity against yeasts. Many yeasts metabolize propionate, and its activity against bacteria, with the exception of *Bacillus mesentericus*, is marginal (Sofos and Busta, 1992; Doores, 1993). In addition to microbial species, antimicrobial activity is affected by product pH. Similar to other lipophilic acid preservatives, the antimicrobial activity increases at pH values approaching its pKa value of 4.9, with a maximum pH of usefulness at 6.0. The antimicrobial activity against bacteria and molds may be reversed by β-alanine, which may indicate that microbial inhibition involves interference with synthesis of β-alanine (Doores, 1993). Other proposed mechanisms of antimicrobial activity are similar to those for other lipophilic acid preservatives, including interference with nutrient transport and inhibition of enzyme systems (Eklund, 1980; Sofos and Busta, 1992).

C. Toxicological Properties

Propionic acid and its salts, calcium and sodium propionate, are classified as GRAS when used at concentrations not exceeding the amount reasonably needed to achieve the intended effect. Propionic acid is described in the *Food Additives Handbook* (Lewis, 1989) as "poison by intraperitoneal route; moderately toxic by ingestion, skin contact and intravenous routes; a corrosive irritant to eyes, skin and mucous membranes; flammable liquid; emitting acrid smoke and irritating fumes when heated to decomposition." Sodium propionate is also described as an allergen. The oral LD_{50} for propionic acid in rats is 3500 mg/kg. Doses of propionic acid causing severe rabbit skin and eye irritations are 495 mg and 990 μg, respectively. The subcutaneous mouse LD_{50} for sodium propionate is 2100 mg/kg, and the skin rabbit LD_{50} is 1640 mg/kg (Lewis, 1989). The intravenous mouse LD_{50} for propionic acid is 625 mg/kg body weight. The oral rat LD_{50} values for calcium and sodium propionate are 3340 and 5100 mg/kg body weights, respectively. The corresponding rat intravenous LD_{50} values are 580–1020 and 1380–3200 mg/kg body weight (Doores, 1993). The Food and Agriculture Organization has set no limit on the ADI for humans for propionic acid and its sodium, potassium, and calcium salts.

As a lipophilic acid, propionate is expected to be metabolized like other fatty acids in the mammalian body. Amounts as high as 1% may be present in Swiss-type cheeses with no adverse effects on consumers. No adverse effects were detected in the health of rats fed diets with levels of up to 5% propionate for periods of time up to one year (Chichester and Tanner, 1972; Doores, 1993).

V. ESTERS OF *PARA*-HYDROXYBENZOIC ACID

A. Chemical Properties and Uses

Esters of p-hydroxybenzoic acid [$C_6H_4(OH)COOH$] used as antimicrobial agents in cosmetics, pharmaceutical and food products include methyl, ethyl, propyl, butyl, and heptyl esters, also known as parabens, paracepts, or PHB esters. They are available as ivory-to-white, free-flowing powders, and their properties are similar to those of benzoic acid. In contrast to benzoic acid, however, their solubility in water is higher and decreases with increasing number of carbon atoms in the ester group. Solubility in oil, ethanol, and propylene glycol increases with more atoms in the ester group. The compounds are stable in air and resistant to cold and heat and steam sterilization. All parabens are odorless except for the methyl ester, which has a faint characteristic odor (Chichester and Tanner, 1972; Parker, 1992; Sofos and Busta, 1992; Davidson, 1993).

The parabens permitted for use in foods in the United States are methyl, propyl, and heptyl esters. Common applications involve use of a combination of methyl and propyl parabens at ratios of 2–3:1. These combinations take advantage of respective solubilities and antimicrobial properties and are used in concentrations of 0.05–0.1%. For application, the compounds may be dissolved in room temperature or warm water, ethanol, propylene glycol, or in the food. Products in which parabens have been used, or at least tested, as antimicrobial agents include bakery products, cheeses, soft drinks, beer, wines, jams, jellies, preserves, pickles, olives, syrups, and fish products. Potential taste problems, high solubility in lipids, and cost may be limiting factors in the use of parabens as antimicrobial agents in foods (Chichester and Tanner, 1972; Lück, 1980; Robach, 1980; Sofos and Busta, 1980, 1992; Jermini and Schmidt-Lorenz, 1987; Davidson, 1993).

B. Antimicrobial Properties

Parabens exert antimicrobial activity against yeasts, molds, and bacteria. Microbial inhibition increases with alkyl chain length. The antimicrobial activity of branched chain esters is low. Yeasts and molds are more sensitive to inhibition than bacteria, especially the gram-negative species. Genera of microorganisms inhibited by parabens include *Alternaria, Aspergillus, Penicillium, Rhizopus, Saccharomyces, Bacillus, Staphylococcus, Streptococcus, Clostridium, Pseudomonas, Salmonella, Vibrio,* etc. (Robach and Pierson, 1978; Lück, 1980; Sofos and Busta, 1980, 1992; Draughon et al., 1982; Fung et al., 1985; Payne et al., 1989; Davidson, 1993).

Use of parabens is advantageous in high-pH products because of their high pKa (8.5) value. Depending on cost, pH, and flavor, they may also be used in combination with benzoic acid, especially in products with slightly acidic pH values. Parabens are preferred, however, in higher-pH foods where other antimicrobial agents are ineffective (Sofos and Busta, 1992).

Inhibition of microbial growth by parabens has been attributed to interference with nutrient transport functions (Eklund, 1980). Other effects attributed to parabens include inhibition of bacterial spore germination, respiration, protease secretion, and DNA, RNA, and protein synthesis (Nes and Eklund, 1983; Venugopal et al., 1984; Sofos and Busta, 1992).

C. Toxicological Properties

The methyl and propyl parabens are listed as GRAS in the United States, while the heptyl ester is also approved for use in malt beverages and noncarbonated soft drinks. The ethyl and butyl esters are also approved for use in some countries (Chichester and Tanner, 1972; Sofos and Busta, 1992). The *Food Additives Handbook* (Lewis, 1989) describes the ethyl and methyl esters as "moderately toxic by ingestion and intraperitoneal routes; experimental teratogen and mutagen; when heated to decomposition it emits acrid smoke and fumes." The oral mouse LD_{50} for the ethyl ester is 3 g/kg body weight. In general, the LD_{50} doses range from 180 to 8000 mg/kg body weight, depending on the compound, animal, and route of administration (Lück, 1980; Sandmeyer and Kirwin, 1981; Sofos and Busta, 1992; Davidson, 1993). The acceptable daily intake is 10 mg/kg body weight. Other toxicity data for the ethyl ester include intraperitoneal mouse LD_{50} of 520 mg/kg, oral rat TDL_o of 45,600 mg/kg for 8–15 days during pregnancy, causing teratogenic effects, cytotoxic to hamster fibroblasts at 250 mg/L, and mutagen for *Escherichia coli* at 10 mmol/L. The methyl ester has an oral dog LD_{50} of 3000 mg/kg body weight, and it is cytotoxic to hamster lungs at 125 mg/L/27 hours (Lewis, 1989).

In dogs, parabens cause acute myocardial depression and hypotension, but the effect is noncumulative. Subchronic testing at 500 mg methyl paraben per kg body weight in rabbits over 6 days had no toxic activity, while the dose of 3500 mg was toxic (Lück, 1980). Feeding rats diets with 2% of methyl and propyl parabens for 96 weeks caused no changes in weight gain and histology, but the 8% level retarded growth. Concentrations as high as 5% have caused no skin irritation in humans. The parabens are believed to be absorbed in the intestines, from which travel to the kidney and the liver, where the ester bond is hydrolyzed, resulting in *p*-hydroxybenzoic acid, glucuronic acid esters, or sulfates, most of which are excreted by the body (Chichester and Tanner, 1972; Lück, 1980; Sandmeyer and Kirwin, 1981; Davidson, 1993).

VI. SULFUR DIOXIDE AND SULFITES

A. Chemical Properties and Uses

Sulfur dioxide (SO_2) is one of the oldest antimicrobial agents, used as a fumigant in products such as wines (Banks et al., 1987; Sofos and Busta, 1992). The compound is a colorless, nonflammable gas or liquid under pressure, with a suffocating, pungent odor. When dissolved in the water of foods, it yields sulfurous acid and its ions, because it is soluble in water. The amount of ions increases with decreasing pH values. In addition to sulfur dioxide gas, sulfite salts, such as sodium sulfite (Na_2SO_3), potassium sulfite (K_2SO_3), sodium metabisulfite ($Na_2S_2O_5$), and potassium metabisulfite ($K_2S_2O_5$) may be used as preservatives. The sulfite salts are more convenient to use because they are available as dry materials, which, when dissolved in water, form sulfurous acid, bisulfite (HSO_3^-), and sulfite ($SO_3^=$) ions. During storage, however, the available sulfur dioxide in the dry salts decreases due to oxidation, which is higher in moist environments. Stability increases from sulfites to bisulfites and metabisulfites (Chichester and Tanner, 1972; Sofos and Busta, 1992; Ough, 1993a). The dissociation constants for sulfur dioxide are 1.76 and 7.20, and their reactivity has been discussed by Ough (1993a).

The sulfiting agents are used as antimicrobial agents in several food products, including wines, dehydrated fruits and vegetables, fruit juices, pickles, salads, syrups, meat, and fish products. In the United States their use in meat products is not permitted because they can destroy thiamine and may restore the color of old meat, which would mislead consumers (Tompkin et al., 1980; Sofos and Busta, 1992). In addition to antimicrobial activity, they are useful in foods for their antioxidant and reducing properties, which inhibit enzymatic and nonenzymatic browning reactions.

Use of sulfites in wine-making destroys the naturally occurring microbial flora before addition of the desirable fermentation yeast. Additional effects in the wine industry include decontamination of equipment, inhibition of bacteria spoilage, and activity as antioxidant and clarifying agents. The concentration used ranges from 0.005 to 0.01%, depending on condition of grapes, type of wine, pH, sugar concentration, and contamination. Use of sulfites in wines is often combined with addition of sorbate (Sofos, 1989). Excessive amounts of sulfites result in off-flavors and product discoloration in products such as fruits, where they control molds (Chichester and Tanner, 1972; Sofos, 1989; Sofos and Busta, 1992; Ough, 1993a).

B. Antimicrobial Properties

The antimicrobial activity of sulfites against yeasts, molds and bacteria is selective, with certain species being more sensitive to inhibition than others (Sofos and Busta, 1992). Bacteria are generally more sensitive to inhibition than yeasts and molds (Chichester and Tanner, 1972). The major groups of microorganisms that are of interest, relative to the antimicrobial activity of sulfites, are acetic acid– and malolactic acid–producing bacteria, fermentative and spoilage yeasts, and molds involved in spoilage of fruits (Ough, 1993a). The *Acetobacter* bacteria are inhibited through reaction of sulfur dioxide with cysteine and thiamine. In addition, sulfites inhibit lactic acid–producing bacteria of the genera *Lactobacillus, Pediococcus,* and *Leuconostoc* in wines. Sodium metabisulfite has also inhibited growth of *Clostridium botulinum* in canned pork (Tompkin et al., 1980). There is evidence, however, that sulfur dioxide is more effective against gram-negative than gram-positive bacteria (Ough, 1993a).

In wine-making, sulfites inhibit or inactivate wild yeasts present in grape juice. Susceptibility of yeasts to sulfites, however, is variable with genera, with the fermentative *Saccharomyces* generally being resistant to inhibition. Sulfites are also useful as mold inhibitors in fruits such as grapes.

The undissociated sulfurous acid is 100–1000 times more inhibitory than sulfite and bisulfite ions against microorganisms. In addition to pH, antimicrobial activity is affected by concentration, sulfur dioxide binding, and duration of contact (Sofos and Busta, 1992). Being highly reactive, sulfur dioxide reacts with cell components, such as proteins, enzymes, vitamins, cofactors, nucleotides, nucleic acids, and lipids, producing inhibitory or lethal effects (Woodzinski et al., 1978; Clark and Takacs, 1980; Lück, 1980). As a lipid prooxidant, sulfur dioxide may interfere with membrane functions, while by cleaving disulfide bonds of proteins, it changes enzyme conformation and activity (Sofos and Busta, 1992).

C. Toxicological Properties

Sulfur dioxide and sulfites are GRAS substances, but levels of application are restricted to 0.035% in wines. Higher levels result in undesirable flavors, and sulfites are not permitted in foods considered as sources of the vitamin thiamine, because they inactivate the nutrient (Chichester and Tanner, 1972; Daniel, 1985; Walker, 1988; Sofos and Busta, 1992; Ough, 1993a).

The LD_{50} doses for sulfites vary with animal species and route of administration and are 130–675 mg/kg of body weight for mice, 115–2000 mg/kg for rats, 65–300 mg/kg for rabbits, 95 mg/kg for hamsters, and 244 mg/kg for dogs (Ough, 1993a). Sulfur dioxide is included in the "extremely hazardous substances" list of the Environmental Protection Agency (EPA). According to the *Food Additives Handbook* (Lewis, 1989), the safety profile of sulfur dioxide is described as "a poison gas; moderately toxic experimentally by inhalation; mildly toxic to humans by inhalation; experimental tumorigen and teratogen; causing human systemic effects by inhalation, such as pulmonary vascular resistance, respiratory depression and other pulmonary changes; affecting mostly the upper respiratory tract and bronchi; may cause edema of the lungs or glottis and respiratory paralysis; a corrosive irritant to eyes, skin and mucous membranes; levels of 0.04–0.05% are immediately dangerous to life, with levels of 0.005–0.01% being considered as maximum permissible for exposures of 30–60 minutes; excessive exposures to high concentrations can be fatal; reacts with water or steam to produce toxic and corrosive fumes; when heated to decomposition, it emits toxic fumes of SO_x." Sodium sulfite is described as "poison by intravenous and subcutaneous routes; moderately toxic by ingestion and intraperitoneal routes; when heated to decomposition it emits very toxic fumes of Na_2O and SO_x." Sodium bisulfite is listed as "poison by intravenous and intraperitoneal routes; moderately toxic by ingestion; a corrosive irritant to skin, eyes and mucous membranes; and allergen." The description of sodium metabisulfite includes "poison by intravenous route; moderately toxic by parenteral route; and experimental reproductive effects." Additional toxicity data are listed by Lewis (1989).

Ingestion of sulfites at levels present in foods does not result in accumulation in the body because they are rapidly oxidized to sulfate and excreted in the urine. Sublethal, but higher than tolerable, doses (e.g., 62 mg/kg body weight) of sulfur dioxide have resulted in physiological changes in rats, including polyneuritis, bleached incisors, visceral organ atrophy, bone marrow atrophy, renal tubular caste, limited growth, and spectacle eyes (Sofos and Busta, 1992). When it comes in contact with the eyes, as highly soluble in fat, sulfur dioxide is absorbed and penetrates the cornea, causing deep keratitis and iritis (Ough, 1993a).

Levels of sulfur dioxide above 33 mg/L of air can cause severe distress or death when inhaled by sensitive individuals (Amadur, 1975). This is due to pulmonary dysfunction, which is manifested as pulmonary edema, lung hemorrhage, and visceral congestion, as well as coughing, lacrimation, and sneezing (Ough, 1993a). Chronic symptoms include hypertrophy of goblet cells and mucous glands and lungs (NAS, 1978). Individuals working in old sugar beet–processing plants are at risk of being overexposed to sulfur dioxide (Ough, 1993a).

Ingested levels of sulfur dioxide of 30–100 mg/kg body weight per day, depending upon species, were declared as causing no toxic effects (Select Committee on GRAS Substances, 1976). The acceptable daily intake established by the Joint FAO/WHO Committee (1974) is 0.7 mg sulfur dioxide/kg body weight per day. In addition, the Select Committee on GRAS substances (1976) indicated that the estimated human consumption of 0.2 mg/kg body weight per day was not a hazard to human health (Ough, 1993a). These findings were reexamined and endorsed by the FDA (1985). The FDA report also indicated that sulfur dioxide decreased the mutagenic activity of other substances, even though some studies found it to be mutagenic on bacteria (De Giovanni-Donnelly, 1985). In general, no mutagenic, teratogenic, or carcinogenic effects were reported for sulfur dioxide in studies using rats and mice (Wedzicha, 1984; Ough, 1993a).

Sulfites, however, have been associated as triggering asthma attacks and other acute allergenic responses, some of which are life threatening or fatal in a small number of susceptible asthmatic humans (Ough, 1993a). It appears that most asthmatics are hypersensitive to sulfites present in medical preparations or foods (Gunnison, 1981; FDA, 1983; Gunnison and Jacobsen, 1987; Gunnison et al., 1987). A major problem has been use of sulfites as agents to maintain freshness in salads and fruits served in restaurants and in wines (Martin et al., 1986; Ough, 1993a). The FDA (1985) has published lists of foods and beverages containing sulfites and the estimated average daily human intake from each product. They range from none in some dried fruits to 3.68 mg per capita per day in some wines (Ough, 1993a). This has resulted in restrictions in their use as food preservatives, labeling requirements, and concerns about foods sold without labels, such as salads in restaurants, which may be treated with sulfites to prevent browning (Walker, 1985; FDA, 1986a,b, 1988, 1990; Anonymous, 1986; Sofos and Busta, 1992).

VII. CARBON DIOXIDE

A. Chemical Properties and Uses

Carbon dioxide (CO_2) is a gas that solidifies at $-78.5°C$, forming dry ice. As a gas, it is colorless, odorless, and noncombustible with an acidic odor and flavor. In addition to dry ice, it is commercially available as a liquid under pressure (58 kg per cm^2). The gas is highly soluble in water (171% at $0°C$), and it forms carbonic acid in the liquid phase of foods (Clark and Takacs, 1980; Sofos and Busta, 1992).

In addition to its use as an antimicrobial agent, carbon dioxide is useful as an aerating, carbonation, cooling, leavening, pH control, processing aid, and propellant agent (Lewis, 1989). Products preserved or treated with carbon dioxide include carbonated beverages, vegetables, fruits, meat, poultry, fish, and wines. As dry ice, it is useful in the low-temperature storage and transportation of products. As it sublimes, it generates gas, which then inhibits microbial growth. As a component of controlled or modified atmospheres in storage of fruits and vegetables, it delays respiration and ripening and inhibits growth of yeasts and molds. In carbonated soft drinks and mineral waters, carbon dioxide serves not only as an effervescing agent, but also as an inhibitor of microbial growth. In beer and ale, it inhibits oxidative changes (Sofos and Busta, 1992).

B. Antimicrobial Properties

The antimicrobial activity of carbon dioxide depends on concentration, types of microorganisms, water activity, and temperature of storage. As these factors vary, carbon dioxide may exert no effect, stimulate growth, inhibit growth, or be lethal to microorganisms (Enfors and Molin, 1978; Clark and Takacs, 1980; Davidson et al., 1983; Foegeding and Busta, 1983; Sofos and Busta, 1992). At high concentrations, carbon dioxide inactivates microorganisms or at least increases their log phase and generation time. Low concentrations may enhance bacterial spore germination and growth. The inhibitory action increases linearly as concentrations increase to up to 25–50% in the atmosphere, but increases in inhibitory activity at higher concentrations are only slight.

Inhibition of bacteria by carbon dioxide is variable, while molds are generally sensitive and yeasts usually resistant (Davidson et al., 1983; Sofos and Busta, 1992). The gram-negative psychrotrophic bacteria are more sensitive to carbon dioxide than are gram-positive species. Thus, storage of products such as meats and fish under reduced oxygen and increased carbon dioxide modified atmospheres should inhibit aerobic spoilage organisms and encourage growth of lactic acid bacteria (Rowe, 1988; Baker and Genigeorgis, 1990). There is a concern, however, whether pathogens will outgrow spoilage organisms and render products unsafe for human consumption, while they still appear unspoiled, under the modified atmosphere package (Genigeorgis, 1985; Post et al., 1985; Garcia et al., 1987; Hintlian and Hotchkiss, 1987).

C. Toxicological Properties

Inhalation of 30–60% carbon dioxide in the presence of 20% oxygen can cause death to animals, while exposure of humans to atmospheres of more than 10% results in unconsciousness (Lück, 1980; Sofos and Busta, 1992). Also, inhalation of small amounts over extended periods of time may be dangerous. Exposure of male mice to a mixture of 1.8:1.0 of air-carbon dioxide for 6 hours reduced the area and breadth of the head and of the midpiece of live spermatozoa in the vase deferentia. A total exposure of 26.5 hours over 6 days reduced conception rates, but the number of offspring produced per litter were normal (Mukherjee and Singh, 1967). When used according to good manufacturing practices, however, the compound is listed as GRAS.

In the *Food Additives Handbook* (Lewis, 1989), carbon dioxide is described as "an asphyxiant, experimental teratogen; causing experimental reproductive effects; causing burns as dry ice; causing ignition and explosion of dusts of magnesium, aluminum, manganese, chromium, and some magnesium-aluminum alloys; reacting vigorously with oxides, several salts or ions; being incompatible with acrylaldehyde, aziridine, metal acetylides and sodium peroxide."

VIII. OTHER ANTIMICROBIAL AGENTS

A. Dimethyl and Diethyl Dicarbonates

Dimethyl dicarbonate (DMDC) has a molecular weight of 134.09, and its solubility in water is 3.65%. The compound is a colorless liquid of fruity flavor (Lewis, 1989;

Sofos and Busta, 1992; Ough, 1993b). It is a mold and yeast inhibitor useful in wines, where it is permitted for use at the maximum level of 0.02% (Lewis, 1989). DMDC, as well as diethyl dicarbonate (DEDC), hydrolyzes to methanol, or ethanol, and carbon dioxide in water solutions, especially in acidic environments. DEDC has a molecular weight of 162.16 and is soluble in alcohols, esters, and hydrocarbons. Its activity is against yeasts and bacteria, but its use in foods and wines is prohibited in the United States; it may be used in some countries as a wine preservative (Chichester and Tanner, 1972; Lewis, 1989; Sofos and Busta, 1992; Ough, 1993b).

In addition to wines, legal uses of DEDC as a sterilant in the past included beverages, fruit juices, and beer. Banning was due to products of hydrolysis and decomposition, such as methanol and ethyl carbonate. DMDC may still be used as a yeast inhibitor in wines at levels no to exceed 0.02%. The Expert Committee on Food Additives of the FAO/WHO of the United Nations has recommended that human daily intakes of ethyl carbonate not exceed 10 µg. Ethyl carbonate is a carcinogen formed from reactions of DEDC with ammonia (Sofos and Busta, 1992). The *Food Additives Handbook* (Lewis, 1989) describes DMDC as "poison by ingestion and intraperitoneal routes; irritating to eyes, mucus membranes and skin when concentrated; emitting acrid smoke and fumes when heated to decomposition." The oral LD_{50} doses are 850 and 2027 mg/kg body weight for rats and mice, respectively. The intraperitoneal LD_{50} dose for rats is 100 mg/kg (Lewis, 1989). Additional information on the toxicology of DEDC has been presented by Ough (1993b).

B. Epoxides

Ethylene (C_2H_4O) and propylene (C_3H_6O) oxides are cyclic ethers with one oxygen atom linked to two adjacent carbon atoms of the same chain (Davidson et al., 1983; Sofos and Busta, 1992). Ethylene oxide exists as a colorless, noncorrosive gas at room temperature, which liquefies at 10.8°C and freezes at -111.3°C (Sofos and Busta, 1992; Hugo and Russell, 1992; Christensen and Kristensen, 1992). The compound is flammable and at concentrations exceeding 0.07%, it has an etherlike odor. When mixed at levels of 10–20% with 80–90% carbon dioxide it becomes nonflammable. Low concentrations of ethylene oxide, however, are explosive. Generally, it is safer for use when mixed with carbon dioxide or other gases.

Ethylene oxide gas can penetrate, without damage, most organic materials, which makes it useful in the sterilization of heat sensitive materials. The compound has been used to decontaminate several dried products, including dried fruits, potato flour, corn, wheat, barley, dried eggs, gums, gelatin, and cereals. In addition, both epoxides have been used to decontaminate equipment, spices, and other heat-sensitive materials. Their application in spices has been noteworthy. Inactivation of microorganisms in spices depends on concentration, temperature, relative humidity, and ease of penetration. Epoxides are effective against yeasts, molds, and insects, but less active against bacteria. The antimicrobial action of both epoxides is due to their alkylating properties and depends on humidity and ease of penetration (Clark and Takacs, 1980; Davidson et al., 1983).

The safety profile of ethylene oxide in the *Food Additives Handbook* (Lewis, 1989) indicates that it is "poison by ingestion, intraperitoneal, subcutaneous, intravenous and possibly other routes; moderately toxic by inhalation; suspected human carcinogen; experimental carcinogen, tumorigen, neoplastigen and teratogen; causing human systemic effects by inhalation, such as convulsions, nausea, vomiting, olfactory and pulmonary changes; causing experimental reproductive effects; human skin irritant; experimental eye irritant; irritant to mucous membranes of respiratory tract; high concentrations causing pulmonary edema." The subcutaneous and oral LD_{50} doses for rats are 187 and 72 mg/kg body weight, respectively. Additional toxicity data are listed by Lewis (1989).

In general, ethylene oxide is highly toxic and carcinogenic, even at levels (0.005–0.01%) below its odor threshold (0.07%). When in contact with the skin, it causes blister formation. In foods, it can form nonvolatile and toxic ethylene glycol and ethylene chlorhydrin. Upon treatment, however, the epoxides are removed from the food by evacuation and gentle heating (Davidson et al., 1983; Sofos and Busta, 1992).

The other epoxide, propylene oxide, is less active as a sterilant and less penetrating than ethylene oxide. The properties of both compounds are similar, but higher amounts of propylene oxide are needed for the same antimicrobial effect. Propylene oxide is also less toxic than ethylene oxide. One of its degradation products is propylene glycol, which is an approved food additive (Sofos and Busta, 1992).

C. Hydrogen Peroxide

Hydrogen peroxide (H_2O_2), or hydrogen dioxide, is a colorless, water-miscible, heavy liquid or a crystalline solid at low temperatures (Davidson et al., 1983; Lewis, 1989; Sofos and Busta, 1992). It is an oxidizing and bleaching agent with antimicrobial properties. It is very unstable and decomposes readily to form water and oxygen. Its decomposition, as well as antimicrobial activity, increases at higher temperatures.

It is approved for use as an antimicrobial, bleaching, oxidizing, preservative, and starch modifying agent (Lewis, 1989). Products in which it has been used include milk, dried eggs, corn syrup, distilling materials, starch, instant tea, tripe, whey, wine, vinegar, and packaging materials. Specific uses of hydrogen peroxide include treatment of milk with 0.5% for manufacture of cheeses with unheated milk, addition of egg whites for pasteurization at lower temperatures, and treatment of cartons or containers for aseptically processed foods (Sofos and Busta, 1992).

The antimicrobial activity of hydrogen peroxide is derived from its oxidizing properties, and it depends on concentration, pH, temperature, and exposure time (Smith and Brown, 1980; El-Gendy et al., 1980; Stevenson and Shafer, 1983). When used in foods, the compound decomposes rapidly or is inactivated by heat or by addition of catalase, which catalyzes formation of water and oxygen.

In addition to its use as an additive, hydrogen peroxide is also produced by lactobacilli in foods. In certain foods it may act not only as a direct antimicrobial agent, but also by reacting with thiocyanate to form the lactoperoxidase system (Banks et al., 1986; Daeschel, 1989).

Hydrogen peroxide is allowed for use in cheese making, whey processing, and other applications (Davidson et al., 1983; Lewis, 1989; Cords and Dychdala, 1993). In the *Food Additives Handbook* (Lewis, 1989), it is described as "moderately toxic by inhalation, ingestion and skin contact; corrosive and irritant to skin, eyes and mucous membranes; experimental tumorigen and suspected carcinogen; very powerful oxidizer; very irritating to body tissues." The oral mouse LD_{50} dose is 2 g/kg body weight, and the skin rat LD_{50} is 4060 mg/kg body weight (Lewis, 1989). Certain studies have indicated that it may be mutagenic and carcinogenic (Davidson et al., 1983; Melo Filho and Meneghini, 1984).

D. Products of Microbial Metabolism

In addition to chemical additives, certain compounds produced by microorganisms have exhibited antimicrobial activity. Some of these have been approved for use in food preservation, while others have only been proposed or tested as antimicrobial agents. Such substances include various antibiotics, bacteriocins, and other compounds, including lactic acid, hydrogen peroxide, and diacetyl (Hurst, 1981; Katz, 1983; Sofos and Busta, 1992; Katz and Brady, 1993; Hurst and Hoover, 1993; Davidson and Doan, 1993; Hoover, 1993).

In the 1950s and 1960s, antibiotics were tested extensively for use as antimicrobial agents in foods, but their application was later restricted or prohibited (Marth, 1966; Fukusumi, 1972). The only antibiotic still remaining in use in some countries is natamycin (pimaracin) (Davidson and Doan, 1993). The compound is approved for use as a mold inhibitor in cheese in some countries. Its rat LD_{50} doses are 5–10, 5000, 250, and 1500 mg/kg by the intravenous, subcutaneous, intraperitoneal, and oral routes, respectively. Additional information on the toxicology of natamycin is presented by Davidson and Doan (1993).

The reason for the discontinuation of the use of antibiotics as antimicrobial agents in foods was the potential development of antibiotic-resistant strains of microorganisms. If such strains colonize the digestive tract of humans and animals, then the antibiotics used for therapeutic purposes may become ineffective. Development of resistant strains from continuous use of antibiotics in foods at sublethal concentrations would reduce their future value as antimicrobial agents (Franco et al., 1990; Sofos and Busta, 1992).

Polypeptide bacteriocins were studied extensively in the 1980s for their potential to be used as natural antimicrobial agents in foods. The compounds are produced by bacteria and constitute a heterogeneous group of substances with variable antimicrobial activity, mode of action, and chemical properties (Klaenhammer, 1988; Daeschel, 1989; Montville, 1989; Gombas, 1989; Hansen et al., 1989; Sofos and Busta, 1992). Many bacteriocins are produced by lactic acid bacteria involved in food fermentations. Being polypeptides, they are considered safe, but their future as antimicrobial agents in foods is unknown.

The only microbially produced polypeptide that has been approved for use in certain cheeses is nisin (Hurst, 1981; Hurst and Hoover, 1993). Nisin preparation ($C_{143}H_{230}N_{42}O_{37}S_7$) is derived from *Streptococcus* (now *Lactococcus*) *lactis* Lancefield Group N and is approved for use as an antimicrobial agent in pasteurized cheese spreads in the United States at a maximum level of 0.025%. The only safety concern listed in the *Food Additives Handbook* is that "when heated to decomposition it emits acrid smoke and irritating fumes" (Lewis, 1989). Since lactococci are used in dairy fermentations, the compound should be naturally present in some of these products (Delves-Broughton, 1990).

Another antimicrobial agent that is derived by microorganisms and may be found in foods is ethyl alcohol (C_2H_6O), which is a clear, colorless liquid with a fragrant odor and burning taste. In the United States, ethyl alcohol may be used as an antimicrobial agent on pizza crusts prior to baking, at levels not to exceed 2% (Lewis, 1989; Sofos and Busta, 1992). Its antimicrobial activity is derived from its ability to denature proteins in the protoplast of the cells or through a reduction in water activity (Shapero et al., 1978).

Ethyl alcohol is classified as GRAS, but its safety profile in the *Food Additives Handbook* describes it as "moderately toxic to humans by ingestion; mildly toxic by inhalation and skin contact; experimental tumorigen and teratogen; moderately toxic experimentally by intravenous and intraperitoneal routes; causing human systemic effects when taken by ingestion and subcutaneous routes, including sleep disorders; hallucinations, distorted perception; convulsions, motor activity changes, ataxia, coma, antipsychotic, headache, pulmonary changes, alteration in gastric secretion, nausea or vomiting, other gastrointestinal changes, menstrual cycle changes and body temperature decrease; changes in female fertility index; toxic effects on newborn; mutagen; and eye and severe skin irritant." The oral LD_{50} dose for rats is 7060 mg/kg body weight. Other toxicity data are presented by Lewis (1989). In general, consumption of 200–400 ml of pure alcohol in a short period of time is hazardous for humans. Levels of 40–80 ml daily over long periods of time may be tolerable, but continuous use may lead to damage of the liver, where it is metabolized (Sofos and Busta, 1992).

E. Sanitizers

Chemical sanitizers used in the food industry are not permitted for direct use in foods, but they may be present in products indirectly when they are used to disinfect equipment surfaces and utensils, animal carcasses, or udders of milk-producing animals (Cords, 1983; Cords and Dychdala, 1993). The common sanitizers used in food-processing operations include halogens (e.g., chlorine and chlorine compounds and iodophors) and surface-active agents (e.g., quaternary ammonium compounds, acid-anionic surfactants, and amphoteric surfactants). Since these compounds are not used directly in foods, they are discussed only briefly. Use of chlorine as a disinfectant in drinking water has been criticized because it may react with organic matter to form carcinogenic trihalomethane compounds. Use of iodophor sanitizers at recommended levels should not be deleterious to human health. For more information on the chemical, antimicrobial, and toxicological properties of sanitizers, see Cords (1983) and Cords and Dychdala (1993).

IX. SUMMARY

Antimicrobial agents are necessary to extend the shelf life and combat pathogenic microorganisms of perishable food products. Use of antimicrobial agents is controlled and regulated by the health authorities of various countries, and their safety must be proven before they are approved for incorporation into food products. Commonly used antimicrobial agents in the United States include lipophilic acids, such as sorbic, benzoic, and propionic acids and their salts, esters of *p*-hydroxybenzoic acid, sulfur dioxide and sulfites, carbon dioxide, and certain other compounds of lesser application. As with every chemical agent, when administered at sufficiently high doses, almost all of these compounds can be toxic to laboratory animals or humans. At concentrations employed in foods and under conditions of good manufacturing practices, however, they are considered safe and useful as antimicrobial agents.

REFERENCES

Amadur, M. D. (1975). Air pollutants. In *Toxicology: The Basic Sciences of Poisons*, L. J. Casarett and J. Doull (eds.). Macmillan, New York, pp. 527–554.

Anonymous. (1986). Sulfites in foods—press conference report. *Food Technol. 40* (9):48–50.

Arya, S. S., and Thakur, B. R. (1988). Degradation of sorbic acid in aqueous solutions. *Food Chem. 29*:41–49.

Baker, D. A., and Genigeorgis, C. (1990). Predicting the safe storage of fresh fish under modified atmospheres with respect to *Clostridium botulinum* toxigenesis by modeling length of the lag phase of growth. *J. Food Prot. 53*:131–140.

Banks, J. G., Board, R. G., and Sparks, N. H. C. (1986). Natural antimicrobial systems and their potential in food preservation in the future. *Biotech. Appl. Biochem. 8*:103–147.

Banks, J. G., Nychas, G. J., and Board, R. G. (1987). Sulphite preservation of meat products. In *Preservatives in the Food, Pharmaceutical and Environmental Industries*, R. B. Board, M. C. Allwood, and J. G. Banks (eds.). Society for Applied Bacteriology Technical Series No. 22. Blackwell Scientific Publications, Oxford, pp. 17–33.

Beuchat, L. R. (1981). Influence of potassium sorbate and sodium benzoate on heat inactivation of *Aspergillus flavus*, *Penicillium puberulum* and *Geotrichum candidum*. *J. Food Prot. 44*:450–454.

Blocher, J. C., and Busta, F. G. (1985). Multiple modes of inhibition of spore germination and outgrowth by reduced pH and sorbate. *J. Appl. Bacteriol. 59*:469–478.

Chichester, D. F., and Tanner, F. W. (1972). Antimicrobial food additives. In *Handbook of Food Additives*, 2nd ed., T. E. Furia (ed.). CRC Press, Boca Raton, FL, pp. 115–184.

Chipley, J. R. (1993). Sodium benzoate and benzoic acid. In *Antimicrobials in Foods*, 2nd ed., P. M. Davidson and A. L. Branen (eds.). Marcel Dekker, New York, pp. 11–48.

Christensen, E. A., and Kristensen, H. (1992). Gaseous sterilization. In *Principles and Practice of Disinfection, Preservation and Sterilization*, 2nd ed., A. D. Russell, W. B. Hugo and G. A. J. Ayliffe (eds.). Blackwell Scientific Publications, London, pp. 557–572.

Clark, D. S., and Takacs, J. (1980). Gases as preservative. In *Microbial Ecology of Foods*, Vol. I, *Factors Affecting Life and Death of Microorganisms*. International Commission on Microbiological Specifications of Foods. Academic Press, New York, pp. 170–192.

Concon, J. M. (1988). Food additives. In *Food Toxicology, Part B: Contaminants and Additives*. Marcel Dekker, Inc., New York, pp. 1249–1311.

Cords, B. R. (1983). Sanitizers: halogens and surface-active agents. In *Antimicrobials in Foods*, A. L. Branen and P. M. Davidson (eds.). Marcel Dekker, New York, pp. 257–298.

Cords, B. R., and Dychdala, G. R. (1993). Sanitizers: halogens, surface-active agents, and peroxides. In *Antimicrobials in Foods*, 2nd ed., P. M. Davidson and A. L. Branen (eds.). Marcel Dekker, New York, pp. 469–538.

Daeschel, M. A. (1989). Antimicrobial substances from lactic acid bacteria for use as food preservatives. *Food Technol. 43* (1):164–167.

Daniel, J. W. (1985). Preservatives. In *Food Toxicology—Real or Imaginary Problems?*, G. G. Gibson and R. Walker (eds.). Taylor and Francis, London, pp. 229–237.

Davidson, P. M. (1993). Parabens and phenolic compounds. In *Antimicrobials in Foods*, 2nd ed., P. M. Davidson and A. L. Branen (eds.). Marcel Dekker, New York, pp. 263–306.

Davidson, P. M., and Doan, C. H. (1993). Natamycin. In *Antimicrobials in Foods*, 2nd ed., P. M. Davidson and A. L. Branen (eds.). Marcel Dekker, Inc., New York, pp. 395–408.

Davidson, P. M., Post, L. S., Branen, A. L., and McCurdy, A. R. (1983). Naturally occurring and miscellaneous food antimicrobials. In *Antimicrobials in Foods*, A. L. Branen and P. M. Davidson (eds.). Marcel Dekker, New York, pp. 371–419.

De Giovanni-Donnelly, R. (1985). The mutagenicity of sodium bisulfate on base-substitution of *Salmonella typhimurium*. *Teratogenesis, Carcinogenesis Mutagenesis 5*:195–203.

Delves-Broughton, J. (1990). Nisin and its uses as a food preservative. *Food Technol. 44* (11):100–117.

Deuel, H. J., Jr., Alfin-Slater, R., Weil, C. S., and Smyth, H. F., Jr. (1954a). Sorbic acid as a fungistatic agent for foods. 1. Harmlessness of sorbic acid as a dietary component. *Food Res. 19*:1–12.

Deuel, H. J., Jr., Calbert, C. E., Anisfeld, L., McKeehan, H., and Blunder, H. D. (1954b). Sorbic acid as a fungistatic agent for foods. II. Metabolism of β-unsaturated fatty acids with emphasis on sorbic acid. *Food Res. 19*:13–19.

Dickens, F., Jones, H. E. H., and Waynforth, H. B. (1968). Further tests on the carcinogenicity of sorbic acid in the rat. *Br. J. Cancer 22*:762–768.

Doores, S. (1993). Organic acids. In *Antimicrobials in Foods,* 2nd ed., P. M. Davidson and A. L. Branen (eds.). Marcel Dekker, New York, pp. 95–136.

Draughon, F. A., Sung, S. C., Mount, J. R., and Davidson, P. M. (1982). Effect of the parabens with and without nitrite on *Clostridium botulinum* toxin production in canned pork slurry. *J. Food Sci. 47*:1635–1637, 1642.

Edinger, W. D., and Splittstoesser, D. F. (1986a). Production by lactic acid bacteria of sorbic alcohol, the precursor of the geranium odor compound. *Am. J. Enol. Vitic. 37*:34–38.

Edinger, W. D., and Splittstoesser, D. F. (1986b). Sorbate tolerance by lactic acid bacteria associated with grapes and wine. *J. Food Sci. 51*:1077–1078.

Eklund, T. (1980). Inhibition of growth and uptake processes in bacteria by some chemical food preservatives. *J. Appl. Bacteriol. 48*:423–432.

Eklund, T. (1983). The antimicrobial effect of dissociated and undissociated sorbic acid at different pH levels. *J. Appl. Bacteriol. 54*:383–389.

Eklund, T. (1985). The effect of sorbic acid and esters of p-hydroxybenzoic acid on the protonmotive force in *Escherichia* coli membrane vesicles. *J. Gen. Microbiol. 131*:73–76.

El-Gendy, S. M., Nassib, T., Abed-El-Gellel, H., and Nanafy, N-El-Hoda. (1980). Survival and growth of *Clostridium* species in the presence of hydrogen peroxide. *J. Food Protect. 43*:431–432, 434.

El-Shenawy, M. A., and Marth, E. H. (1988). Sodium benzoate inhibits growth of or inactivates *Listeria monocytogenes*. *J. Food Protect. 51*:525–530.

Enfors, S.-O., and Molin, G. (1978). The influence of high concentrations of carbon dioxide on the germination of bacterial spores. *J. Appl. Bacteriol. 45*:279–285.

Foegeding, P. M., and Busta, F. F. (1983). Effect of carbon dioxide, nitrogen and hydrogen gases on germination of *Clostridium botulinum* spores. *J. Food Protect. 46*:987–989.

Food and Drug Administration (FDA). (1983). Sulfites in foods and drugs. *FDA Drug Bull. 13* (2):11–12.

Food and Drug Administration (FDA). (1985). *The Reexamination of the GRAS Status of Sulfiting Agents*. FDA 223-83-2020. Life Sci. Res. Office Fe. Am. Soc. Exp. Biol., Bethesda, MD.

Food and Drug Administration (FDA). (1986a). Sulfiting agents; revocation of GRAS status of use on fruits and vegetables intended to be served raw to consumers. *Fed. Reg. 51* (131):25012.

Food and Drug Administration (FDA). (1986b). Food labeling, declaration of sulfiting agents. *Fed. Reg. 51* (131):25012.

Food and Drug Administration (FDA). (1988). Sulfiting agents; affirmation of GRAS status. *Fed. Reg. 53* (243):51065.

Food and Drug Administration (FDA). (1990). Sulfiting agents; revocation of GRAS status for use on "fresh" potatoes served or sold unpackaged and unlabeled to consumers. *Fed. Reg. 55* (51):9826.

Franco, D. A., Webb, J., and Taylor, C. E. (1990). Antibiotic and sulfonamide residues in meat: Implications for human health. *J. Food Protect. 53*:178–185.

Fukusumi, E. (1972). Preservatives in the future. Properties and uses. *Shokuhin Kogyo 15*:40–45.

Fung, D. Y. C., Lin, C. C. S., and Gailani, M. B. (1985). Effect of phenolic antioxidants on microbial growth. *CRC Crit. Rev. Microbiol. 12* (2):153–183.

Garcia, G. W., Genigeorgis, C., and Lindroth, S. (1987). Risk of growth and toxin production by *Clostridium botulinum* nonproteolytic types B, E and F in salmon fillets stored under modified atmospheres at low and abused temperatures. *J. Food Protect. 50*:330–336.

Gaunt, I. F., Butterworth, K. R., Hardy, J., and Gangolli, S. D. (1975). Long-term toxicity of sorbic acid in the rat. *Food Cosmet. Toxicol. 13*:31–45.

Genigeorgis, C. A. (1985). Microbial and safety implications of the use of modified atmospheres to extend the storage life of fresh meat and fish. *Internat. J. Food Microb. 1*:237–251.

Gombas, D. E. (1989). Biological competition as a preserving mechanism. *J. Food Safety 10*:107–117.

Guest, D., Katz., G. V., and Astill, B. D. (1982). Aliphatic carboxylic acids. In *Patty's Industrial Hygiene and Toxicology*, 3rd ed., G. D. Clayton and F. E. Clayton (eds.). Wiley, New York, pp. 4901–4987.

Gunnison, A. F. (1981). Sulphite toxicity: a critical review of *in vitro* and *in vivo* data. *Food Cosmet. Toxicol. 19*:667–682.

Gunnison, A. F., and Jacobsen, D. N. (1987). Sulfite: Hypersensitivity, a critical review. *CRC Crit. Rev. Toxicol. 17* (3):185.

Gunnison, A. F., Sellakumar, C. D., and Snyder, E. A. (1987). Distribution, metabolism and toxicity of inhaled sulfur dioxide and endogenously generated sulfite in the respiratory tract of normal and sulfite oxidase-deficient rats. *J. Toxic. Environ. Health 21*:141–162.

Hansen, J. N., Banerjee, S., and Buchman, G. W. (1989). Potential of small ribosomally synthesized bacteriocins in design of new food preservatives. *J. Food Saf. 10*:119–130.

Hartman, P. E. (1983). Review: Putative mutagens and carcinogens in foods, II: Sorbate and sorbate-nitrite interactions. *Environ. Mutagen. 5*:217–222.

Hendy, R. J., Hardy, J., Gaunt, I. F., Kiss, I. S., and Butterworth, K. R. (1976). Long-term toxicity studies of sorbic acid in mice. *Food Cosmet. Toxicol. 14*:381–386.

Hintlian, C. B., and Hotchkiss, J. H. (1987). Comparative growth of spoilage and pathogenic organisms on modified atmosphere-packaged cooked beef. *J. Food Prot. 50*:218–223.

Hinton, D. M., Brouwer, E. A., Vocci, K. J., Joshi, A., Yang, G., and Ruggles, D. I. (1981). Pilot studies on the membrane toxicity and chemical reactivity of combinations of sorbates and nitrite in a processed food. *Fed. Proc. 40*:878.

Hoover, D. G. (1993). Bacteriocins with potential for use in foods. In *Antimicrobials in Foods*, 2nd ed., P. M. Davidson and A. L. Branen (eds.). Marcel Dekker, Inc., New York, pp. 409–440.

Hugo, W. B., and Russell, A. D. (1992). Types of antimicrobial agents. In *Principles and Practice of Disinfection, Preservation and Sterilization*, 2nd ed., A. D. Russell, W. B. Hugo and G. A. J. Ayliffe (eds.). Blackwell Scientific Publications, London, pp. 7–88.

Hurst, A. (1981). Nisin. In *Advances in Applied Microbiology*, Vol. 27, D. Perlman and A. I. Laskin (eds.). Academic Press, New York, pp. 85–123.

Hurst, A., and Hoover, D. G. (1993). Nisin. In *Antimicrobials in Foods*, 2nd ed., P. M. Davidson and A. L. Branen (eds.). Marcel Dekker, New York, pp. 369–394.

Jermini, M. F. G., and Schmidt-Lorenz, W. (1987). Activity of Na-benzoate and ethyl-paraben against osmotolerant yeasts at different water activity values. *J. Food Prot.* 50:920–927.

Joint FAO/WHO Expert Committee on Food Additives. (1974). *Toxicological Evaluations of Certain Food Additives with a Review of General Principles and of Specifications.* 17th Rep., Food and Agriculture Organization of the United Nations, Rome, p. 40.

Jung, R., Cojocel, C., Müller, W., Böttger, D., and Lück, E. (1992). Evaluation of the genotoxic potential of sorbic acid and potassium sorbate. *Food Chem. Toxicol.* 30:1–7.

Kalbag, S. S., and Palekar, A. G. (1988). Sodium benzoate inhibits fatty acid oxidation in rat liver: effect on ammonium levels. *Biochem. Med. Metab. Biol.* 40:133.

Kao, J., Jones, C. A., Fry, J. R., and Bridges, J. W. (1978). Species differences in the metabolism of benzoic acid by isolated hepatocytes and kidney tubule fragments. *Life Sci.* 23:1221.

Katz, S. E. (1983). Antibiotic residues and their significance. In *Antimicrobials in Foods*, A. L. Branen and P. M. Davidson (eds.). Marcel Dekker, New York, pp. 353–370.

Katz, S. E., and Brady, M. S. (1993). Antibiotic residues in foods and their significance. In *Antimicrobials in Foods*, 2nd ed., P. M. Davidson and A. L. Branen (eds.). Marcel Dekker, Inc., New York, pp. 571–596.

Kimble, C. E. (1977). Chemical food preservatives. In *Disinfection, Sterilization, and Preservation*, S. S. Block (ed.). Lea & Febiger, Philadelphia, pp. 834–858.

Klaenhammer, T. R. (1988). Bacteriocins of lactic acid bacteria. *Biochimie* 70:337–349.

Kubota, K., Horai, Y., Kushida, K., and Ishizaki, T. 1988. Determination of benzoic acid and hippuric acid in human plasma and urine by high-performance liquid chromatography. *J. Chromatogr.* 425:67.

Leistner, L. (1985). Hurdle technology applied to meat products of the shelf stable product and intermediate moisture food types. In *Properties of Water in Foods*, D. Simators and J. C. Multon (eds.). Martinus Nijhoff Publishers, Dordredt, The Netherlands, pp. 309–329.

Lewis, R. J., Sr. (1989). *Food Additives Handbook*. Van Nostrand Reinhold, New York.

Liewen, M. B., and Marth, E. H. (1985). Growth and inhibition of microorganisms in the presence of sorbic acid: a review. *J. Food Protect.* 48:364–375.

Lück, E. (1976). Sorbic acid as a food preservative. *Int. Flavors Food Additives* 7 (3):122–124, 127.

Lück, E. (1980). *Antimicrobial Food Additives, Characteristics, Uses, Effects*. Springer-Verlag, Berlin.

Marth, E. H. (1966). Antibiotics in foods—naturally occurring, developed and added. *Residue Rev.* 12:65–161.

Martin, L. B., Nordlee, J. A., and Taylor, S. L. (1986). Sulfite residues in restaurant salads. *J. Food Prot.* 49:126–129.

Mason, P. L., Gaunt, I. F., Hardy, J., Kiss, I. S., Butterworth, K. R., and Gangolli, S. D. (1976). Long-term toxicity of parasorbic acid in rats. *Food Cosmet. Toxicol. 14*:387.

Melo Filho, A. C., and Meneghini, R. (1984). *In vivo* formation of single-strand breaks in DNA by hydrogen peroxide is mediated by the Haber-Weiss reaction. *Biochim. Biophys. Acta 781*:56–63.

Montville, T. J. (1989). The evolving impact of biotechnology on food microbiology. *J. Food Saf. 10*:166–173.

Mukherjee, A., Giri, A. K., Talukder, G., and Sharma, A. (1988). Sister chromatid exchanges and micronuclei formation induced by sorbic acid and sorbic acid-nitrite *in vivo* in mice. *Toxicol. Lett. 42*:47–53.

Mukherjee, D. P., and Singh, S. P. (1967). Effect of increased carbon dioxide in inspired air on the morphology of spermatozoa and fertility of mice. *J. Reprod. Fert. 13*:165–167.

Münzer, R., Guigas, C., and Renner, H. W. (1990). Re-examination of potassium sorbate and sodium sorbate for possible genotoxic potential. *Food Chem. Toxicol. 28*:397–401.

National Academy of Sciences (NAS). (1978). *Sulfur Oxides*. National Research Council, Committee on Sulfur Oxides, National Academy of Science, Washington, DC, pp. 130–179.

National Academy of Sciences (NAS). (1982). *Alternatives to Current Use of Nitrite in Foods*. National Academy Press, Washington, DC.

Nes, I. F., and Eklund, T. (1983). The effect of parabens on DNA, RNA and protein synthesis in *Escherichia coli* and *Bacillus subtilis*. *J. Appl. Bacteriol. 54*:237–242.

Ough, C. S. (1993a). Sulfur dioxide and sulfites. In: *Antimicrobials in Foods*, 2nd ed., P. M. Davidson and A. L. Branen (eds.). Marcel Dekker, New York, pp. 137–190.

Ough, C. S. (1993b). Dimethyl dicarbonate and diethyl dicarbonate. In *Antimicrobials in Foods*, 2nd ed., P. M. Davidson and A. L. Branen (eds.). Marcel Dekker, New York, pp. 343–368.

Parker, M. S. (1992). Preservation of pharmaceutical and cosmetic products. In *Principles and Practice of Disinfection, Preservation and Sterilization*, 2nd ed., A. D. Russell, W. B. Hugo, and G. A. J. Ayliffe (eds.). Blackwell Scientific Publications, London, pp. 335–350.

Payne, K. D., Rico-Munoz, E., and Davidson, P. M. (1989). The antimicrobial activity of phenolic compounds against *Listeria monocytogenes* and their effectiveness in a model milk system. *J. Food Protect. 52*:151–153.

Plakas, S. M., and James, M. O. (1990). Bioavailability, metabolism, and renal excretion of benzoic acid in the channel catfish (*Ictalurus punctatus*). *Drug Metab. Dispos. 18*:552.

Post, L. S., Lee, D. A., Solberg, M., Furgang, D., Specchio, J., and Graham, C. (1985). Development of botulinal toxin and sensory deterioration during storage of vacuum and modified atmosphere packaged fish fillets. *J. Food Sci. 50*:990–996.

Robach, M. C. (1980). Use of preservatives to control microorganisms in food. *Food Technol. 34* (10):81–84.

Robach, M. C., and Pierson, M. D. (1978). Influence of *p*-hydroxybenzoic acid esters on the growth and toxin production of *Clostridium botulinum* 10755A. *J. Food Sci. 43*:787–789.

Robach, M. C., DiFate, V. G., Adam, K., and Kier, L. D. (1980a). Evaluation of the mutagenicity of sorbic acid-sodium nitrite reaction products produced in bacon-curing brines. *Food Cosmet. Toxicol. 18*:237–240.

Robach, M. C., Owens, J. L., Paquette, M. W., Sofos, J. N., and Busta, F. F. (1980b). Effects of various concentrations of sodium nitrite and potassium sorbate on nitrosamine formation in commercially prepared bacon. *J. Food Sci. 45*:1280–1284.

Ronning, I. E., and Frank, H. A. (1987). Growth inhibition of PA3679 caused by stringent-type response induced by protonophoric activity of sorbic acid. *Appl. Environ. Microbiol. 53*:1020–1027.

Ronning, I. E., and Frank, H. A. (1988). Growth response of putrefactive anaerobe 3679 to combinations of potassium sorbate and some common curing ingredients (sucrose, salt, and nitrite), and to noninhibitory levels of sorbic acid. *J. Food Protect. 51*:651–654.

Rowe, M. T. (1988). Effect of carbon dioxide on growth and extracellular enzyme production by *Pseudomonas fluorescens* B52. *Int. J. Food Microbiol. 6*:51–56.

Salmond, C. V., Knoll, R. G., and Booth, I. R. (1984). The effect of food preservatives on pH homeostasis in *Escherichia coli. J. Gen. Microbiol. 130*:2845–2850.

Sandmeyer, E. E., Kirwin, C. J., Jr. (1981). Esters. In *Patty's Industrial Hygiene and Toxicology*, 3rd ed., G. D. Clayton and F. E. Clayton (eds.). Wiley and Sons, New York, pp. 2259–2412.

Sax, N. I., and Lewis, R. J., Jr. (1989). *Dangerous Properties of Industrial Materials*, 7th ed. Van Nostrand Reinhold, New York.

Select Committee on GRAS Substances. (1976). *Evaluation of the Health Aspects of Sulfiting Agents as Food Ingredients.* Report SCOGS-15 Bureau of Foods, Food and Drug Administration, Department of Health, Education and Welfare, Washington, DC, pp. 1–25.

Shapero, M., Nelson, D. A., and Labuza, T. P. (1978). Ethanol inhibition of *Staphylococcus aureus* at limited water activity. *J. Food Sci. 43*:1467–1469.

Shtenberg, A. J., and Ignat'ev, A. D. (1970). Toxicological evaluation of some combinations of food preservatives. *Food Cosmet. Toxic. 8*:369–380.

Smith, Q. J., and Brown, K. L. (1980). The resistance of dry spores of *Bacillus subtilis* var. *globibii* (NCIB 80958) to solutions of hydrogen peroxide in relation to aseptic packaging. *J. Food Technol. 15*:169–179.

Sofos, J. N. (1981). Nitrite, sorbate and pH interaction in cured meat products. In *Proceedings of the 34th Annual Reciprocal Meat Conference.* National Live Stock and Meat Board, Chicago, pp. 104–120.

Sofos, J. N. (1989). *Sorbate Food Preservatives.* CRC Press, Boca Raton, FL.

Sofos, J. N., and Busta, F. F. (1980). Alternatives to the use of nitrite as an antibotulinal agent. *Food Technol. 34* (5):244–251.

Sofos, J. N., and Busta, F. F. (1981). Antimicrobial activity of sorbate. *J. Food Protect. 44*:614–622.

Sofos, J. N., and Busta, F. F. (1992). Chemical food preservatives. In *Principles and Practice of Disinfection, Preservation and Sterilization*, 2nd ed., A. D. Russell, W. B. Hugo, and G. A. J. Ayliffe (eds.). Blackwell Scientific Publications, London, pp. 351–397.

Sofos, J. N., and Busta, F. F. (1993). Sorbic acid and sorbates. In *Antimicrobials in Foods*, 2nd ed., P. M. Davidson and A. L. Branen (eds.). Marcel Dekker, New York, pp. 49–94.

Sofos, J. N., Busta, F. F., and Allen, C. E. (1979a). Sodium nitrite and sorbic acid effects on *Clostridium botulinum* spore germination and total microbial growth in chicken frankfurter emulsions during temperature abuse. *Appl. Envir. Microb. 37*:1103–1109.

Sofos, J. N., Busta, F. F., and Allen, C. E. (1979b). Botulism control by nitrite and sorbate in cured meats: a review. *J. Food Protect. 42*:739–770.

Sofos, J. N., Busta, F. F., Bhothipaksa, K., Allen, C. E., Robach, M. C., and Paquette, M. W. (1980). Effects of various concentrations of sodium nitrite and potassium sorbate on *Clostridium botulinum* toxin production in commercially prepared bacon. *J. Food Sci. 45*:1285–1292.

Sofos, J. N., Pierson, M. D., Blocher, J. C., and Busta, F. F. (1986). Mode of action of sorbic acid on bacterial cells and spores. *Int. J. Food Microb. 3*:1–17.

Statham, J. A., and McMeekin, T. A. (1988). The effect of potassium sorbate on the structural integrity of *Aeromonas putrefaciens*. *J. Appl. Bacteriol.* *65*:469–476.

Stevenson, K. E., and Shafer, B. D. (1983). Bacterial spore resistance to hydrogen peroxide. *Food Technol.* *37* (11):111–114.

Tanaka, K., Chung, K. C., Hayatsu, H., and Kada, T. (1978). Inhibition of nitrosamine formation *in vitro* by sorbic acid. *Food. Cosm. Toxicol.* *16*:209–215.

Thabrew, I. M., Babunmi, E. A., and French, M. R. (1980). Metabolic fate of carbon-14-labeled benzoic acid in protein-energy deficient rats. *Toxicol. Lett.* *5*:363.

Tompkin, R. B., Christiansen, L. N., and Shaparis, A. B. (1980). Antibotulinal efficacy of sulfur dioxide in meat. *Appl. Envir. Microbiol.* *39*:1096–1099.

Venugopal, V., Pansare, A. C., and Lewis, N. F. (1984). Inhibitory effect of food preservatives on protease secretion by *Aeromonas hydrophila*. *J. Food Sci.* *49*:1078–1081.

Walker, R. (1985). Sulphiting agents in foods: some risk/benefit considerations. *Food Addit. Contam.* *2*:5–24.

Walker, R. (1988). Toxicological aspects of food preservatives. In *Nutritional and Toxicological Aspects of Food Processing*, R. Walker and E. Quarttrucci (eds.). Taylor and Francis, London, pp. 25–49.

Walker, R. (1990). Toxicology or sorbic acid. *Food Add. Contam.* *7*:671–676.

Warth, A. D. (1977). Mechanism of resistance of *Saccharomyces bailli* to benzoic, sorbic and other weak acids used as food preservatives. *J. Appl. Bacteriol.* *43*:215–230.

Warth, A. D. (1985). Resistance of yeast species to benzoic and sorbic acids and to sulfur dioxide. *J. Food Protect.* *48*:564–569.

Warth, A. D. (1988). Effect of benzoic acid on growth yield of yeasts differing in their resistance to preservatives. *Appl. Envir. Microb.* *54*:2091–2095.

Warth, A. D. (1989). Relationships among cell size, membrane permeability, and preservative resistance in yeast species. *Appl. Envir. Microb.* *55*:2995–2999.

Wedzicha, B. L. (1984). Toxicology. In *Chemistry of Sulphur Dioxide in Foods*. Elsevier Applied Science Publishers, London, pp. 312–365.

Woodzinski, R. S., Labeda, D. P., and Alexander, M. (1978). Effect of low concentrations of bisulfic-sulfite and nitrite on microorganisms. *Appl. Envir. Microb.* *35*:718–723.

Index

CPSIA information can be obtained
at www.ICGtesting.com
Printed in the USA
LVHW061032101222
734958LV00005B/71